Taraprasad Das
PremNandhini Satgunam
Editors

Ophthalmic Diagnostics

Technology, Techniques, and Clinical Applications

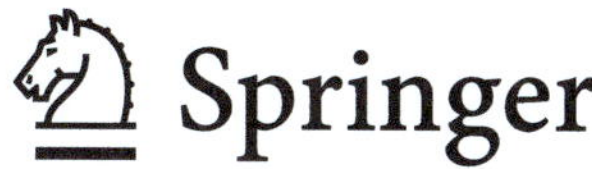

Editors
Taraprasad Das
Anant Bajaj Retina Institute, Srimati Kanuri Santhamma Centre for Vitreoretinal Diseases, Kallam Anji Reddy Campus
L V Prasad Eye Institute
Hyderabad, Telangana, India

PremNandhini Satgunam
Brien Holden Institute of Optometry and Vision Sciences and Prof. Brien Holden Eye Research Centre
L V Prasad Eye Institute
Hyderabad, Telangana, India

ISBN 978-981-97-0140-7 ISBN 978-981-97-0138-4 (eBook)
https://doi.org/10.1007/978-981-97-0138-4

This Springer imprint is published by the registered company Springer Nature Singapore Pte Ltd.
The registered company address is: 152 Beach Road, #21-01/04 Gateway East, Singapore 189721, Singapore

To

My patients who encouraged me to interpret the test reports in their clinical context.

TD

****

Several teachers came together to make this book a reality. I dedicate this book to all these teachers, and to the future teachers.

PN

Foreword 1

The ocular system is highly intricate, complex and involves not only the globe of the eye itself, but also its neural connections with the brain and surrounding muscular tissue. In order to perceive visual information of the highest quality, all ocular components are required to function harmoniously together. Consequently, examination approaches of the eye are required to meet an equivalent level of sophistication. Several sub-specialties have developed within ophthalmology; however, alongside some highly specific examination tools, key underlying examination techniques form the basis for standardized assessments of visual function and delivery of eye care. Thus, to provide an accurate diagnosis, clinicians must be well-versed in the fundamental techniques of ocular examination and be aware of any significant new and upcoming technologies within the field. While technological advancements allow for more detailed imaging and assessment of the eye as well as the opportunity to gain a deeper understanding of the underlying pathophysiology of disease states, these also present unique challenges as these additional tools must be integrated into standard practice.

This book, *Ophthalmic Diagnostics: Technology, Techniques, and Clinical Applications* by Taraprasad Das and PremNandhini Satgunam, contains 35 unique chapters, each contributed by expert authors, covering both basic and clinical aspects of ophthalmic diagnosis, as well as novel and recent investigational techniques. Cumulatively, the contents bring together a valuable collection of skills and techniques for accurately diagnosing pathologic conditions. This is a useful reference tool for all professionals involved in the eye care sector: medical, nursing, optometry, orthoptics, and vision science.

In modern clinical practice, virtually all parts of the eye can be examined from a functional, pathologic, or biometric perspective. These are highly interrelated and synergized; a suite of testing procedures and multimodal imaging techniques is often required to understand the patient thoroughly. Visual acuity has long been the standard parameter to measure visual function and indicate the presence of ocular pathology; however, visual acuity scores alone often have limited real-world applicability. Contrast sensitivity, visual fields, stereopsis, color vision, and ocular alignment also need to be considered for a broader assessment of the visual function of patients in the real world. Additionally, visual acuity will be significantly influenced by the optical state of the eye, and this requires accurate measures of refraction to be obtained. Aside from its clinical use, information from refraction can be translated into functional benefits for the patient by prescribing and dispensing corrective spectacles. While technological advancements tend toward eliminating examiner bias through automated objective measures, examination via retinoscopy remains an invaluable skill, particularly for assessments in remote environments and in children and patients with intellectual disabilities.

To identify pathologies, slit lamp biomicroscopy is the core technique used to observe structures in the anterior segment of the eye. This has founded other viewing techniques, such as gonioscopy and fundoscopy. Since the advent of film and flash photography in the nineteenth century, numerous imaging modalities are now available to document pathologic conditions from the surface of the eye to the retina and optic nerve. Optical coherence tomography (OCT) is the fundamental modern-day imaging device which offers insights into almost every layer and tissue plane of the eye for both practitioners in the clinic and surgeons in the operating room. Further advancements in OCT capabilities have allowed finer segmentation on a cellular level as well as non-invasive visualization of the array of blood vessel networks located between the retina and the choroid. Earlier compromises between imaging speed, resolution, and invasiveness are significantly less apparent, contributing to a more detailed investigation with less patient burden.

On a global scale, cataract formation has been the most significant contributor to blindness, particularly in developed countries. In ophthalmic practice, cataract assessment is routine and a fundamental surgical indication for ophthalmologists. Biometry with current technologies and optimized lens formulas can now account for complex optics to provide accurate and convenient measurements, minimizing errors across a broad range of eyes. However, ultrasound techniques remain a reliable technique in the clinic to overcome the challenges of dense cataract and ocular media opacity, which hinder standard optical-based measures.

While the identification of ocular diseases and improvement of visual function is often the main intent of conducting ocular examinations, deeper insights can be gained as ocular pathology, alignment, and function can be the manifestations of systemic diseases, including diabetes, trauma, inflammatory and autoimmune conditions, as well as neurological defects. Testing pupillary responses is a core medical skill that assesses the optic nerve and higher neurological function. Electrophysiology has been able to differentiate, diagnose, and understand several rare inherited retinal degenerations using the principles of neuronal activity.

Naturally, the culmination of technological advancements opens the door to future novel applications. Tele-ophthalmology is evolving to become a vital solution for delivering ophthalmic and optometric healthcare to remote areas. The development of smartphone-based ophthalmic imaging is one of the key drivers allowing this to be implemented more efficiently with minimal economic burden; however, it requires a lot of support from healthcare systems.

A wide spectrum of eye care professionals in early and established careers will find this book a most valuable resource in the clinical care of patients.

Andrew Chang
AM, MBBS, PhD, FRACS

Medical Director, Sydney Retina Clinic,
Sydney, NSW, Australia

Head of Ophthalmology, Sydney Eye Hospital,
Sydney, NSW, Australia

Clinical Associate Professor, Sydney University,
Sydney, NSW, Australia

Conjoint Professor, Discipline of Surgery, UNSW
Sydney, NSW, Australia

Foreword 2

The field of eye care—optometrists, ophthalmologists, students, and residents alike—will benefit from this outstanding book, which provides a comprehensive, detailed description of the current state of ophthalmic diagnostics. The book is extraordinarily well organized, enabling the eye care practitioners to access the information they need for a specific patient. Likewise, the new student can start at the beginning and move through to the most current technology that makes our jobs as eye doctors easier.

Superbly curated by Drs. Taraprasad Das and PremNandhini Satgunam, the authors, have obviously worked hard on their state-of-the-art contributions. The effort and care taken by the many contributing authors is evident on every page. All are to be congratulated for the important contribution to the ophthalmic literature.

First, the book's chapters cover the traditional components of the eye examination, starting with the basics of assessing vision and refractive error. The reader will be able to extend the information on how to measure a patient's most fundamental visual function, blur, into the art of prescribing eyeglasses and optical dispensing.

The reader can then learn (or refresh their memory) on quantifying the binocular vision system, pupillary reactions, visual field, and colour vision.

And then the true, novel value of this textbook emerges. Chapters on the most current technology that enhances our ability to perform eye examinations are included. They cover smartphone-based imaging, cataract grading and imaging, microperimetry, and adaptive optics. The chapter on optical coherence tomography will be particularly valuable to the new student or resident.

As dean of The Ohio State University College of Optometry in Columbus, Ohio, United States, I calculated the number of eye examinations one cohort of optometry students will perform during their careers. If I conservatively figure the average optometrist practices for 30 years and sees 10 patients per day, 240 working days each year, a cohort of 70 graduating optometrists will be entrusted with 5,040,000 pairs of eyes!

I anticipate this book will be consulted early in students' and residents' careers and often when they enter eye care practice and continue to examine those five million patients. In the end, their patients will be the real beneficiaries of these authors' hard work.

Karla Zadnik

Dean and Glenn A. Fry Professor in
Optometry and Physiological Optics
The Ohio State University College of Optometry
Columbus, OH, USA

Interim Dean
The Ohio State University College of Public Health
Columbus, OH, USA

Preface

With the advent of technology, "time flies" at speed, sometimes even faster than light.

Just within the lifetime of three generations, we have seen how clunky telephones that were once only found in the houses of the elite are now sleek devices that are owned by almost everyone. Every single profession has been touched and turned around, sometimes even upside down, by these changing waves of technology.

Health care, including eye care, is no exception to this. Many instruments have become obsolete and outdated, and some have disappeared into oblivion. Yet, some are indispensable and have stood the test of time, showing that old is indeed gold.

The world has become smarter, often due to the "smart gadgets" in most people's hands in the form of phones. With this mini-computer called the smartphone, one can do wonders. Many Apps have been developed for various tests that were once expensive and found exclusively within the sanctorum of big institutes. These technologies have broken barriers, blurred borders, and provided even private practitioners in rural settings with advanced diagnostic tools. While some of these smart devices and Apps may not stand the test of time, some are robust and would evolve into better, faster, and more importantly, more accurate versions. Although the choices available are sometimes overwhelmingly many, a little research can often identify the correct smart tools and instruments to suit one's needs.

Given the drastic changes and many choices in diagnostic tools available today, a compilation of information on new and old diagnostic tools must be created. Such a compilation can help clinical practitioners to remain updated and avoid becoming outdated in their clinical practice. Within the clinical practice of eye care, which includes optometry, ophthalmology, and opticianry, the most rapid changes occur in the area of diagnostics. It is an area where tools, devices, instruments, and newer techniques keep evolving to improve eye care practices.

Therefore, consolidating all this information into a comprehensive book is a real need. In fact, as a ready, go-to handbook, it will be of immense help to any student, clinician, or researcher in eye care. This is the prime motivation for putting this book together.

Although some commercial product names are mentioned in this book, the editors (and authors) are not endorsing or promoting any product. Since some of the descriptions of the techniques are drawn from the individual author's scope of practice, we are hopeful that the diverse and global cast of authors will provide a plethora of viewpoints that will be valuable to anyone involved in eye care anywhere in the world.

We are immensely grateful to these contributing authors, who took the time to share their wisdom and clinical pearls with us. Additionally, we also thank the science editor, Anusha Krishnan, PhD, and the content editor, Ms. Neerja Padmanabhan, from Springer Nature, for their help.

The book title reads *Technology, Techniques, and Clinical Application*. The aspirational goals of this book are to briefly explain the scientific principles of various diagnostic tools and techniques, provide an easy-to-follow protocol to execute specific techniques, and explain the clinical applications of these techniques. In essence, this book attempts to fill the "why" gaps in "what we do" in ophthalmic diagnosis wherever possible. We have also included information on newer tools, innovations, and techniques. In addition, the sequence of chapters in this book follows the sequence of clinical tests that are normally followed during an eye examination. However, very specialized or sophisticated techniques have not been included. Instead, this book focuses on generalized and commonly used techniques. We have also included a section on tele-eye health, as the SARS CoV 2 pandemic has taught us that this form of service delivery is not only possible but could also encourage eye care-seeking behaviour in rural areas; in addition, we feel that tele-eye health can and will change the future of eye care delivery. As we write this, we feel that all of us in the eye care sector must rise to face the challenges of the future, where eye care can be accessed with a click of a button or a swipe of a finger. We need to be ready.

This book is written with the desire to keep pace with the changing times. Although we are aware that many of the techniques documented in this book may become outdated shortly, we believe that this book will still be useful to eye care practitioners everywhere. Although every chapter provides a historical perspective on the techniques and instruments discussed in it, the question of whether this book describes the history of the eventual past or educates us on the practice of the future is something only time can tell.

However, one must start somewhere to ride the wave of development for better eye care.

We hope that the readers of this book enjoy this ride!

Hyderabad, Telangana, India — Taraprasad Das
Hyderabad, Telangana, India — PremNandhini Satgunam

Contents

Contributors

Afra Abdussamad, DNB GMR Varalakshmi Campus, L V Prasad Eye Institute, Vishakhapatnam, India

Vedvati Hemant Albal, MD Shri Nathmal Singhvi Jadhavbhai Glaucoma Services, Sankara Nethralaya Medical Research Foundation, Chennai, India

Deepak Kumar Bagga, PhD Institute for Vision Rehabilitation, Kallam Anji Reddy Campus, L V Prasad Eye Institute, Hyderabad, India

Sayan Basu, MS Shantilal Shanghvi Cornea Institute, Kallam Anji Reddy Campus, L V Prasad Eye Institute, Hyderabad, India

Shrikant R. Bharadwaj, BSopt, PhD Brien Holden Institute of Optometry and Vision Sciences, Prof. Brien Holden Eye Research Centre, L V Prasad Eye Institute, Hyderabad, India

Muna Bhende, MS Medical Research Foundation, Sankara Nethralaya, Chennai, India

Nandini Bothra, MD Govindram Seksaria Institute of Dacryology, Kallam Anji Reddy Campus, L V Prasad Eye Institute, Hyderabad, India

Michelle Buckland, OD, MS The Ohio State University College of Optometry, Columbus, OH, USA

Priya R. Chandrasekaran, DNB, FRCS Singapore National Eye Centre, Singapore Eye Research Institute, Singapore, Singapore

Gemmy Cheung, MD Singapore National Eye Centre, Singapore Eye Research Institute, Singapore, Singapore

Jay Chhablani, MD Department of Ophthalmology, University of Pittsburgh, Pittsburgh, PA, USA

Paul A. Constable, PhD Flinders University, College of Nursing and Health Sciences, Caring Futures Institute, Adelaide, SA, Australia

Prajakta Dandekar, DNB, FICO Shantilal Shanghvi Eye Institute, Mumbai, India

Taraprasad Das, MD, FRCS Anant Bajaj Retina Institute, Srimati Kanuri Santhamma Centre for Vitreoretinal Diseases, Kallam Anji Reddy Campus, L V Prasad Eye Institute, Hyderabad, Telangana, India

Debarati Dasgupta, DNB Greater Lions Eye Hospital, Siliguri, India

Rashmi Deshmukh, MS, DNB, FRCS Shantilal Shanghvi Cornea Institute, Kallam Anji Reddy Campus, L V Prasad Eye Institute, Hyderabad, India

Nick Fogt, OD, PhD The Ohio State University College of Optometry, Columbus, OH, USA

Suganeswari Ganesan, DNB Medical Research Foundation, Sankara Nethralaya, Chennai, India

Kara R. Grimes, MSc New York Medical College, New York, USA

Prashant Gupta, MS Kallam Anji Reddy Campus, L V Prasad Eye Institute, Hyderabad, India

Shikha Gupta, MD Dr. Rajendra Prasad Centre for Ophthalmic Sciences, AIIMS, New Delhi, India

Viney Gupta, MD, MBA Dr. Rajendra Prasad Centre for Ophthalmic Sciences, AIIMS, New Delhi, India

Amithavikram R. Hathibelagal, PhD Brien Holden Institute of Optometry and Vision Sciences, Prof. Brien Holden Eye Research Centre, L V Prasad Eye Institute, Hyderabad, India

Graham E. Holder, PhD, FARVO Department of Ophthalmology, Yong Loo Lin School of Medicine, National University of Singapore, Singapore, Singapore

Ninan Jacob, MD Kode Venkatadri Chowdary Campus, L V Prasad Eye Institute, Vijayawada, India

Benjamin Jastrzembski, MD University of California, Davis, Sacramento, CA, USA

Sanil Joseph, MHA, MSc Lions Aravind Institute of Community Ophthalmology, Aravind Eye Care System, Madurai, India

Anahita Kate, MS Kode Venkatadri Chowdary Campus, L V Prasad Eye Institute, Vijayawada, India

Ramesh Kekunnaya, MD, FRCS Child Sight Institute, Jasti V Ramanamma Children's Eye Care Center, Kallam Anji Reddy Campus, L V Prasad Eye Institute, Hyderabad, India

Sardar M. Khan, DO Gullapalli Pratibha Rao International Centre for Advancement of Rural Eye Care, L V Prasad Eye Institute, Siddipet, India

Mona Khurana, MD Shri Nathmal Singhvi Jadhavbhai Glaucoma Services, Sankara Nethralaya, Medical Research Foundation, Chennai, India

Deepika Kommanapalli, MC (Optom), MPhil Faculty of Health, Social Care and Education, Anglia Ruskin University, Cambridge, UK

Mounica Sai Konda, MS Institute of Ophthalmic Sciences, AIG Hospitals, Hyderabad, India

Ashwini Kulkarni, DNB Kode Venkatadri Chowdary Campus, L V Prasad Eye Institute, Vijayawada, India

Timothy Y. Y. Lai, MD Department of Ophthalmology and Visual Science, The Chinese University of Hong Kong, Faculty of Medicine, Pok Fu Lam, Hong Kong

Dennis S. C. Lam, MD International Eye Research Institute of The Chinese University of Hong Kong, Shenzhen, China

C-Mer International Eyecare Group, Hong Kong, China

Oliver R. Marmoy, DClinSci, MSc Great Ormond Street Hospital for Children NHS Foundation Trust, London, UK

GOS-ICH University College London, London, UK

Srikanth Maseedupalli, M Optom The Standard Chartered-LVPEI Academy for Eye Care Education, L V Prasad Eye Institute, Hyderabad, India

Sashwanthi Mohan, DNB Medcare Eye Centre, Dubai and Rajan Eye Care Hospital, Chennai, India

Sujoy Mukherjee, MSc(Optom) Mithu Tulsi Chanrai Campus, L V Prasad Eye Institute, Bhubaneswar, India

Somasheila I. Murthy, MD, FRCS Shantilal Shanghvi Eye Institute, Mumbai, India

Shanmuganathan Nagarajan, BSc, MBA Remidio Innovative Solutions Pvt Ltd, Bengaluru, India

Mekhla Naik, MD Shantilal Shanghvi Eye Institute, Mumbai, India

Kalpa Negiloni, PhD Remidio Innovative Solutions Pvt Ltd, Bengaluru, India

Maneck Nicholson, MS, FRCS Shantilal Shanghvi Eye Institute, Mumbai, India

Debananada Padhy, MSc(Optom) Gullapalli Pratibha Rao International Centre for Advancement of Rural Eye Care, L V Prasad Eye Institute, Hyderabad, India

Srikanta K. Padhy, MD Anant Bajaj Retina Institute, Mithu Tulsi Chanrai Campus, L V Prasad Eye Institute, Bhubaneswar, India

Sourav Pal, Ph.D Forus Health Pvt. Ltd., Bengaluru, India

Gayathri J. Panicker, MS Sri Ramachandra Institute of Higher Education and Research, Chennai, India

Arnav Panigrahi, MD Dr. Rajendra Prasad Centre for Ophthalmic Sciences, AIIMS, New Delhi, India

K. Gowri Pratinya, DNB Kallam Anji Reddy Campus, L V Prasad Eye Institute, Hyderabad, India

Niladri B. Puhan, Ph.D Indian Institute of Technology Bhubaneswar, Bhubaneswar, India

Aparna Raghuram, OD, PhD Boston Children's Hospital/Harvard Medical School, Boston, MA, USA

Aparna Rao, MD, FRCS, Ph.D Kallam Anji Reddy Campus, L V Prasad Eye Institute, Hyderabad, India

Divya Parthasarathy Rao, MS Remidio Innovative Solutions Inc., Glen Allen, VA, USA

Srinivas K. Rao, MD, FRCS Darshan Eye Care and Surgical Centre, Chennai, India

Suryasnata Rath, MD, FRCS Mithu Tulsi Chanrai Campus, L V Prasad Eye Institute, Bhubaneswar, India

Pallavi Ray, MD Mithu Tulsi Chanrai Campus, L V Prasad Eye Institute, Bhubaneswar, India

Avik K. Roy, MS Mithu Tulsi Chanrai Campus, L V Prasad Eye Institute, Bhubaneswar, India

Swapnali Sabhapandit, MS Institute of Ophthalmic Sciences, AIG Hospitals, Hyderabad, India

Niroj Kumar Sahoo, MD, DNB Anant Bajaj Retina Institute, Kode Venkatadri Chowdary Campus, L V Prasad Eye Institute, Vijayawada, India

PremNandhini Satgunam, BSOpt, MS, PhD Brien Holden Institute of Optometry and Vision Sciences, Prof. Brien Holden Eye Research Centre, L V Prasad Eye Institute, Hyderabad, Telangana, India

Supriya Sharma, DNB, FICO Shantilal Shanghvi Eye Institute, Mumbai, India

Ramyashri Shastry, MD Drishti Eye Centre, Hyderabad, India

Jenil Sheth, MD Shantilal Shanghvi Eye Institute, Mumbai, India

Swati Singh, MS Kallam Anji Reddy Campus, LV Prasad Eye Institute, Hyderabad, India

Anand Sivaraman, PhD Remidio Innovative Solutions Pvt, Bengaluru, India

Sanjeev P. Srinivas, MD Darshan Eye Care and Surgical Centre, Chennai, India

Rebecca Sumalini, BSc, PhD Institute of Vision Rehabilitation, Kallam Amji Reddy Campus, L V Prasad Eye Institute, Hyderabad, India

Meenakshi Swaminathan, MD Sri Ramachandra Institute of Higher Education and Research, Chennai, India

Simon K. H. Szeto, MD Department of Ophthalmology and Visual Science, The Chinese University of Hong Kong, Faculty of Medicine, Pok Fu Lam, Hong Kong

Bhoomi Thakkar, MD Mithu Tulsi Chanrai Campus, L V Prasad Eye Institute, Bhubaneswar, India

Margaret Woodhouse, PhD School of Optometry and Vision Sciences, Cardiff University, Cardiff, UK

Visual Acuity: High Contrast and Low Contrast

1

Rebecca Sumalini
and PremNandhini Satgunam

1.1 Introduction

There are many components of vision. These include visual acuity, contrast sensitivity, visual fields, 3D vision, motion perception, etc. Of all these components, the most important component is visual acuity, the ability of the eye to resolve and perceive small targets. There are various methods and ways to measure this resolution capacity of the eye. All these methods use black letters on a white background. Ironically, none of the real-world scenes and scenarios appear in black and white. The visual function that is more relevant to the real-world scenario is contrast sensitivity. Contrast sensitivity is the ability of the eye to detect the dimmest target and largely depends on the background (for example, a white bead placed on a white tabletop has poorer contrast than a gray bead on a white tabletop). This ability of the eye to distinguish the contrast of the target against the background is also related to the size of the object. If this ability is mapped for different target sizes, we arrive at the contrast sensitivity function (CSF). Interestingly, high-contrast visual acuity (or visual acuity) is only a single-point measurement within the CSF (see Sect. 2.3.2). Yet, we mostly draw conclusions and correlate patients' complaints and functional vision difficulties (e.g., identifying faces, pouring water into a cup) with the visual acuity value. Unfortunately, measures of contrast sensitivity have been mainly restricted to low-vision practice or research. However, for those patients whose symptoms are not explained through the "regular" visual acuity, measuring contrast sensitivity or low-contrast visual acuity may be insightful.

This chapter gives an equal importance to visual acuity, contrast sensitivity, and low-contrast visual acuity. The importance of these measurements, with commonly used and commercially available tests, is discussed. Some special scenarios in which the conventional measurements are difficult are also discussed, with available alternate options.

1.2 History

1.2.1 Visual Acuity Tools

The origin of standardized visual acuity testing dates back to 1862 by the Dutch ophthalmologist Hermann Snellen; this test is widely known

R. Sumalini
Institute of Vision Rehabilitation, Kallam Amji Reddy Campus, L V Prasad Eye Institute, Hyderabad, India
e-mail: rebecca@lvpei.org

P. Satgunam (✉)
Brien Holden Institute of Optometry and Vision Sciences, Prof. Brien Holden Eye Research Centre, L V Prasad Eye Institute, Hyderabad, Telangana, India
e-mail: premnandhini@lvpei.org

T. Das, P. Satgunam (eds.), *Ophthalmic Diagnostics*, https://doi.org/10.1007/978-981-97-0138-4_1

as the Snellen chart [1]. The most commonly used notation for visual acuity is the Snellen fraction (e.g., 20/20 or 6/6), a format easily understood by all clinicians and researchers. The numerator is the test distance, and the denominator is the distance from which the letter should be visible. Therefore, visual acuity of 20/200 indicates what is visible from 200 feet to a normally sighted individual, is only visible from a closer distance of 20 feet to someone with visual impairment. The Snellen acuity chart, despite its wide use, has several limitations. These include an unequal number of letters in each acuity line, unequal size progression of optotypes between acuity lines, unequal spacing between the letters, and reliability concerns. To address these shortcomings, the logMAR chart was developed in 1976 by Ian Bailey and Jan Lovie-Kitchin [2]. The chart had a uniform number of letters, uniformly spaced progression, and proportionate spacing between the letters.

In 1982, the National Eye Institute used the Sloan letter set (i.e., non-serif letters) and logMAR principles as described by Bailey and Lovie [2] and produced the current "gold-standard" ETDRS chart (Early Treatment of Diabetic Retinopathy Study) (Fig. 1.1, left) [3]. In addition to English letters, several other optotypes have been developed for individuals unfamiliar with English optotypes, such as letters of different languages (e.g., Chinese [4], Arabic [5], Hindi [6]), LEA symbols ((named after the inventor Lea Hyvarinen) [7]) (Fig. 1.1, middle), tumbling E [8], and Landolt C charts [9]. The recent computer-based visual acuity measurement tool, COMPlog (Fig. 1.1, right) [10] has several advantages such as ease of use, easy maintenance, and the ability to shuffle between and within optotypes whenever required.

Based on the preferential-looking principle, grating acuity tests are the tests of choice for preverbal/non-verbal individuals. Robert Fantz first described the principle in 1965 [11]. The currently used Teller acuity cards-II (Fig. 1.2, left) is a modified prototype of the same after several iterations. A handful of grating acuity tests are available (such as Keeler acuity cards and LEA gratings paddle), including the app-based grating acuity test, such as the Peekaboo Vision application (Fig. 1.2, right) [12].

Near visual acuity is a valuable measurement given that most of our day-to-day activities involve several near tasks such as reading, writing, and household chores (including cooking), to name a few. Jaeger cards were first developed by the Austrian ophthalmologist Eduard Jaeger in 1854 for checking near visual acuity [13]. The text size of the reading text progresses from 0.37 to 2.5 mm [14]. These cards have been discontinued because of a lack of standardization [15]. In 1980, Ian Bailey and Jan Lovie-Kitchin developed the Bailey–Lovie word reading charts (Fig. 1.3); these consisted of random words with a logarithmic progression of lines.

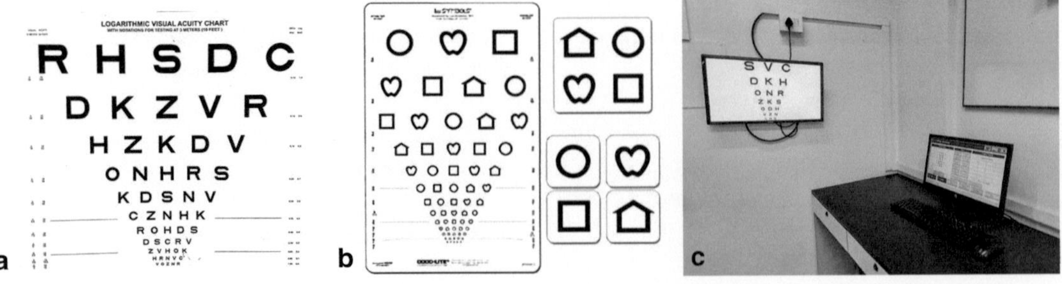

Fig. 1.1 Recognition acuity tests: (left) ETDRS chart, (middle) LEA symbols, and (right) COMPlog electronic chart. *ETDRS* early treatment of diabetic retinopathy study, *COMPlog* computerized logarithmic test

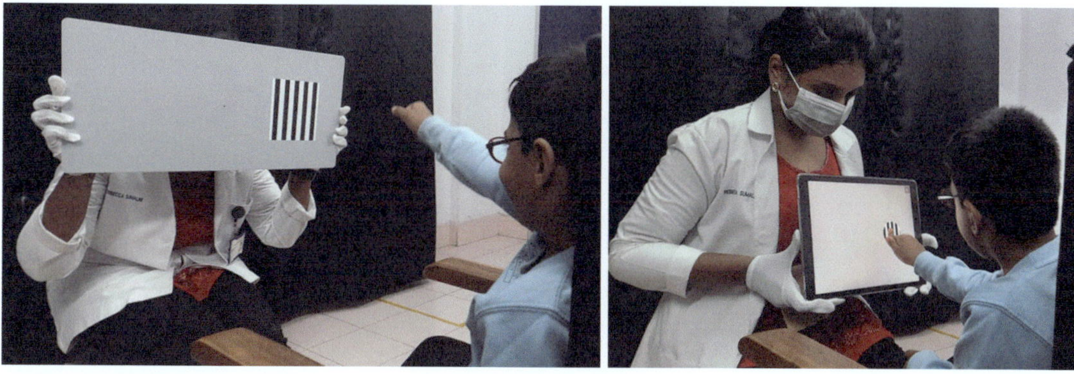

Fig. 1.2 (left) Grating acuity assessment using teller acuity cards-II (without testing stage) and (right) the Peekaboo Vision application

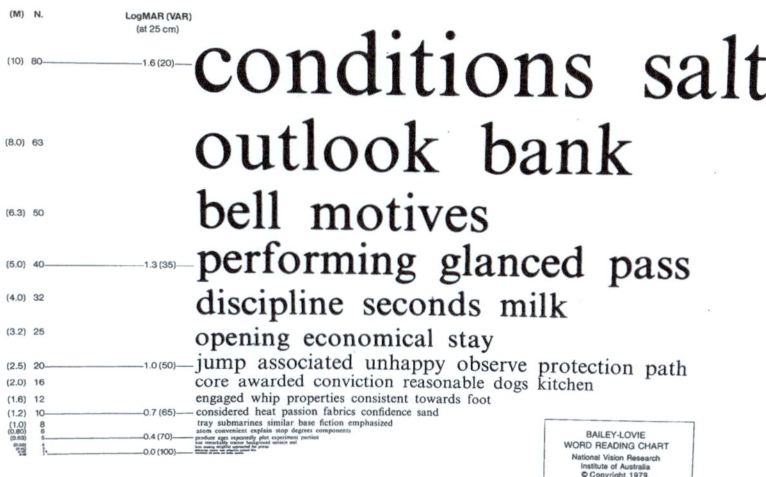

Fig. 1.3 The Bailey–Lovie word reading chart

1.2.2 Contrast Sensitivity Tools

Contrast sensitivity testing was first demonstrated in 1978 using Arden gratings and consisted of varying spatial frequencies and contrast levels. Based on similar principles, the functional acuity contrast test, first described by Arthur Ginsburg, consists of sine wave gratings of varying spatial frequencies and contrast levels [16]. The most popularly known contrast sensitivity test, the Pelli–Robson contrast sensitivity chart, was developed by DG Pelli, JG Robson, and AJ Wilkins; they published the design of this chart in 1988 [17]. In the Pelli–Robson contrast sensitivity chart (Fig. 1.4), English letters in triplets with fixed spatial frequency (i.e., constant size) vary in contrast levels. The optotype size subtends 2.8° at 1 m (~20/672) (appropriate for patients with visual impairment), which is equivalent to 20/224 at 3 m (~2.67 CPD [cycles per degree]) (recommended testing distance). The logCS was comparable at these two testing distances [18]. This chart measures contrast sensitivity from 0.00 to 2.25 logCS range. The higher the logCS, the better the contrast sensitivity. The chart has good repeatability of ±0.15 log units in young and older adults [19].

In addition, there are several commercially available contrast sensitivity tools using various targets such as pictures (hiding Heidi contrast

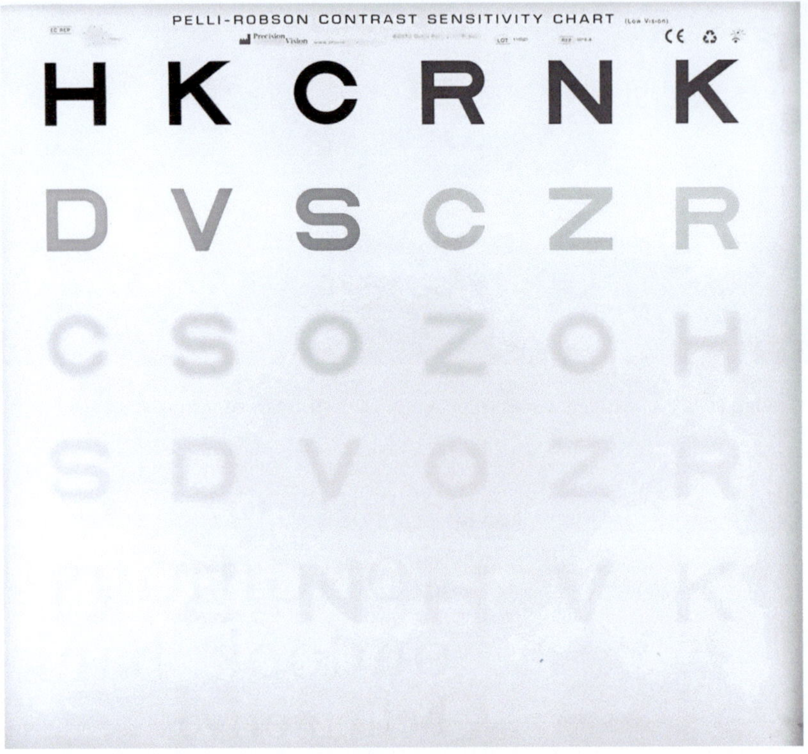

Fig. 1.4 The Pelli–Robson contrast sensitivity chart placed in a lightbox

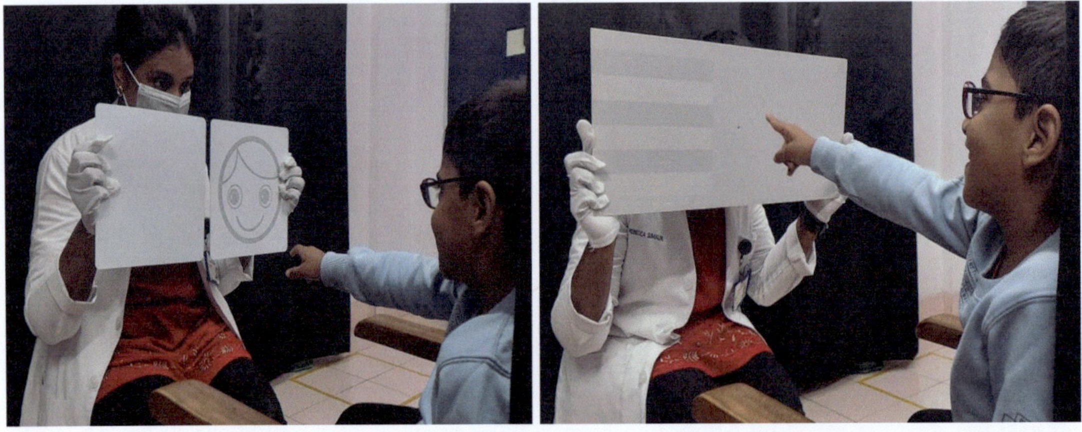

Fig. 1.5 Contrast sensitivity assessment using (left) the hiding Heidi low-contrast face test and (right) Ohio contrast cards

sensitivity test) (Fig. 1.5, left), gratings (Cambridge low-contrast gratings, Ohio contrast cards [20] (Fig. 1.5, right), letters (Mars letter contrast sensitivity test) [21], and circles (spot checks) [22].

1.3 Underlying Concept

1.3.1 Distance Visual Acuity

Visual acuity is the resolution capacity of an eye. The resolution capacity is the smallest gap an eye can detect between two objects. This gap would subtend an angle at the nodal point of the eye. Therefore, the smallest angle resolved by the eye is its visual acuity (Fig. 1.6). Any angle or separation smaller than this would result in a single blurred object instead of two distinct objects. The smallest visual angle a human eye could resolve is about 1′ (1 min of arc) (see Box 1.1) [23].

As seen in Fig. 1.6, two black lines with a white separation will require a minimum of 3 photoreceptors to resolve it. One photoreceptor detects one dark line, another photoreceptor detects the white space, and a third adjacent photoreceptor detects the other dark line. If we consider one dark line and the white space as one cycle, then two dark lines separated by a white space will have 1.5 cycles. Therefore, to resolve 1.5 cycles, three photoreceptors (i.e.,) double the cycles are required. This limit of how many minimum photoreceptors are required to resolve an object is called the Nyquist limit. This is a borrowed concept from signal processing in electronics. If we consider the eye a device to capture and process light signals, the minimum number of photoreceptors required will be twice the spatial frequency (cycles per degree or CPD). Hence, to resolve 10 cycles, 20 photoreceptors are needed. Given this, and with the anatomical limi-

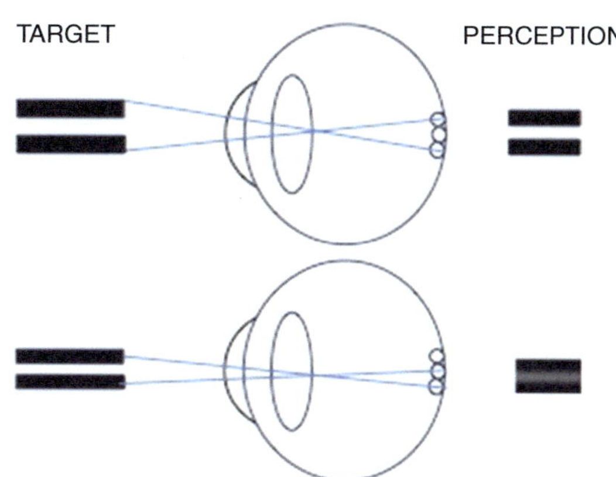

Fig. 1.6 An illustration of the minimum angle of resolution (MAR) to discern a black-and-white grating. A minimum of three photoreceptors are required to see the grating target (top panel). If the grating subtends a smaller angle than the MAR, then a blurred blob of the grating is seen, which makes it indiscernible (lower panel)

Box 1.1 An Example Computation of Minimum Angle of Resolution (MAR)

Let us consider a visual acuity chart calibrated for 6 meters.

The height of the 6/6 or 20/20 optotype is 0.875 cm or ~0.00875 m

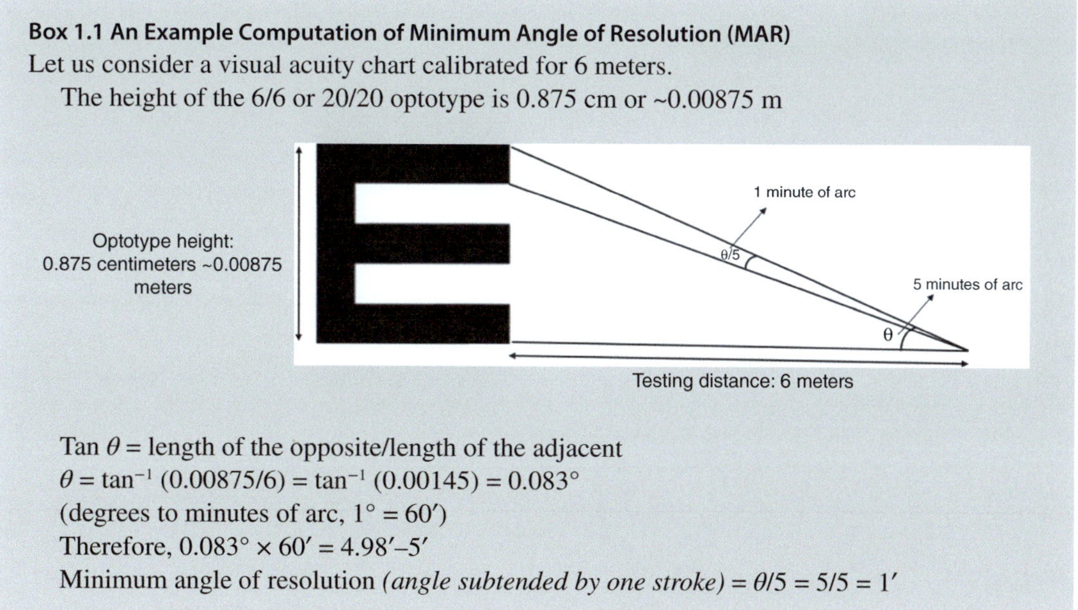

Tan θ = length of the opposite/length of the adjacent

$\theta = \tan^{-1}(0.00875/6) = \tan^{-1}(0.00145) = 0.083°$

(degrees to minutes of arc, $1° = 60'$)

Therefore, $0.083° \times 60' = 4.98'–5'$

Minimum angle of resolution *(angle subtended by one stroke)* = $\theta/5 = 5/5 = 1'$

tation of how many photoreceptors can be packed into the fovea, along with neural and optical limitations, the maximum resolution capacity of the eye is usually around 30 CPD. This spatial frequency corresponds to a visual acuity of 20/20 (or 6/6). The math for this is shown in the calculation in Box 1.2 with a 20/40 optotype as an example. It must be noted that acuity better than 20/20 (or 6/6) is also possible depending on an individual's neural and optical factors. In the periphery, the packing of the photoreceptors is not dense, and the morphology of the cones in the periphery is wider than those in the foveal region. Also, more rods are interspersed in the periphery. All these contribute to poorer visual acuity in the periphery [24].

1.3.2 Near Visual Acuity

The resolution capacity of the eye remains the same for both distant and near objects. The only difference between distance and near vision is that the crystalline lens needs to accommodate for near vision. This is because light rays from a near source are divergent, unlike those from distant objects, for which parallel light rays reach the eye. Hence, to negate the diverging light rays, the lens increases the plus power by becoming more biconvex, a process called accommodation. In younger individuals, a good distance acuity should also be reflected as good near acuity. If not, accommodative issues should be considered or ruled out. In individuals closer to their

Box 1.2: An Example Computation for Converting the Snellen Fraction to Cycles Per Degree and Cycles Per Degree to Snellen Fraction

Snellen fraction to cycles per degree

Let us consider a 6/12 or 20/40 optotype. In this, each stroke subtends 2 minutes of arc and therefore 1 cycle (black and white region) = 4 min of arc

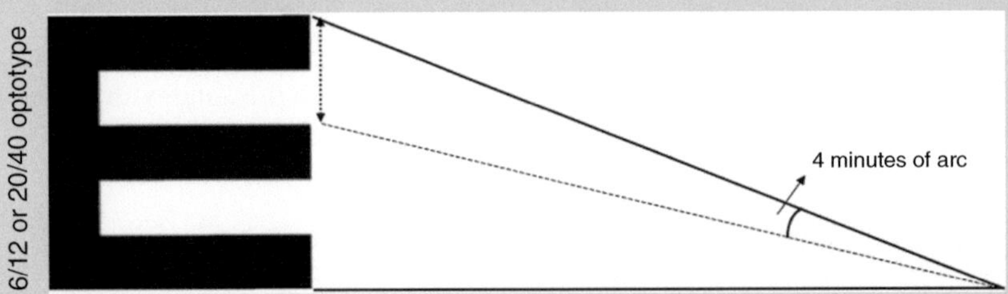

as 1° = 60′ (minutes of arc)

(1 cycle/4′) × (60′/1°) = 15 cycles per degree (CPD)

Therefore 20/40 = ~15 CPD

Cycles per degree to Snellen fraction

Let us consider the resolution acuity of 15 CPD. Since 15 cycles are in 1°, therefore one cycle's angle of subtense is

(1 cycle/15 cycles/degree) × (60′/1°) = 4′

In 1 cycle, we have 4′ since there are 2 strokes in one cycle,

Minimum angle of resolution of one stroke = 4′/2 = 2′

Therefore, the Snellen denominator = 2′ = x/20; x = 40

Hence, 15 CPD ~20/40

fourth decade of life (40 years), decreased accommodative amplitude may cause a reduction in near acuity (presbyopia). An appropriate near addition will restore the near visual acuity in such patients. However, in some instances, children may also have accommodative disorders, with or without good near visual acuity. These children may also require near addition [25, 26].

In other instances, where an accommodative disorder is not present, central opacity could be responsible for the reduction in near acuity. This is because of the pupillary miosis at near vision, and the effect of a central opacity, especially those closer to the nodal point (e.g., posterior polar cataract), could be more profound. Sometimes, binocular vision disorders like convergence insufficiency could cause a disturbance in reading. In some instances, pupillary miosis can cause an increased depth of focus, and that could result in better near visual acuity, with minimal or no near addition, even in the presbyopic age-group (e.g., use of pilocarpine in older adults for glaucoma could result in good near visual acuity).

1.3.3 Contrast

Contrast sensitivity is closely related to real-world visual functioning. Individuals with reduced contrast sensitivity at middle-to-low spatial frequencies were found to have difficulty in day-to-day tasks such as face recognition, identifying road signs and objects placed in common places, e.g., on an office desk, etc. [27]. In a large retrospective study of 1000 patients visiting a low-vision clinic, close to 50% of them with better than 20/60 presenting distance visual acuity, reported difficulty in face recognition [28]. In another large prospective study (n = 1113) on individuals with different ocular conditions, such as age-related macular degeneration, cataract, glaucoma, and retinitis pigmentosa, the contrast sensitivity tests provided valuable information in addition to visual acuity tests in the early detection of the disease [29].

Contrast sensitivity and low-contrast acuity are two different terms; therefore, care should be taken not to use them interchangeably. As discussed earlier, only the CSF gives a complete picture of the individual's contrast sensitivity across varying spatial frequencies; currently, CSF can be measured using tests such as the Functional Acuity Contrast Test (FACT) [30] and quick CSF [31].

1.3.3.1 Low-Contrast Visual Acuity

Similar to high-contrast visual acuity (HCVA), low-contrast visual acuity (LCVA) also tests the resolution of the eye but at contrast levels lower than the HCVA. The HCVA (or simply visual acuity) charts have a contrast level closer to 100%. Contrast levels usually tested for LCVA typically include 10% contrast, as in the Bailey–Lovie low-contrast visual acuity charts. At this level of contrast (i.e., at 10%), the expected reduction in visual acuity is by 2 lines earlier than that in HCVA [32]. The level of visual acuity reduction for different levels of contrast can be understood from the CSF (see Sect. 2.3.2). The factors that affect HCVA also affect LCVA. The blur circles formed due to refractive error impede the low-contrast acuity much more than the high-contrast acuity [33].

1.3.3.2 Contrast Sensitivity Function and Contrast Sensitivity

The CSF measures sensitivity to different contrast levels at different spatial frequencies. It is an inverted U-shaped function. The area under this function is where our visibility for different object sizes and contrasts lies. Every object or contrast outside this curve will be invisible to our eyes. Making those objects visible would require magnification or contrast enhancement, or both.

HCVA is a horizontal measurement in the CSF along the x-axis at 100% contrast value. LCVA is a horizontal measurement in the CSF along the x-axis at a 10% contrast value. The contrast is held constant in both these measures, and the spatial frequency is changed. Contrast sensitivity measure, on the other hand, is a vertical measurement where the spatial frequency (x-axis) is held constant, and only contrast is changed

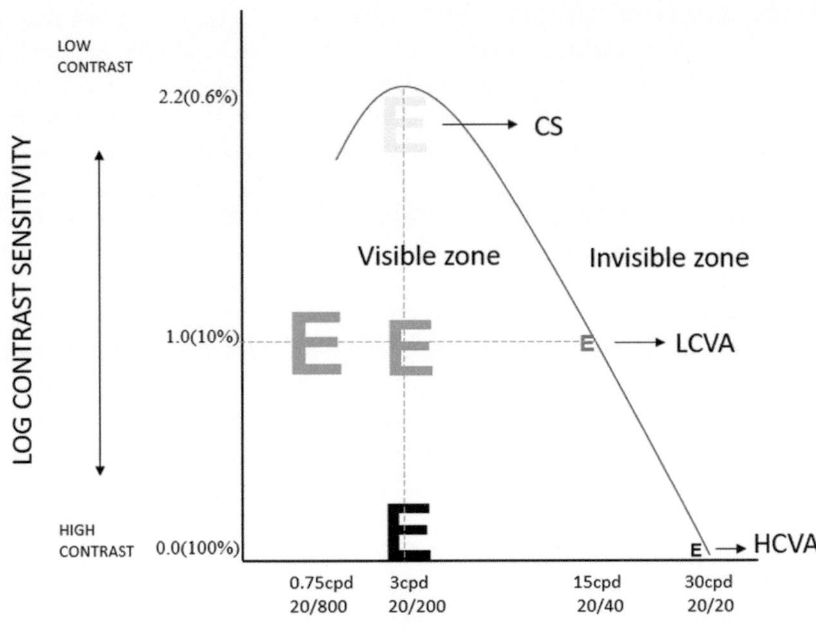

Fig. 1.7 An illustration of the contrast sensitivity function (CSF). On the *x*-axis are the different spatial frequencies denoted in cpd (cycles per degree) and Snellen fractions. Contrast values vary along the *y*-axis. *CS* contrast sensitivity, *LCVA* low-contrast visual acuity, *HCVA* high-contrast visual acuity

along the *y*-axis. At the lowest contrast (~1% contrast), the human eye can only see a target size of about 20/200 (or 6/60). This is the peak of the CSF (Fig. 1.7).

The high spatial frequency cut-off in CSF is the HCVA or visual acuity limit of the patient. This cut-off is determined by the photoreceptor density that also determines the resolution. The roll-off at the low spatial frequency end of the CSF is due to lateral inhibition of the receptive fields. A receptive field is the extent to which a stimulus can trigger neuronal firing within the neuron. Beyond this, the firing would decrease or cease. The ganglion receptive fields have a center-surround configuration. The center could get stimulated for an ON response, while the peripheral gets stimulated for an OFF response (ON-center, OFF-surround) or vice versa. A target big enough to fall within the center would stimulate a receptive field. However, if the target is too big (as in the low spatial frequencies), it falls on both the center and surround, cancelling the stimulation (lateral inhibition). This is why very low-spatial frequencies are also not visible.

Generally, when a reference to "contrast sensitivity" is made, it refers to the maximum peak in the CSF function. The height of this function is usually between 2 and 4 cpd; this corresponds to an acuity value of 20/200 (6/60) for 3 cpd. This value indicates the lowest contrast that can be detected. The maximum sensitivity (or lowest threshold) of the human eye is about 1% for a target at 20/200 (6/60) size.

1.4 Technique

Visual acuity is the first test most clinicians would do after obtaining a thorough patient history. This test should be treated as sacrosanct, and enough time should be given to take a proper measure without rushing and adapting shortcuts (e.g., only showing single letters in an electronic chart). Ideally, thresholding should be done to find the potential visual acuity of a person. There have to be 5 letters shown for each acuity level (i.e., in LogMAR style charts). This would ensure that crowding is uniformly maintained in the different levels of acuity.

Thresholding means that 50% of the time, the person is right in their response. The conventional stopping criteria for visual acuity is 3 or more mistakes in a line with 5 letters. Every letter read is valuable information to record, especially in determining improvement with an intervention in randomized clinical trials. It will be important to note such minor details (e.g., $20/20^{+1}$ or $20/20^{-2}$). Depending on the history, one could decide on which line to start to measure visual acuity. If no complaints are mentioned, one could directly show the 20/32 or 20/25 line and ask the patient to read from there. If difficulty in vision is reported, one could start from 20/200 level and ask the patient to read the first letter. If read correctly, the patient can be asked to read only the first letter in each line, essentially going down the chart, till they miss a letter, at which time, the patient should be asked to read the line above fully. This would save time and help reach the visual acuity threshold quickly.

Observe how fast the letters are read; if these are missed systematically on the left/right side, it could indicate a visual field defect. Similarly, people with age-related macular degeneration may have to fixate eccentrically to read. While patients with tunnel vision, like in retinitis pigmentosa or glaucoma, should be oriented to the location of the chart to be able to read and should also be given sufficient time to read. Patients unfamiliar with English letters can be shown alternate optotypes such as region-specific optotypes, symbols, pictures, tumbling E, and Landolt C.

Box 1.3 Examples of Visual Acuity Conversions for Different Distances in the Metric and Non-metric Systems

Example 1: If a patient reads a 6/60 optotype calibrated for 6 m at a 1-m testing distance, then the acuity will be 1/60, equivalent to 6/360 (obtained by multiplying the numerator and the denominator by 6).

Example 2: If a patient cannot read a 20/796 optotype on a COMPlog system calibrated for 20 feet. The patient can be asked to move closer (to 10 feet); therefore, a 20/796 optotype at 10 feet will be 10/796, equivalent to 20/1592 (obtained by multiplying the numerator and denominator by 2).

1.4.1 Measuring Acuity in Individuals with Vision Impairment

In the case of patients whose visual acuity cannot be recorded at standard testing distances such as 3, 4, and 6 m due to visual impairment, closer testing distances should be considered. Recording acuity by finger counting and hand movement should be avoided as much as possible, as they are not standardized or repeatable measures. When shorter testing distances are used, it is important to perform appropriate conversions (see Box 1.3).

Best corrected distance visual acuity is an important visual function (in addition to the peripheral visual field); it is considered for categorizing vision impairment and providing social benefits based on nation-specific acts and regulations. The different categories of vision impairment as per the International Classification of Diseases-11 (ICD-11) [34] are summarized in Table 1.1. There could be a wider variability in the test–retest of visual function parameters in individuals with vision impairment due to factors such as adaptation to illumination levels, disease progression, and psychosocial states. Therefore, the patient should be given adequate time to respond during testing [35].

Charts such as the Berkeley Rudimentary Vision Test (BRVT) (Fig. 1.8) can be used to quantify visual acuity in individuals with severe to profound visual impairment. The acuity range measured using the BRVT is 1.40–2.60 logMAR (i.e., 20/500–20/8000) in a single tumbling E

Table 1.1 Categories of vision impairment as per the International Classification of Diseases-11 (ICD-11) [34]

Category of vision impairment	Distance visual acuity range
Mild vision impairment	Worse than 6/12–6/18
Moderate vision impairment	Worse than 6/18–6/60
Severe vision impairment	Worse than 6/60–3/60
Blindness	Worse than 3/60
Near vision impairment: worse than N_6 or 8M at 40 cm	

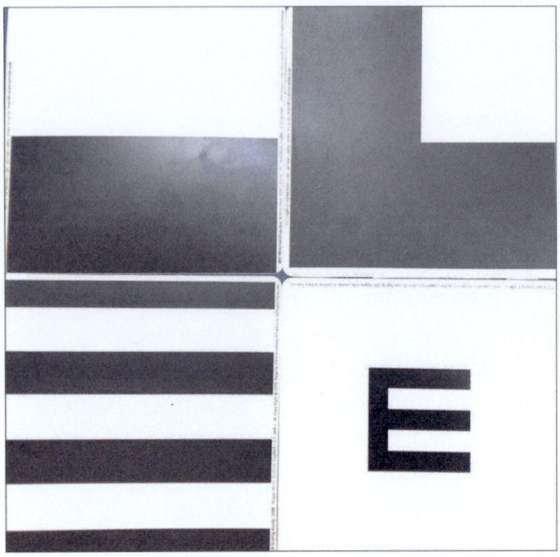

Fig. 1.8 The Berkeley Rudimentary Vision Test (BRVT)

chart. For the grating acuity, the range is 2.30–2.90 logMAR (i.e., 20/4000–20/16,000), and for the white-field projection (including hemifield and quad-field), the logMin = 3.2 for testing spatial localization; for a basic visual function test called the black-white discrimination (BWD), the logMin = 3.5 [36]. Note logMin (not logMAR) values given are arbitrary values as per the specifications of the test card. If the patient's visual acuity is unrecordable with any of the measures discussed above, projection of rays (in all 4 quadrants) and perception of light should be documented.

1.4.2 Measuring Visual Acuity in Children

Visual acuity testing is vital for detecting amblyopia. Therefore, it is important to avoid single-line and single-optotype testing. Test results with full chart vs. single line and single optotype can be variable, with the acuity estimates of the latter two techniques over-estimating visual acuity in amblyopia compared to the entire chart [37].

Visual acuity measurement in children can prove to be tricky. The optotypes should be shuffled while checking monocular acuity, and rechecking the same acuity line may lead to issues as children are likely to memorize the letters. In case of unavailability of an extra acuity chart, the letters could be asked to be read randomly or in reverse order. This problem is prevented in electronic visual acuity charts.

The choice of visual acuity tools in children cannot always be limited to chronologically age-appropriate tests. In such cases, alternate testing tools/techniques should be explored. For example, if a 10-year-old girl diagnosed with Down syndrome cannot respond verbally to letter optotypes, she can be asked to copy the letters (alternate technique), or testing with symbols/picture optotypes can be considered (alternate testing tools). Grating/resolution acuity tests are popularly used among infants, young children, children, and individuals with special needs, although acuities obtained using resolution and recognition acuity tests may not be comparable [38].

In using grating acuity tests (e.g., Teller acuity cards-II), it is important to mask the clinician to the location of the grating to avoid clinician bias. Firstly, the child's verbal/non-verbal response (finger pointing or based on eye movement) should be recorded by the clinician, and then the location of the grating should be checked on the card to judge whether it is a correct or incorrect response. For thresholding purposes, 2 of 3 correct criteria are suggested. When using grating paddles such as LEA grating paddles (Fig. 1.9), it is important to move both the paddles (plain and the grating) equally to avoid movement-initiated eye movement.

The chart used should also be documented, and if possible, the same chart should be used in the follow-up visit as well, as the acuities obtained with various tests may not be comparable [39, 40]. Good documentation is essential for an appropriate clinical interpretation of the acuity measure (e.g., progression with intervention). When documenting grating acuity, the cycles per centimeter (CPCM) should be converted to CPD (Box 1.4).

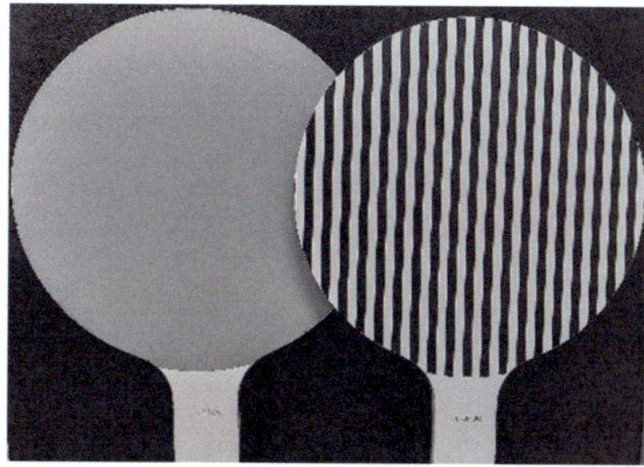

Fig. 1.9 LEA grating paddles

> **Box 1.4: An Example Computation to Convert Cycles Per Centimeter to Cycles Per Degree**
> (at 57 cm, 1 cm = 1° of visual angle; therefore, at 57 cm, CPCM~CPD)
> For e.g., 10 CPCM at 38 cm = (38/57) × 10 = 6.66 CPD
> (*CPCM* cycles per centimeter, *CPD* cycles per degree)
> CPD = (testing distance/57) × CPCM

1.4.3 Measuring Near Visual Acuity

In near visual acuity measurement (ideal to record in "M" or "N" notation), it is important to mention the testing distance, chart, and illumination used for recording the acuity. While testing individuals with visual impairment, testing distance helps to determine the magnification required for near assistive devices. In addition to room illumination, extra illumination, when used, should be documented as well, as patients with impaired contrast sensitivity may have better near acuity with extra illumination. For individuals unfamiliar with words, alternate tools such as isolated letter charts, numbers (Fig. 1.10), symbols, tumbling E, and Landolt C should be considered for measurement purposes.

1.4.4 Contrast Acuity and Contrast Sensitivity

The assessment of LCVA is similar to that for HCVA, with the same thresholding criteria (3 of 5 optotypes). Assessment of LCVA at 2.5% was reported to help detect certain ocular conditions such as optic neuritis [41] and multiple sclerosis [42] and for a few occupational requirements, such as those for pilots [43]. However, in the clinic, the LCVA is conventionally assessed at 10% contrast, and HCVA is assessed at 95–100%, as most of the functional visual tasks are within this range of contrast. Reduction of acuity at 10% contrast sensitivity is important as it would mean a tenfold loss of contrast sensitivity than the normal measure of approximately 1%, which causes disabling effects in regular activities [44]. A decline of 2 or more lines in LCVA (recorded at 10% contrast sensitivity) compared to the high-contrast visual acuity is considered a clinically meaningful difference and can have functional implications [32]. This is commonly observed in individuals with vision impairment, who are then advised to use appropriate contrast-enhancing measures such as using appropriate illumination and maintaining good target and background contrast in regularly accessed stations (such as office desks, kitchen counters, etc.). In ocular conditions, such as albinism, aniridia, and a few retinal dystrophies, filters and tints are recommended to reduce glare and enhance contrast.

First, measuring binocular contrast sensitivity is suggested to quickly understand the patient's visual concerns in regular clinical practice. Care should be taken to shuffle the optotypes or show different ones to avoid the bias likely to occur due to memorizing them.

Card-based acuity and contrast charts can undergo wear and tear due to extensive usage in the clinics and should be regularly replaced. Using the charts with utmost care is important to avoid incorrect readings. Gloves should be used

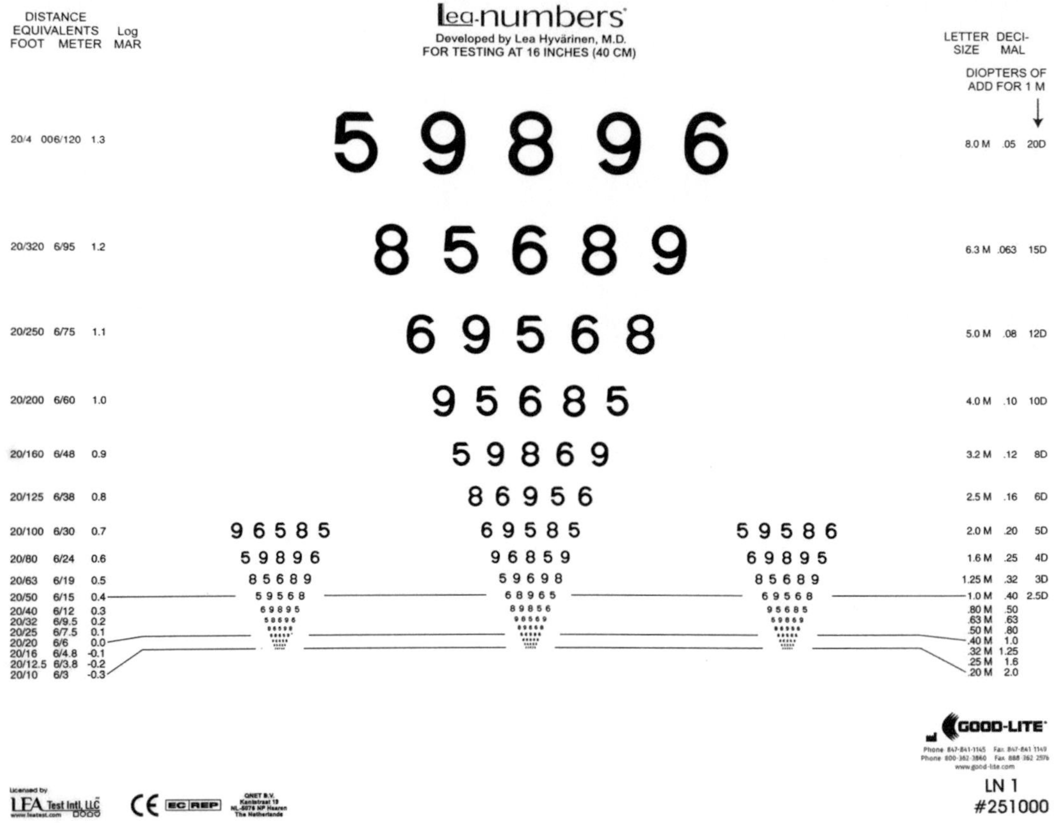

Fig. 1.10 The LEA numbers near visual acuity chart

particularly when handling charts used to assess contrast sensitivity or low-contrast visual acuity, as the discoloration of the charts can make the low-contrast stimuli more challenging to resolve, thereby underestimating the patient's contrast values.

1.5 Conclusion

High- and low-contrast visual acuity and contrast sensitivity measures are useful screening parameters to help the clinician understand the patient's complaints. They are also important outcome measures to quantify the effectiveness of any intervention or to understand the disease progression. Inadequate awareness of the techniques used to measure these visual function parameters among clinicians can lead to errors in documentation and intervention. Although these are commonly noted as quick measures, appropriate thresholding techniques should be used while recording to avoid over/underestimating the same. Vulnerable groups such as children (particularly those with special needs) and individuals with visual impairment are likely to need extra time and care, as there could be a wider test–retest difference in their visual function parameters owing to the severity of the condition and overall developmental delays.

Acknowledgments We thank Ms. Shakthi Pradheepa for her help with the figures.

Funding Funding Hyderabad Eye Research Foundation, Hyderabad, India.

Disclosure None.

References

1. Snellen H. Test-types for determination of the acuteness of vision, vol. 44. Utrecht: van de Weijer; 1862. p. 520.
2. Bailey IL, Lovie JE. New design principles for visual acuity letter charts. Am J Optom Physiol Optic. 1976;53(11):740–5.
3. Ferris FL 3rd, Kassoff A, Bresnick GH, Bailey I. New visual acuity charts for clinical research. Am J Ophthalmol. 1982;94(1):91–6.
4. Woo G, Lo P. A Chinese word acuity chart with new design principles. Singap Med J. 1980;21(5):689–92.
5. Al-Mufarrej MM, Abo-Hiemed FA, Oduntan AO. A new Arabic distance visual acuity chart. Optom Vis Sci. 1996;73(1):59–61.
6. Datta S, Varadharajan S, Mazumdar D, et al. Construction and validation of LEA Hindi chart: a multicenter study. Optom Vis Sci. 2020;97(5):351–9.
7. Hyvarinen L, Nasanen R, Laurinen P. New visual acuity test for pre-school children. Acta Ophthalmol. 1980;58(4):507–11.
8. Taylor HR. Applying new design principles to the construction of an illiterate E chart. Am J Optom Physiol Optic. 1978;55(5):348–51.
9. Pointer JS, Gilmartin G, Larke JR. The evolution of the broken ring visual acuity test figure. J Am Optom Assoc. 1980;51(8):741–5.
10. Laidlaw DAH, Tailor V, Shah N, et al. Validation of a computerised logMAR visual acuity measurement system (COMPlog): comparison with ETDRS and the electronic ETDRS testing algorithm in adults and amblyopic children. Br J Ophthalmol. 2008;92(2):241–4.
11. Fantz RL. Visual perception from birth as shown by pattern selectivity. Ann N Y Acad Sci. 1965;118(21):793–814.
12. Sumalini R, Satgunam P. Grating acuity tests for infants, young children and individuals with disabilities: a review of recent advances. Semin Ophthalmol. 2022;38:76.
13. Runge PE. Eduard Jaeger's test-types (Schrift–Scalen) and the historical development of vision tests. Trans Am Ophthalmol Soc. 2000;98:375–438.
14. Blesi M, Wise BA, Kelley-Arney C. Medical assisting administrative and clinical competencies. Cengage Learning; 2011.
15. Colenbrander A, Runge P. Can Jaeger numbers be standardized. Invest Ophthalmol Vis Sci. 2007;48(13):3563.
16. Kaur K, Gurnani B. Contrast sensitivity. In: StatPearls. Treasure Island (FL): StatPearls Publishing; 2023. https://www.ncbi.nlm.nih.gov/books/NBK580542/.
17. Pelli DG, Robson JG, Wilkins AJ. The design of a new letter chart for measuring contrast sensitivity. Clin Vis Sci. 1988;2(3):187–99.
18. Njeru SM, Osman M, Brown AM. The effect of test distance on visual contrast sensitivity measured using the Pelli–Robson chart. Transl Vis Sci Technol. 2021;10(2):32.
19. Elliott DB, Sanderson K, Conkey A. The reliability of the Pelli–Robson contrast sensitivity chart. Ophthalmic Physiol Opt. 1990;10(1):21–4.
20. Hopkins GR 2nd, Dougherty BE, Brown AM. The Ohio contrast cards: visual performance in a pediatric low-vision site. Optom Vis Sci. 2017;94(10):946–56.
21. Arditi A. Improving the design of the letter contrast sensitivity test. Invest Ophthalmol Vis Sci. 2005;46(6):2225–9.
22. Anderson HA, Mathew AR, Cheng H. Evaluation of the SpotChecks contrast sensitivity test in children. Ophthalmic Physiol Opt. 2023;43(1):64–72.
23. Kniestedt C, Stamper RL. Visual acuity and its measurement. Ophthalmol Clin N Am. 2003;16(2):155–70. v
24. Volpe NJ. Adler's physiology of the eye: clinical application. J Neuro-Ophthalmol. 2004;24(4):348.
25. Satgunam P, Datta S, Sumalini R. Near vision in individuals with down syndrome: a vision screening study. Eye (Lond). 2019;33(8):1254–60.
26. Nandakumar K, Leat SJ. Bifocals in children with down syndrome (BiDS)—visual acuity, accommodation and early literacy skills. Acta Ophthalmol. 2010;88(6):e196–204.
27. Owsley C, Sloane ME. Contrast sensitivity, acuity, and the perception of 'real-world' targets. Br J Ophthalmol. 1987;71(10):791–6.
28. Rubin GS, Schuchard RA, editors. Does contrast sensitivity predict face recognition performance in low-vision observers? Noninvasive assessment of the visual system. Nevada: Optica Publishing Group; 1990.
29. Xiong Y-Z, Kwon M, Bittner AK, et al. Relationship between acuity and contrast sensitivity: differences due to eye disease. Invest Ophthalmol Vis Sci. 2020;61(6):40.
30. Ginsburg AP. A new contrast sensitivity vision test chart. Optom Vis Sci. 1984;61(6):403–7.
31. Lesmes LA, Lu ZL, Baek J, Albright TD. Bayesian adaptive estimation of the contrast sensitivity function: the quick CSF method. J Vis. 2010;10(3):17–21.
32. Mowry EM, Loguidice MJ, Daniels AB, et al. Vision related quality of life in multiple sclerosis: correlation with new measures of low and high contrast letter acuity. J Neurol Neurosurg Psychiatry. 2009;80(7):767–72.
33. Johnson CA, Casson EJ. Effects of luminance, contrast, and blur on visual acuity. Optom Vis Sci. 1995;72(12):864–9.
34. Blindness and Vision Impairment: Definitions. https://www.who.int/news-room/fact-sheets/detail/blindness-and-visual-impairment. Accessed 4 July 2023.
35. Bittner AK, Ibrahim MA, Haythornthwaite JA, et al. Vision test variability in retinitis pigmentosa and psychosocial factors. Optom Vis Sci. 2011;88(12):1496–506.

36. Bailey IL, Jackson AJ, Minto H, et al. The Berkeley rudimentary vision test. Optom Vis Sci. 2012;89(9):1257–64.
37. Morad Y, Werker E, Nemet P. Visual acuity tests using chart, line, and single optotype in healthy and amblyopic children. J AAPOS. 1999;3(2):94–7.
38. Friedman DS, Munoz B, Massof RW, et al. Grating visual acuity using the preferential-looking method in elderly nursing home residents. Invest Ophthalmol Vis Sci. 2002;43(8):2572–8.
39. Anstice NS, Jacobs RJ, Simkin SK, et al. Do picture-based charts overestimate visual acuity? Comparison of kay pictures, lea symbols, HOTV and Keeler logMAR charts with Sloan letters in adults and children. PLoS One. 2017;12(2):e0170839.
40. Sumalini R, Satgunam P, Subramanian A, Conway M. Clinical utility of 'Peekaboo Vision' application for measuring grating acuity in children with down syndrome. Br Ir Orthopt J. 2022;18(1):18–26.
41. Park SH, Park CY, Shin YJ, et al. Low contrast visual acuity might help to detect previous optic neuritis. Front Neurol. 2020;11:602193.
42. Balcer L, Raynowska J, Nolan R, et al. Validity of low-contrast letter acuity as a visual performance outcome measure for multiple sclerosis. Mult Scler J. 2017;23:135245851769082.
43. Hyvarinen L. LEA contrast sensitivity. https://www.leatest.com/sites/default/files/pdf/ContrastSensitivity.pdf. Accessed 29 June 2023.
44. Leat SJ, Legge GE, Bullimore MA. What is low vision? A re-evaluation of definitions. Optom Vis Sci. 1999;76(4):198–211.

2 Autorefraction: Objective Estimation of Refractive Error

Shrikant R. Bharadwaj

2.1 Introduction

Uncorrected refractive error is the leading cause of visual impairment and one of the most common causes of avoidable blindness globally [1, 2]. Inaccurately corrected refractive errors also lead to undesirable consequences such as suboptimal visual resolution, asthenopia, binocular vision anomalies, and amblyopia in children; all of these adversely affect the individual's quality of life and daily activities [3–5]. Therefore, screening for uncorrected refractive errors and accurate correction is vital in eye care [6]. Identifying and correcting such errors in a typical eye examination are a two-step process, commonly designated as "objective" and "subjective" refraction. Objective refraction involves the eye care practitioner estimating the refractive error of the eye through one of several "objective" techniques, while subjective refraction involves refining the refractive error estimates to optimize the patient's vision by eliciting "subjective" responses from the patient. The endpoint of objective refraction is typically used as the starting point of subjective refraction. This chapter will focus on specific automated techniques commonly used in objective refraction. Retinoscopy, the present-day gold standard for objective refraction, against which all other autorefractors are compared will be discussed along with subjective refraction techniques in other chapter(s) of this book.

Several techniques have been developed over the years to objectively estimate the eye's spherocylindrical refractive error [7, 8]. Given the automated nature of refractive error estimation, sans the intervention of a human observer, this technology has come to be broadly referred to as "autorefraction," and the instrumentation associated with autorefraction is referred to as "autorefractors." This chapter will focus briefly on the measurement techniques used in these autorefractors, their accuracy, vis-à-vis, retinoscopy, repeatability, and their scope of use in tertiary eye care settings versus mass screening of uncorrected refractive error in public health settings. Given the intended purpose of this book as a ready reckoner for optometrists and ophthalmologists about the different technologies involved in automated refraction, only broad overviews of these technologies will be provided. For specific technical details on the relative performance of different autorefractors, the readers are referred to the recent publications by Padhy et al. [7] and Venkataraman et al. [8].

S. R. Bharadwaj (✉)
Brien Holden Institute of Optometry and Vision Sciences, Prof. Brien Holden Eye Research Centre, L V Prasad Eye Institute, Hyderabad, India
e-mail: bharadwaj@lvpei.org

T. Das, P. Satgunam (eds.), *Ophthalmic Diagnostics*, https://doi.org/10.1007/978-981-97-0138-4_2

2.2 Technology

2.2.1 Measurement Principle of Autorefractors

Autorefraction technology may be categorized into several types based on instrument design and measurement principles (Table 2.1). Each technology has advantages and disadvantages that determine its accuracy, precision, and utility in tertiary-level care or mass screening in public health endeavors. Depending on the instrument design, autorefractors can be categorized as: (1) those that measure the refractive status of each eye separately (monocular techniques) or of both eyes simultaneously (binocular techniques), (2) those that control for the accommodative status of the eye by allowing presentation of real-world targets through an open-field viewing design or those that "fog" the stimulus using a closed-field viewing design, and (3) those that use the entire pupil area for estimation of refractive error or those that use only the central pupil for estimation of refractive error. These autorefractors use one of several measurement principles, including wavefront analysis, Scheiner disc principle, best

Table 2.1 Detailed characteristics of currently available common refractive error measurement techniques

Characteristics	Retinoscopy	Open/closed-field autorefractors	Wavefront-based autorefractors	Photorefractors
Working principle	Foucault knife-edge	Scheiner pupil | ray deflection | best-focus	Wavefront aberrometry	Eccentric infrared photorefraction
Operating range	No specific operating range	+22 D to −25 D for sphere and ±10.00 D for cylinder	±10.00 D for sphere and ±6.00 D for cylinder	±7.50 D for sphere and ±3.50 D for cylinder
Invasiveness of measurement	Non-invasive Measurements performed from a distance	Non-invasive Participant stabilized on forehead rest	Device touches the face for measurement	Non-invasive Measurements are performed from a distance
Portability	Portable	Table-top	Portable	Portable
Measurement time	Measurement takes time	~5 measurements per second	~10 measurements per second	<1 s per measurement
Fixation distance	Distant target	Near target with simulated distance viewing	Distant target	Distant target
Pupil size dependence	Measurements become challenging with pupil miosis	Stable measurements for pupil diameter up to 2 mm	Measurement accuracy may vary with pupil diameter	Measurement accuracy decreases with pupil miosis
Binocular viewing/ measurements	Viewing can be binocular, but the measurement is monocular	Only monocular viewing and measurements	Only monocular viewing and measurements	Viewing and measurement can be binocular
Participant cooperation	Needs limited cooperation Useful in challenging cases	Participant cooperation is essential for reliable measurements	Participant cooperation is critical for reliable measurements	Needs limited cooperation Useful in challenging cases
Examiner training	Examiner training is time-consuming	Examiners can be trained within a short time	Examiners can be trained within a short time	Examiners can be trained within a short time
Near-triad measurements	Only measurement of accommodation is possible	Only measurement of accommodation is possible (in closed-field, only the measure of refractive error is possible)	Only measurement of accommodation is possible	Near-triad can be measured in sync with each other
Examples of commercial devices	Welch Allyn 18245 Elite HPX Streak Retinoscope	Nidek TONOREF™ III | HandyRef-K | Shin-Nippon NVision-K 5001	E-see | Visionix Eye Refract | WaveAnalyzer 700	Welch Allyn Spot Vision Screener | PlusoptiX A12C

Data on operating ranges and measurement time are obtained from the manufacturer-prescribed user manual of each instrument. Table adapted from Padhy et al. [7]

focus principle, proprietary rotary prism technology (i.e., ray-deflection), and photorefraction.

Autorefractors dependent on wavefront analysis typically shine a coherent light source in the infrared wavelength into the eye and capture the light reflected from the retina onto a Shack–Hartmann-based wavefront sensor. The sensed wavefront, at the level of the eye's pupil, is then broken down into component Zernike polynomials from which the sphero-cylindrical refractive error is calculated [9]. The lower-order aberration of defocus ($Z_{2,0}$) corresponds to the spherical refractive error, while the cylindrical error of the eye is computed from a combination of the defocus and the two astigmatism terms [vertical astigmatism ($Z_{2,2}$) and oblique astigmatism ($Z_{2,-2}$)] terms of the Zernike polynomial series [9]. The readers are referred to the excellent review on the topic of clinical applications of wavefront-based refraction by Bruce and Catania [10] for details on the measurement of the eye's wavefront aberrations and the Zernike polynomial-based representation of the eye's wavefront aberrations (the *Z*-notation stated above) and the various dependencies of the eye's wavefront aberration profile (e.g., pupil diameter, viewing distance) [10].

Autorefractors that use Scheiner's disc principle essentially perform the same measurement as the wavefront-based technique, with the exception that the reflected light from the retina is converted into a diplopic image using Scheiner's pupil. In addition, the dioptric position of the sensor within the autorefractor where the diplopic components converge to become a single image is considered as the refractive error of the eye. The orientation of Scheiner's pupil is changed to estimate the refractive error of the eye across different meridians to compute the astigmatic refractive error of the eye. Autorefractors relying on the ray deflection technique, in principle, work similarly to the previous technology, but given the proprietary nature of this technology, the exact details of its operation remain unknown. Likewise, autorefractors, relying on the best focus technique, attempt to determine the conjugate focus of an internal target in different meridians to determine the sphero-cylindrical refractive error of the eye.

Photorefractors (also called photoscreeners [11]) determine the spherocylindrical refractive error by sending in infrared light from a series of LEDs placed slightly eccentrically from the camera aperture and analyzing the pattern of luminance profile formed across the pupil by the light reflected from the retina (Fig. 2.1a). An emmetropic eye has a uniform pattern of luminance across the pupil, while those with refractive errors tend to have a graded profile, the orientation of which is dependent on whether the light is focused in front of the retina (myopia) or behind the retina (hypermetropia) (see example of luminance profile with induced myopia in Fig. 2.1b). This luminance profile is quantified using standard linear regression analysis and converted into units of diopters (*D*) using a defocus calibration factor (Fig. 2.1c). The luminance profile formed across the pupil and, hence, the refractive error estimated by the photorefractor depends on several factors, such as the overall light intensity reflected off the retina, the pupil diameter, and the subject's ethnicity [12, 13]. All these limit the operating range of the photorefractor and make the refractive error estimates prone to large inter-individual and inter-ethnic variations (Fig. 2.1c, d) [12, 13].

All these autorefractor designs are available as tabletop or handheld designs that determine their portability. As an aside, some autorefractors also come with the advantage of being able to estimate additional ocular parameters that are associated with the refractive error of the eye (e.g., pupillary diameter and vergence eye position as part of the near-triad keratometry to estimate corneal curvature and axial length measurements to determine the source of the uncorrected refractive error).

2.2.2 Relative Advantages/Disadvantages of Different Autorefractors

Each autorefractor design has certain advantages over the others and may be useful in specific settings or for particular populations (Table 2.1). For instance, photorefraction can rapidly obtain

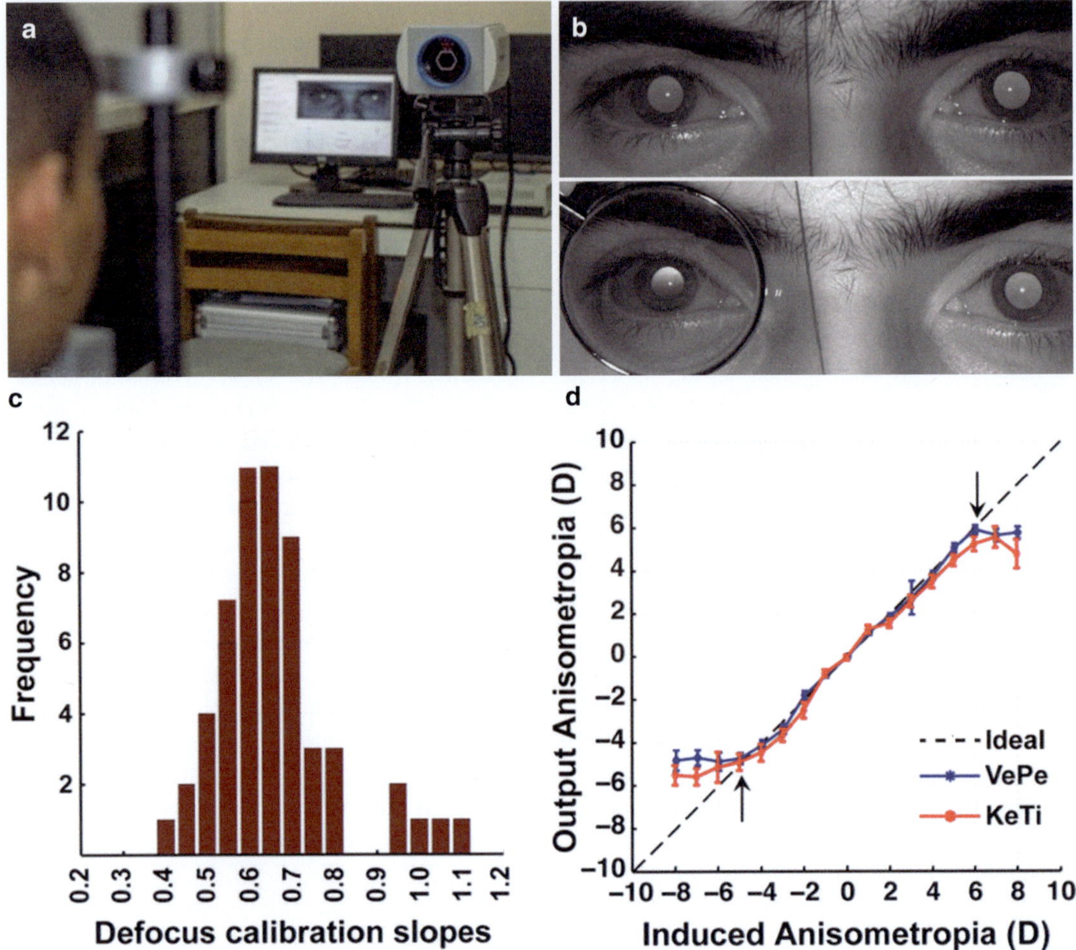

Fig. 2.1 An eccentric infrared photorefractor used for estimating the eye's refractive error (Panel **a**). The infrared light that is mounted eccentric to the camera aperture is seen in this panel. The luminance profile across the pupil in a representative emmetropic subject without (top panel) and with (bottom panel) induced refractive error (Panel **b**). The pupil was uniformly illuminated at the baseline, while the luminance profile gradually changed from bright to dark from the top to the bottom of the pupil, with induced myopia in the right eye (bottom panel). The slope of this luminance profile is calibrated into diopters—the defocus calibration slope. The intersubject variability in the defocus calibration slope may induce variability in the refractive error measurements of photorefraction (Panel **c**). The refractive error (anisometropia) measured by the photorefractor was plotted as a function of the induced refractive error (anisometropia) for two representative subjects (Panel **d**). The vertical arrows in this panel indicate the values where the refractive error measurements saturate, reflecting the operating range of the photorefractor

simultaneous estimates of refractive error from both eyes and the near-triad from a remote distance; this is advantageous when scanning infants, children, and special-needs populations, where cooperation may be limited (Table 2.1, Fig. 2.1a). Variability in the defocus calibration profile and the operating range of the photorefractor (Fig. 2.1c, d) limit its utility as an accurate and precise device for estimating the objective refractive error of the eye. This technology is, therefore, confined to being mainly used as a screening tool for refractive errors in a public health setting [11]. However, photorefractors are useful in research settings that investigate the near-triadic properties of the visual system [14, 15], and have more recently also been used to identify ocular refractive pathologies like keratoconus [16] and spasm of near reflex [17].

Much like photorefraction, autorefraction technologies based on wavefront aberrometry also use the entire pupil to determine the refractive error status of the eye [7, 8]. Due to the inherent dependence of wavefront aberrometry on pupil size, these autorefractors have built-in technologies that estimate pupil diameter and scale the wavefront measurements to that pupil diameter. The refractive error estimates, therefore, may vary slightly depending on the pupil size. Given that this technology estimates several orders of wavefront errors of the eye, they may be more useful in estimating the refractive error in people with highly aberrated optics (e.g., eyes with keratoconus or post-corneal transplantation). However, this remains a theoretical possibility for now, and additional scientific evidence must be gathered to support or refute this possibility.

Autoreflectors based on the Scheiner disc, best focus, or ray-deflection principles only utilize the central pupil to measure refractive error [7, 8]. These become the choice of measurement for patients with high refractive errors outside the operating range of other techniques, with high accuracy and repeatability (Table 2.1). The ability of technology to control the accommodative status of the eye to minimize instrument myopia and reveal the maximum hyperopic refractive error has been subject to intense scientific investigation. In general, technologies within this domain that have an open-field viewing design have been shown to exert better control over the accommodative state of the eye relative to their counterparts with closed-field designs that attempt to minimize the impact by using blurred fixation stimuli with a linear perspective. However, the refractive error output from these autorefractor designs is quite sensitive to patient alignment and typically requires them to be positioned in a chinrest for reliable measurements. This tends to make the design bulky and demanding, thus limiting its portability and utility in infants, children, and individuals with special needs. Further, autorefractors within this domain are monocular, cannot measure the vergence status of the eye, and do not come with algorithms that can measure the pupil size (although such a measurement is theoretically possible). While open-field autorefractors were traditionally used in research settings that required accurate control over the accommodative demand [18], more recently, they have also gained popularity in measuring the peripheral refraction of the eye [19], a critical component in the management of myopia and its progression [20].

2.3 Clinical Applications

2.3.1 Accuracy and Precision Considerations

The aforementioned advantages of any autorefractor technology are contingent on the technology producing accurate and repeatable measurements. Accuracy is the closeness of the technique's estimate of the parameter of interest (refractive error, in this case) to a gold standard value [21, 22]. Simultaneously, repeatability (also called reliability or precision) is the variability in estimating the given parameter over repeated measurements [21, 22]. Repeatability also reflects the measurement technique's ability to discriminate one value of the given parameter from another—the higher the precision, the better the discriminant capability [21, 22]. For screening purposes, an allowance for measurement accuracy can be made so that the device's sensitivity and specificity in identifying a predetermined level of refractive error are not compromised. For diagnostic settings, the accuracy of measurements is more critical as these become the starting point for subjective refraction or, in some challenging cases where subjective refraction is not possible, and the refractive error correction is based entirely on the objective refraction value (e.g., young children or mentally challenged individuals). For both settings, high measurement repeatability is desirable to increase faith in the outcome measures.

Comparative analyses of accuracy and repeatability across different autorefraction techniques obtained from the same cohort of subjects provide critical input on one technique's performance against others, enabling evidence-based justification of their utility as a starting point for subjective refraction in the clinic and/or as a screening tool for refractive errors in public health settings. Two recent studies—Padhy et al. [7] and Venkataraman et al. [8]—systematically addressed this issue and found similar results. On an average, none of the autorefractors showed larger biases in the estimates of spherical and cylindrical refraction relative to retinoscopy, but there was significant inter-technique variability in the results (Fig. 2.2). The estimate of refractive error by an autorefractor could differ from retinoscopy by as much as ±2.5 D for the spherical component and by as much as ±1 D for the astigmatic component (Fig. 2.2) [7]. Surprisingly, this difference does not seem to be impacted by the patient's age [7], as one would expect from younger children with stronger accommodative tendencies [23]. The inter-session repeatability of refractive error estimates was within ±1 D and ±0.75 D in the spherical and astigmatic components, respectively, across all measurement techniques [7]. Photorefraction showed marginally poorer repeatability than the other techniques (Fig. 2.3) [8]. Open-field autorefractors and closed-field autorefractors with an inbuilt fogging mechanism showed better accuracy and precision than those that did not incorporate such a mechanism [8]. However, the inter-session repeatability of the measurement techniques was smaller than the inter-instrument repeatability, indicating that some of the variability shown

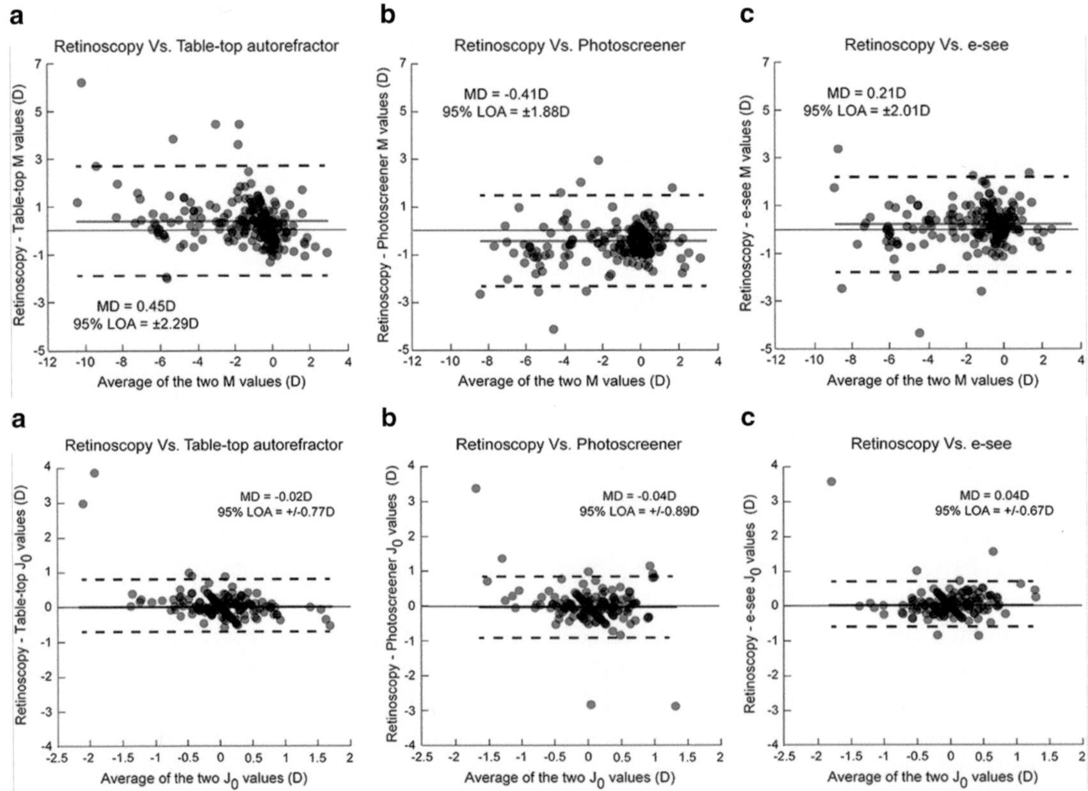

Fig. 2.2 Bland–Altman type plots of the agreement in M (top panels) and J_0 (bottom panels) power vector values between the three autorefractor designs and retinoscopy evaluations in this study (see Sect. 2.3.2 for details of power vector analysis). The solid dashed lines in each panel indicate the mean difference (MD) and the 95% limits of agreement (LOA). The numerical values of these parameters are also indicated in each panel. The negative values along the abscissa of each panel indicate myopic refraction. The positive and negative values along the ordinate of each panel indicate an overestimation and underestimation bias by a given autorefractor relative to retinoscopy. (Figure adapted from Padhy et al. [7])

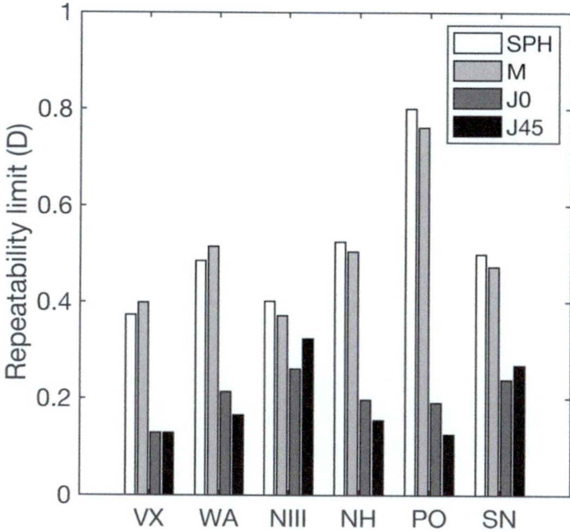

Fig. 2.3 Repeatability of M, J_0, and J_{45} power vector components obtained across different autorefractor designs (see Sect. 2.3.2 for details of power vector analysis). *SPH* sphere, *M* spherical equivalent, J_0, and J_{45} cylindrical vector components, *VX* eye refract, *WA* WaveAnalyzer 700, *NIII* TONOREF™ III, *NH* handheld ref./keratometer Handy Ref-K, *PO* PlusoptiX A12C, *SN* NVision-K 5001. (Figure adapted from Venkataraman et al. [8])

above in Fig. 2.2 occurs genuinely due to the autorefractor technology mis-estimating the eye's spherocylindrical refractive error. Since the cohort in both studies had regular refractive errors, the accuracy and precision in estimating the oblique and irregular astigmatism components remain to be fully evaluated. Such an investigation will offer important insights into the utility of autorefractor technology for estimating the refractive errors of eyes with complicated optics (e.g., keratoconus).

2.3.2 Legitimate Representation of Sphero-Cylindrical Refraction

This section is not unique to the estimation of the eye's refractive error by autorefractors; it applies to the representation of sphero-cylindrical refraction in general, as estimated by retinoscopy, autorefractors, and subjective refraction or corrections applied to the eye using spectacles or contact lenses. This section is motivated by the routine errors observed in the representation of sphero-cylindrical refraction while comparing between instruments, describing longitudinal data obtained from patients, describing the impact of optical/surgical interventions on the eye's optical power, or while comparing the sphero-cylindrical refractions of two cohorts of patients (e.g., keratoconus vs. healthy controls). Consider a scenario where the patient's refractive error is +2.00 DS/−1.00 DC × 70° on the first visit and +2.50 DS/−2.00 DC × 30° on the second visit. Clearly, the spherical equivalent of refraction (1.50 D) remains the same between the two visits. However, making inferences about a change in the astigmatic component of the two refractions is less straightforward because there is an alteration in both the magnitude and axis of the astigmatism. Often, an inference about the change in astigmatism is arrived at by simply comparing their magnitudes while ignoring their axes. This is incorrect because astigmatism is a vector inherently defined by its magnitude and axis. It is more legitimate to compare the magnitudes of astigmatism when they are referenced to the same axis. Several mathematical formulations have been derived to achieve this, notably including the power vector analysis by Thibos et al. [24] and vector decompensation analysis by Alpins et al. [25] and Harris et al. [26]. The former analysis will be briefly described here; readers interested in a deeper understanding of this topic are urged to read the abovementioned citations.

The power vector analysis breaks down any sphero-cylindrical refraction into three terms: M, J_0, and J_{45}, the equations for which are noted below (Eqs. 2.1–2.3) [24]. The term M corresponds to the traditional spherical equivalent of refraction that represents the overall refractive error of the eye, the correction of which will move the Conoid of Sturm onto the retina. The terms J_0 and J_{45} correspond to the cross-cylinder astigmatism terms of Jackson's cross-cylinder lens, the correction of which will collapse the Conoid of Sturm into a point image on the retina. The J_0 component represents the equivalent astigmatic power along the 90° and 180° axes, while the J_{45} component represents the same along the 45° and 135° axes. Eyes with regular with- or against-the-rule astigmatism will have non-zero values only for the J_0 component, while those with oblique astigmatism will have non-zero values for both, the J_0 and J_{45} components. Effectively, an astigmatic vector along any axis is now referenced to two standard cross-cylinder axes, enabling them to be compared meaningfully. For the two patient visits noted above with oblique astigmatisms, the J_0 and J_{45} terms will be −0.38 D and +0.32 D, respectively, for the first visit and +0.50 D and +0.86 D, respectively, for the second visit. It is now meaningful to surmise that astigmatism has indeed increased in the second visit of the patient relative to the first visit, even while the spherical equivalent of refraction has remained unaltered.

$$M(D) = \text{spherical component} + (\text{cylindrical component} / 2) \quad (2.1)$$

$$J_0(D) = (-\text{Cylindrical component} / 2) \times \cos(2\theta) \quad (2.2)$$

$$J_{45}(D) = (-\text{Cylindrical component} / 2) \times \sin(2\theta). \quad (2.3)$$

The reverse, i.e., reconstructing the magnitude and axis of astigmatism from the J_0 and J_{45} power vector terms, is easily possible by applying the formulae shown in Eqs. (2.4) and (2.5) [24].

$$\text{Cylinder component} = -2 \times \sqrt{\left[(J_0)^2 + (J_{45})^2\right]} \quad (2.4)$$

$$\text{Axis of astigmatism} = ½ \times \operatorname{atan}(J_{45} / J_0). \quad (2.5)$$

2.3.3 Impact of Measurement Wavelength on the Accuracy of Autorefraction

While the measurement technique may vary across autorefractors, one common factor is the wavelength of light used for estimating the refractive error. All autorefractors, without exception, use infrared light to estimate the refractive error of the eye. This is in contrast to retinoscopy, which uses visible light. Given the ability of infrared light to penetrate deeper into tissues vis-à-vis visible light [27], the plane of reflection of the input light source is likely to be from the retino-choroidal junction for infrared light, while it may be from the vitreoretinal junction for visible light. Assuming that the average thickness of the retina in humans is ~250 μm, the difference in the plane of reflectance between visible and infrared light will translate into approximately 0.5 D of variation in the refractive power of the eye [28]. This value scales inversely with the eye's axial length, resulting in up to 2 D of error in refractive power estimation for infants [28]. This error, popularly known as the "small eye artifact," will result in autorefractors overestimating myopia by ~0.5 D and ~2.0 D in adults and infants, respectively, relative to retinoscopy [28]. While the quantum of over/underestimation of refractive error will obviously depend on the thickness of the retina, the axial length of the eye, and the wavelength of infrared light used, clinicians should appreciate the existence of the small eye artifact and factor this into the subjective refraction techniques they pursue to finalize the refractive error correction prescribed to the patient.

2.4 Technique

2.4.1 General Guidelines for Obtaining Measurements Using Autorefractors

Most autorefractors are straightforward "point and shoot" devices that can be operated by minimally trained technicians following a quick orientation session. The general steps involved in obtaining measurements using these devices involve: (1) aligning the patient to the optical axis of the measurement device, which is easier when the device has a built-in chin/forehead rest than handheld devices; (2) ensure clear focus of the pupil; (3) offer clear instructions to the patient to stably fixating on the visual target, avoid blinking during the measurements, and relax their focus as much as possible; and (4) obtain multiple measurements of the eye's refractive error to ensure reliable results.

In this general context, the following points may be considered to optimize the obtained measurements. Most monocular measurement devices involve the patient looking through a narrow turret and fixate on a target projected inside this turret. Once the patient achieves this, the examiner must align the measurement graticule along the horizontal and vertical axes to the patient's pupil and avoid spurious measurements from misaligned optics. The measurement system may also be moved back and forth from the patient to ensure appropriate focus; optimal focus may be determined automatically by the instrument (e.g., the measurement graticule turning from red to green), or it may be qualitatively judged by the examiner noticing the sharpest focus of the first Purkinje image and/or the surrounding iris tissue. The examiner must take additional care when using binocular measurement devices like the open-field autorefractor or the photorefractor, for the chances of device misalignment are greater with these devices vis-à-vis their monocular counterparts. For the open-field autorefractor, even while viewing is binocular, the measurement is made monocularly, and all aforementioned cautionary steps should be followed for optimal measurements. For the hand-held photorefractor, it is important that the device is placed on an axis with the patient's face and centered around the mid-point between the two eyes. Care must be exercised to ensure that the images of both eyes are visible in the designated measurement window of the photorefractor and that each eye is equidistant from the edges of this measurement window.

Recent studies on the spasm of near reflex, a binocular vision dysfunction characterized primarily by pseudo-myopic refraction [29, 30], have demonstrated large short-term variations in the refractive error status of the eye (Fig. 2.4a–c) [15, 17]. Such fluctuations have been deemed a sensitive non-cycloplegic marker for this dysfunction [15, 17]. While these were identified in the research laboratory using a dynamic photorefractor with a high temporal sampling rate (50 Hz) [15, 17], they could also be identified in routine clinics by taking repeated measurements of refraction using a standard autorefractor. Many autorefractors default to taking multiple measurements, the average of which is deemed as the sphero-cylindrical refractive error of the patient. In addition to noting this mean value, the examiner should also pay attention to the variations in the refractive power over repeated measurements to identify conditions like the spasm of the near reflex. This dysfunction can then be cross-verified through a vacillating reflex in retinoscopy, and a final diagnosis may be made through cycloplegic refraction.

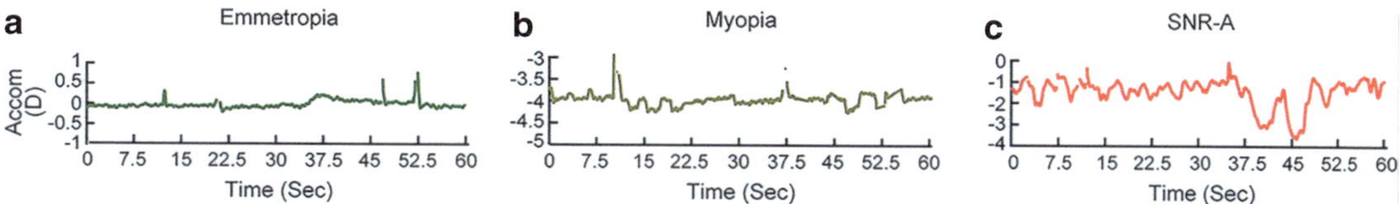

Fig. 2.4 Raw data of the accommodative responses during steady fixation plotted as a function of time in a representative emmetropic and myopic control subject (Panels **a**, **b**) and a patient with the accommodation variant of the spasm of near reflex (SNR-A, Panel **c**). The accommodative responses of the controls show minor fluctuations in the refractive error of the eye arising from microfluctuations of accommodation [31]. In contrast, the fluctuations of accommodation are significant in a patient with a spasm of near reflex. Note that the *y*-axis scales are different in panels (**a**–**c**): each tick mark represents 0.5 D of change in refractive error in Panels (**a**) and (**b**), while it represents 1 D of change in refractive error in Panel (**c**). (Figure adapted from Bharadwaj et al. [17])

2.5 Can Autorefractors Replace Retinoscopy in Clinical Practice?

With the evolution of autorefractor technology combined with artificial intelligence and machine learning models in predicting the eye's sphero-cylindrical refractive error [32], is it time to bid adieu to retinoscopy as an objective refraction technique? After all, the accuracy and precision of refractive error estimation using retinoscopy is an art in itself, potentially requiring several years of practice [21, 22]. The current evidence on the performance of autorefractors, independent of their design and operating principle, is that they work with good accuracy and precision for regular sphero-cylindrical refractive errors. Their performance in hyperopes and children with strong accommodative tendencies becomes sub-optimal, and their performance in individuals with complicated optics has not been evaluated yet. In all these cases, retinoscopy remains the preferred technique for estimating the eye's sphero-cylindrical refractive error. Therefore, eye care institutions/hospitals and training programs should continue to invest in experienced retinoscopists and training in retinoscopy, even while autorefractors may replace/supplement retinoscopy for estimating the uncorrected refractive error in routine cases.

2.6 Conclusions

Autorefractors vary significantly in their measurement principles and instrument design, and they continue to evolve in their technology and measurement accuracy/repeatability. Automated refraction shows minimal bias and good short-term repeatability, relative to retinoscopy. However, the inter-instrument variability can be as large as ±2.0 D for spherical error and ±1.0 D for cylindrical error in select cases. Autorefractors based on Scheiner disc, best focus, or ray deflection principles are well-suited for routine objective refraction in the clinic. They are less suited for eye screenings owing to their bulky designs. Although photorefraction shows poorer repeatability than other autorefractors, it may be used for mass screening due to the portability of the instrument and its ability to measure both eyes simultaneously. Open-field autorefractor designs offer better control over the eye's accommodative status and may be useful for estimating the peripheral refraction of the eye. Refractive errors calculated using autorefractors may be slightly biased in the myopic direction relative to retinoscopy, owing to the infrared light used for the estimation. Such a bias may be larger in children than adults. Astigmatism is a vectorial quantity and their magnitudes cannot be compared without considering the axes. Vector decompensation techniques must be adopted for legitimate comparison of astigmatic values. Finally, while autorefractors may replace retinoscopy for refractive error estimation in routine cases, the latter remains the gold standard for patients with strong accommodative tendencies (e.g., the pediatric population), complicated optics, certain disease conditions and media opacities where autorefractions may be out of bounds or produce erroneous results.

Funding Hyderabad Eye Research Foundation.

Disclosure None.

References

1. Bourne RRA, Flaxman SR, Braithwaite T, et al. Magnitude, temporal trends, and projections of the global prevalence of blindness and distance and near vision impairment: a systematic review and meta-analysis. Lancet Glob Health. 2017;5(9):e888–97.
2. Hashemi H, Fotouhi A, Yekta A, et al. Global and regional estimates of prevalence of refractive errors: systematic review and meta-analysis. J Curr Ophthalmol. 2018;30(1):3–22.
3. Coles-Brennan C, Sulley A, Young G. Management of digital eye strain. Clin Exp Optom. 2019;102(1):18–29.
4. Heus P, Verbeek JH, Tikka C. Optical correction of refractive error for preventing and treating eye symptoms in computer users. Cochrane Database Syst Rev. 2018;4(4):CD009877.
5. Kidd Man RE, Fenwicick EK, Sabanayagam C, et al. Prevalence, correlates, and impact of uncorrected presbyopia in a multiethnic Asian population. Am J Ophthalmol. 2016;168:191–200.

6. Tahhan N, Papas E, Fricke TR, et al. Utility and uncorrected refractive error. Ophthalmology. 2013;120(9):1736–44.
7. Padhy D, Bharadwaj SR, Nayak S, et al. Does the accuracy and repeatability of refractive error estimates depend on the measurement principle of autorefractors? Transl Vis Sci Technol. 2021;10(1):2.
8. Venkataraman AP, Brautaset R, Dominguez-Vicent A. Effect of six different autorefractor designs on the precision and accuracy of refractive error measurement. PLoS One. 2022;17(11):e0278269.
9. Thibos LN, Applegate RA, Schwiegerling JT, et al. Standards for reporting the optical aberrations of eyes. J Refract Surg. 2002;18(5):S652–60.
10. Bruce AS, Catania LJ. Clinical applications of wavefront refraction. Optom Vis Sci. 2014;91(10):1278–86.
11. Ferreira A, Vieira R, Maia S, et al. Photoscreening for amblyopia risk factors assessment in young children: a systematic review with meta-analysis. Eur J Ophthalmol. 2023;33(1):92–103.
12. Bharadwaj SR, Sravani NG, Little JA, et al. Empirical variability in the calibration of slope-based eccentric photorefraction. J Opt Soc Am A Opt Image Sci Vis. 2013;30(5):923–31.
13. Sravani NG, Nilagiri VK, Bharadwaj SR. Photorefraction estimates of refractive power varies with the ethnic origin of human eyes. Sci Rep. 2015;5:7976.
14. Bharadwaj SR, Candy TR. Cues for the control of ocular accommodation and vergence during postnatal human development. J Vis. 2008;8(16):14–6.
15. Bharadwaj SR, Roy S, Satgunam P. Spasm of near reflex: objective assessment of the near-triad. Invest Ophthalmol Vis Sci. 2020;61(8):18.
16. Patel AM, Kumar P, Vaddavalli PK, et al. The value of eccentric infrared photorefraction in evaluating keratoconus. Optom Vis Sci. 2022;99(10):763–73.
17. Bharadwaj SR, Ravisankar C, Roy S, Satgunam P. Fluctuations of steady-state accommodation is a marker for screening spasm of near reflex. Transl Vis Sci Technol. 2021;10(11):9.
18. Anderson HA, Glasser A, Stuebing KK, Manny RE. Minus lens stimulated accommodative lag as a function of age. Optom Vis Sci. 2009;86(6):685–94.
19. Fedtke C, Ehrmann K, Holden BA. A review of peripheral refraction techniques. Optom Vis Sci. 2009;86(5):429–46.
20. Erdinest N, London N, Lavy I, et al. Peripheral defocus and myopia management: a mini-review. Korean J Ophthalmol. 2023;37(1):70–81.
21. Bharadwaj SR, Malavita M, Jayaraj J. A psychophysical technique for estimating the accuracy and precision of retinoscopy. Clin Exp Optom. 2014;97(2):164–70.
22. Goss DA, Grosvenor T. Reliability of refraction—a literature review. J Am Optom Assoc. 1996;67(10):619–30.
23. Major E, Dutson T, Moshirfar M. Cycloplegia in children: an optometrist's perspective. Clin Optom (Auckl). 2020;12:129–33.
24. Thibos LN, Wheeler W, Horner D. Power vectors: an application of Fourier analysis to the description and statistical analysis of refractive error. Optom Vis Sci. 1997;74(6):367–75.
25. Alpins NA. A new method of analyzing vectors for changes in astigmatism. J Cataract Refract Surg. 1993;19(4):524–33.
26. Harris WF, Evans T, van Gool RD. Quantitative analysis of eyes and other optical systems in linear optics. Ophthalmic Physiol Opt. 2017;37(3):347–52.
27. Delori FC, Pflibsen KP. Spectral reflectance of the human ocular fundus. Appl Opt. 1989;28(6):1061–77.
28. Glickstein M, Millodot M. Retinoscopy and eye size. Science. 1970;168(3931):605–6.
29. Roy S, Bharadwaj SR, Patil-Chhablani P, Satgunam PN. Spasm of near reflex: a comprehensive management protocol and treatment outcomes. J AAPOS. 2021;25(3):162 e1–6.
30. Hyndman J. Spasm of the near reflex: literature review and proposed management strategy. J Binocul Vis Ocul Motil. 2018;68(3):78–86.
31. Charman WN, Heron G. Microfluctuations in accommodation: an update on their characteristics and possible role. Ophthalmic Physiol Opt. 2015;35(5):476–99.
32. Hernandez CS, Gil A, Casares I, et al. Prediction of manifest refraction using machine learning ensemble models on wavefront aberrometry data. J Optom. 2022;15(Suppl 1):S22–31.

3 Retinoscopy

Deepak Kumar Bagga
and J. Margaret Woodhouse

3.1 Introduction

Retinoscopy is a manual, objective method of evaluating the refractive status of an individual's eye. Accurate, objective refraction can significantly reduce the time taken for subjective refraction. It is an essential eye testing procedure for young children, people with disabilities, dementia, etc., and who may not be able to co-operate for autorefraction and may be unable to respond to subjective refraction. Retinoscopy is useful in many ways as, in addition to refraction, it also provides information about optical aberrations and media opacity. Retinoscopy is performed using a retinoscope, which emits a line or "streak" of light into a patient's eye; the reflection of this light is used to gauge refraction objectively. Spot retinoscopy, which employs a circle of light, is less commonly used. This chapter describes the fundamental techniques of streak retinoscopy.

3.2 History

In the mid-nineteenth century, several attempts were made to measure the refractive status of the eye by observing the shadows cast within a person's eye; these were called "shadow tests." The development of retinoscopy is illustrated in Table 3.1. For further details on historical perspectives, readers can refer to published texts [1, 2].

D. K. Bagga (✉)
Institute for Vision Rehabilitation, Kallam Anji Reddy Campus, L V Prasad Eye Institute, Hyderabad, India
e-mail: dkbagga@lvpei.org

J. M. Woodhouse
School of Optometry and Vision Sciences, Cardiff University, Cardiff, UK
e-mail: Woodhouse@cardiff.ac.uk

T. Das, P. Satgunam (eds.), *Ophthalmic Diagnostics*, https://doi.org/10.1007/978-981-97-0138-4_3

Table 3.1 Evolution of retinoscopy

Year	Contributors	Evolution of retinoscopy
1859	Sir William Bowman	Described an objective technique for detecting astigmatism in keratoconus using an ophthalmoscope for the first time
1873	Ferdinand Cuignet[a]	Used a simple mirror ophthalmoscope to assess refractive errors qualitatively by observing the movement of reflex and described it as "keratoscopie"
1880	Henry parent	Used lenses to determine refractive errors and coined the term "retinoscopie"; however, later changed it to "skiascopie" (skia means shadow)
1903	Alexander Duane	Introduced the use of cylindrical lenses for retinoscopy in astigmatic errors
1920	Jack C. Copeland[b]	Devised a bulb that produced linear beams of light and additional features for a rotating bulb, changing the direction of light beam—The streak retinoscope

[a]Ferdinand Cuignet is acknowledged as the "father" of retinoscopy
[b]Jack C. Copeland as the "father" of streak retinoscopy

3.3 Equipment

3.3.1 Retinoscope

Historically, the early retinoscope designs had a plane/concave mirror with a peephole in the center for the examiner to view the movement of light reflected from the patient's retina, known as the "reflex." While performing retinoscopy, a candle, or later an incandescent bulb, was used as a light source. The light source would be positioned above the patient's head, and the retinoscope's mirror would direct light into the patient's eye. The examiner observed the shape, intensity, and direction of movement of the reflex in the patient's pupil to estimate the refractive status. Later, spot retinoscopes were developed with an inbuilt light source, increasing the convenience and portability of retinoscopes. These self-illuminated retinoscopes opened the opportunity for community eye health programs as they could be carried to locations without electricity.

Jack C. Copeland developed the first streak retinoscope by accident. While Copeland was using a spot retinoscope, it fell to the floor, damaging its bulb filament; the damaged filament produced a linear reflex and was the first streak retinoscope. Later, Copeland improved the instrument and described various techniques for using the streak retinoscope. Given Copeland's contribution, he is considered the "father" of streak retinoscopy.

3.3.2 Description of a Streak Retinoscope (Fig. 3.1)

Peephole: The first component in the observation system of a retinoscope is a peephole. The examiner observes the characteristics of the reflex in a patient's pupil through the peephole in the mirror.

Sleeve/collar: Up/downshifts of the sleeve allow changes in the vergence of the light rays leaving the retinoscope, and its rotation changes the orientation of the light beam to observe the reflex in different meridians. In most retinoscopes, the sleeve at the bottom position provides divergent rays, and when above, the para-stop provides convergent rays (Fig. 3.2a, c).

Para-stop: This is a mechanical guide for the sleeve position, wherein the emitted rays from

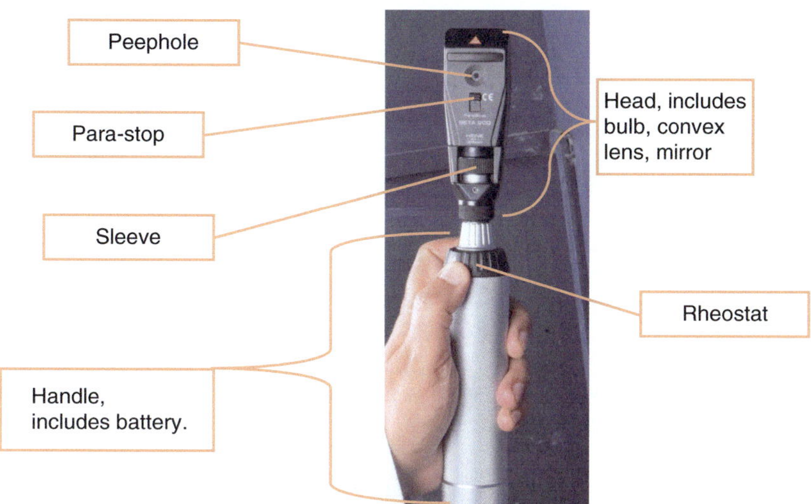

Fig. 3.1 Streak retinoscope

the retinoscope are parallel. Some clinicians prefer using a para-stop to ensure that they use the plane mirror effect during the retinoscopy (Fig. 3.2b).

Rheostat: This is a variable resistor that is used to control the brightness level and to turn on the instrument.

Groove/magnetic cards: Target cards are accessories for dynamic retinoscopy fixation and can be attached through the groove in the Heine Beta 200 retinoscope (HEINE Optotechnik GmbH & Co. KG, Germany). However, in the Welch Allyn retinoscope (Welch Allyn Inc. Corporate Headquarters, New York), the head's magnetic logo allows placing these dynamic retinoscopy cards.

Battery: The power system for a retinoscope includes rechargeable or replaceable batteries. There are also retinoscopes with power cables that can be directly plugged into an electric power supply for turning on their illumination system.

3.3.3 Trial Lens Set/Phoropter

In addition to a retinoscope, a phoropter or, a range of trial lenses, and a trial frame are needed to perform retinoscopy. For high refractive errors (>5 D), it is important to note the vertex distance. Therefore, a trial frame that allows measuring the vertex distance of lenses must be preferred. Key features of the phoropter include adjustable interpupillary distance, pantoscopic tilt, and high-contrast labeling of the axis on the outermost cell. For refraction in infants, clinicians may prefer using lens racks.

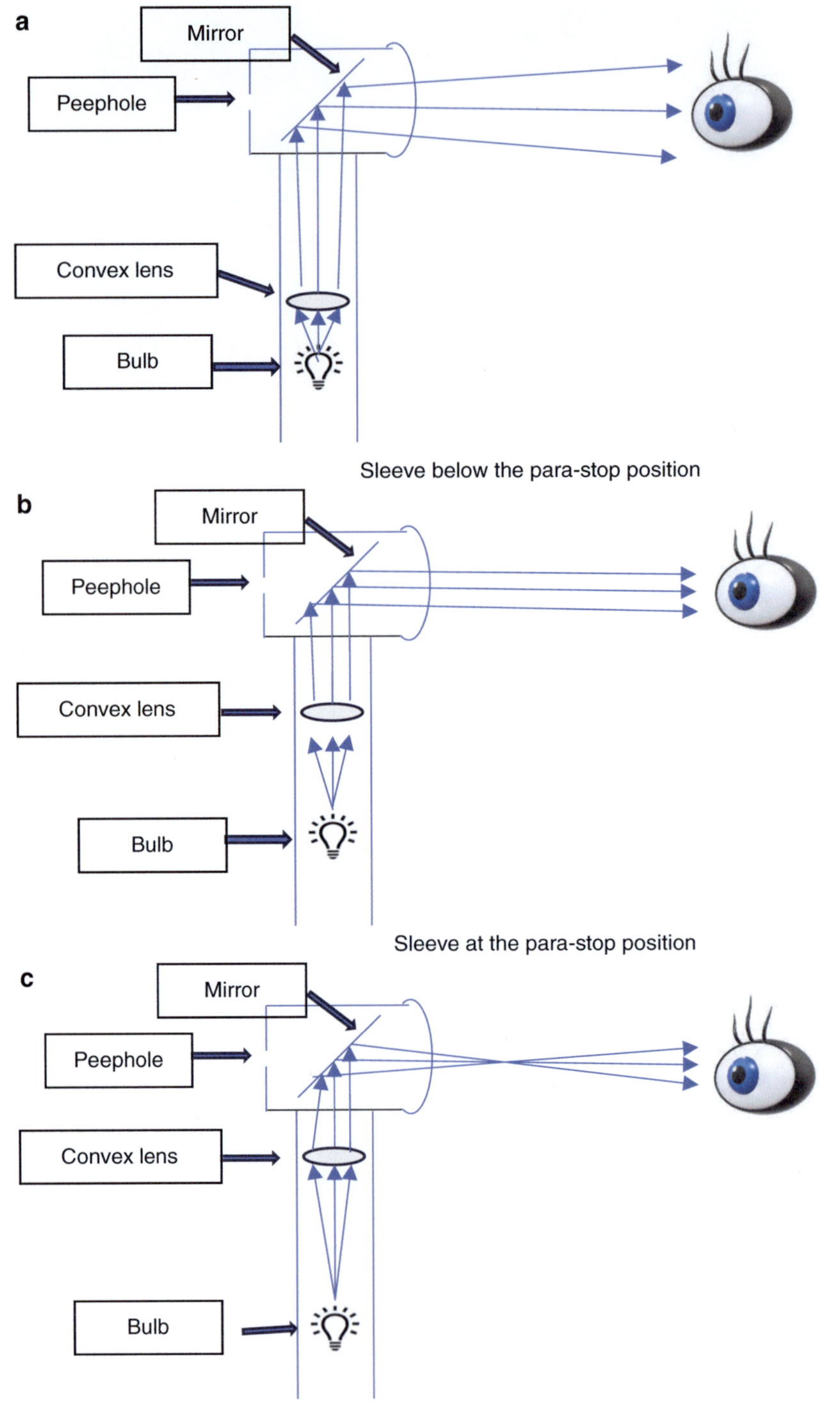

Fig. 3.2 (**a**) The sleeve is at the bottom position, and the light source (bulb) is positioned at a shorter distance than the principal focus of the lens, producing divergent rays. (**b**) The sleeve is at the para-stop position, and the light source is positioned at the principal focus point of the convex lens, causing emergent rays to run parallel. This is the plane mirror effect. (**c**) The sleeve-up position is where the distance between the light source (bulb) is more than the focal length of the convex lens, causing convergent emerging rays. If the emerging convergent rays focus at a point before entering the patient's eye, it is considered the concave mirror effect. In this effect, the observed movement of reflex will be reversed from those observed during retinoscopy with the plane mirror effect

3.4 Basic Principles

During retinoscopy, the examiner uses a combination of trial lenses to bring the far point of the patient's eye to their test distance. Since the examiner works quite close to the patient, the patient is rendered artificially myopic. The examiner can then derive the refractive error by adjusting the lens power to account for the induced myopia. This means adding minus power (or subtracting plus power) equivalent to the dioptric value of the examiner's working distance (see examples).

Example 1

In a person with emmetropia, the strength of the convex lens corresponds to the working distance that will bring the person's far point from infinity to the test distance (Fig. 3.3a, b) [1].

Example 2

In a person with myopia, the far point is located at a finite distance (Fig. 3.4a) [1]. If a −2.50 D concave lens brings the far point to 66.67 cm (Fig. 3.4b), and the net refractive error will be obtained by adding the working distance correction (−1.50 D). Therefore, this person has −4.00 D myopia {−2.5 D + (−1.50 D)}.

Example 3

In another case, the examiner observes the end point of retinoscopy with a +3.50 D spherical convex lens at 66.67 cm (Fig. 3.5a, b) [1]. This case will have hypermetropia of +2.00 D {+3.50 D −1.50 D (compensation for working distance)}.

Some practitioners prefer to begin retinoscopy by putting an appropriate convex lens (in the above examples, this would be +1.50 D) in the trial frame before checking the reflex. In the end, the lens is simply removed to give the final correction. This lens, known as the working distance lens, adds extra weight and reflections and takes up room in the trial frame, so it is best avoided, and a simple calculation, as above, can be carried out.

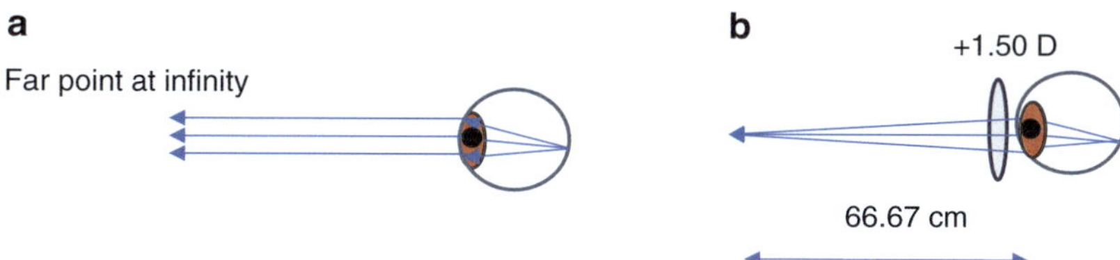

Fig. 3.3 (**a**) In an emmetropic eye, the retina and infinity are conjugate foci. (**b**) Placing a +1.50 D sphere lens in trial frame brings the far point to 66.67 cm (100/1.5 = 66.67 cm)

Fig. 3.4 (**a**) In a myopic eye, the far point is within a finite distance. (**b**) Placing a −2.50 D spherical concave lens in a trial frame brings the far point to 66.67 cm

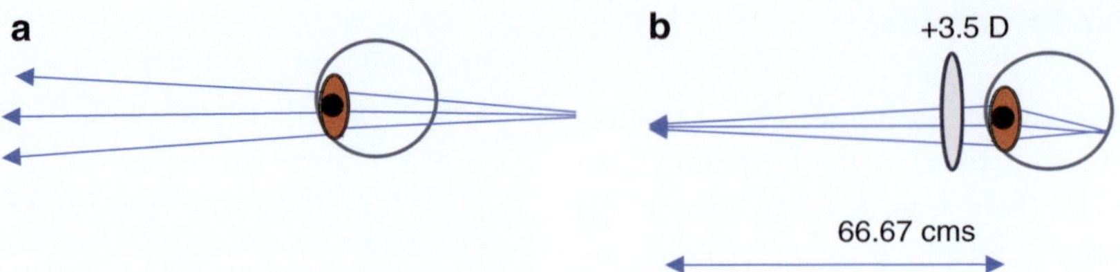

Fig. 3.5 (**a**) In hypermetropic eyes, the far point is behind the eye. (**b**) A convex lens is used to obtain the end point of retinoscopy in cases with hypermetropia. The magnitude of hypermetropia is determined by subtracting the power corresponding to the test distance

A working distance lens also restricts the examiner to remain at a fixed distance during retinoscopy. Once close to the endpoint, experienced practitioners sometimes find it useful to vary the working distance to find the neutral reflex rather than make minor changes to the lenses and then subtract the appropriate sphere power for the final working distance. This speeds up the process but does require the practitioner to have a precise perception of distances.

3.5 Essentials of Retinoscopy

3.5.1 Reflex

When performing retinoscopy, the examiner moves the streak light beam across the patient's eye perpendicular to the streak, with the sleeve/collar at its lowest position (divergent beam). This light beam creates an illuminated patch on the patient's retina, and this light reflects and emerges after passing through the optical system. During the retinoscopy, the examiner observes the image of this illuminated patch in the pupillary area, referred to as the reflex (Fig. 3.6).

The beam of light seen outside the pupillary area on the patient's face is referred to as the intercept. During retinoscopy, the examiner observes the following characteristics of the reflex to estimate the refractive error:

1. Thickness in relation to the intercept.
2. Brightness: a brighter reflex suggests low refractive error, and a dull reflex suggests high refractive error.
3. The movement of the reflex in relation to the intercept—"with" or "against" (Figs. 3.7 and 3.8).
4. Speed of reflex: the speed of the reflex motion in relation to the movement of the streak indicates the magnitude of the refractive error. A "slow" speed indicates high refractive error, and a "fast" speed indicates low refractive error. Therefore, near the endpoint of retinoscopy, the relative speed of the reflex increases significantly [3].

3.5.2 Endpoint of Retinoscopy

The endpoint of retinoscopy is a "neutral reflex," that is, a reversal of the reflex's movement. The endpoint can be quickly confirmed by moving the retinoscope slightly further away from the patient to produce an "against" movement and closer to produce a "with" movement. The endpoint is, therefore, a transition from one to the other.

3.5.3 Astigmatism

The lenses that neutralize the movement in astigmatism will differ in the two principal meridians. The examiner turns the sleeve/collar to align the reflex with the intercept in one meridian and neutralizes the movement. Then, the examiner turns the streak 90° to the opposite meridian and uses cylindrical lenses aligned along the streak to neutralize the movement. If the examiner chooses to work with a plus cylinder, the least plus/most

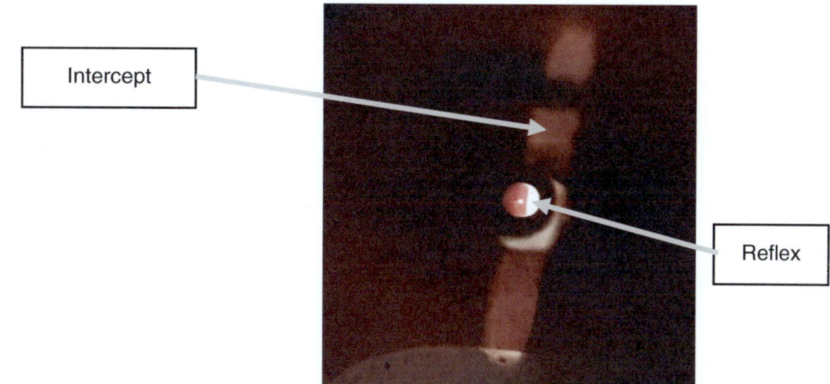

Fig. 3.6 Reflex and intercept

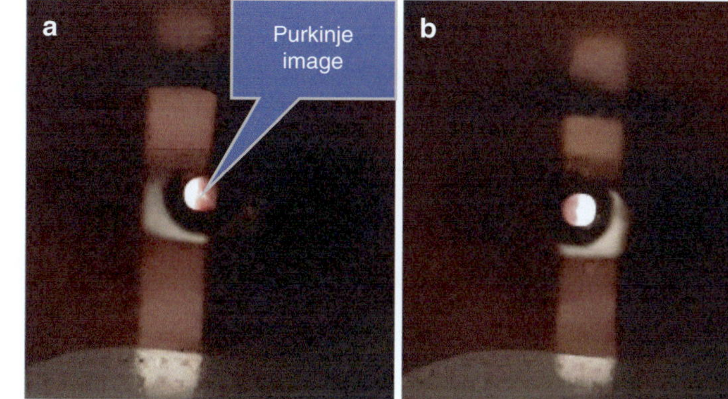

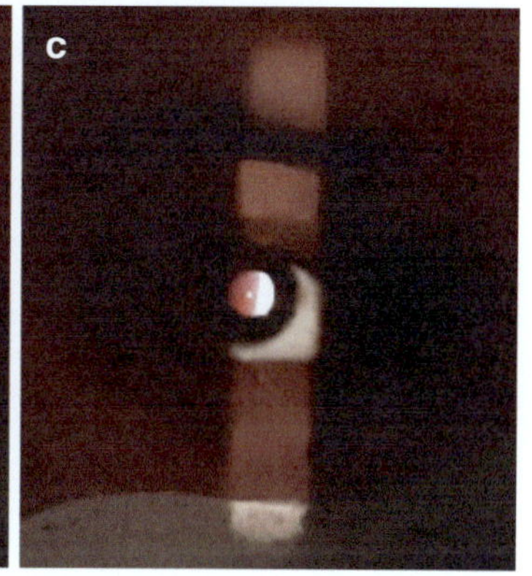

Fig. 3.7 Images captured from a retinoscopy video demonstrate the intercept and reflex moving in the same direction when the streak is moved from the patient's right to their left side. (**a**) The intercept and reflex are both seen on the right side of the Purkinje image. (**b**, **c**) Show the change in position of reflex as intercept moves toward patient's left. Both intercept and reflex are in the same direction, left of the Purkinje image. A "with" reflex is neutralized with a plus spherical lens. It indicates hypermetropia, or myopia of power less than the working distance equivalent

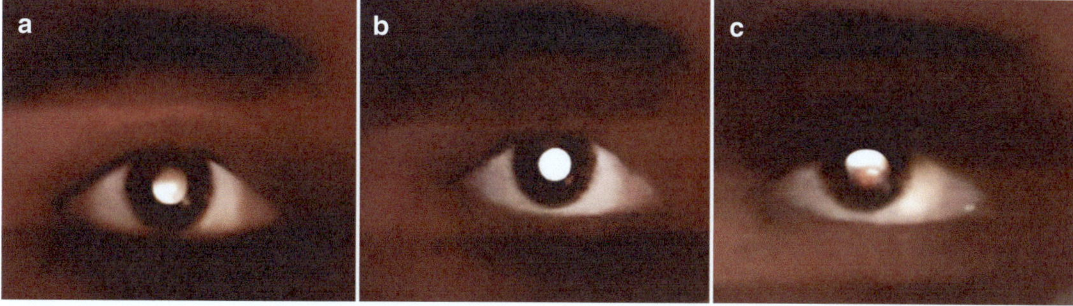

Fig. 3.8 The above images illustrate the "against" movement of the reflex, this time with a horizontal streak moving downwards. In the first image (**a**), the reflex can be seen at the lower edge of the pupil. The reflex moves up as the light beam (intercept) moves down in the third image (**c**). The reflex has moved in the opposite direction—this is known as "against reflex." Panel (**b**) shows the reflex in the center of the pupil when the intercept is in the mid-position vertically. The "against" reflex indicates myopia, and the endpoint of retinoscopy is achieved by placing the appropriate concave lenses

minus meridian is neutralized first. If the examiner prefers to work with a minus cylinder, the most plus/least minus meridian is first neutralized.

3.5.4 Alignment

The best alignment would be refracting along the patient's visual axis. Therefore, the examiner checks for the first Purkinje image while the patient is asked to look toward the distance target. If this image is in the center of the pupil, it indicates good alignment (Fig. 3.9).

Note that the Purkinje image cannot be considered for reference in patients with eccentric viewing, such as patients with Stargardt's disease or macular degeneration. In these cases, the examiner should refract in the patient's adapted viewing position.

The patient usually has both eyes open during retinoscopy, but in the case of strabismus, it may be necessary to cover the fixing eye to ensure the deviated eye takes up fixation and is aligned. Otherwise, refracting patients with both eyes open may assist the examiner in maintaining good alignment. The patient's right eye should be refracted using the examiner's right eye and vice versa to avoid parallax errors.

3.5.5 Controlling Accommodation

In conventional or "static" retinoscopy, the patient fixates on a target at a distance (6 m or 20 ft), thus encouraging relaxed accommodation. To minimize accommodation, the fixation target should be large (e.g., a 6/60 letter or picture for children). Relaxed accommodation can be further encouraged by "fogging" (blurring with plus/+ve lenses) the eye not under the test. For young hypermetropes with active accommodation, it may be useful to fog with a plus lens that is 2.00 D greater than their previous prescription.

Other forms of retinoscopy, including cycloplegic and Mohindra, will be discussed later (Sect. 3.8.1). These techniques control accommodation by different means, but the underlying principles of retinoscopy remain the same.

3.5.6 Ambient Light

Retinoscopy is a darkroom procedure. Reducing the ambient light helps by increasing the patient's pupil size and relaxing the accommodation. In addition, the dark room improves the examiner's ability to perceive the reflex by enhancing the contrast.

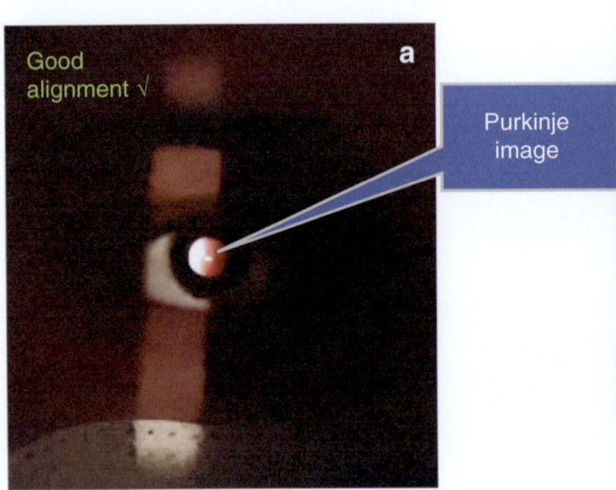

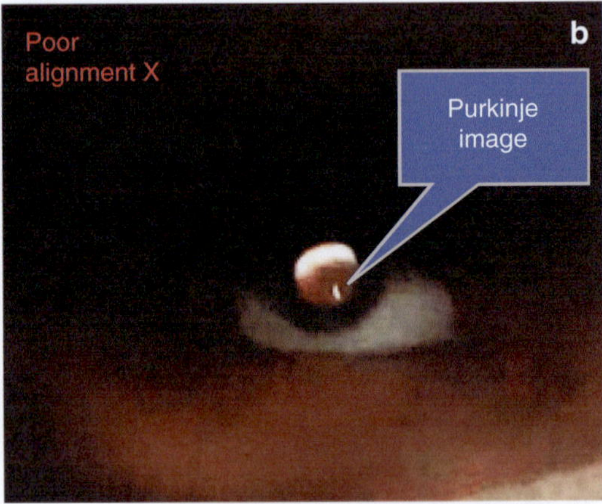

Fig. 3.9 Images reflecting (**a**) good and (**b**) poor alignment based on the location of the Purkinje image observed during retinoscopy. The examiner can change their position vertically and horizontally to ensure appropriate alignment during the retinoscopy

Table 3.2 Centimeters to D conversion scale

Working lens power in diopter (D)	33.33	20	10	5	2.5	2	1.25	1
Test distance in cm	3	5	10	20	40	60	80	100

3.5.7 Use of Brightness Controls

The rheostat of a streak retinoscope helps control the brightness of the light beam. An appropriate brightness level provides adequate visibility of reflex for the examiner without causing glare for the patient. There are a few ocular conditions where patients may experience significant intolerance to light, such as achromatopsia, congenital glaucoma, or aniridia. In these cases, if the media (cornea, lens, and vitreous) are clear and the examiner can observe at a low brightness level, the brightness can be adjusted to a level the patient can tolerate. In contrast, in some cases with media opacification, using the maximum brightness may help visualize the characteristics of the reflex.

3.5.8 Working Distance and Spherical Errors in Retinoscopy

Table 3.2 shows the centimeters (cm) to diopter (D) conversion scale and represents the test distance and corresponding working lens correction. It shows that the examiner must be precise about their working distance correction for shorter test distances. This is because even a small change at a shorter working distance accounts for a large dioptric change. For a working distance of 50 cm or longer, a minor incorrect estimation of the working distance may not make a clinically significant error (over 0.25 D). The other advantage of using a longer working distance is to encourage the patient to relax their accommodation, as some patients might intermittently look at the retinoscope's light or the examiner's face. A shorter working distance will stimulate proximal accommodation, adding inaccuracies in measuring the refractive errors.

While there are advantages to using longer working distances (≥50 cm), there are special situations, such as a miotic pupil or media opacity, where the examiner may need to use a shorter test distance.

3.6 Estimation of Refractive Errors

At the outset of retinoscopy, estimating the approximate refractive error is very useful so that the first lens inserted brings the reflex close to the endpoint.

3.6.1 When the Observation Is an "Against" Movement of the Reflex

As the far point in a myopic eye is within a finite distance, it is easy to estimate the magnitude of myopia. Simply reduce the test distance to observe the first noticeable "with" and then move back to the first noticeable "against"; between these two points lies the far point. Estimate the distance between the point of reversal and the patient's eye and convert it to D. For example, if the point of reversal was observed at 20 cm, the person would have 5.00 D myopia.

3.6.2 When the Observation Is a "with" Movement of the Reflex

The "enhancement" technique helps estimate the strength of the "with" reflex up to about 5 D [1]. The examiner slowly moves the sleeve position to vary positive vergence and achieve an enhanced reflex (thinnest, sharpest, and brightest) while remaining in the plane mirror effect of retinoscopy (i.e., not reversing the movement). If the examiner needs to apply the maximum positive vergence (moving the sleeve upwards to its furthest) possible in the plane mirror effect to enhance the reflex, it represents +5.00 D or more. If the sleeve at the bottom-most position itself provides the enhanced reflex, then it means about +0.5 D. For estimating the magnitude of hypermetropia for the complete range between +0.5 D and +5.0 D, the examiner needs to consider the beam width that produces the enhanced reflex and interpret it in relation to the difference between the two extreme sleeve positions. Figure 3.10 demonstrates how the width of the beam (intercept) guides the estimate of the magnitude of hypermetropia.

3.6.3 Estimating and Confirming the Axis of Astigmatic Error

Three commonly used techniques for estimating the axis of astigmatic error are (1) thickness, (2) break, and (3) skew phenomena [1].

Thickness phenomena: The examiner must observe the change in the thickness of the reflex when observing the reflex across different meridians. The direction providing the thinnest, brightest, and sharpest reflex is the axis for the plus cylinder (Fig. 3.11). The thickness phenomenon is best observed when refracting the eye using

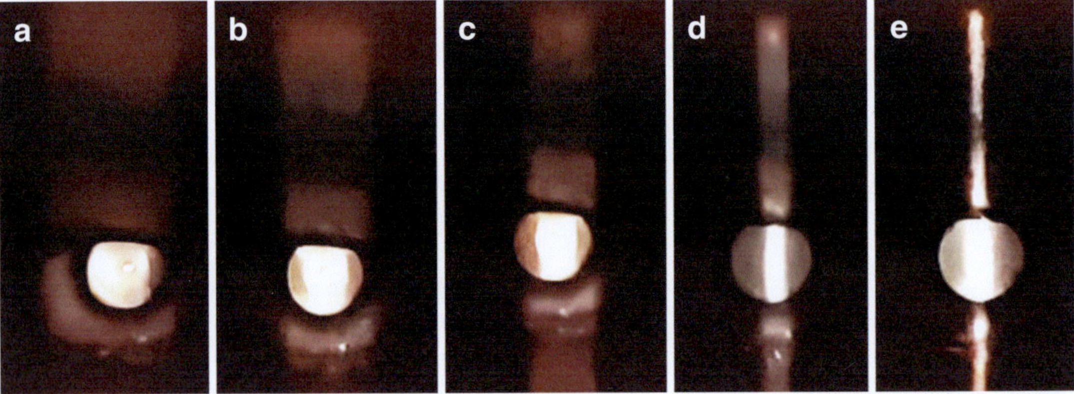

Fig. 3.10 The above figures illustrate the change in thickness, brightness, and sharpness of the reflex as the sleeve is moved up {Panel (**a**) (sleeve at the bottom most position) to panel (**e**) (sleeve position upwards with maximum convergence, in plane mirror)}. This change in sleeve position causes a change in the vergence of the rays entering the eye. In the enhancement technique, hypermetropia is estimated by the width of the intercept that produces enhanced reflex (thinnest, brightest, and sharpest). Panel (**d**) is an enhanced reflex, and the estimate for this case will be +3.50 D

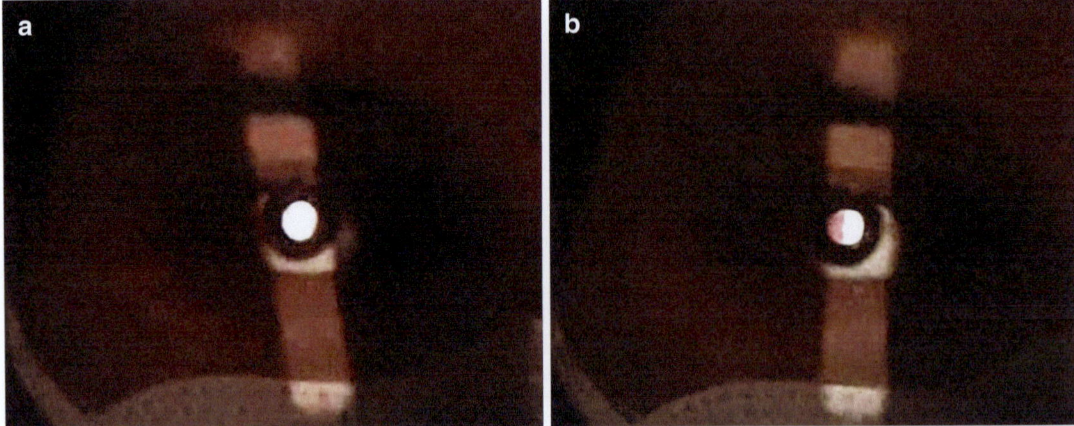

Fig. 3.11 Thickness phenomenon: Panel (**a**) illustrates a thicker reflex than panel (**b**), as the streak is not aligned to the correct axis in panel (**a**)

plus cylinders, as it would be most readily visualized using the enhancement technique described above (Sect. 3.6.2). If the examiner wishes to use minus cylinders, the method can be used with the sleeve at its highest, thus reversing the reflex to "with" and moving it downwards to enhance the reflex.

Break phenomena: The examiner observes the direction of the reflex in relation to the direction of the intercept. In astigmatic errors, a break will be observed as an angle between the intercept (the light beam of streak) and reflex when the intercept is not aligned with one of the principal meridians of astigmatism (Fig. 3.12).

Skew phenomenon: A skew phenomenon is observed in the dynamic movement of the reflex in relation to the direction of the light beam of a streak (the intercept). When the intercept is off-axis/not aligned to the principal meridians of astigmatic error, the intercept and reflex move in different directions, called the skewing phenomena. Therefore, the axis of the cylindrical lens will be in a direction in which the reflex and intercept move in the same direction.

The **straddling technique** allows the examiner to confirm the cylindrical axis once a cylindrical lens is placed in the trial frame. First, a correcting cylindrical lens is placed in the trial frame based on the estimations obtained using the thickness, break, and skewing phenomena. If the estimated axis is incorrect, an orientation difference (break and skew) between the three components: the retinoscope streak (intercept), cylindrical lens markings, and reflex will be observed. This difference can be best visualized at 45° away from the axis of the cylindrical lens placed in the trial frame (Fig. 3.13). The orientation of the axis must be adjusted until all three align [1]. When the orientation of the axis is correct, straddling will show similar characteristics (thickness, brightness, and movement) of reflex at 45° to either side. If not, these characteristics will differ, as shown in Fig. 3.13. Particularly for the movement of the reflex, one side of the straddle could show a "with" reflex while on the other side, an "against" movement can be observed.

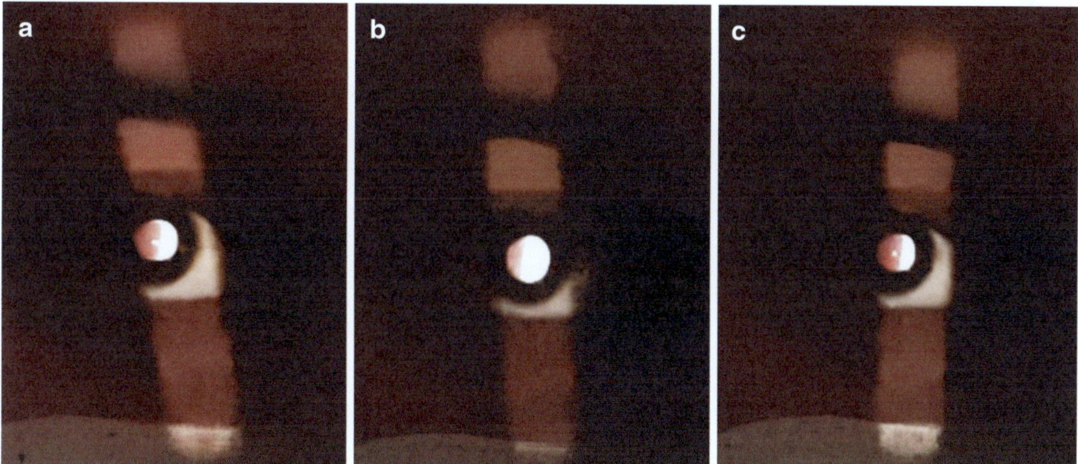

Fig. 3.12 Demonstration of the break phenomenon. There is a distinct angle, called the "break" between the intercept and the direction of reflex, in all three examples (Fig. 3.12a–c). The break will disappear if the streak in panel (**c**) is moved slightly to 85°, the true axis

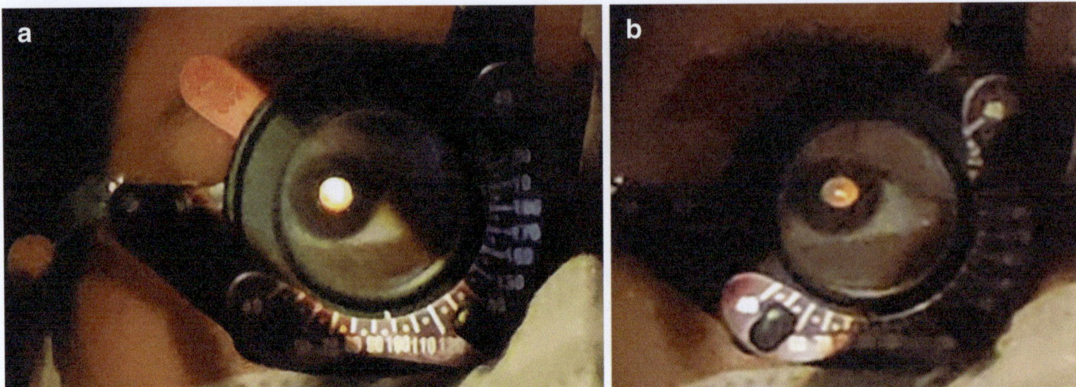

Fig. 3.13 Straddling technique: In Fig. (**a**), the axis of a convex cylindrical lens is placed at 95°. The observations at 140° (**a**) and 50° (**b**) reveal the difference in thickness, brightness, and movement of reflex (not appreciated in a static picture), indicating the inaccurate placement of the astigmatic lens

3.6.4 Finalizing the Magnitude of Astigmatism

When the reflex movement has been neutralized with a cylindrical lens at the correct orientation, it is important to check the opposite (sphere) meridian again. It is all too easy for the examiner to inadvertently change the working distance slightly between neutralizing the sphere and moving on to correct astigmatism. When comparing the movement of reflex across all meridians, it should move (or remain neutral) in the same way.

3.7 Tips for Performing Retinoscopy (Table 3.3)

Table 3.3 Tips for performing retinoscopy in complex conditions

Conditions posing challenges	Recommendations
Nystagmus	Keep the retinoscope still and allow the patient's eye movements to replace the retinoscope movements. Concentrate on observing the movement of reflex to determine "with" or "against," when the patient's eye is directed in the appropriate direction
Media opacity	Reduce the test distance, try dimming room lights further, and use the maximum brightness of the retinoscope
Accommodation	Contralateral (fellow eye) fogging. In the testing eye, begin with over plus lens to get an "against" reflex and reduce to neutral
Multiple reflexes—different zones in the pupillary area showing different refractive errors	Focus on the central 2–3 mm zone, close to the Purkinje image, and ignore the reflexes seen in the periphery
Central shadow	Refract the immediate next zone to the shadow
Miotic pupil	Reduce working distance and room illumination
Subluxated lens (example: Marfan's syndrome)	Refract the zone closer to the Purkinje image; it may be possible to refract both aphakic and phakic zones. Later, improvement in the visual acuity should be assessed monocularly and binocularly to decide the spectacle prescription
Reflection from trial lenses	Use of trial lenses with anti-reflection coatings; in the case of planoconcave lenses, flip the lens with a concave surface facing the patient; this will reduce the size of the annoying reflections
High refractive errors	When the reflex is close to neutral, it appears bright and has crisp movement. In contrast, a reflex far from the neutral is dim, wide, and slow. In high refractive errors, it can be challenging to determine the movement, and inexperienced examiner can sometimes assume neutrality because there is no apparent movement. Moving the retinoscope further and closer does not produce the "against" and "with" movements that confirm neutrality. If the reflex is difficult to interpret, simply holding up a high-power plus and minus lens will quickly help since one will reveal a brighter reflex, and the other will worsen matters

3.8 Special Techniques

3.8.1 Cycloplegic and Mohindra Retinoscopy

Static retinoscopy, as described above, controls accommodation by asking the patient to fixate on a distant target, fogging the fellow eye, etc. The static technique may be inappropriate for some patients, particularly young children or people with learning disabilities, who cannot reliably maintain fixation at a distance.

Cycloplegic retinoscopy eliminates accommodation by using cycloplegic eye drops that temporarily paralyze the ciliary muscles. Once the cycloplegic eye drops have taken effect, the patient can directly fixate the retinoscope light, with the advantage that the refraction is now conducted on the visual axis, and the examiner can use her/his preferred eye. The disadvantage (apart from patient discomfort and time for instillation and drug action) is that cycloplegic drugs also dilate the pupils, giving rise to aberrations and making the retinoscopy reflex more challenging to interpret [4].

Mohindra retinoscopy uses the phenomenon known as "tonic accommodation" or "empty field myopia" [4, 5]. It is conducted in total darkness apart from the retinoscopy light, which is dimmed as much as possible. Eyes in darkness adopt a stable, small amount of accommodation. The patient fixates on the retinoscope light, and refraction is carried out as normal. However, occluding one eye is a recommended exception to cut out convergence cues that might trigger accommodation. The working distance allowance is modified to allow for the small amount of accommodation the patient adopts in the dark [5]. According to research studies, [6] to obtain the same refraction as under cycloplegia and for a working distance of 50 cm, the examiner should deduct 0.75 D for an infant under 2 years, 1.00 D for a child aged 2 and over, and 1.25 D for a young adult. Unfortunately, there are no guidelines for the age at which the examiner changes from child-appropriate to adult-appropriate deductions. Since the difference between the two is only 0.25 D, this is probably trivial. Mohindra has the advantages of being non-invasive and allowing other visual functions, such as accommodation, to be assessed after refraction.

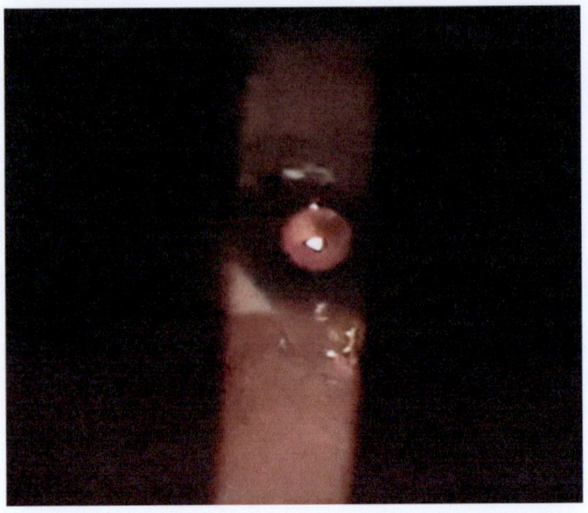

Fig. 3.14 A central shadow seen in the retinoscopy reflex due to posterior subcapsular opacity in the lens

3.9 Additional Observations

The retinoscopy reflex can provide additional information and indicate eye disorders causing a change in the pupil size, shape, color of reflex, scissors/irregular reflex, a shadow in reflex, or invisible reflex. Media opacities/disturbances (such as early keratoconus) can be much easier to spot with a retinoscope than with other means so that appropriate examinations can be carried out (Fig. 3.14). Retinal disturbances, such as detachment and coloboma, can be seen in the different colorations of the retinoscopy reflex, especially as the patient looks around. In patients with severe disabilities, the ability to fixate can be assessed with a retinoscope.

3.10 Comparison Between Autorefraction and Retinoscopy

Both retinoscopy and autorefraction have their own merits and belong in a state-of-the-art eye examination room. Table 3.4 provides a quick comparison of the key parameters of both techniques to enable clinicians to determine when to use retinoscopy, autorefraction, or both.

Table 3.4 Comparing retinoscopy and autorefraction

Parameter	Autorefraction	Retinoscopy
Cost of equipment	Expensive	Less expensive
Cost of refraction	Less expensive	Expensive (considering the time taken to perform the test)
Accuracy	Reasonably accurate findings in most cases, irrespective of the skills of the examiner	Completely depends on the skills of the examiner
Suitability	In most cases, with normal pupil size and simple refractive errors. However, autorefraction may show an error in measuring complex refractions, such as high refractive errors, eyes with nystagmus, large eccentric fixation, or miotic pupils Suitable for able-bodied, confident, and compliant patients	Suitable for all patients irrespective of age and abilities/disabilities. Can be used in most of the complex cases of high refractive errors, such as 20D of astigmatism or 50D of myopia, and a large variety of challenges; application of estimation techniques, such as direct retinoscopy or enhancement, and can provide a useful starting point for subjective refraction

3.11 Conclusion

Retinoscopy is essential for all eye care professionals involved in refractive correction. In cases where subjective refraction is not possible (for example, children and people with special needs), inconsistent or non-availability of autorefraction values (cases with uveal coloboma, aniridia, or irregular cornea), and high refractive errors where large variability may be observed in different methods, retinoscopy by an experienced eye care service provider can be the only way of determining the refractive correction. In addition to providing information about the refractive status, examiners can identify other ocular findings, such as posterior subcapsular cataracts, vitreous opacities, and spherical aberrations. Retinoscopy has two major limitations: one, it is dependent on the skills of the professional; two, it could take a longer time to perform than an autorefractor-based examination. Despite these limitations, this is one of the important objective methods to measure refractive errors in all, including the vulnerable and challenging cases.

Finally, reading about retinoscopy might motivate the reader, but unless the reader practices the various techniques step by step and multiple times, it may not help the reader and those waiting to get an appropriate refractive correction. Therefore, practice is essential to improve refractive corrections to make the patient see clearly.

Funding Hyderabad Eye Research Foundation.

Disclosure **None.**

References

1. Corboy JM. The retinoscopy book: an introductory manual for eye care professionals. Slack Incorporated; 2003.
2. Bennett AG. An historical review of optometric principles and techniques. Ophthalmic Physiol Opt. 1986;6(1):3–21.
3. Bennett A, Rabbetts R. Clinical visual optics, vol. 62. London: Butterworths; 1984. p. 924.
4. Benjamin WJ. Borish's clinical refraction-E-book. Elsevier Health Sciences; 2006.
5. Mohindra I. A technique for infant vision examination. Optom Vis Sci. 1975;52(12):867–70.
6. Saunders KJ, Westall CA. Comparison between near retinoscopy and cycloplegic retinoscopy in the refraction of infants and children. Optom Vis Sci. 1992;69(8):615–22.

4 Prescribing Spectacles

PremNandhini Satgunam

4.1 Introduction

Vision is a collective process of optics, physiology, and visual perception at the higher centers of the brain. To achieve clear vision, all these processes must be intact. Imperfect optics, resulting in refractive error, can be alleviated through a pair of spectacles. However, all the processes that contribute collectively toward vision also determine the final spectacle prescription for a patient. As a result of this complex interplay and physiological variabilities, the same patient examined by the same examiner may end up with different spectacle prescriptions on two separate occasions. This variability must be kept in mind, especially while changing earlier spectacles. Determining a spectacle prescription is a collaborative effort, involving both the examiner and the patient. Truly, prescribing a pair of spectacles is both an art and a science. Science is learned, and art comes with practice. This chapter aims to give tips on both science and craft.

P. Satgunam (✉)
Brien Holden Institute of Optometry and Vision Sciences, Prof. Brien Holden Eye Research Centre, L V Prasad Eye Institute, Hyderabad, Telangana, India
e-mail: premnandhini@lvpei.org

4.2 Background

The procedure for prescribing spectacles is called subjective refraction. The "subjectivity" in this involves factors related to the patient (e.g., their tolerance of blur) and the examiner (e.g., their technique). Because of this subjectivity, spectacles cannot be prescribed directly to a patient based solely on the autorefractor or the retinoscopic value. In a study that evaluated the patient's tolerance to spectacles prescribed based on autorefraction and subjective refraction done by an optometrist, the latter was more tolerable [1]. Patient–clinician communication is important to dispense the appropriate spectacles. A systematic review and meta-analysis found that about 16% of spectacles non-tolerance resulted from poor communication [2].

The first step toward giving a spectacle prescription, before subjective refraction, is good objective refraction. Readers can refer to Chap. 3 in this book for objective refraction. A list of good references [3–7] for prescribing spectacles is also put together at the end of this chapter. In addition, guidelines for spectacle prescription, especially for children (considering the risk of amblyopia), are also available from the websites of different professional organizations (including Ophthalmology and Optometry) [8, 9]. There are several tools and techniques that can be used for subjective refraction. Not all of these are described in this chapter. Only those techniques

T. Das, P. Satgunam (eds.), *Ophthalmic Diagnostics*, https://doi.org/10.1007/978-981-97-0138-4_4

that are commonly used and can be easily adopted by an individual practitioner will be discussed. This chapter will also describe only the trial frame refraction used most commonly in the author's country of practice. However, these techniques and logic can be easily adapted to phoropter refraction as well.

4.3 Principle

The fundamental goal of a spectacle prescription is to provide clear visual acuity to a person at all viewing distances. To achieve this, the far point of the person should be conjugate with optical infinity. With the spectacles, one should be able to see clearly at far distance with nil accommodative effort and at all other closer distances with optimal accommodative effort (before presbyopia sets in). In the attempt to abolish accommodation for distance, the most common philosophy followed for spectacle prescription is "minimum minus for maximum visual acuity and maximum plus for maximum visual acuity." This can be modified as "optimal correction (plus or minus) for maximum visual acuity with nil visual stress." Visual stress can be reduced or eliminated when we consider other factors of binocular vision status for prescribing spectacles.

For example, in the presence of an exodeviation, with a hyperopic refractive error and a high AC/A (accommodative convergence/accommodation) ratio, a little under-correction of the plus power can be considered if a good control for exodeviation is achieved without compromising visual acuity and stressing the accommodative system. The lag of accommodation over the subjective acceptance in this scenario can be checked to ensure that it is within the tolerable limit (+0.25 D to +0.75 D). Such a spectacle prescription would achieve optimal correction, maximal visual acuity, and minimal visual stress. Of course, this could be a rare event. The conventional principle would work in most instances, but in exceptional situations, the spectacle prescription can be modified to alleviate the signs and symptoms of the patient. Therefore, there is no one correct method/technique to prescribe spectacles. Yet, we will be discussing the broad guidelines and techniques here.

4.4 Technique

The first step toward spectacle prescription starts with history, followed by measurement of visual acuity (distance and near), objective refraction, and eventually, subjective refraction for distance and then near viewing. The near visual acuity check is typically done at a 40 cm viewing distance. For those in the presbyopic age-group or those whose near visual acuity is not optimal, a near addition is prescribed to improve the near acuity.

Proper patient history matters in subjective refraction. If a patient is very comfortable with their earlier spectacles and simply wants to change their frame, it still requires performing good refraction. However, the final spectacle prescription should be close enough, if not similar, to their earlier spectacle correction, especially if the visual acuity is good for both distance and near with their current spectacles. If very different, it requires careful examination and perhaps cycloplegic refraction. In one study, about 10% of patients with non-tolerance to their new spectacles had adaptation issues even when the refraction was correct [2]. Sometimes, some people may not tolerate even a ±0.50 D difference in spherical error [10]. Errors of refraction were the leading cause (47%) for spectacles non-tolerance [10]. Hence, it will be important to learn the technique carefully to minimize this error.

It is good to remember the following important points before subjective refraction.

1. Age of the patient matters in how we start the subjective refraction. For pre-presbyopic adults and young children, a good starting point is to leave the working lens (typically +1.50 DS) and start fogging (actually defogging).
2. A general rule of thumb is for every 0.25 DS (or 0.50 DC) change, one-line visual acuity improvement should be expected [11, 12].

This rule of thumb, however, depends on other factors like pupil size, and blur adaptation of the patient, etc. Nevertheless, this rule helps check the correlation between uncorrected visual acuity and refractive error.

3. For example, if a young person has a logMAR visual acuity of 20/200, to improve to 20/20, which is about 10 lines in the logMAR chart, a refractive error of −2.50 DS could be expected. On the other hand, a refractive error of −6.00 DS appears unrealistic for that level of visual acuity.
4. In the above case, other factors, such as squinting/squeezing the eyes by the patient to read or spasm of near reflex [13], should be considered.
5. This said, sometimes there can be outliers who have reasonably good visual acuity despite having a high astigmatic error (e.g., 3.00 DC). This could have resulted from better blur interpretation with one clear meridian (especially, vertical clarity can still help read English optotypes than a vertical blur) [12].
6. It will also be necessary to closely observe the time taken and the ease with which patients read the letters with or without spectacles. Look also beyond the patient's verbal response; look for the patient's body language, facial frowns, head tilts, etc.
7. Particularly in non-verbal patients, looking for these signs becomes even more important in deciding whether the final spectacle prescription should or should not be given.
8. Some patients can be finicky or sensitive to any axis change they are not used to. So, check the axis in their previous prescription before changing it and make sure it warrants a change.
9. Cycloplegic refraction is advisable for children, first-time spectacle wearers, patients with asthenopic symptoms, sometimes patients with pre-presbyopia, and in those when visual acuity, objective, and subjective refraction are not correlating.
10. PMT (post-mydriatic test) or, more appropriately, PCT (post-cycloplegic test) visit will be indicated if there is a major change from the previous spectacle prescription or if the subjective acceptance and cycloplegic objective refraction are very different. Else, the spectacle prescription can be finalized in one visit itself.

The spectacle correction for ametropia is divided into a spherical and cylindrical correction. Considerations for anisometropic correction (see Sect. 4.4) and presbyopia correction (Sect. 4.5) are also discussed.

4.4.1 Spherical Correction

Spherical correction is fairly straightforward for patients with myopia or hyperopia, as long as the patient's accommodation is without large (>0.50 D) fluctuations and is able to relax fully. Fogging should be done for children and young adults. It is also done for those with asthenopic symptoms with good visual acuity (regardless of age). Patients with high hyperopia and lower myopic errors can also show accommodative fluctuations and would need fogging. Fogging is a must for over-corrected (over-minus) myopic patients as well. Pre-presbyopes with mild myopic or hyperopic refractive error will also benefit from fogging.

Spectacle prescription is challenging in people with hyperopic correction, especially with active accommodation (children and young adults). Different age-groups of children and magnitudes of ametropia have different guidelines for prescribing spectacles [6]. The Vision in Preschoolers–Hyperopia in Preschoolers (VIP–HIP) study group [14, 15] and a systematic review [16] showed increasing evidence for the need to prescribe hyperopic correction for children, especially when there are concerns in academic performance. For example, the child may have 20/20 visual acuity, but the refractive error could be +5.00 DS; in such cases, it will be necessary also to do a dynamic retinoscopy and determine the lag of accommodation. Remember, children spend most of their time doing near and intermediate tasks. Hence, while they may have good accommodation momentarily to read a chart (distance and near), they may be unable to sustain their accommodation for longer periods.

In an esodeviation, full correction of the hyperopic refractive error is mandatory. But even in the absence of esodeviation, if the lag of accommodation is high (>+0.75 D), the child may benefit from a spectacle prescription. Normative lag for different accommodative stimuli for children has been studied [17]. This would be helpful when considering closer working distance for young children since their Harmon distance (the distance between the elbow and the knuckle) is smaller. Also, in children with special needs (e.g., Down syndrome), it would be important to check for their lag of accommodation, and some children may need a near reading addition as well [18, 19].

For patients who cannot relax their accommodation, techniques such as the Borish delayed subjective test [20] will be useful. Briefly, this test requires regular subjective refraction, and then a negative relative accommodation (NRA) procedure is done to relax the accommodation. In NRA, plus lenses in the steps of +0.25 DS are added binocularly till the patient reports a sustained blur of the reading material held at 40 cm. Post this procedure, the patient looks at the distance visual acuity chart, 20/20 line with the NRA value. The examiner then defogs until the patient can again read that line. Through this procedure, the patient can accept additional plus power. For patients who cannot accept their hyperopic correction initially, it is important to educate them about their spectacle prescription and inform them that they may have to change their spectacles later (after 3–6 months). During this time, the patient would be able to relax their accommodation with their new spectacles and, in their subsequent visit(s), may easily accept a higher or their full hyperopic correction (see Case 1). In some ophthalmology practices, homatropine hydrobromide (2%) eye drops are prescribed, and higher (or full) hyperopic spectacle prescription is given to aid the spectacle adaptation process.

As a clinical note, if leaving a patient with maximum plus, ensure the binocular acuity is at least one line better than 20/20 (i.e., 20/16 or −0.1 LogMAR). This assures that the patient can easily adapt to their plus spectacle correction without many complaints of distance blur. A similar check can also be done in myopic correction (minimum minus). Also, check for correlations with axial length (A-scan measurements) in cases of high refractive errors.

Case 1

A 31-year-old male had a history of intermittent blurring of vision and dry eyes while working on the computer for the past 5 years. He was prescribed spectacles and lubricating eye drops but was still symptomatic. He was advised to undergo psychological counselling since there was no reason to explain his blurred vision.

Visual acuity with his spectacle prescription: RE: −0.25 DS (20/20, N6); LE: plano (20/20, N6). Dry Retinoscopy: RE: +0.50 DS; LE: +0.25 DS; Cycloplegic retinoscopy and acceptance: RE: +2.00 DS (20/25); LE: +1.75 DS (20/25 + 2). He was called for the post-cycloplegic visit and was first prescribed +0.75 DS (20/20 − 2) for each eye. After 2 months, his spectacles were changed to +1.50 DS (20/20 + 3) in each eye. He was more comfortable with the new spectacles and was less symptomatic for his computer work from then on.

4.4.2 Cylindrical Correction

Cylindrical correction is given for astigmatism. In astigmatism, the two principal meridians in the eye have different refractive errors. As a result of this, instead of a single point (stigma), an elongated ellipse (a-stigma) is seen. This ellipse is the conoid of Sturm, and the clearest image within this zone is the circle of least confusion. A perfect refractive correction should aim to collapse this conoid of Sturm to a clear point that will be focused on the retina. An indication for a cylindrical correction will be evident when the patient reads letters like “V” as “Y” or “O” as “Q,” etc.

It is generally easier to adapt to spherical correction than cylindrical errors. However, when the cylindrical correction is large (>1.00 DC), patients quickly appreciate the clarity this correction provides and easily adapt to this. For the first-time spectacle wearer, the cylindrical spectacle correction's accuracy for both the magnitude of the power and the axis of the correcting cylindrical lens is crucial. Patients who adapt to a wrong axis may later have difficulty accepting the correct axis and may prefer the cylinder axis oriented to their previous spectacle correction.

There are different types of astigmatism; these include:

1. With-the-rule astigmatism: refractive power of the vertical meridian is higher than the horizontal meridian (e.g., K-readings: 44.70 D @106 and 41.80 D @16, (Fig. 4.1).
2. Against-the-rule-astigmatism: refractive power of the horizontal meridian is higher than the vertical meridian (e.g., −2.00 DS/−3.00 DCx90).
3. Oblique astigmatism: The principal meridians are within 120°–150° and 30°–60° in an oblique direction (e.g., −2.00 DS/−3.00 DCx40).
4. Regular astigmatism: The principal meridians are perpendicular to each other (e.g., 44.00 D @20 and 47.00 D @110).
5. Irregular astigmatism: The principal meridians are not perpendicular to each other (e.g., 44.00 D @30 and 47.00 D @90); this can be seen in keratoconus or corneal opacities post trauma.
6. Simple myopic astigmatism: only one of the principal meridians has a myopic refractive error; the other is focused on the retina (e.g., plano/−1.00 DCx90).
7. Compound myopic astigmatism: both the principal meridians are in front of the retina (e.g., −2.00 DS/−1.00 DCx60).
8. Simple hyperopic astigmatism: only one of the principal meridians has a hyperopic defocus; the other is focused on the retina (e.g., +0.50/−0.50 DCx90 = plano/+0.50 DCx180).
9. Compound hyperopic astigmatism: both the principal meridians are focused behind the retina (e.g., +1.00 DS/−0.50 DCx100 = +0.50 DS/+0.50 DCx10).
10. Mixed astigmatism: one of the principal meridians has a hyperopic defocus while the other has a myopic defocus (e.g., +3.00 DS/−5.00 DCx20 = −2.00 DS/+5.00 DCx110).

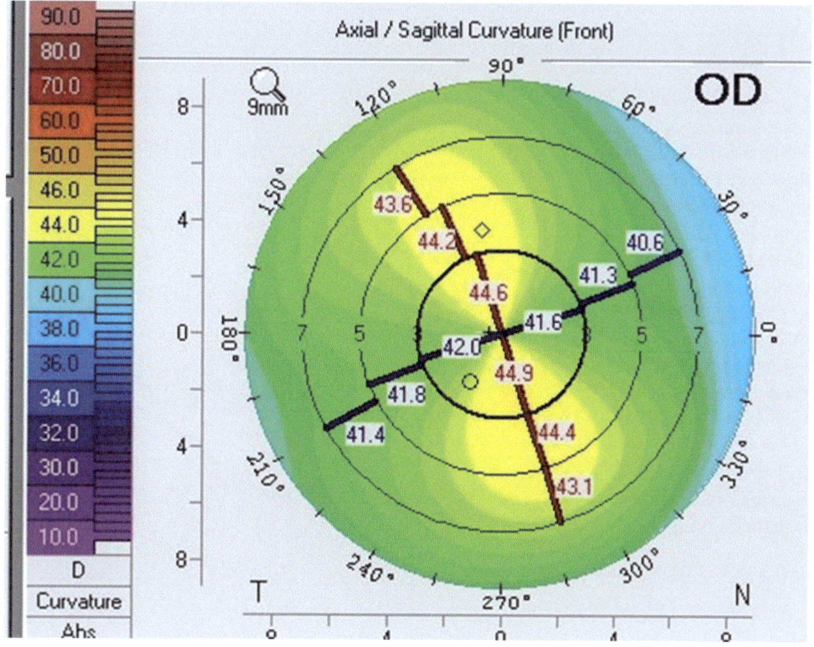

Fig. 4.1 Corneal topography of a patient who has with-the-rule, regular astigmatism. The vertical meridian has higher power than the horizontal meridian. The correcting cylinder for this patient was −3.00 DCx15°

The above examples are given using keratometric readings or spectacle corrections in both minus and plus cylinder forms to provide a broad understanding of the astigmatism presentations. However, we usually prescribe and dispense the spectacles for astigmatic correction in a minus cylinder. As a convention, "@" indicates the corneal power in that meridian in keratometric readings. While "x" is used to indicate the correcting cylinder axis in the spectacle prescription. This axis will be perpendicular to the corneal meridian with higher power for the minus cylinder. For example, 44.00 D@90/45.00 D@180 can have a sphero-cylindrical correction as plano/−1.00 DCx90. The vertical corneal meridian will form the horizontal focal line and vice versa with the horizontal corneal meridian (forms the vertical focal line). It will be important to keep this understanding as we learn further about correcting astigmatism (see also Fig. 4.2).

The steps for prescribing cylindrical spectacle correction are as follows:

1. First, refine the spherical refractive error through fogging when appropriate.
2. If there is no improvement in visual acuity upon further addition of spherical lenses (more minus or less plus), then introduce the cylinder power. The introduction of cylinder power is similar to the spherical fogging technique. The initial cylinder axis position is based on the objective refraction value.
3. A 0.50 DC increase in power should improve the visual acuity by one line. When a reasonable amount of acuity is achieved (i.e., about 20/63 or better), axis and power refinement can be fine-tuned further by using JCC (Jackson's Cross Cylinder). The JCC procedure is explained below.
4. A keratometer and topography can also help determine cylinder power and axis. It is also a recommended procedure to detect any corneal pathologies like keratoconus.

JCC helps in the refinement of the power and axis of the cylinder. It is good for finer refinement. If large changes are expected, rechecking the objective refraction or using topography for confirmation would be ideal.

JCC has two cylinders of equal magnitude and opposite signs (plus and minus) aligned perpendicular to each other and is available in different powers such as ±0.25 D, ±0.50 D, ±0.75 D, and even ±1.00 D. When the visual acuity is very good, even the smallest blur can be detected; choose the lower denomination of the JCC for those patients. For those with poorer visual acuity, a higher denomination can be used. Usually, red dots/lines indicate minus cylinder and white (or black or green) indicates plus cylinder.

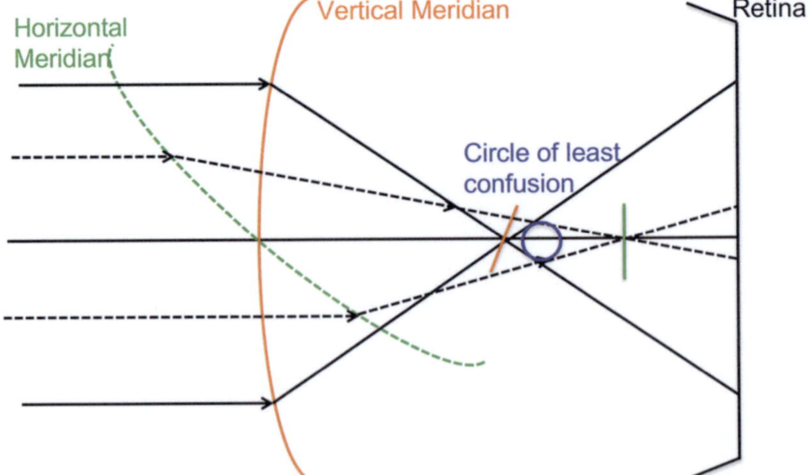

Fig. 4.2 Illustration of compound myopic astigmatism. Note that the linear distance is not equally spaced in the conoid of Sturm, hence the circle of least confusion appears closer to one image than the other. The horizontal corneal meridian (dotted green lines) forms the vertical image (solid green line). Similarly, the vertical corneal meridian forms the horizontal image

However, it is always better to verify this before starting the JCC procedure. The spherical equivalent of JCC is always zero. The technique is explained below.

4.4.3 Jackson's Cross Cylinder (JCC) Technique

1. JCC is used after arriving upon the best sphero-cylinder correction.
2. The procedure is done without any fogging lens. The patient is asked to look at a line that is two lines above their best visual acuity (e.g., if 20/20 is the best acuity, the patient can look at a 20/30 line).
3. First step is to refine the axis. For this, the JCC handle is held parallel to the correcting cylinder axis (Fig. 4.3a).
4. The patient is asked to view two positions by straddling the JCC back and forth and to report "if 1 is better than 2 or vice-versa or if both are equally blurred."
5. The endpoint is when the patient says, "both are equally blurred" or "both positions are bad, and removing it is good."
6. Sometimes the patient may say the letters slant in one direction in position 1 and the opposite direction in the other position. This is also a good indication that the axis is correct.
7. If the patient prefers one position over the other, move the correcting minus cylinder toward the minus cylinder position in JCC. The first step size can be large (10°), and in the subsequent refinement, it can be smaller (5°) when the direction to move the minus cylinder changes. The endpoint to achieve is step 5 above.
8. Next, cylinder power is refined. The cylinder (indicated by dots/lines) in the JCC is kept parallel to the cylinder axis in the trial frame (Fig. 4.3b). The JCC is then straddled between the two positions. The endpoint to achieve is step 5.
9. If the patient prefers one position over the other, change the cylinder power accordingly. For example, if minus power is preferred, increase the magnitude of the minus cylinder power and, at the same time, add plus sphere power (half of the cylinder value) to maintain the spherical equivalent. Vice versa for plus cylinder power increase (i.e., the minus sphere will be added).
10. For example, if a patient has −1.00DS/−0.50DCx90, if with JCC the patient prefers −0.50 DC, the resultant power in the trial lens should be −0.75DS/−1.00DCx90.

JCC refinement aims to put the circle of least confusion on the retina. This is why the endpoint is "both views are equally blurred," and upon removing the JCC, the patient reports the clarity is much better if the correct power and axis are achieved (Fig. 4.4). This is because, for an already clear point on the retina, the JCC expands the conoid of Sturm with the circle of least confu-

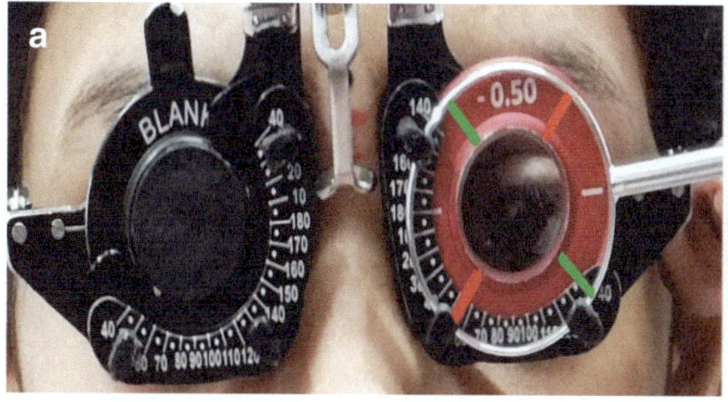

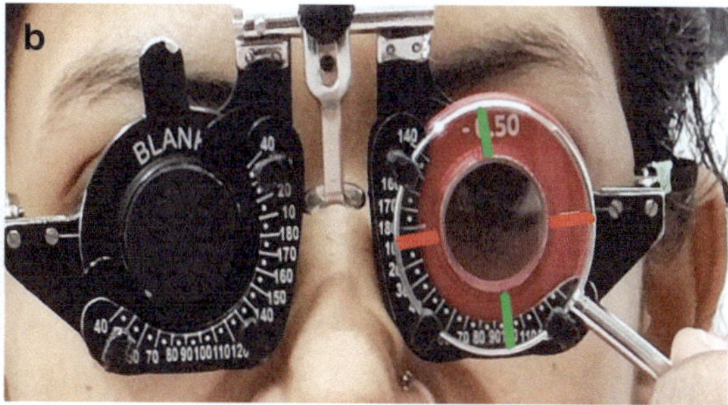

Fig. 4.3 JCC (Jackson's cross cylinder) technique depicted for (**a**) axis refinement: the handle of the JCC is held parallel to the cylinder axis and (**b**) power refinement: the axis markings of the JCC is held parallel to the cylinder axis. The two JCC axes are drawn in red (minus) and green (plus) thick lines in this picture for better illustration

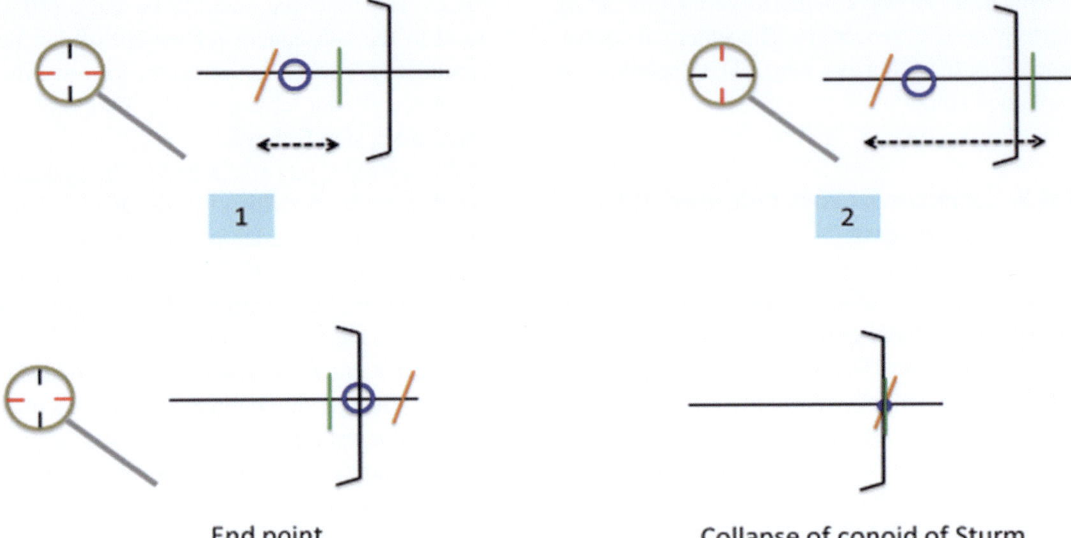

Fig. 4.4 Illustration of the JCC technique. Two positions (1&2 [blue boxes]) are shown to the patient by flipping the JCC. The blur circles are smaller in position 1 than 2 (upper panel). Accordingly, the power or axis is adjusted (see text for description). The procedure continues until the endpoint is reached, which places the circle of least confusion on the retina (lower panel, left image). The patient would report equal blur upon flipping the JCC at this position. Upon removal of the JCC, a clear image is formed on the retina (lower panel, right image)

sion on the retina. In positions 1 and 2, the two principal meridians simply straddle around the circle of least confusion, giving the perception of equally blurred. The conoid collapses upon removal of the JCC. Thus, the patient appreciates the clarity on JCC removal.

Generally, the cylindrical axis and power in both eyes tend to be symmetrical. It is easier to adapt to a symmetrical axis in both eyes. However, occasionally an asymmetrical value can also be observed. Sometimes asymmetrical cylindrical errors are found in accommodative stress such as spasm or accommodative excess. In such patients, a cylinder power of −0.50DCx50 in only one eye and a plano in the other eye (for example) would disappear in cycloplegic refraction. Hence apply caution to prescribe an oblique axis, even if there is a slight improvement in visual acuity, and the patient prefers it. Perform a cycloplegic refraction (especially for first-time spectacles wearers). This said, cases of astigmatism in very different axes between the two eyes, while very rare, can still be encountered (for example, the cylinder axis in one eye is 90°, and the other eye is 170°).

In those patients with presbyopia who are uncomfortable with their spectacle correction only for near vision, do near refraction to check for any axis variation in the cylindrical power. In very rare instances, there might be an axis change. If the magnitude of the cylinder is high, even a small change in axis can also cause a lot of visual disturbance. Consider giving separate spectacles for distance and near in such cases. In some patients with high astigmatism (corneal), the quality of vision obtained with Rigid Gas Permeable (RGP) contact lenses (CLs) will be superior to the spectacle correction. Encourage these patients to give CLs a try. Sharp visual acuity can be a good motivation for them to switch and be compliant with CLs.

4.4.4 Astigmatic Fan and Stenopic Slit

Astigmatic fan, clock dial charts, rotating T chart, etc., can be used to determine the axis of the cylinder. The fundamental principle of all these tests is similar. Hence only the astigmatic fan test will

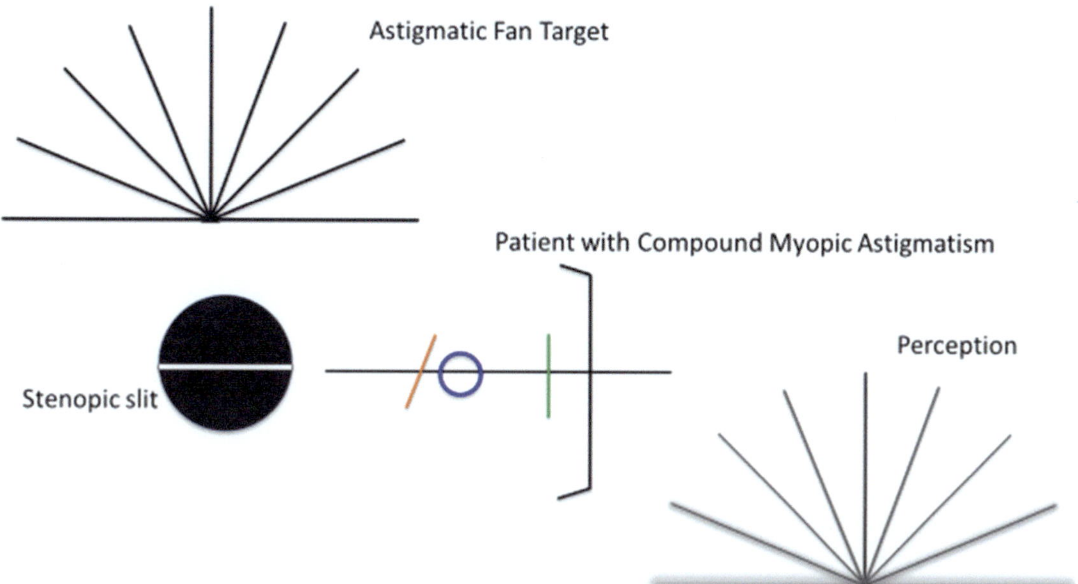

Fig. 4.5 Illustration of an astigmatic fan chart viewed by a patient with compound myopic, with-the-rule astigmatism. Therefore, the vertical line (green) formed by the horizontal meridian has the least myopic power and is closer to the retina. Therefore, the patient perceives this line as sharper, and the horizontal line is the most blurred. A stenopic slit oriented in the horizontal direction would cut the blurred circles formed by the vertical meridian (horizontal line), and in that position, the patient would say the image appears clear. The correcting minus cylinder for this patient will be ×180°

be explained with an example (Fig. 4.5). The test can be done with a weak fogging lens; that way, the principal meridians are both kept in front of the retina. Else, accommodative fluctuations can make it difficult to interpret the result, and the patient response may be variable. The patient is asked to look at all the lines and to pick one line that appears the darkest, blackest, and sharpest. The chosen line (say, for example, 90°) is formed by the least myopic meridian (or low refractive power) of the eye (i.e., 180°). Therefore, the most myopic meridian is perpendicular to this (i.e., 90°). The correcting minus cylinder axis should be perpendicular (i.e. 180°) to the most myopic meridian. So, an easy way to remember this is to give the minus cylinder perpendicular to the line chosen to be the darkest, blackest, and sharpest.

A stenopic slit is a handy tool that can help find the axis for irregular astigmatism due to corneal pathologies and where retinoscopy and keratometry are difficult to perform. This procedure can also be done with a weak fogging lens. A stenopic slit can be considered as an elongated pinhole. The orientation of the slit where better clarity of the chart (visual acuity chart can be shown) is obtained will be the minus cylinder axis position. This is because the orientation of the slit isolates the meridian position that gives the best clarity (say 40°). The most blurred position, therefore, could be perpendicular to this meridian (130°). Hence to correct that meridian, a minus cylinder oriented in the same location as the stenopic slit (40°) can improve the clarity.

4.4.5 Duochrome Test

After arriving at the refractive correction for each eye, the duochrome test (Fig. 4.6) is done as the endpoint of the monocular subjective refraction procedure. Duochrome (also referred to as bichrome) test works on the principle of chromatic aberration. Therefore, the test can also be administered to those with a color deficiency. In this test, the red band that has a longer wavelength will be focused behind the retina. The green band

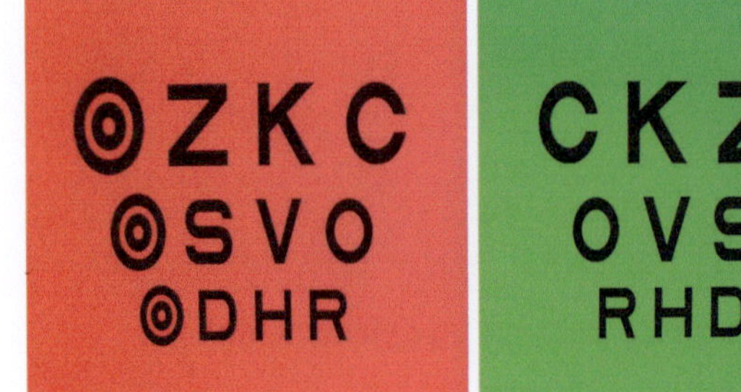

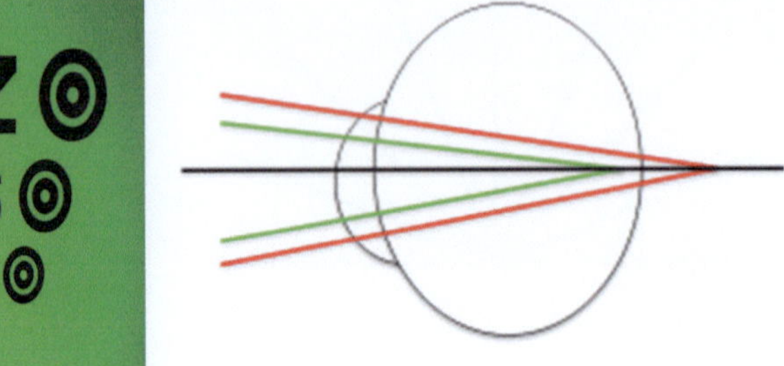

Fig. 4.6 Duochrome test. If the accommodation is optimally relaxed and with appropriate refractive error correction, the images from the red and green background will be formed behind and in front of the retina, respectively, thus giving a perception of both being equally clear

that has a shorter wavelength will be focused in front of the retina. Therefore, the black letters on these colored backgrounds will appear equally clear if the refractive correction is optimal plus or minus. Else, letters or symbols on the green background will appear darker and sharper in case of overcorrection for myopia or under-correction for hyperopia. It would be vice versa for overcorrection of hyperopia and under-correction of myopia, i.e., letters or symbols on red will be darker or sharper. The ideal is to achieve balance or leave the patient slightly red better so as not to stress the accommodative system. An important check to make here is in cases of spasm of near reflex with the accommodative component; the patient may always report red better, no matter how much more minus power is added. Therefore, checking on reversal for the response is a good habit. That is, the patient is expected to report "green better" when extra minus power is added (under-correction of hyperopia or overcorrection of myopia) and to say "red better" when extra plus is added (overcorrection of hyperopia or under-correction of myopia). Such a reversal response indicates that the accommodation system is not on overdrive, and the patient is consistent with their response and has understood the test.

4.4.6 Binocular Balancing

Most of the routine subjective refraction would stop after the monocular duochrome check. Upon finalizing the spectacle power, the patient is allowed to view the visual acuity chart binocularly. As a good practice, the patient should be shown the chart with their old spectacles and the new correction. This would help the patient to appreciate the difference in clarity and to decide on changing the spectacles.

For some patients, especially those with asthenopic symptoms, those who are not happy with their spectacle correction, etc., it would be better to perform a few additional tests to give them a comfortable pair of spectacles. One such additional test is binocular balancing. This test aims to balance the accommodation (not visual acuity) between both eyes. In those patients who do not have equal visual acuity, a couple of lines above the acuity level of the worst eye can be used. Different methods can be used to achieve binocular balancing. This includes prism dissociation, alternate occlusion, and duochrome with prism dissociation. There is also the Turville Infinity Balance (TIB); however, unlike the other methods, which are dissociating fusion, this method provides a peripheral fusion lock and allows monocular viewing only for central viewing. For this reason, this test is included under "binocular refraction," which provides a bit more naturalistic viewing to balance the accommodation. Please also refer to the text Primary Care Optometry for details of other methods [21]. Prism dissociation technique will be explained below.

The prism dissociation test can be a quick and handy test to do for binocular balancing. While

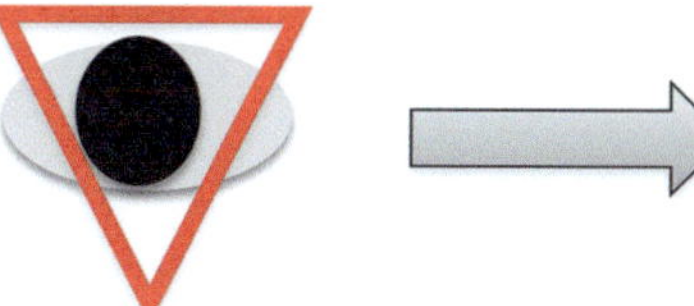

Fig. 4.7 Binocular balancing using prism dissociation test. Prisms base down (image perceived up) and base up (image perceived down) are placed in front of the eyes. Patient is asked to report which chart appears clearer. A power of +0.25 DS is added to that eye that views the clear chart

the alternate occlusion is the easiest, where each eye is occluded alternately and quickly to compare the images in each eye, it may not be a very efficient test. The act of occluding one eye itself can result in some accommodative fluctuations. As an extreme example, a report of a case of spasm of accommodation has been noted in a patient only when one eye is occluded [22]. Prism dissociation can be done using the prism lenses in the trial box and does not need any other equipment.

Dissociating prisms (4PD base down and 5PD base up) can be placed in each eye (Fig. 4.7). This way, there will be an equal luminance level for both eyes, as opposed to placing the prism only in one eye. The unequal prisms are chosen only because the trial box has a single prism for a given power denomination. Vertical dissociation is easier, as horizontal vergence eye movements can easily overcome horizontal dissociation. After arriving at the monocular subjective endpoint, the procedure is done with little fog (each eye can be added +0.50 DS or +0.75 DS). The fogging lens will reduce the acuity by about 2 or 3 lines. The patient is instructed to look at that line and to report whether the top or the bottom chart appears clearer. To the eye that reports the chart to be clear (base down prism will form an image above and vice versa for base up), a +0.25 DS can be added. If both look equally clear, the procedure is stopped. If the clarity flips to the other eye, the +0.25 DS can be removed and taken as accommodation being equalized. If the same eye image is still reported to be clear, another +0.25 DS is added till an equal or reversal endpoint is achieved. After reaching the endpoint, prisms are removed, and binocular defogging is done. A prescription that allows the patient to read 20/20 or better is given. Under binocular viewing, accommodation can be relaxed more.

4.5 Anisometropia

The steps involved in giving the spherical and cylindrical correction for anisometropic patients are relatively similar. However, in anisometropia, it will be important to check for the effects of aniseikonia and tolerance to the new spectacle correction. Adaptation time should be given with the new spectacle prescription in the trial frame to ensure the patient can tolerate the difference. A difference of more than 2.5 D should be checked for binocular fusion for both near and distance with the Worth Four Dot Test. However, it must

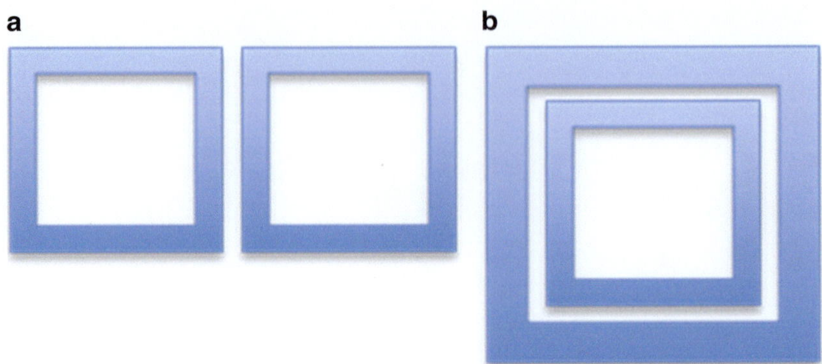

Fig. 4.8 Examples of (**a**) typical double vision (horizontal diplopia) as could arise from horizontal strabismus. (**b**) Double vision in the case of aniseikonia could appear as "front and back" or one image inside the other

be noted that the "double" reported by the patient in anisometropia arises from aniseikonia. Hence this "double" is not similar to that observed in strabismus (Fig. 4.8).

If the patient cannot tolerate it, then the difference in anisometropia should be reduced to a tolerable level. This would involve reducing the refractive correction in the more anisometropic eye. However, better solutions should aim at reducing aniseikonia (contact lenses) or anisometropia (refractive surgery for adults). In younger children, high anisometropic refractive errors can lead to amblyopia. Thus, giving the full refractive correction for both the dominant and amblyopic eye would be important. This is specifically true in the case of hyperopic refractive error (see Case 2).

Case 2

A 12-year-old boy presented for eye testing for the first time. His visual acuity was 20/20 and 20/125 in the right and left eye, respectively. His refractive error was +0.50 DS and +5.00 DS in the right and left eye, respectively. His subjective acceptance was plano (20/20) and +4.00 DS (20/80). His cycloplegic retinoscopy showed +2.50 DS and +6.50 DS, respectively. In PCT, with fogging, he accepted +1.25 DS (20/30) and +5.00 DS (20/100). In a 1-month follow-up visit, the visual acuity improved to 20/20–2 and 20/50 in the right and left eyes, respectively. The aim here is to give appropriate correction and not hesitate in giving the correction, even if the acuity is lower on the first examination. The initial blurred vision in the right eye would disappear if the patient could tolerate and adapt well to the appropriate spectacle correction.

4.6 Presbyopia Correction

The most common practice of giving the near addition power is by age. The easy-to-remember formula is [age/10]−3. For example, a 55-year-old person will be given an addition of +2.5 DS ([55/10]−3). In a large majority of cases, this formula works well. The other methods to prescribe the near addition depend on the accommodation amplitude, dynamic retinoscopy, fused cross cylinder, near duochrome, and measuring positive and negative relative accommodation. It has been shown that going by age gave a good estimation for the near addition when all methods were compared [23].

A large majority of the patients adapt to their new prescription by adjusting their working distances as well. The incipient presbyope, however, tends to hold the reading material far away and would expect the same working distance with the new spectacles due to habit. In a few cases, where they strongly prefer a particular working distance or in cases of over-zealously corrected hypermetropia for distance, simply giving an addition by the age criteria alone can be troublesome. Hence prescribing near addition should be undertaken with care. It is mandatory to check the range of the near working distance with the near addition, ensuring that it falls within the comfort range of the patient's habitual viewing distances.

Generally, a range from 35 to 60 cm should be very comfortable. The philosophy for near addition is the opposite of the prescribing pattern for distance visual acuity; i.e., the lowest plus power that gives the maximum comfortable near working distance is prescribed for near addition. Also, remember that when increasing the plus power for distance, it would be necessary to check the near addition and range carefully and not simply go by the age criteria (Case 3).

Case 3

A 50-year-old female, accountant by profession complained of blurring for near vision. She had never worn any spectacles before. Her dry retinoscopy showed minimal hyperopic correction. She was given +1.50 DS for near vision. The patient returned after a week; she reported discomfort with reading but felt better with the spectacles for distance viewing. Upon cycloplegic retinoscopy, she was found to have +1.50 DS for distance. She read 20/20 both with and without her distance correction. Duochrome was red better only with her spectacle correction; without it, green was better. Her spectacles were changed to a distance correction of +1.50 DS and a reading addition of +1.25 DS, which gave her a comfortable range. The learning point here is to do cycloplegic refraction even in older individuals who could still have active accommodation. Note this lady has never worn any reading correction till 50 years of age, in spite of having hyperopic correction for distance. In such individuals, near addition should not be based on age, especially after fully correcting their hyperopic error for distance.

4.7 Conclusion

Prescribing spectacles through subjective refraction is an art. With practice and experience, each clinician carves out their practice pattern and gets a sense of what would work best for their patient. The end goal of subjective refraction is to give a comfortable 20/20 vision. It is important to remember this, or else if the goal is only to get the patient to read the last line, it could end up in unnecessary over-minus or under-plus in spectacle correction. Understanding the occupational visual needs of the person is equally important to determine the appropriate spectacle prescription. There are a few more specialty prescriptions that could incorporate relieving prisms, size lenses, yoke prisms, etc., that are beyond the scope of this book. The topics discussed here should help a general clinician understand the fundamental concepts for arriving at a regular spectacle prescription encountered in a day-to-day clinic.

Funding Hyderabad Eye Research Foundation, Hyderabad, India.

Disclosure None.

References

1. Strang NC, Gray LS, Winn B, et al. Clinical evaluation of patient tolerance to autorefractor prescriptions. Clin Exp Optom. 1998;81(3):112–8.
2. Bist J, Kaphle D, Marasini S, et al. Spectacle non-tolerance in clinical practice—a systematic review with meta-analysis. Ophthalmic Physiol Opt. 2021;41(3):610–22.
3. Milder B, Rubin ML. The fine art of prescribing glasses. Triad Publishing Company; 1991.
4. Wilkson ME. Sharpen your subjective refraction technique. Rev Optom. 2016;58–65. https://www.reviewofoptometry.com/CMSDocuments/2016/1/SharpenYourSubjectiveRefractionTechnique.pdf.
5. Cantor LB, Rapuano CJ, George AC. Clinical optics basic and clinical science course. Am Acad Ophthalmol. 2019;61(713):385.
6. Leat SJ. To prescribe or not to prescribe? Guidelines for spectacle prescribing in infants and children. Clin Exp Optom. 2011;94(6):514–27.

7. Rosenfield M, Logan N. Optometry: science, techniques and clinical management. 2nd ed. Elsevier; 2009.
8. Collins N, Garratt S. Preferred practice pattern. Am Acad Ophthalmol. 2012:49.
9. American Optometric Association. Comprehensive pediatric eye and vision examination. 2017;10–39. https://www.aoa.org/AOA/Documents/Practice/Management/Clinical/Guidelines/EBO/Guidelines/Comprehensive/Pediatric/Eye/and/Vision/Exam.pdf.
10. Freeman CE, Evans BJW. Investigation of the causes of non-tolerance to optometric prescriptions for spectacles. Ophthalmic Physiol Opt. 2010;30(1):1–11.
11. Westheimer G. Scaling of visual acuity. Arch Ophthalmol. 1979;97:327–30.
12. Atchison DA, Mathur A. Visual acuity with astigmatic blur. Optom Vis Sci. 2011;88(7):798–805.
13. Roy S, Bharadwaj SR, Patil-Chhablani P, et al. Spasm of near reflex: a comprehensive management protocol and treatment outcomes. J AAPOS. 2021;25(3):162.e1–6. https://doi.org/10.1016/j.jaapos.2021.02.010.
14. Kulp MT, Ciner E, Maguire M, et al. Uncorrected hyperopia and preschool early literacy: results of the vision in preschoolers-hyperopia in preschoolers (VIP–HIP) study. Ophthalmology. 2016;123(4):681–9.
15. Ciner EB, Kulp MT, Maguire MG, et al. Visual function of moderately hyperopic 4- and 5-year-old children in the vision in preschoolers—hyperopia in preschoolers study. Am J Ophthalmol. 2016;170:143–52. https://www.sciencedirect.com/science/article/pii/S0002939416303634.
16. Mavi S, Chan VF, Virgili G, et al. The impact of hyperopia on academic performance among children: a systematic review. Asia Pac J Ophthalmol (Philadelphia, Pa). 2022;11(1):36–51.
17. McClelland JF, Saunders KJ. Accommodative lag using dynamic retinoscopy: age norms for school-age children. Optom Vis Sci. 2004;81(12):929–33.
18. Satgunam P, Datta S, Sumalini R. Near vision in individuals with down syndrome: a vision screening study. Eye (Lond). 2019;33(8):1254–60.
19. Al-Bagdady M, Stewart RE, Watts P, et al. Bifocals and Down's syndrome: correction or treatment? Ophthalmic Physiol Opt. 2009;29(4):416–21.
20. Borish IM. Comments on a "Delayed subjective" test. Optom Vis Sci. 1945;22(9):433. https://journals.lww.com/optvissci/Fulltext/1945/09000/COMMENTS_ON_A__DELAYED_SUBJECTIVE__TEST_.5.aspx.
21. Grosvenor TP. In: Falk K, editor. Primary care optometry. 5th ed. Butterworth Heinemann Elsevier; 2007.
22. Rutstein RP. Accommodative spasm in siblings: a unique finding. Indian J Ophthalmol. 2010;58(4):326–7.
23. Antona B, Barra F, Barrio A, et al. Comparing methods of determining addition in presbyopes. Clin Exp Optom. 2008;91(3):313–8.

5 Optical Dispensing

Srikanth Maseedupalli

5.1 Introduction

Optical dispensing is an essential component of refractive error correction. In optical dispensing, various tools and devices are used for precise eye measurements to dispense accurate eyewear prescriptions. These measurements are crucial in assessing visual needs, determining lens parameters, and ensuring optimal vision correction. This chapter will look into the common tools used for optical dispensing and describe their usage.

5.2 Tools, Devices, Machines, and Instruments in Optical Dispensing

Tools are handheld or manually operated objects to assist in performing specific tasks such as frame adjustments, lens cleaning, and minor repairs. Devices measure a particular parameter (e.g., a lens clock). Machines are mechanical devices to perform specific tasks, such as lens edging, surfacing, etc. Instruments are specialized tools used to obtain precise measurements for scientific, technical, or medical purposes (Fig. 5.1c). An automated lensometer is an example of an instrument.

S. Maseedupalli (✉)
The Standard Chartered-LVPEI Academy for Eye Care Education, L V Prasad Eye Institute, Hyderabad, India
e-mail: srikanthm@lvpei.org

T. Das, P. Satgunam (eds.), *Ophthalmic Diagnostics*, https://doi.org/10.1007/978-981-97-0138-4_5

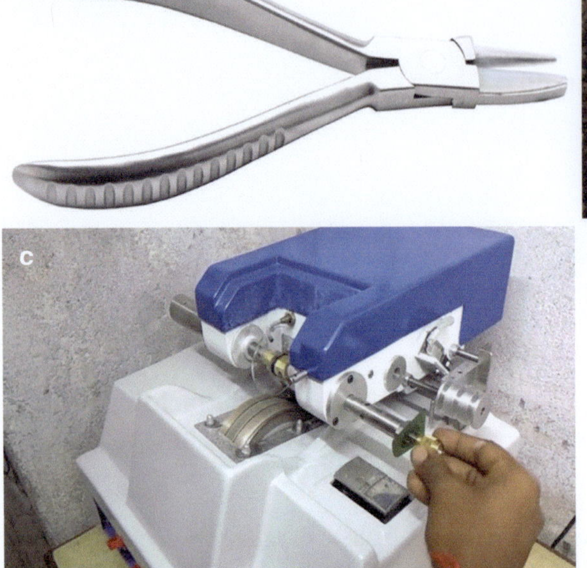

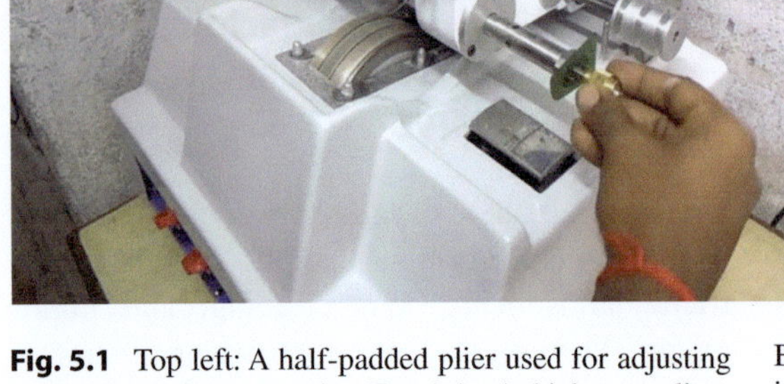

Fig. 5.1 Top left: A half-padded plier used for adjusting the spectacle frame temples. Top right: A thickness caliper used for measuring the thickness of an ophthalmic lens. Bottom: A semiautomated edging machine used for shaping the lens and fixing it in a spectacle frame

5.3 Manual Lensometer

This measures spherical and cylindrical lens power (Fig. 5.2).

The different parts of the lensometer are as follows: [1].

The eyepiece: Allows the user to view the lens and measurements.

The lens holder: Holds the lens in position during measurement.

Power drum: Allows for fine adjustments to accurately measure the lens's power. It is rotated to bring the mires (green lines) into focus.

The axis wheel: Used to adjust the axis of cylindrical lenses. It enables the alignment of the mires with the appropriate axis markings on the protractor.

Reticule or protractor: Provides a scale for measuring the axis of cylindrical lenses.

5.3.1 Guide to Using a Lensometer

Step I: Focusing the eyepiece: [1] makes the reticule, or protractor, appears clear with distinct lines. Start by turning the eyepiece anticlockwise, and while looking through it, rotate clockwise until the reticule lines are sharply visible.

Step II: Noting the instrument error: [2]. There are two kinds of instrument errors.

(a) The *power error* of the instrument can affect the accuracy of lens measurements. Begin by rotating the power drum to the "zero" reading and observe whether the mires (green lines) are clear and distinct. If they are, the instrument has no power error, and you can proceed to the next step (Step b). If the mires are not clear, adjust the power drum until

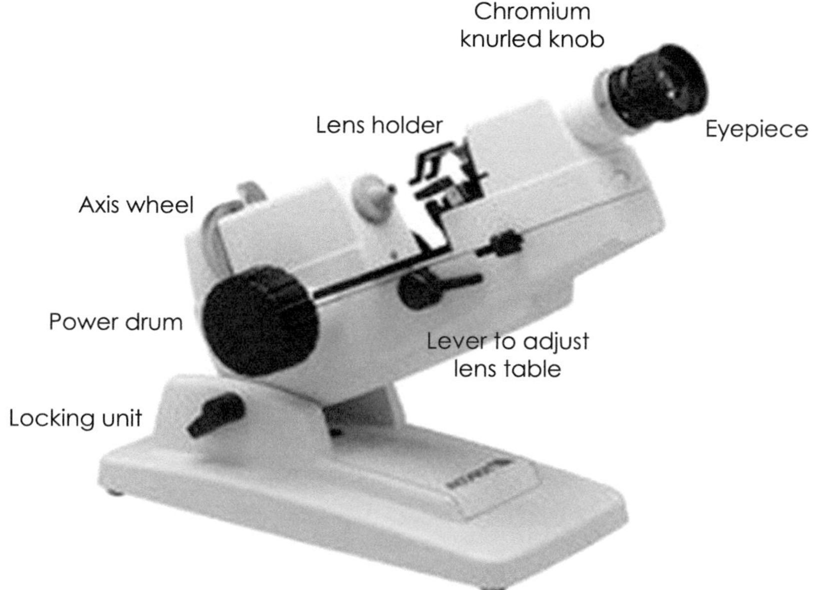

Fig. 5.2 Lensometer

they become sharp. Note the reading at which the mires appear clear (e.g., mires clear at +0.25). This indicates an error of +0.25 DS. To obtain the correct lens power, subtract 0.25 from the reading.

Example 1
If the reading is +1.50 DS, then after correction, it would be (+1.50 to −0.25) = +1.25 DS.

Example 2
For sphero-cylindrical values, only correct the spherical component. For a reading of +1.75 DS/−0.75 DC × 180, after correction, it would be +1.50 DS/−0.75 DC × 180.

(b) The *axis error* is applicable only when the lens has cylindrical power. Set the axis to "zero" by rotating the axis wheel and check whether the horizontal mires coincide with the 180° on the protractor. If they align, proceed to Step 3. If the mires do not align, rotate the axis wheel to align the mires with the 180° line on the protractor and note the axis reading.

Example 1
If the axis shows 6°, it means it is displaying 6° more than required. To correct this, subtract 6° from the reading while determining the lens power.

Example 2
If the prescription reads +2.00 DS/−1.00 DC × 120°, the correct axis would be 114°. Thus, the final prescription would be +2.00 DS/−1.00 DC × 114°).

Step III: Checking the Power of a Single-Vision Lens (Fig. 5.3a)

(a) **Spherical power**: For single-vision lenses, position the lens with the back surface against the lens stop without tilt. Rotate the power drum until the mires are clear and perpendicular to each other. Once the mires appear clear and distinct, write down the reading as the spherical power.

Example: The mires are clear and distinct, and the power reads as −3.00 D. Write this as the spherical component.

(b) **Cylindrical lenses: Example −3.00 DS/−1.50 DC × 130°**. If you cannot focus both the mires on a single go (Fig. 5.3, bottom left), it indicates a cylinder lens. In this case, focus the mires in one meridian and align the axis to ensure clear, distinct, and continuous lines, the power reads as −3.00 D (Fig. 5.3, bottom center). Note the reading as the spherical power, I.

Next, rotate only the power drum to focus the perpendicular mires.

The perpendicular mires focus at −4.50 D (Fig. 5.3, bottom right). Write this as II.

Calculate the cylindrical power by finding the difference between the two powers (II—I; −4.50 − (−3.00) = −1.50). The cylindrical power is −1.50, labeled as III.

Note the angle at which the mires for −4.50 D are aligned by looking through the eyepiece, not relying on the axis wheel. If the mires are aligned at 130°, write this as the axis (IV).

Thus, the power of the lens should be **written as I/III × IV**, i.e., −3.00 DS/−1.50 DC × 130°.

5.3.2 Important Notes

1. The technique described here is one of many. Optometrists may use alternative methods based on their preferences and expertise.
2. Placing the lens back surface against the lens stop is necessary to determine the back vertex power, particularly for single-vision lenses [1].

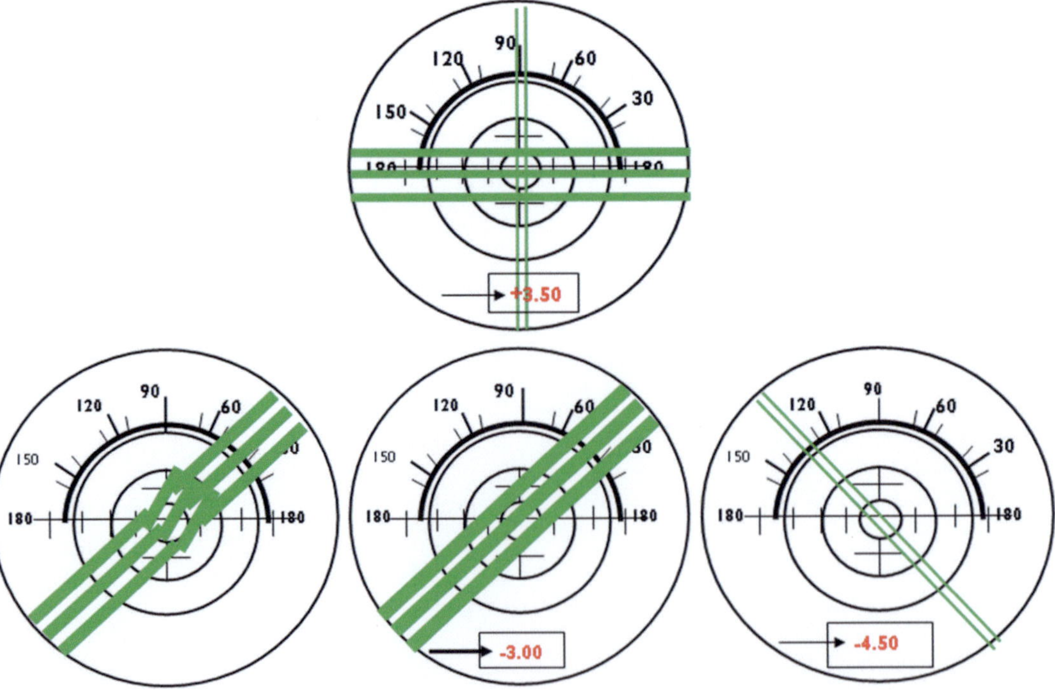

Fig. 5.3 Top: the focused vertical and horizontal mires, power reads as +3.50 DS. Bottom: left: misaligned mires, center; center: aligned mires at −3.00 D; and right: perpendicular mires aligned at −4.50 D

3. For bifocals, the measurement of the *add* power depends on whether it is altered on the front or back surface [1]. If altered on the front surface (glide your finger through the surfaces, the addition is on the side where you feel a bump or ledge in the transition from distance to near zone; if smooth, it is a fused bifocal that is always on the front surface), subtract the distance back vertex power from the near front vertex power in each meridian to determine the bifocal addition.
4. Exercise caution when dealing with high minus lenses, as they may appear as single-vision lenses but could be progressive addition lenses, especially when combined with a low near addition. Check the power in the upper and lower nasal portion of the lens. Check if there is a difference of at least 0.75; it could be a progressive addition lens. You can also look for the engravings on the temporal side of the lens that would indicate it as a progressive addition lens.
5. If you cannot bring the mires to the center of the circle in the lensometer, the lens may have a grounded prism incorporated during lens manufacturing. The base is always toward the direction of the displaced mires, and the magnitude can be read from the graticule. The first circle accounts for 0.5 prism diopter and the next one is 1.0 prism diopter, and each circle from there on accounts for one prism diopter.
6. Similarly, mires may not be aligned at the center when checking the near power for bifocal lenses when there is a significant amount of distance power, usually above 3.00 D.

5.4 Geneva Lens Measure

The Geneva Lens Measure (GLM) is a valuable device used in optical dispensing to measure the surface dioptric power of lenses, [1]. It is a mechanical dial indicator; by understanding the calibration process and following the power determination techniques, optical professionals can accurately measure the surface dioptric power of lenses. This knowledge is essential for providing accurate prescriptions and ensuring effective vision correction.

5.4.1 GLM Calibration

The calibration of the GLM ensures accurate power measurements (Fig. 5.4). Follow these steps for calibration:

Step 1: Placement: place the GLM on a flat surface, ensuring that all three pegs touch the surface. Avoid applying pressure on the device during calibration.

Step 2: Calibration reading: if the GLM is calibrated, the pointer will read zero. If the pointer does not read zero, error compensation is necessary. If it shows an error of +0.25 D, subtract 0.25 D from the final reading or vice versa.

5.4.2 Power Determination

One must recognize the front and back surfaces before determining the power. The front surface refers to the surface facing away from the eye. The back surface refers to the surface facing the eye.

Step 1: Proper positioning: hold the GLM so that the central peg aligns with the optic center of the lens. Ensure that the peg is perpendicular to the lens surface [1].

Step 2: Readings in different meridians: note the GLM readings in at least four different merid-

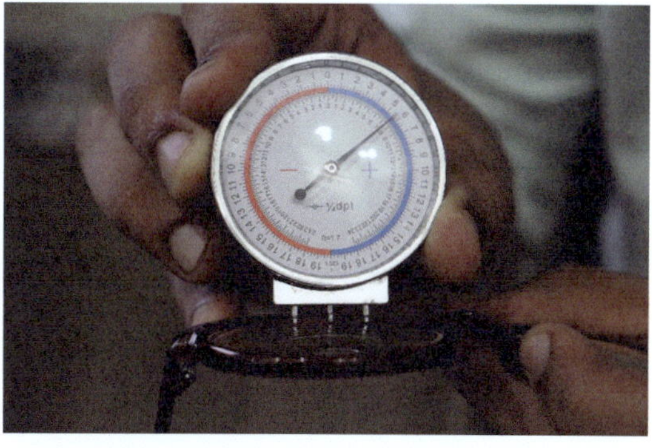

Fig. 5.4 Geneva lens measure— measuring the front surface of an ophthalmic lens

ians of the lens. Compare the readings to see if there are any differences [1].

Step 3: Spherical surface determination: the lens surface is spherical if the GLM readings remain unchanged in all meridians. Spherical lenses have the same power in all meridians.

Step 4: Toric surface determination: if the GLM readings vary across meridians, the lens surface is cylindrical (or toric). Note the highest and lowest GLM readings and their corresponding meridians. Toric lenses have two principal meridians with different powers.

Approximate Power Calculation. In some cases, it is necessary to calculate the approximate power of a lens. The following formula can be used:

Approximate Power = Front Surface Power + Back Surface Power.

5.5 Thickness Caliper—Measuring Lens Thickness

A thickness caliper is used to measure the thickness of lenses (Fig. 5.5). The thickness of a lens is crucial for proper frame fitting and lens aesthetics.

5.5.1 Calibration of the Thickness Caliper

Calibration ensures accurate measurements. Follow these steps for calibration:

Step 1: Merge the end points: close the jaws of the caliper until the two endpoints touch each other. The caliper should read zero when the endpoints are merged.

Step 2: Error compensation: there is an error if the caliper does not read zero after merging the endpoints. To compensate for the error, adjust the caliper screw (one of the tips) to bring the reading to zero while both tips touch each other. Seek assistance or consult a supervisor if needed.

5.5.2 Measuring Thickness

Follow these steps to measure:

Step 1: Positioning: hold the thickness caliper perpendicular to the lens surface you wish to measure. Ensure that the caliper is stable and appropriately aligned.

Step 2: Reading: use the jaws (tips) of the caliper to measure the thickness. The outer short lines typically have increments of 0.05 mm. The

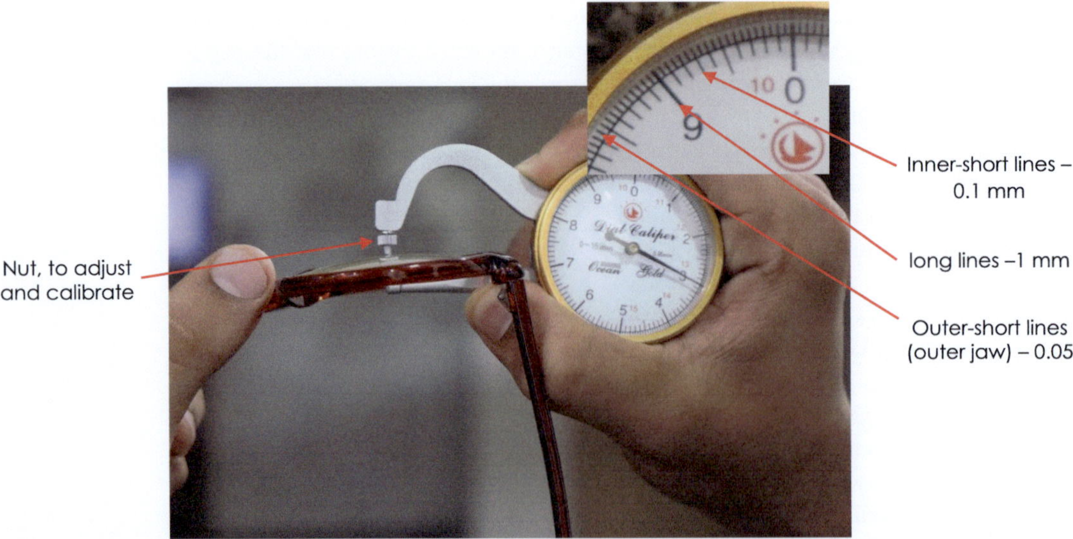

Fig. 5.5 The thickness caliper is used for measuring the central thickness of an ophthalmic lens. The top right insert is the magnified view of the measuring clock

inner short lines usually have increments of 0.1 mm, the longer 0.5 mm, and the longest, 1 mm. Gently close the jaws around the lens edge or center until they lightly touch.

Note the reading.

If the thickness of the lens is more than 9.95 mm, the pointer would meet either at zero point or go beyond one complete rotation, and the readings are indicated in red color.

5.6 Polariscope—Detecting Internal Stress in Transparent Materials

The polariscope or colmascope is an optical inspection device to detect internal stress in transparent materials, including glass, plastics, and synthetic resins (Fig. 5.6). Stress can occur due to external forces or manufacturing processes, and it can affect the structural integrity and optical properties of the material [3].

5.6.1 Procedure for Using the Polariscope

To use the polariscope effectively, follow these steps:

Step 1: Setup: position the material to be examined between the two polarized lenses of the polariscope. Ensure the material is placed against a light source, such as a backlight, for optimal visibility.

Step 2: Observation: look through the polariscope at the material against the light source. Observe the patterns and colors displayed by the material.

5.6.2 Interpreting Patterns and Colors

Different materials and types of stress will exhibit distinct patterns and colors when viewed through the polariscope. Here are some common observations:

Birefringence: materials such as glass, plastics, and synthetic resins that are internally stressed will show patches or bands of color when viewed through the polariscope.

Injection molded lenses: color fringes may be observed at the center of the lens.

Thermally toughened glass lenses: birefringence may be noted throughout the lens.

Polycarbonate lenses: birefringence may be observed (Fig. 5.6, right) [4].

Stress from tight frame fit: color fringes can be seen at the portion of the lens tightly fitted into the frame.

Chemically toughened and crown glass lenses: no distinct pattern is typically noticed.

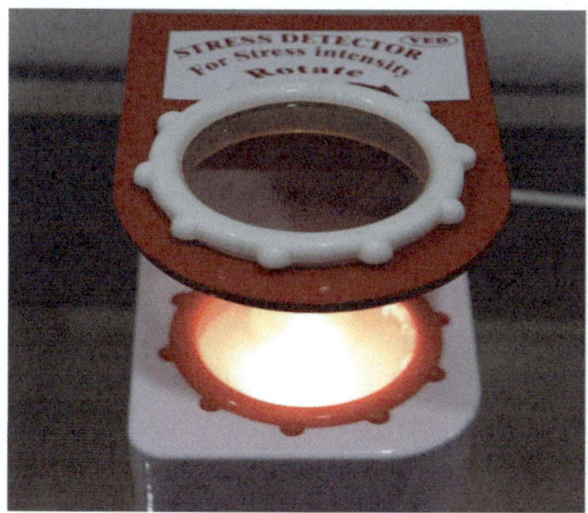

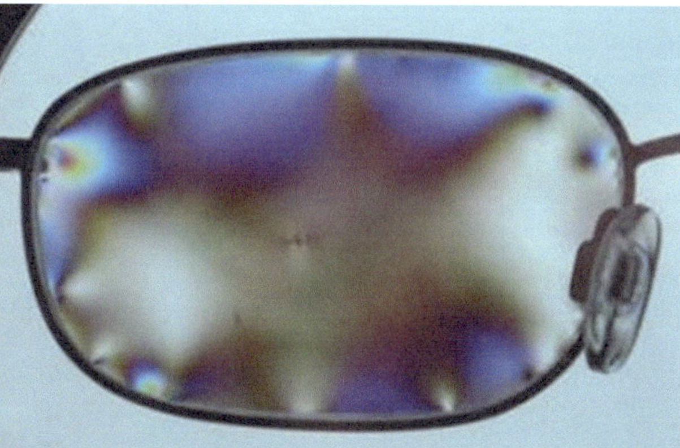

Fig. 5.6 Left: a polariscope; right: view of a polycarbonate lens through a polariscope

5.6.3 Analysis and Evaluation

By interpreting the patterns observed through the polariscope, optical professionals can assess the internal stress level in different materials. For example, if this is present toward the edges of the lens, it indicates that the lenses are fit too tight, and if not modified, the lenses may have warpage and may chip off. If it is in the center, it indicates that the lens is polycarbonate. Patients may not face any visual disturbances, but these affect the mechanics and, in severe cases, influence the quality of vision. Hence, this information is crucial for lens selection, frame fitting, and ensuring the quality and durability of optical products.

5.7 Corneal Reflex Pupillometer—Measuring Pupillary Distance

The corneal reflex pupillometer is a specialized tool to accurately measure pupillary distance (PD) or interpupillary distance (IPD) (Fig. 5.7) [5]. The corneal reflex pupillometer utilizes the reflection of light from the cornea to determine the PD. It comprises a handheld device with a light source and a viewing lens. This measurement is essential for the precise fitting of spectacles and for ensuring optimal visual comfort for patients. Ill-fitting spectacles can result in asthenopia, blurry or distorted vision, and visual discomfort and can influence binocular vision. The eyes must work harder to adjust to the incorrect optical alignment.

PD is the distance between the center of the pupil and the median plane.

IPD is the distance between the two pupil centers.

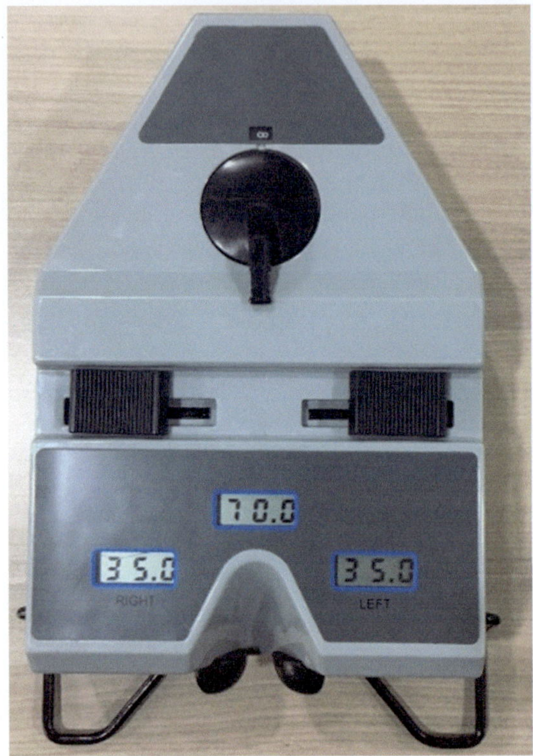

Fig. 5.7 A corneal reflex pupillometer or PD meter

5.7.1 Measuring Pupillary Distance (PD)

Step 1: Preparation: ensure that the patient is comfortable and relaxed and looking straight ahead. Set the pupillometer to measure the PD for an infinite distance.

Step 2: Positioning: hold the pupillometer with the headrest on the patient's face. Align the patient's eyes with the viewing lens of the pupillometer.

Step 3: Activating the light source: activate the light source of the pupillometer, which will create reflections on the patient's corneas.

Step 4: Identifying the pupil centers: direct the patient to focus on a distant target or a specific point. Observe the reflections of the corneal light on each eye through the viewing lens. Identify the centers of the pupils based on the position of the corneal reflections.

Step 5: Measuring PD: move the pupillometer to align the measurement markers with the identified pupil centers. Read the displayed value on the pupillometer, which represents the PD.

The PD measures can also be done quickly in the clinic without a pupillometer.

Step 1: The examiner and the patient should sit at the same eye level.

Step 2: The examiner must be equipped with a simple ruler and a torch for measurement.

Step 3: The examiner closes one of their eyes. For example, let's say the examiner closes right eye.

Step 4: The patient is made to look at the eye that is kept open, which in this case is the examiner's left eye.

Step 5: The light from the torch is directed into the patient's eye for measurement.

Step 6: The zero mark of the ruler is positioned to the patient's right eye corneal reflex (First Purkinje's image).

Step 7: The value on the ruler that aligns with the median plane of the patient's face is read and noted [6]. This reading provides the right eye PD (RE PD) of the patient.

Step 8: Now, the examiner closes left eye and opens right eye.

Step 9: The patient should look into the examiner's right eye.

Step 10: The ruler is read while the zero mark is aligned to the median plane of the patient's face, this time at the corneal reflex of the patient's left eye.

Step 11: This reading provides the left eye PD (LE PD). The torchlight must be shifted from the patient's right eye to their left eye.

Step 12: The measurements for both RE PD and LE PD have been obtained.

Step 13: To find the Interpupillary Distance (IPD), the RE PD and LE PD are added.

Step 14: Note that providing individual eye PD measurements (RE PD and LE PD) is more accurate than providing the IPD.

Step 15: The logic behind this method is that the patient's right eye and left eye align parallel to the examiner's open (opposite) eye, simulating distance viewing.

Step 16: Generally, subtracting approximately 3 mm from the distance IPD approximates the near IPD [6].

5.8 Conclusion

Each of the devices mentioned in this chapter is important for accurate optical dispensing. By being meticulous and using these devices correctly, one could ensure spectacles fit well and provide clear vision.

Funding Hyderabad Eye Research Foundation, Hyderabad, India.

Disclosure None.

References

1. Brooks CW. System for ophthalmic dispensing. 3rd ed. Butterworth-Heinemann; 2007.
2. Fannin TE, Grosvenor TP. Clinical optics. Butterworths; 1987.
3. Alonso J, Gómez-Pedrero JA, Quiroga JA. Modern ophthalmic optics. Cambridge University Press; 2019.
4. Manchikanti N, Maseedupalli S. Birefringence in ophthalmic lenses. Indian J Ophthalmol Case Rep. 2021;1:455.
5. Elliott DB. Clinical procedures in primary eye care. Butterworth Heinemann Elsevier; 2007.
6. Gantz L, Shneor E, Doron R. Agreement and inter-session repeatability of manual and automatic interpupillary distance measurements. J Optom. 2021;14:299–314.

6 Extraocular Muscle Tests and Cover Tests

Aparna Raghuram and Benjamin Jastrzembski

6.1 Introduction

Extraocular muscle (EOM) and cover tests are integral to ophthalmic examinations. These tests allow the clinician to detect the presence or absence of strabismus (ocular misalignment). Additionally, these tests give a wealth of information on both the afferent and efferent function of the eye and may diagnose cranial nerve palsies and even systemic diseases such as myasthenia gravis.

6.2 History

Extraocular muscle movement is described by two eponymous laws: Hering's law of equal innervation and Sherrington's law of reciprocal innervation. Sherrington's law states that a muscle's contraction is accompanied by the relaxation of its antagonist muscle. For example, the contraction of the medial rectus muscle is accompanied by the relaxation of the lateral rectus muscle in the same eye. Charles Sherrington won the 1932 Nobel Prize in Physiology and Medicine for his work on this concept, as well as his work on synapses (a term he coined) and neuronal circuits [1]. Hering's law of equal innervation states that neural impulses to an EOM accompany an equal impulse to its synergistic EOM in the other eye. In other words, the neural impulse to one muscle is yoked to its partner muscle in the other eye. For example, the contraction of the medial rectus in the right eye is yoked to the contraction of the lateral rectus in the left eye, causing the eyes to have a conjugate movement to the left. The concept was developed in 1868 by the German scientist Ewald Hering, who also contributed to understanding color vision and respiratory reflexes [2]. Although these concepts are described as "laws" they have exceptions, such as in Duane's retraction syndrome.

6.3 Technology

The equipment to perform most EOM and cover tests in the clinical setting are simple: a fixation target, loose prisms and/or prism bars, and a simple occluder. Additional equipment, including Maddox rod lenses, red and green color filter lenses, a synoptophore, and a prism flipper, may sometimes be used. Maddox rods in trial frames are used to quantify cyclotorsion. A synoptophore is a mechanical instrument that allows for the subjective and objective measurement of strabismus and assessment of retinal correspon-

A. Raghuram
Boston Children's Hospital/Harvard Medical School, Boston, MA, USA
e-mail: aparna.raghuam@childrens.harvard.edu

B. Jastrzembski (✉)
University of California, Davis, Sacramento, CA, USA
e-mail: benjast@ucdavis.edu

T. Das, P. Satgunam (eds.), *Ophthalmic Diagnostics*, https://doi.org/10.1007/978-981-97-0138-4_6

dence and stereoacuity [3]. In addition to these mechanical instruments, software is also available to measure strabismus.

6.4 Technique

6.4.1 Motility and Versions

In general, the first EOM test to be performed is the motility test to check for the movements of both eyes. The patient is asked to follow a target, such as the examiner's index finger, in all directions of gaze. Although the task is easily performed by a conscious, cooperative, and neurotypical patient, cooperation may be aided in children and those with cognitive impairments by using a toy to encourage attention. The head may be gently held to prompt eye movement rather than head movement in these cases. Normal, full versions (conjugate movements) of the eyes consist of unimpeded movement in all directions of gaze, with both eyes moving in the same direction (Fig. 6.1). Under Hering's Law, a pair of partner muscles, one from each eye, primarily drive the movement of the eyes in each of the six diagnostic positions of gaze (Fig. 6.2). Normal vergences refer to coordinated eye movement in

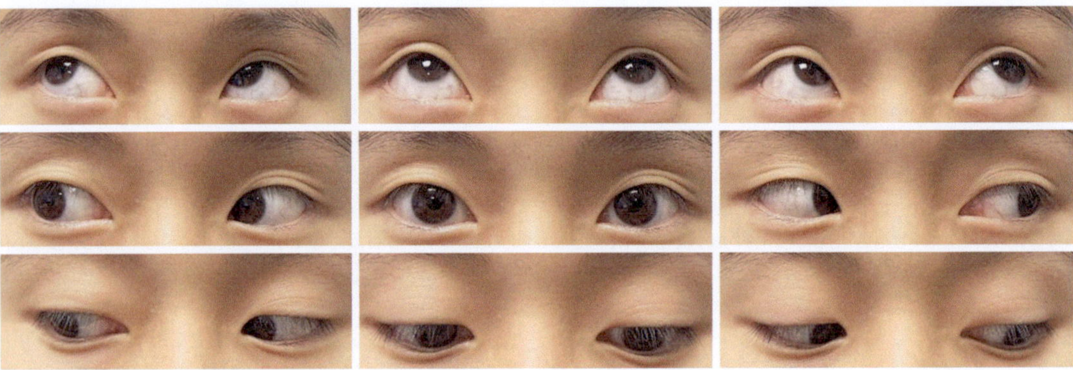

Fig. 6.1 The cardinal positions of gaze

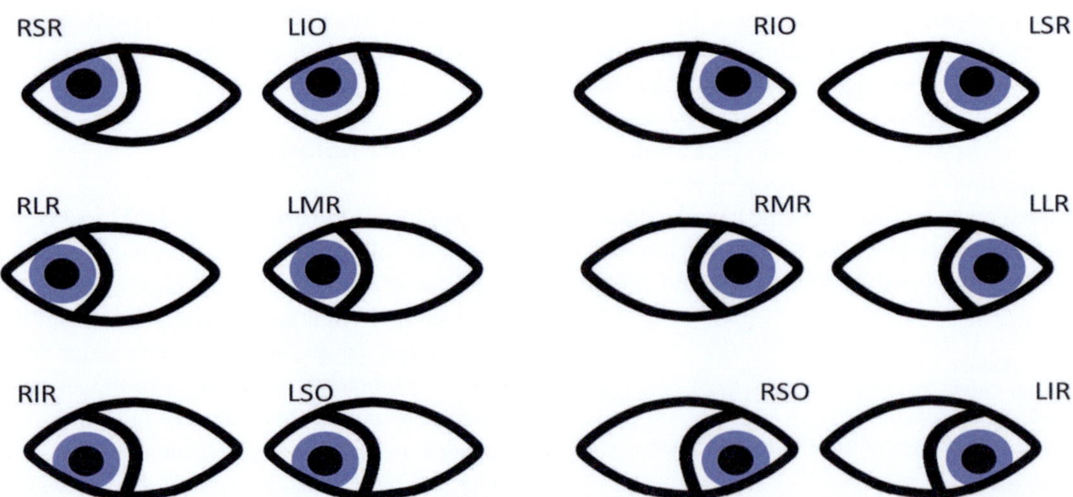

Fig. 6.2 The six diagnostic positions of gaze. *RSR* right superior rectus, *RLR* right lateral rectus, *RIR* right inferior rectus, *LIO* left inferior oblique, *LMR* left medial rectus, *LSO* left superior oblique, *RIO* right inferior oblique, *RMR* right medial rectus, *RSO* right superior oblique, *LSR* left superior rectus, *LLR* left lateral rectus, *LIR* left inferior rectus

different directions (disconjugate movements) to achieve fixation on a near or distant target.

If the versions and vergences are full, there is no indication for further extraocular muscle testing during most eye examinations. Normal versions and vergences typically demonstrate that the cranial nerves serving the EOMs are functioning as expected, that the brain stem nuclei of the cranial nerves and the higher level central nervous system visual processing centers are intact, that each eye has at least some vision, that there are no gross abnormalities of the orbit (e.g., a large mass or a fracture) restricting movement, and the EOMs themselves are functioning. Given the number of processes required for normal EOM motility, the EOM motility test may be considered a "vital sign" of the eye examination, analogous to a heart rate or blood pressure measurement in the general medical examination.

However, on an initial EOM motility test, it can be easy to miss subtle underaction or overaction in motility. Notably, Sherrington's law of reciprocal innervation dictates that not only is EOM underaction abnormal, but overaction of an EOM is abnormal as well. Therefore, in the setting of the strabismus or neuro-ophthalmology clinic, or when there is concern about an abnormality of the EOMs, additional testing beyond the fundamental EOM motility test is indicated.

6.4.2 Ductions

A reasonable second test to perform after the testing of EOM versions is the test of EOM ductions with one eye open and the other eye covered, especially when abnormalities are detected in the versions testing. Ductions are defined as the movement of a single, isolated eye, in contrast to the versions, which refer to movements with both eyes open. The terms used to describe the duction movements of a single eye are supraduction, infraduction, abduction (away from the nose in the horizontal), adduction (towards the nose), incyclotorsion (incycloduction), and excyclotorsion (excycloduction). Each of the six extraocular muscles has a primary action described with this terminology, and the superior and inferior muscles have secondary and tertiary actions (Table 6.1).

Duction testing may be useful to highlight subtle underaction that may be difficult to observe with version testing, especially when an overaction is the most obvious finding on version testing. For example, a patient with a partial VI (abducens) cranial nerve palsy of the right eye, when observed with both eyes open, may show obvious overaction of adduction in the left eye due to Hering's Law and little to no limitation in abduction of the right eye. With the right eye closed, ductions of the left eye will be normal, and with the left eye closed, ductions of the right eye may demonstrate a subtle abduction deficit.

6.4.3 Ocular Alignment

Abnormalities in ocular alignment are categorized as heterotropia (tropia) or heterophoria (phoria). A tropia is a misalignment of the eye that occurs without disassociation and may be observed with both eyes open. It may be constant or intermittent. A phoria is a latent misalignment observed only after breaking fusion between the eyes. Observation of a phoria is most commonly observed by covering an eye to break fusion. In

Table 6.1 Actions of the extraocular muscles

Muscle	Primary action	Secondary action	Tertiary action
Medial rectus	Adduction	–	–
Lateral rectus	Abduction	–	–
Superior rectus	Elevation	Intorsion	Adduction
Inferior rectus	Depression	Extorsion	Adduction
Superior oblique	Intorsion	Depression	Abduction
Inferior oblique	Extorsion	Elevation	Abduction

Adapted from Table 1.1 of Rowe (2012) [3]

other words, the phoria is observed when the brain does not have normal afferent input from the eyes to maintain ocular alignment.

Clinically, the terms heterotropia or heterophoria are infrequently used. Rather, the strabismus is named based on the direction of misalignment. An esodeviation, either an esophoria or esotropia, is defined as a deviation toward the nose; an exodeviation, either an exophoria or exotropia, is defined as a deviation away from the nose; a hypertropia or hyperphoria as a deviation upwards or cranial; and a hypotropia or hypophoria as a deviation downwards or caudal.

Given that fixation depends on vision, all tests that measure ocular alignment should be performed with the patient's best possible correction in place.

6.4.3.1 Tests Based on the Light Reflex

The next tests to perform are the Hirschberg and Krimsky tests, which estimate the patient's strabismus, if present. In the Hirschberg test, a penlight is directed at the patient's open eyes from a distance of about 1/3 of a meter, and the clinician characterizes any deviation of the corneal light reflex to estimate the strabismus. Alternatively, a flash photograph may provide analogous information. Many eyes with normal alignment may appear slightly exotropic on Hirschberg testing due to a small nasal displacement of the corneal light reflex. This normal, slightly exotropic appearance is due to the temporal location of the fovea in relation to the center of the pupil; it is referred to as a positive angle kappa. In these cases, cover testing will demonstrate normal alignment—also called orthophoria. In the Krimsky test, a penlight is shone at the patient's open eyes from a distance of about 1/3 of a meter. A loose prism or prism bar is placed over the deviated eye to center the corneal reflex. If the prism is placed over the fixating eye to center the deviating eye's corneal reflex, it is called the Modified Krimsky test. Using the dimmest light possible is advisable as a bright penlight may be dissociative for some people. Since the Hirschberg and Krimsky tests do not interfere with fixation, they only measure tropia, not phoria.

6.4.3.2 Cover Tests

Cover testing provides a more accurate characterization of strabismus than Hirschberg and Krimsky testing. However, eyes with the best corrected visual acuity worse than 20/200 will not be able to fixate on a target reliably enough to make cover testing useful. In these situations, the Hirschberg and Krimsky tests must be relied on. The patient must also cooperate with cover testing by actively fixating on the target of interest. It is important for the examiner to encourage the patient to actively fixate on the object and be aware that poor cooperation may lead to misleading results, especially in children who may find cooperation challenging.

The cover test begins with covering the fixating eye or eye with better vision with an occluder and observing any movement of the other, weaker eye. The occlusion interrupts afferent input from the stronger eye, and the brain is forced to switch fixation to the weaker eye. This is the cover test. The refixation movement of the weaker eye reveals the direction of strabismus: an observed movement away from the nose is an esodeviation, and a movement toward the nose is an exodeviation. The speed of refixation reflects the vision in the weaker eye as well as the attention of the patient. An eye with poor vision or a patient with impaired attention or cognition will have slower refixation. The magnitude of the tropia may be quantified by adding a plastic prism in the visual plane over the weaker eye as the occluder is placed over the stronger, fixating eye. The magnitude of the prism required to eliminate all refixation movement in the weaker eye quantifies the tropia. This test is called the *simultaneous prism and cover test* (SPCT).

If the vision is equal or close to it in both eyes, the cover test should be repeated with the occluder placed on each eye. The tests are also typically repeated in the primary position, with the eyes fixating on a near (1/3 m) or distant (6 m) target and in the secondary directions of gaze at a distance. If no refixation movement is observed on the cover test, then no tropia is present, although a phoria may exist.

To quantify a phoria, the *prism and alternate cover test* (PACT) is performed. In this test, the occluder is alternated between the two eyes, and a prism is placed over the weaker eye to neutralize any refixation movement. The prism diopters measured in the PACT test are the sum of the deviation combining both the phoria and tropia. The expected normal deviation range for distance is 1 Δ exophoria ±2 Δ and for near 3 Δ exophoria ±3 Δ [4]. If no tropia were observed previously with the cover test, the measurement would quantify the phoria only. When the prism is placed over the stronger eye during the PACT, the measurement is called the primary deviation. If the prism is instead placed over the weaker eye, the measurement is referred to as the secondary deviation. The secondary deviation is always larger than the primary deviation. The PACT is frequently repeated in multiple directions of gaze at a distance. Incomitance in the angle of deviation (i.e., a difference in the measured prism diopters of strabismus in different directions of gaze) is an important clue for paretic strabismus secondary to cranial nerve palsy. For example, a patient with a right VI (abducens) cranial nerve palsy will show an esotropia, greater in the right gaze than in the left gaze, and this incomitance will be revealed by testing with the PACT in multiple directions of gaze.

If the magnitude of the deviation is so large that one prism is insufficient the prisms may be stacked in the same direction on a single eye or a single prism may be placed over each eye, which is preferable. Similarly, if a vertical and horizontal strabismus exists, a horizontal prism may be placed over one eye and a vertical prism over the other. In these cases, the use of multiple prisms should be noted in the documentation. As the deviation becomes larger, the accuracy of the measurement decreases.

6.4.4 Vergence Testing

Vergence describes two eyes moving in opposite directions (disconjugate eye movements). Detailed vergence testing informs us on how well the eyes are working together [4–10]. Convergence is defined as the vergence when both eyes move toward the nose, and divergence is away from the nose. Supravergence describes when one eye moves upwards relative to the other, and infravergence is when one eye moves downwards relative to the other. Appropriate refractive correction should be worn before vergence testing begins.

6.4.4.1 Near Point of Convergence

To assess vergence, start by measuring the maximum ability of the eyes to converge by determining the near point of convergence (NPC). In this test, an accommodative target size two steps larger than the maximum resolvable size is recommended (typically, a 20/30 single letter or vertically aligned letters is/are used) (Fig. 6.3a). The target is placed approximately 60 cm from the eyes and moved at about 1 cm per second closer toward the eyes. The patient is asked to maintain focus on the target, to keep the target single, and to report when it splits into two. The distance from the middle of the forehead to the point when the target can no longer be perceived as single is recorded as the NPC "break" in cms. Next, the target is moved back along the midline to where fusion is recovered; that is, the target becomes single. This distance is recorded as "recovery." A "break" measure of 6 cm or less is normal in children, adolescents, and young adults [7, 8]. It is important to note that the reference point of measure is from the middle of the forehead (Figs. 6.3a, b and 6.4a). If NPC is measured from the lateral canthus or tip of the nose as a reference, it cannot be compared to the 6 cm cut-off as it will lead to an overestimation or underestimation. When measured from the lateral canthus, the NPC can be, on average, 1–2 cm more than when measured from the forehead [5]. Variability in human anatomy and morphology across gender, race, and ethnicity can also affect the normal range. Measuring from the tip of the nose should be avoided due to significantly higher variability in nose sizes across the population.

Sometimes, the patient may not report the target doubling due to suppression. In that instance, the examiner notes when fusion is lost by keenly observing one eye drifting out. This objectively measures the "break" (Fig. 6.4b). When the patient is unable to report a doubling of the target due to strong suppression, the test can be repeated

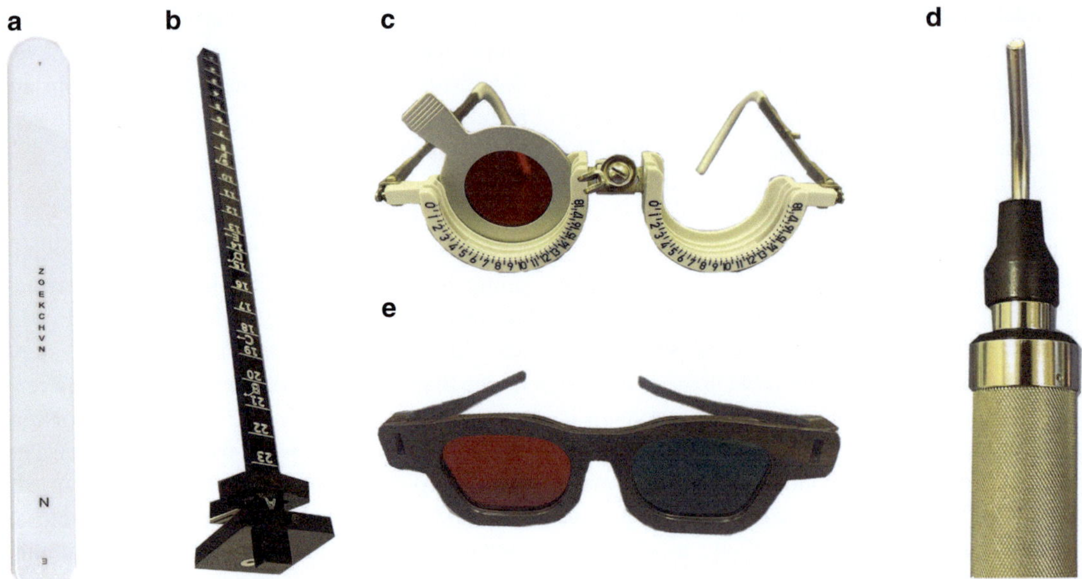

Fig. 6.3 Tools for measuring the near point of convergence. (**a**) A near fixation stick with a vertical row of letters; (**b**) a near point rule to place between forehead and measure distance; (**c**) a red lens; (**d**) a transillumination light; (**e**) a pair of red and green glasses

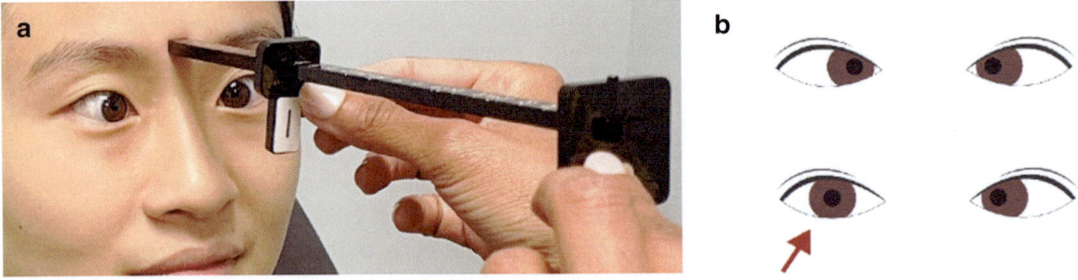

Fig. 6.4 Measuring the near point of convergence. (**a**) An example of how the test is performed; (**b**) an objective measure (red arrow) of when fusion is broken is noted as a break on the "near point" of convergence testing

with a red lens (Fig. 6.3c) placed in front of one eye and room lights dimmed or switched off. A penlight (Fig. 6.3d) is moved toward the eyes, and the patient is asked to report when they see two separate lights, one red and one yellow. A red/green glass (Fig. 6.3e) can also be used instead of just a red lens, and the patient would be asked to report when they see the light split into red and green lights [7]. If convergence is limited due to poor accommodation, the test can be repeated with a +1.00 DS lens on a trial frame or held over the patient's glasses, and the NPC test can be repeated with an accommodative target. If the test results improve with the +1.00 DS lenses, this suggests that the accommodative system was the driver of the convergence deficit.

6.4.4.2 Fusional Vergence Ranges

Next, we measure fusional vergence ranges, which estimate how much the eyes can move horizontally (converge and diverge) and vertically (move up or down) while maintaining single vision. Prism bars are introduced while the patient looks at a 20/40 or 20/30 letter size target for distance and near vision testing, respectively. Vertically aligned letters of the same letter sizes

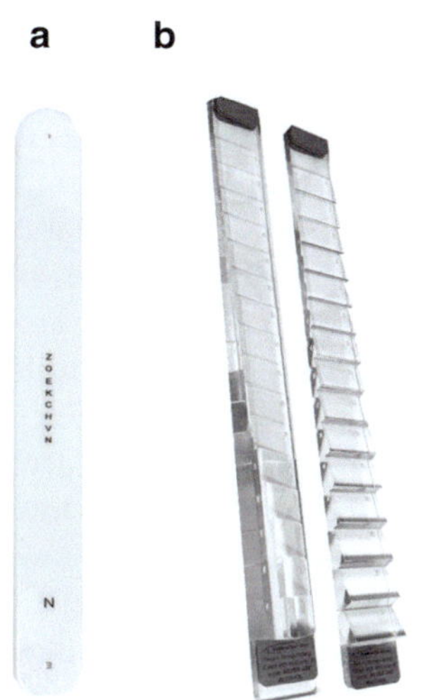

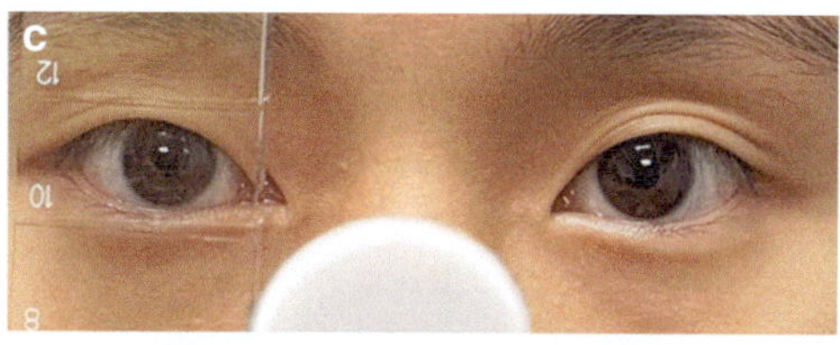

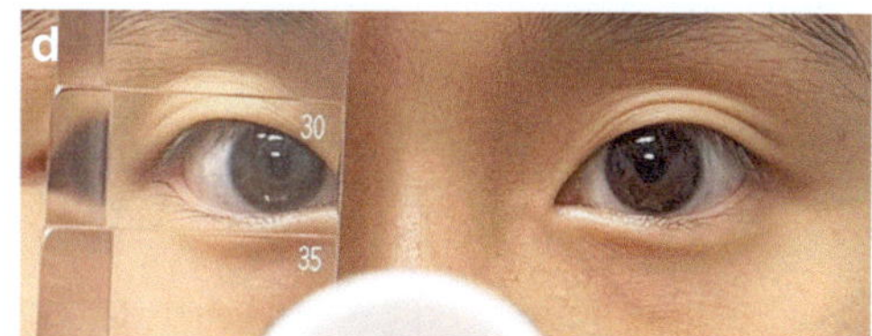

Fig. 6.5 Fusional ranges testing: (**a**) the fixation target used for testing; (**b**) the horizontal and vertical prism bars used for testing; (**c**) a demonstration of the fusional divegence range limit; (**d**) a demonstration of the fusional convergence range limit

(Fig. 6.5a) for horizontal ranges and horizontally aligned letters for vertical ranges or a single letter are ideal targets.

6.4.4.2.1 Horizontal Vergence

For horizontal fusional ranges, a prism bar with a base-in configuration (Fig. 6.5c; the wide edge of the prism is closer to the nose) is placed before one eye, and its strength is increased at 2 prism diopters per second. At the 20-prism diopter level, the rate of diopter change increases to 5 prism diopters per second. This is due to a preset dioptric change of a prism bar. The patient is first asked to report when the target gets blurry when it splits into two (double, horizontally separated), and when it returns to a single target. These findings are recorded as blur, break, and recovery in prism diopters. Some patients may not report blur or report blur and break at the same time. The divergence amplitude is the prism diopter recorded at blur or break (when blur is not reported).

Note: When testing divergence amplitude for distance with adequately corrected refractive error, we do not expect "blur" to be reported as accommodation is fully relaxed. The steps are repeated with a prism bar in the base-out (Fig. 6.5d; the wide edge of the prism is away from the nose) direction to record the convergence amplitude. The results are noted as convergence ranges/divergence ranges, distance/near, and blur/break/recovery in prism diopters [4–10].

Mechanism of action: When the prism bar is oriented in the base in a direction in front of either the right or left eye, the light rays bend toward the base of the prism, shifting the image viewed, nasally, away from the fovea. For the visual system to see the target as a single image, the eye must diverge to land the fovea to where the image is displaced. When the eye reaches its threshold, and the patient cannot diverge his/her eyes any further, the patient will perceive the target doubling or being seen as two.

When the prism bar is oriented in the base-out direction before the right or left eye, the light rays bend toward the base of the prism, shifting the image viewed temporally away from the fovea. For the visual system to see the viewed target as single, the eye must converge to land the fovea where the image is displaced. When the eye reaches its threshold, and the patient cannot converge his/her eyes any further, the patient will perceive the target doubling or being seen as two.

When measured at a distance, the influence of accommodation is minimal, but the interplay of accommodation with vergence cannot be discounted at near-testing distances. Retinal disparity, that is, dissimilar images on the fovea, drives fusional vergence. When testing near the fixed distance, using letters as targets and making the patient call out the letters helps to keep accommodation under control. However, accommodation can be driven along with fusional vergence to keep the target clear and single. On horizontal fusional vergence testing, if the patient reports a "blur," that is the point till which fusional vergence has helped drive control; following this, accommodative vergence primarily drives control until the target splits into two and fusion can no longer be maintained.

Expected values for adolescent and young adults for distance: divergence range (prism diopters Δ): break = 5–9 and recovery = 3–5; convergence range (Δ): blur = 7–11, break = 15–23, and recovery = 8–12. For near divergence range (Δ): blur = 11–15, break = 19–23, and recovery = 10–16; convergence range (Δ): blur = 14–20, break = 18–24, and recovery = 7–15 [4, 11–14].

6.4.4.2.2 Vertical Ranges

A prism bar with the base up or down is placed before one eye and moved 1 prism diopter per second to measure vertical ranges. The patient is asked to report when the target splits into two (double, vertically separated), and the prism power is lowered in magnitude to record when the target returns to being single. The break is recorded as right infravergence or left supravergence when the prism is placed base up before the right eye and right supravergence or left infravergence when the prism is placed base down before the right eye.

Note: supravergence in one eye is equivalent to infravergence in the other eye.

Mechanism of action: When a vertical prism is placed before one eye, for example, base down before the right eye, the light rays bend toward the base of the prism, shifting the image below the fovea in the right eye relative to the left eye. To maintain single vision, the right eye must move upwards (toward the apex of the prism) to bring the image back to the fovea (supravergence) and maintain single vision. When the base-up prism is placed in front of the right eye, the light rays bend toward the base of the prism, shifting the image above the fovea in the right eye relative to the left eye. To maintain single vision, the right eye must move downwards (toward the apex of the prism) to bring the image back to the fovea (infravergence) and maintain single vision.

The influence of accommodation is not expected for vertical fusional ranges; hence, patients do not report blur and only report double when fusion is not maintained. The expected values for both supravergence and infravergence for distance and near vision are approximately 2–4 Δ for the break and 1–3 Δ for the recovery [4].

6.4.4.3 Efficiency of the Vergence System

The vergence facility is a nuance test to assess the efficiency or flexibility of the vergence system. A 12-prism base-out and a 3-prism base-in flippers are used for testing. Testing is done for both distance and near vision using a single or vertical column of letters (20/40–20/30 size) (Fig. 6.6a,

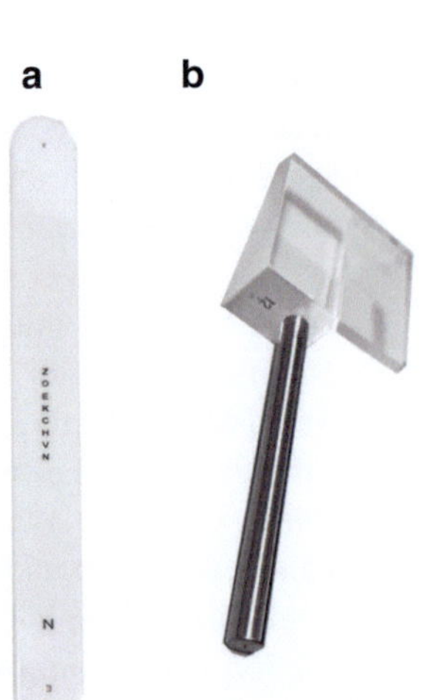

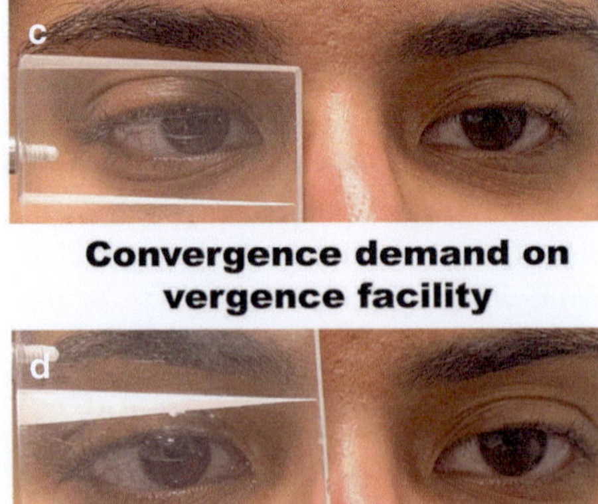

Fig. 6.6 Vergence facility testing. (**a**) A fixation stick with a vertical column of letters used for testing; (**b**) 12-prism base-out and 3-prism base-in wedge; (**c**) the eyes' response to a convergence demand (12-prism base-out); and (**d**) the eyes' response to a divergence demand (3-prism base-in)

b). The test provides information on the eye's ability to move with ease from a convergence (base-out prism), demand to a divergence (base-in prism), demand (net change of 15-prism diopters), and vice versa (Fig. 6.6c, d). The goal is to see how well the system can cope with the real-world demands of viewing different distances, such as directing attention from a whiteboard to a book. The prism flipper is alternated between 12-prism base-out and 3-prism base-in, and the patient is asked to report when the fixated target appears single and clear (in focus). One cycle indicates the ability to clear both the base-out and the base-in prism. The number of cycles in 1 min is recorded. The normal range expected for both distance and near in adolescent and young adults is 12 ± 3 cycles per minute [4, 15].

6.5 Clinical Application and Interpretation

The techniques described in Sect. 6.3 may be applied to virtually any scenario in pediatric ophthalmology, neuro-ophthalmology, optometry, binocular vision, vision therapy, and orthoptic clinics.

Case 1

A 21-month-old girl presented to the eye clinic for eye misalignment. Her eyes had been observed to cross inward since at least 4 months of life. She was a twin, born at 34 weeks gestation, and had a gastrostomy tube to improve her nutrition. Her twin sibling did not have any strabismus. Her ophthalmic examination indicated a normal ability to fix and follow a target of interest with each eye, normal pupils, normal anterior segment, and normal dilated fundus examination. Her cycloplegic refraction showed age-appropriate hypermetropia of +2.50 in each eye. Her extraocular motility examination demonstrated bilateral underaction of the superior obliques and associated overaction of the inferior obliques. On initial version testing, she had difficulty fully abducting each eye due to cross-fixation. However, on duction testing, each eye abducted normally. Krimsky testing was used to estimate the heterotropia, as cover testing could not be reliably performed as she was quite fearful of the examiner, which is typical for her age. Krimsky testing showed an esotropia of 45 Δ by one examiner and an esotropia of 40 Δ by a second examiner. The toddler was diagnosed with infantile esotropia and scheduled for bilateral inferior oblique myectomies and bilateral medial rectus recessions. After the surgery, her alignment was orthotropic by Krimsky testing, and her mother volunteered without prompt that her gross motor skills had improved. Her mother reported that the toddler's walking was steadier and more confident the day following the surgery.

Case 2

A 3-year-old girl presented to the eye clinic as the family noted that her left eye had been turning outwards since age two. Her ophthalmic examination indicated 20/30 vision using Lea symbols in the right and left eye, 50s of stereopsis with Randot circles, near point of convergence at 6 cm when the left eye loses fusion and drifts out, normal pupils, normal anterior segment, and a normal dilated eye exam. Cycloplegic refraction showed age-appropriate hypermetropia of +2.00 in each eye. Her extraocular motility demonstrated mild inferior oblique overaction of 1+ in both eyes. Ductions in each eye were normal. The cover test revealed intermittent exotropia of 30 Δ for distance vision and 25 Δ for near vision with moderate control. She was diagnosed with intermittent exotropia and was recommended to have strabismus surgery to maintain binocularity.

She had a bilateral lateral rectus recession of 6.5 mm. Six months post-surgery, she had small recurrent intermittent exotropia measured by cover test as 14 Δ for distance vision and 18 Δ at near vision with good control. For a year following surgery, recurrent intermittent exotropia continued to be observed with poor control and ill-sustained near point of convergence. She was referred to have a visual function examination to see if eye exercises could improve her control of the deviation.

On examination of her oculomotor function on the cover test, she had a 12 Δ constant left exotropia for distance vision and 14 Δ intermittent exotropia at near vision. The near point of convergence receded at 19 cm, with the left eye drifting out. Positive fusional ranges at the near break at 6 and recovery at 0, indicating poor convergence ranges. Near vergence facility revealed an inability to clear the 12 Δ convergence demand flipper. She was recommended to work on some gross convergence exercises with a Brock string or just with an interesting target to focus on. As she continued to follow up, a loose prism for convergence training for both near and distance was also added. About 18 months post-surgery, she continued to have residual intermittent exotropia for distance and near vision at about 14 Δ, but with improved control for both distance and near vision. Her near point of convergence improved to a 7 cm break and 9 cm recovery with an accommodative target. At a distance, the positive fusional convergence ranges were break at 14 Δ and recovery at 12 Δ. For divergence ranges, the break was at 8 Δ and recovery at 2 Δ. For near convergence, the ranges were 16 Δ for break and 14 Δ for recovery; divergence ranges were 18 Δ for break and 14 Δ for recovery. The vergence facility could be recorded and normalized to 15 cycles per minute for near vision and 11 cycles per minute for distance vision. Eight years after surgery, she continued to have residual intermittent exotropia but with improved control for both distance and near vision. Parents were happy that a second surgery was not required. She continued to make good eye contact, and spontaneous drifting of the left eye out occurred only when she was fatigued.

6.6 Conclusion

Extraocular motility and cover tests are integral to comprehensive eye examinations and are especially useful in neuro-ophthalmologic, strabismic, and non-strabismic binocular vision/visual function contexts. The motility and alignment/cover tests described in this chapter characterize strabismus for diagnosis and surgical planning. In addition, testing of the vergence system provides additional information about how the eyes move together for typical tasks outside of an eye lane. Vergence system information may help determine when strabismus surgery may be unnecessary or guide adjuvant convergence exercises after surgery, as in Case 2. With a bit of practice and minimal equipment, the extraocular motor and cover tests quickly provide an examiner with a host of practical information about the afferent and efferent systems.

Acknowledgments We thank Carissa Wu and Neerali Vyas for assistance with the photographs and figures.

Funding Aparna Raghuram: Boston Children Foundation Discovery Award; Benjamin Jastrzembski: none.

Disclosure None.

References

1. Molnár Z, Brown RE. Insights into the life and work of sir Charles Sherrington. Nat Rev Neurosci. 2010;11(6):429–36.
2. Aminoff MJ, Daroff RB, editors. Encyclopedia of the neurological sciences. 2nd ed. Waltham: Academic Press/Elsevier; 2014. p. 4.

3. Rowe FJ. Clinical orthoptics. 3rd ed. Chichester: Wiley-Blackwell; 2012.
4. Scheiman M, Wick B. Clinical management of binocular vision: heterophoric, accommodative, and eye movement disorders. 3rd ed. Philadelphia: Wolters Kluwer Health/Lippincott Williams & Wilkins; 2008. p. 748.
5. Raghuram A, Cotter SA, Gowrisankaran S, et al. Postconcussion: receded near point of convergence is not diagnostic of convergence insufficiency. Am J Ophthalmol. 2019;206:235–44.
6. Raghuram A, Gowrisankaran S, Swanson E, et al. Frequency of visual deficits in children with developmental dyslexia. JAMA Ophthalmol. 2018;136(10):1089.
7. Scheiman M, Gallaway M, Frantz KA, et al. Nearpoint of convergence: test procedure, target selection, and normative data. Optom Vis Sci. 2003;80(3):214–25.
8. Convergence Insufficiency Treatment Trial Study Group. Randomized clinical trial of treatments for symptomatic convergence insufficiency in children. Arch Ophthalmol. 2008;126(10):1336.
9. Convergence Insufficiency Treatment Trial Group. Manual of procedures. 2023. https://optometry.osu.edu/CITT-manual-procedures.
10. Pediatric Eye Disease Investigator Group. Home-based therapy for symptomatic convergence insufficiency in children: a randomized clinical trial. Optom Vis Sci. 2016;93(12):1457–65.
11. Morgan MW Jr. Analysis of clinical data. Optom Vis Sci. 1944;21(12):477–91.
12. Scheiman M, Wick B. Clinical management of binocular vision: heterophoric, accommodative, and eye movement disorders. 4th ed. Philadelphia: Lippincott Williams & Wilkins; 2014. p. 722.
13. Wajuihian SO. Normative values for clinical measures used to classify accommodative and vergence anomalies in a sample of high school children in South Africa. J Opt. 2019;12(3):143–60.
14. Haines HF. Normal values of visual functions and their application in case analysis. The analysis of findings and determination of normals: part IV. Optom Vis Sci. 1941;18(2):58–73.
15. Gall R, Wick B, Bedell H. Vergence facility: establishing clinical utility. Optom Vis Sci. 1998;75(10):731–42.

7 The Pupil and Pupillary Reflexes

Meenakshi Swaminathan
and Gayathri J. Panicker

7.1 Introduction

A systematic examination of the pupils begins with a thorough patient history. A difference in the size of the pupils (anisocoria) may have been noticed by a friend or a family member, especially in people with light-colored irises. Patients with anisocoria may complain of photophobia, difficulty in focusing, and blurred vision when going from light to dark areas and vice versa. A systematic search of their medical histories and documenting conditions such as migraine and diabetes, if any, is also important [1]. Other points in recording patient history include noting a history of cataract surgery, uveitis, use of dilating or constricting eye drops, exposure to pesticides, use of opiates (which can constrict pupils), and anticholinergics in asthma medications (which can dilate pupils) [2, 3].

The following points must be specially noted while examining the pupils [4].

1. Pupil size: Is it appropriate for the age of the patient? Pupil size can decrease with increasing age.
2. Equality of pupil size: Unequal pupil size is called anisocoria. It is also important to note if the difference is greater in light or dark.
3. Pupil response to light: Is there equal constriction in both eyes in size and velocity?
4. Pupil dilation: Is it equal in both eyes in size and velocity?
5. Response to light and a near target: Do the pupils respond, and is the response equal in both eyes?
6. Presence of afferent pupillary defects.

7.2 Pupil Size Measurement

This is done using a pupil gauge which may be a circular disc or linear scale with increments of 0.1 mm. A handheld pupil camera adds more accuracy to the measurement but is not helpful for pupil measurement in the dark. Infrared video pupillometry overcomes this disadvantage and can capture pupil size in both light and dark conditions [5]. The velocity and latency of the pupillary response can be calculated with software linked to the video input.

7.2.1 Clinical Examination and Interpretation of Anisocoria

Anisocoria is defined as a difference in the pupillary diameter between the eyes of >0.4 mm. The light source used to examine the diameter of the pupil can be normal room light (easy to see the

M. Swaminathan (✉) · G. J. Panicker
Sri Ramachandra Institute of Higher Education and Research, Chennai, India
e-mail: drgjp@sriramachandra.edu.in

T. Das, P. Satgunam (eds.), *Ophthalmic Diagnostics*, https://doi.org/10.1007/978-981-97-0138-4_7

difference in light-colored irises) or a flashlight shone from below, illuminating both pupils equally with the room lights on. This gives an idea of pupillary size in light. To estimate pupillary size in the dark, it is best to dim the room lights and use a flashlight from below to just barely illuminate the field of both eyes to be able to ascertain the pupil size [6].

Anisocoria that is greater in the dark is seen in certain physiological conditions or Horner's syndrome. Many factors influence the pupillary size, such as trauma to the pupillary sphincter or dilator muscle, conditions affecting nerve supply to the iris, and the use of pharmacological agents that dilate or constrict the pupil. Physiological anisocoria is present in about 20% of the population under 17 years of age, and the prevalence increases to 33% in those older than 60 [7].

7.2.2 Pharmacological Tests for Abnormal Pupils

Performing and interpreting pharmacological tests on abnormal pupils for conditions such as Adie's tonic pupil (the pupil constricts better to near than to far light) and Horner's syndrome can aid in diagnosis [8]. However, there are several disadvantages to this approach: (a) the testing conditions must be carefully controlled; (b) the required drugs may not be easily available; (c) tearing, squeezing of eyes, and variable drug penetration can affect the reliability of these tests [4]. The normal pupil of the fellow eye must be used as an internal control for judging the response to these pharmacological agents whenever possible. Therefore, one must always administer the eye drops to both eyes.

Pupillary constriction with diluted pilocarpine (0.0625–0.1%) 30 min after instillation is diagnostic of Adie's tonic pupil. Normal pupils will not constrict at such low concentrations of pilocarpine [9]. In Horner's syndrome, 2–10% cocaine eye drops induce dilatation of the normal pupil after 40–60 min but do not do so in the affected pupil. However, 0.5–1% apraclonidine eye drops cause dilatation of the affected (smaller) pupil but will not affect the normal pupil, resulting in a reversal of anisocoria. Hydroxyamphetamine (5%) eye drops can differentiate between pre-ganglionic and post-ganglionic lesions in proven cases of Horner's syndrome. Dilatation of the affected pupil an hour after application suggests a pre-ganglionic Horner's syndrome; dilatation of the normal pupil, but not of the affected pupil, suggests a post-ganglionic lesion [8, 10]. Phenylephrine (2.5%) eye drops also cause mydriasis of Horner's pupils, which dilates as much as or more than a normal pupil.

7.2.3 Examination of Pupillary Dilation

Dilation lag, or assessment of how quickly the pupils return to their maximal size in the dark, is another important aspect of the pupillary examination. It is guided by sympathetic innervation. To assess pupillary lag, the room lights are turned on very bright and then dimmed to the minimum. Both pupils are observed simultaneously to note how quickly they dilate. The pupils usually reach their maximum size in about 12 s, and the maximum dilation happens in the first 5 s; [11] however, this may take up to 25 s if dilation lag is present. Dilation lag is a sign of sympathetic denervation or Horner's syndrome. Infrared videography is invaluable in capturing dilation lag.

7.3 Pupillary Light Reflex Examination

Examination of pupillary light reflex must ideally be done in a dimly lit room with illumination sufficient to visualize both pupils. The examinee must be instructed to look at a distant target, such as a letter on the distance vision chart at least 3 m away, to avoid unwanted pupillary constriction due to accommodation. The examiner then shines a sufficiently bright focal light from a pen torch onto the pupils 5–10 cm away from the inferotemporal direction (Fig. 7.1) and observes the

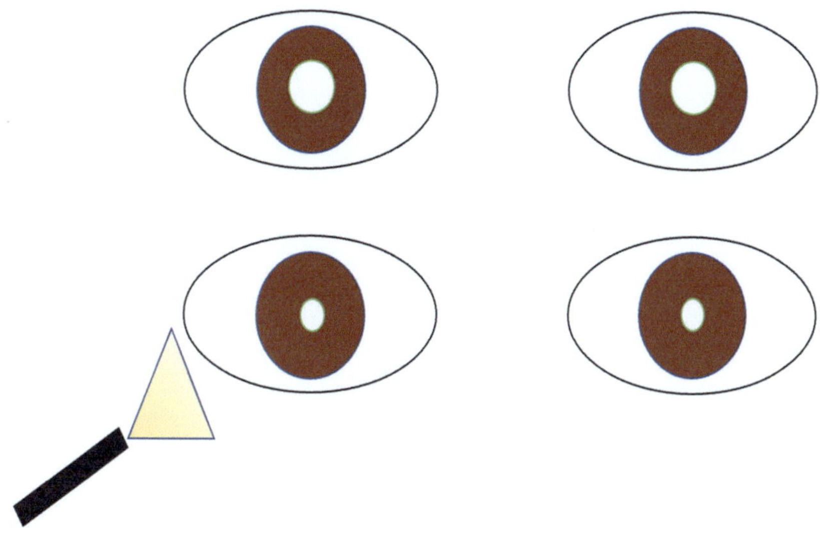

Fig. 7.1 Pupillary constriction response to the light shone on the right eye. The response is seen in the ipsilateral eye (direct light reflex) and contralateral eye (consensual light response)

pupillary response [12]. The light source must not interrupt the patient's fixation as it will induce pupillary constriction due to the near response. Also, using a too-bright or dim light source may mask or miss some abnormal pupillary responses [13, 14].

The pupillary response in the ipsilateral eye, where the light is directed, is termed the "direct light reflex"; the response in the contralateral eye is termed the "consensual light reflex" (Fig. 7.1). Care must be taken to place one of the examiner's hands on the patient's nasal bridge while looking at the consensual response to avoid light from crossing over and falling on the contralateral pupil simultaneously; this can lead to erroneous interpretations. Sometimes, another dim and diffuse light source may be placed below the examinee's face to better observe the consensual reflex, especially in individuals with darker irises [15].

The swinging flashlight test (of Levitan) involves rapid rhythmic to-and-fro swinging of the light source between the two eyes [16]. The light is first shown on one eye for three counts, then swung around to the other eye for three counts, and then swung back. The response of the illuminated pupil is noted as the light is alternated between the two eyes (Fig. 7.2). The speed and number of swinging movements can be varied, but care must be taken that the duration of illumination in each eye and the duration of the swinging movement are equal.

7.3.1 Interpretation of Pupillary Light Reflexes and Swinging Flashlight Test

The light reflex in the pupil is affected in diseases of the anterior part of the afferent limb of the light reflex pathway, i.e., primarily in optic nerve disorders. When the afferent pathway is intact, the pupil constricts briskly and equally in response to light in the ipsilateral (direct light reflex) and the contralateral eye (consensual light reflex) (Fig. 7.1). In an afferent pathway defect, the direct and consensual pupillary response to shining the light on the affected eye will be absent or sluggish. However, the direct and consensual light reflex response of the contralateral eye will be intact (Fig. 7.3). There will be no difference in the pupillary size in afferent pathway defects in ambient light conditions.

When the visual pathway is intact bilaterally, equal pupillary constriction is observed in each eye on the swinging flashlight test (Fig. 7.2). However, when there is an afferent pathway defect, such as optic neuropathy on the one side, there will be apparent dilatation of the affected pupil when light is swung from the normal pupil onto it. This is due to the perceived reduction of input reaching the pretectal region of the midbrain through the abnormal afferent pathway. This is called a relative afferent pupillary defect (RAPD) or Marcus Gunn pupil (Fig. 7.4) [17].

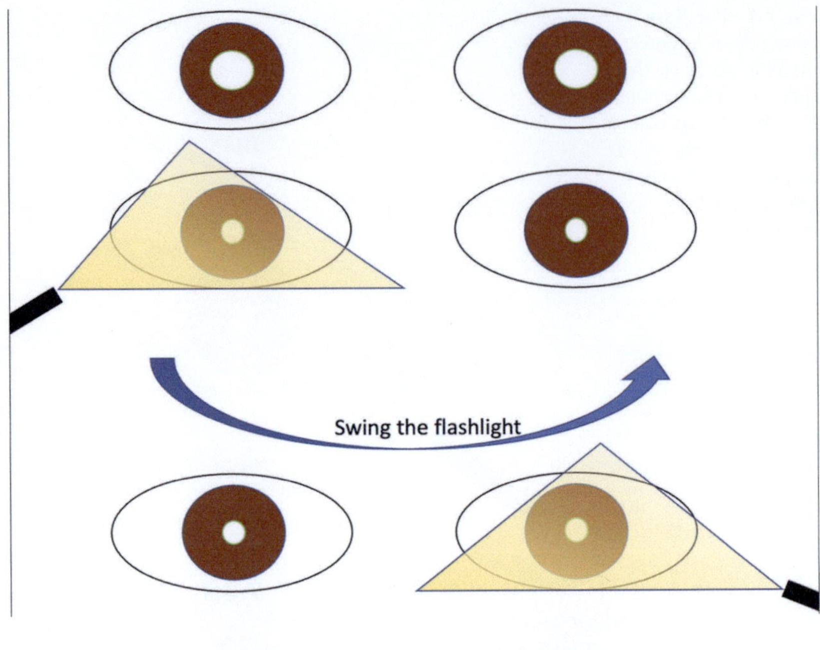

Fig. 7.2 Demonstrating the swinging flashlight test. Pupillary constriction response is equal in each eye, as observed on swinging the light source from one side to the other

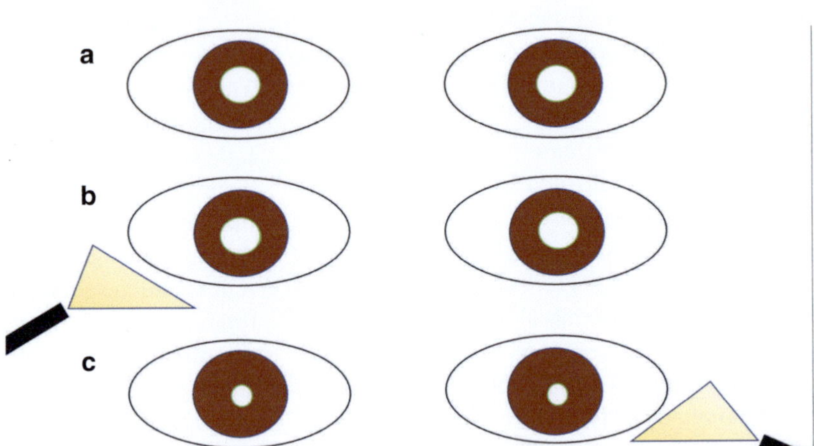

Fig. 7.3 A right-sided afferent pathway defect showing no difference in pupil size in ambient light conditions (**a**) with a reduced direct and consensual light reflex response on shining light on the affected (right) pupil (**b**), while the direct and consensual responses are normal when light is directed on the normal left pupil (**c**)

There are four grades of RAPD.

RAPD grade 1: Mild pupillary constriction followed by greater dilatation (pupillary escape, as described in Marcus Gunn's original description [18]) when light is swung onto the abnormal eye [19].

RAPD grade 2: There is no initial pupillary movement (pupillary stall) followed by dilatation.

RAPD grade 3: The abnormal pupil will dilate immediately.

RAPD grade 4: An amaurotic or deafferented pupil, fixed and dilated [20].

Another method of grading RAPD is by using graded neutral density filters over the normal eye and performing the swinging flashlight test till there is an equal response in both eyes [21]. Bell et al. described a clinical grading system corresponding to the neutral density filter grading of RAPD. In this, grade I is when a weak initial constriction followed by greater re-dilatation occurs; grade II is when an initial stall occurs followed by greater re-dilatation; grade III is when an immediate pupillary dilatation occurs; grade IV is when an immediate pupillary dilatation following prolonged illumination of the good eye for 6 s occurs, and grade V is when an immediate pupillary dilatation with no secondary constriction occurs [22]. However, in common clinical practice, only recording the presence/absence of RAPD is done; usually, grading may not be done.

Given that this is a "relative" test, there must be a significant asymmetry between the visual pathways for a RAPD to manifest, and there can never be a bilateral RAPD, even in bilateral damage to the afferent pathways. In some cases where one pupil is non-reacting due to trauma or efferent damage, a swinging flashlight test can still be done to detect the afferent pupillary defect in the same eye. In this situation, when light is directed on the affected pupil, there will be dilatation of the contralateral normal pupil. This is known as "reverse" RAPD [20] (Fig. 7.5).

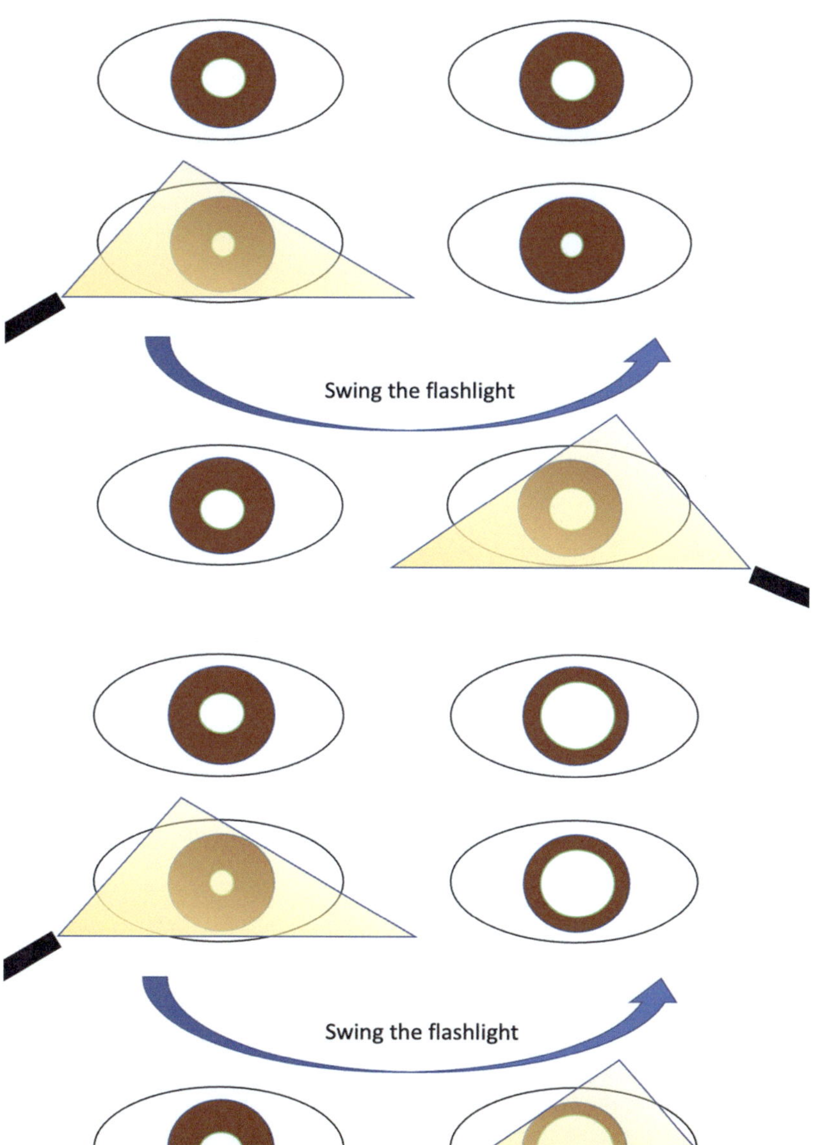

Fig. 7.4 A left relative afferent pupillary defect is where there is paradoxical dilatation of the affected left pupil on swinging the flashlight from the normal right pupil

Fig. 7.5 When the left pupil is non-reacting (e.g., third nerve palsy or traumatic mydriasis) and there is a coexistent left afferent pathway defect, paradoxical dilatation of the normal right pupil is seen when light is swung onto the affected left side; this is known as reverse RAPD

One should suspect a refractive error, amblyopia, media opacity, functional visual loss, or vision loss in the other eye when vision is reduced in one eye and there is no RAPD. Though there are reports of RAPD in a few cases of unilateral amblyopia, it is usually mild (<0.6 log units) and does not correlate with visual acuity. This could be due to visual cortical deficit, which secondarily affects the afferent pathways and the retina in some amblyopes [23]. Hippus, defined as the physiological fluctuation in pupil diameter under constant light conditions, should not be mistaken for a RAPD [24].

7.4 Near Response

Pupillary response to a near target is part of the triad of accommodation and convergence. This is best performed in a fairly well-lit room so that the examiner sees pupils easily. It is advisable not to use any other handheld light source to visualize the pupils, as the pupillary response to light may confuse the picture. An accommodative target with details would be the Ideal target for the patient to look at. It is better to avoid pen, pencil, etc. In a blind patient, the patient's own fingers may be used as a target. The patient is instructed to look at a vision chart located at 3 or 6 meters and then instructed to turn their gaze to the near target briskly while examining the pupillary construction.

7.4.1 Light Near Dissociation

This term describes the condition when the pupillary light response is impaired, but the near response is normal or almost normal. Several causes are known for this, which include blindness from optic nerve or retinal damage, oculomotor nerve paralysis with aberrant regeneration, neurosyphilis, hydrocephalus, pontine tumors, and tonic pupils such as Adie's pupil. Hence it is important to examine for the intact near pupillary response in any patient with impaired light response. It is extremely rare to find the light response is preserved, but the near response is impaired. The commonest cause is not making a good voluntary accommodative effort to the near target by the patient.

7.5 Slit Lamp Examination of the Pupil

The pupils' size, shape, and location must also be examined using a slit lamp to detect the presence of any abnormalities.

1. *Size:* Pupillary size can be measured using a pupil gauge or millimeter rule or on the slit lamp. Normally, the pupils are equal in size, around 3–6 mm in bright light and 4–8 mm in dim light [12]. A difference in pupil size between the two eyes (>0.4 mm) is called anisocoria.
2. *Shape:* The pupils are normally round in shape. Other shapes include festooned pupil, tadpole pupil, keyhole pupil, and irregular or oval pupil. Festooned pupils are seen in iritis, where the posterior synechiae distort the pupil shape; it is more evident after dilatation. Irregular, oval, or slit-like pupils may be congenitally present in anterior segment dysgenesis syndromes or acquired after trauma, surgery, or due to neurological diseases [25]. Tadpole-shaped pupils are seen due to segmental spasms of the iris dilator muscle, which may accompany migraine or ipsilateral Horner's syndrome [26]. Iris coloboma is an inferior or inferonasal notch in the pupil (keyhole appearance), which may be accompanied by chorioretinal colobomas [27].
3. *Location:* The normal pupil is centrally located. Corectopia is a condition where the pupil is eccentric in location. This can be seen in anterior segment dysgenesis syndromes, iridocorneal endothelial syndromes, chronic uveitis, trauma, and postoperatively and congenitally in ectopia lentis et pupillae (corectopia associated with lens subluxation) [25].
4. Congenital anomalies like persistent pupillary membranes may also be seen on the slit lamp. Characteristic spoke-like remnants of the tunica vasculosa lentis are seen across the

pupil. These vary in size and density and are usually visually insignificant [28].

5. The pupillary light reaction can also be tested on the slit lamp by measuring the edge pupillary cycle time [29]. A thin optical slit is placed on the edge of the pupil, which induces pupillary constriction causing the pupil to move out of the slit section. Subsequently, as the illumination decreases, the pupil dilates until the edge again reaches the optical slit. Twenty-five such cycles are timed and noted. The edge pupil cycle time increases in afferent pathway defects [30].
6. *Pupillary movements:* The normal pupil shows small amounts of dilatation and constriction under steady illumination. This constant movement or restlessness of the pupil is called hippus or pupillary unrest. It is more prominent in bright light and younger individuals [31]. Vermiform movements (worm-like movements) and sectoral paralysis (immobility of parts of the pupil) are seen on slit lamp examination of Adie's tonic pupils [32].

7.6 Other Pupillary Phenomena

1. *Westphal–Piltz Reflex:* Pupillary constriction in darkness during sleep is considered normal. This phenomenon is called the Westphal–Piltz reflex. It is thought to be secondary to decreased parasympathetic inhibition [20].
2. *Paradoxical Pupillary Constriction in the dark:* When the lights are turned off, there is initial miosis followed by slow dilatation; this phenomenon is seen in retinal dystrophies like congenital stationary night blindness or achromatopsia. A child with such paradoxical pupillary constriction, poor vision, nystagmus, or a family history of retinal disorders should undergo electroretinography [33].
3. *Tournay's Pupillary Phenomenon:* This refers to pupil dilatation on the abduction of the ipsilateral eye. It is seen in up to 10% of the normal population and is thought to be due to anomalous innervation [34].
4. *Idiopathic Alternating Anisocoria*: It is a rare condition in which the pupils dilate one at a time, alternatingly every few hours [35].

7.7 Conclusion

A thorough examination of the pupils and the pupillary reflexes must be done for every patient visiting an eye clinic. Apart from gaining vital information regarding the integrity of the afferent and efferent limbs of the light reflex pathway, pupil examination can also provide vital clues on several underlying ocular and neurological conditions.

Disclosure None.

References

1. Jacobson DM. Benign episodic unilateral mydriasis. Ophthalmology. 1995;102:1623–7.
2. Murray RB, Adler MW, Korczyn AD. The pupillary effects of opioids. Life Sci. 1983;33:495–509.
3. Weir REP, Whitehead DEJ, Zaid FH, et al. Pupil blown by a puffer. Lancet. 2004;363:1853.
4. Digre KB. Walsh and Hoyt's clinical neurophthalmology. 6th ed.; 2005. pp. 715–38.
5. Wachler BSB, Krueger RR. Agreement and repeatability of infrared pupillometry and the comparison method. Ophthalmology. 1999;106:319–23.
6. Ettinger ER, Wyatt HJ, London R. Anisocoria: variation and clinical observation with different conditions of illumination and accommodation. Invest Ophthalmol Vis Sci. 1991;342:501–9.
7. Lam BL, Thompson HS, Corbett JJ. The prevalence of simple anisocoria. Am J Ophthalmol. 1987;104:69–73.
8. Antonio-Santos AA, Santo RN, Eggenberger ER. Pharmacological testing of anisocoria. Expert Opin Pharmac. 2005;6(12):2007–13.
9. Leavitt JA, Wayman LL, Hodge DO, et al. Pupillary response to four concentrations of pilocarpine in normal subjects: application to testing for Adie tonic pupil. Am J Ophthalmol. 2002;133:333–6.
10. Brown SM, Aouchiche R, Freedman KA. The utility of 0.5% apraclonidine in the diagnosis of Horner syndrome. Arch Ophthalmol. 2003;121:1201–3.
11. Pilley SFJ, Thompson HS. Pupillary "dilation lag" in Horner's syndrome. Br J Ophthalmol. 1975;59:731–5.

12. Elliott DB. Clinical procedures in primary eye care E-book. 5th ed. Elsevier Health Sciences; 2020. p. 205–75.
13. Borchert M, Sadun AA. Bright light stimuli as a mask of relative afferent pupillary defects. Am J Ophthalmol. 1988;106:98–9.
14. Johnson LN. The effect of light intensity on measurement of the relative afferent pupillary defect. Am J Ophthalmol. 1990;109:481–2.
15. Belliveau AP, Somani AN, Dossani RH. Pupillary light reflex. 2022 Jul 25. In: StatPearls [Internet]. Treasure Island (FL): StatPearls Publishing; 2023.
16. Levitan P. Pupillary escape in disease of the retina or optic nerve. Arch Ophthalmol. 1959;62:768–79.
17. Thompson HS, Corbett JJ, Cox TA. How to measure the relative afferent pupillary defect. Surv Ophthalmol. 1981;26:39–42.
18. Cox TA. Pupillary escape. Neurology. 1992;42:1271–3.
19. Enyedi LB, Dev S, Cox TA. A comparison of the Marcus Gunn and alternating light tests for afferent pupillary defects. Ophthalmology. 1998;105(5):871–3.
20. Liu GT, Volpe NJ, Galetta SL. Liu, Volpe, and Galetta's neurophthalmology. 3rd ed. Elsevier; 2019. p. 417–47.
21. Yotharak P, Aui-Aree N. Correlation between clinical grading and quantification by neutral density filter of relative afferent pupillary defect (RAPD). J Med Assoc Thail. 2012;95(Suppl 4):S92–5.
22. Bell RA, Waggoner PM, Boyd WM, et al. Clinical grading of relative afferent pupillary defects. Arch Ophthalmol. 1993;111(7):938–42.
23. Miki A, Iijima A, Takagi M, et al. Pupillography of automated swinging flashlight test in amblyopia. Clin Ophthalmol. 2008;2(4):781–6.
24. Gufoni M, Casani AP. The pupillary (Hippus) nystagmus: a possible clinical Hallmark to support the diagnosis of vestibular migraine. J Clin Med. 2023;12(5):1957.
25. Friedman NJ, Kaiser PK, Pineda R. Massachusetts eye and ear infirmary illustrated manual of ophthalmology. 5th ed. Elsevier Sanders; 2021. p. 267–302.
26. Kawasaki A, Mayer C. Tadpole pupil. Neurology. 2012;79:949.
27. Onwochei BC, Simon JW, Bateman JB, et al. Ocular colobomata. Surv Ophthalmol. 2000;45:175–94.
28. Lee SM, Yu YS. Outcome of hyperplastic persistent pupillary membrane. J Pediatr Ophthalmol Strabismus. 2004;41(3):163–71.
29. Miller SD, Thompson SH. Edge-light pupil cycle time. Br J Ophthalmol. 1978;62:495–500.
30. Sood AK, Mithal S, Elhence A, Maini A. Pupil cycle time. Indian J Ophthalmol. 1985;33(1):41–3.
31. Thompson HS, Franceschetti AT, Thompson PM. Hippus. Semantic and historic considerations of the word. Am J Ophthalmol. 1971;71:1116–20.
32. Sakai T, Shikishima K, Mizobuchi T, et al. Bilateral tonic pupils associated with neurosyphilis. Jpn J Ophthalmol. 2003;47(4):368–71.
33. Barricks ME, Flynn JT, Kushner BJ. Paradoxical pupillary responses in congenital stationary night blindness. Arch Ophthalmol. 1977;95:1800–4.
34. Sharpe JA, Glaser JS. Tournay's phenomenon—a reappraisal of anisocoria in lateral gaze. Am J Ophthalmol. 1974;77:250–5.
35. Bremner FD, Booth A, Smith SE. Benign alternating anisocoria. Neuro-Ophthalmology. 2004;28:129–35.

8 Clinical Measurement of Stereoacuity

Michelle Buckland and Nick Fogt

8.1 Introduction

Depth perception can be derived from both monocular and binocular cues. The term stereopsis, used throughout this chapter, refers to depth percepts from binocular vision. Stereopsis can be used to determine the relative depths of objects and is considered the highest form of binocular cooperation [1]. Stereoacuity is the smallest amount of disparity that results in accurate estimates of relative depth. In this chapter, we discuss many of the clinical tests of stereopsis and stereoacuity currently in use. The methodology of the tests, the normative data from these tests, and the clinical significance of these tests will be described.

8.2 History

Corresponding retinal points are those that have perceptually identical visual directions [2]. For example, in an individual with normal binocular vision, the fovea in one eye corresponds to that in the other eye. Absolute binocular retinal disparity, the stimulus for fusional vergence, is created when an object is at a different distance than that at which an individual is fixating. Relative binocular disparity is created when objects at different distances from the observer project to different sets of retinal coordinates. The relative disparity can be used to recover the relative depths of objects and is relied upon in clinical tests of stereoscopic depth perception or stereoacuity.

While many investigators have contributed to our current understanding of stereoscopic vision, only a few will be mentioned here. For a complete history, see Howard and Rogers [2]. Alhazen described corresponding retinal points. Aguilonius named and provided an early conception of the horopter, now understood as the locus of points in space that projects to corresponding retinal points (Fig. 8.1). Points on the horopter have zero (absolute) disparity. Stereoscopic thresholds for two visual stimuli are increased when these stimuli are moved further from the horopter. Referring to Fig. 8.1, an equation to calculate the angular disparity (n) of an object (in radians) relative to the fixation point is as follows:

$$n = \frac{\mathrm{IPD}^{*}\Delta d}{d^2}$$

where IPD is the interpupillary distance, Δd is the distance between the fixation point (where the eyes are converged) and the object, and d is the distance from the eyes at which the eyes are converged [2].

M. Buckland (✉) · N. Fogt
The Ohio State University College of Optometry, Columbus, OH, USA
e-mail: buckland.14@osu.edu; fogt.4@osu.edu

T. Das, P. Satgunam (eds.), *Ophthalmic Diagnostics*, https://doi.org/10.1007/978-981-97-0138-4_8

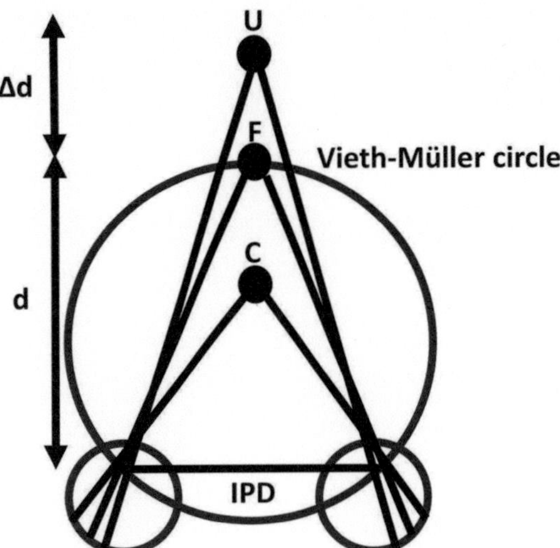

Fig. 8.1 The horopter represented as the Vieth-Müller circle. Point U has uncrossed (absolute) disparity, and point *C* has crossed (absolute) disparity relative to the *F* (fixation point). *IPD* Interpupillary distance

Later, Vieth and Müller independently described the shape of the horizontal horopter as a circle (the Vieth-Müller circle), although empirically, it is known that the shape of the horopter deviates from this circle [2]. Shortly thereafter, Wheatstone developed the mirror stereoscope and demonstrated that binocular disparity results in depth perception. Finally, Bela Julesz developed the random dot stereogram, which eliminates or greatly reduces monocular cues that could otherwise be used to deduce the presence of a disparity. The random dot stereogram (RDS) has been extensively utilized, both, in research studies and in clinical stereopsis testing.

8.3 Types of Stereopsis Tests

Table 8.1 is a list of common commercially available stereoacuity tests. Note that this list is not exhaustive. Included in this table are the test distances and the mode of stereoacuity testing, namely global (cyclopean) and/or local (contour).

For clinical stereopsis testing, there are so-called real depth or physical depth tests that use targets that physically vary in their distance from the observer (e.g., Howard-Dolman stereotest, Frisby stereotest) [3]. The Frisby plates are shown in Fig. 8.2. On the other hand, a second group of commonly used printed tests utilize anaglyphic or polarized stimuli to create dichoptic viewing conditions (e.g., Randot stereotest, Titmus Stereo Fly stereotest, TNO stereotest). The Randot Stereoacuity test is shown in Fig. 8.3. Observers wear red/green or polarized lenses for these tests. It has been suggested that anaglyphic stereotargets may underestimate stereopsis performance compared to polarized stereotargets [4]. The results of real-depth stereotests do not match those of other types of stereotests, and it has been suggested that real-depth tests measure "different aspects of stereoacuity" compared to polarized and anaglyphic tests [5]. Another method to achieve dichoptic viewing is to use (printed) lenticular technology (e.g., Bernell Evaluation of Stereopsis Test (BEST) and Lang I-R and Lang II-R stereotests). In this method, the observer is not required to wear lenses to see the depth in the single stereogram. Finally, a modern method to achieve dichoptic separation of disparate stimuli is to use 3D shutter glasses that alternately occlude the eyes [6].

With these dichoptic viewing techniques, clinical stereotests may assess local (contour) stereopsis, global (cyclopean) stereopsis, or both local and global stereopsis. Local stereopsis is assessed using dichoptic lines or contours displaced from one another to produce a disparity relative to a binocularly fused object near the disparity stimulus. These stimuli contain monocular cues that observers could potentially utilize to detect the relative offset of the monocular images in the disparate stimulus. For example, if an observer were to move their head, motion parallax between the disparate images could provide a cue to the presence of the disparate image [7]. In addition, perfect ocular vergence is not required for tests of local stereopsis. On the other hand, global stereopsis is assessed using random dot stimuli, in which the brain must correlate matching features of a disparate shape or figure embedded in an array of noncorresponding and fused dots or lines [8, 9]. Monocular features of the disparate stimulus are theoretically invisible in random dot

Table 8.1 Common commercially available stereoacuity tests

Test name	Company	Unique feature	Viewing distance	Available disparities	Target type	Technology
Randot Preschool Stereoacuity Test	Stereo Optical	3 booklets	40 cm	800–40″	RDS	Printed Polarized Vectograph
Randot Stereotest (also, a variation including LEA symbols)	Stereo Optical		40 cm	Shapes: 500–250″ Circles: 400–20″ Animals/Shapes: 400–100″	RDS Contour	Printed Polarized Vectograph
Stereo Fly Stereotest/The Fly-S (also, a variation including LEA symbols)	Vision Assessment Corporation (VAC) Stereo Optical		40 cm	House Fly: gross stereopsis Circles: 800–40/20″ Animals/Shapes: 400–100″	Contour	Printed Polarized Vectograph
The Butterfly-S	Vision Assessment Corporation (VAC)		40 cm	Butterfly: 2000–600″ Circles: 400–20″ Shapes: 400–100″	RDS Contour	Printed Polarized Vectograph
Butterfly Test (also, a variation including LEA symbols)	Stereo Optical		40 cm	Butterfly: 2000–700″ Circles: 800–40″ Animals/Shapes: 400–100″	RDS Contour	Printed Polarized Vectograph
Random Dot-S (1, 2)	Vision Assessment Corporation (VAC)		40 cm	Shapes: 500–63″ Circles: 400–12.5″ Shapes children: 400–100″	RDS Contour	Printed Polarized Vectograph
Random Dot 3-S	Vision Assessment Corporation (VAC)		40 cm	Shapes: 900–400″ Circles: 160–12.5″ Shapes: 400–100″ (children)	RDS	Printed Polarized Vectograph
Preschool Assessment of Stereopsis with a Smile (PASS Test)	Vision Assessment Corporation (VAC)	5 versions with various test plates	40 cm	480–30″ depending on the set	RDS	Printed Polarized Vectograph
Lang Stereotests (1-R & 2-R)	Lang Stereotest	Glasses free	40 cm	Lang I-R: 1200–400″, Lang II-R: 600–200″	RDS except Lang II: star viewable monocular (2D)	Lenticular Screen
Bernell Evaluation of Stereopsis Test (BEST)	Bernell Corporation	Glasses free	40 cm	Dinosaur: gross stereopsis Animals: 400–40″	Contour	Lenticular Screen
TNO	Lameris Ootech	Anaglyphic	40 cm	480–60″	RDS	Printed Anaglyph
Frisby Near Stereotest 3 plates	Frisby Stereotests	Disparity dependent on test distance glasses free	30–150 cm	600–5″	Physical Depth	Plate separation of target

(continued)

Table 8.1 (continued)

Test name	Company	Unique feature	Viewing distance	Available disparities	Target type	Technology
The Frisby Pocket Test	Frisby Stereotests	Disparity dependent on test distance glasses free	40–60 cm	340–150″	Physical depth	Plate separation of target
Random Dot E Stereotest	Stereo Optical Vision Assessment Corporation (VAC)	Disparity dependent on test distance	50 cm–16 ft	504″–52″	RDS	Printed Polarized Vectograph
Distance Randot Stereotest	Stereo Optical	2 targets at each disparity	3 M	400–60″	RDS	Printed Polarized Vectograph
Random Dot Distance Test	Vision Assessment Corporation (VAC)		3 M	400–63″	RDS	Printed Polarized Vectograph
Frisby-Davis 2 (FD2)	Frisby Stereotests	Disparity dependent on test distance glasses free	3–6 m	200–5″	Physical Depth	Plate separation of target
Bernell Stereo Test Book	Bernell Corporation	Anaglyphic	40 cm & 3 m	Near Contour: 1500–40″ Far Contour 180–60″ Random Dot: 800–25″	RDS Contour	Printed Anaglyph

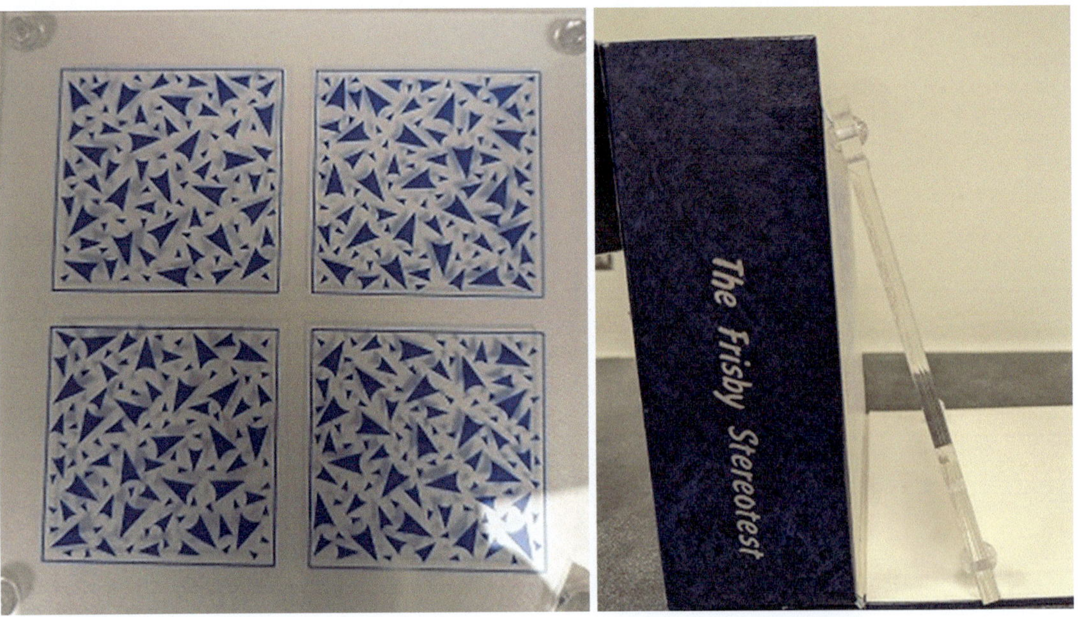

Fig. 8.2 Frisby Near Stereotest

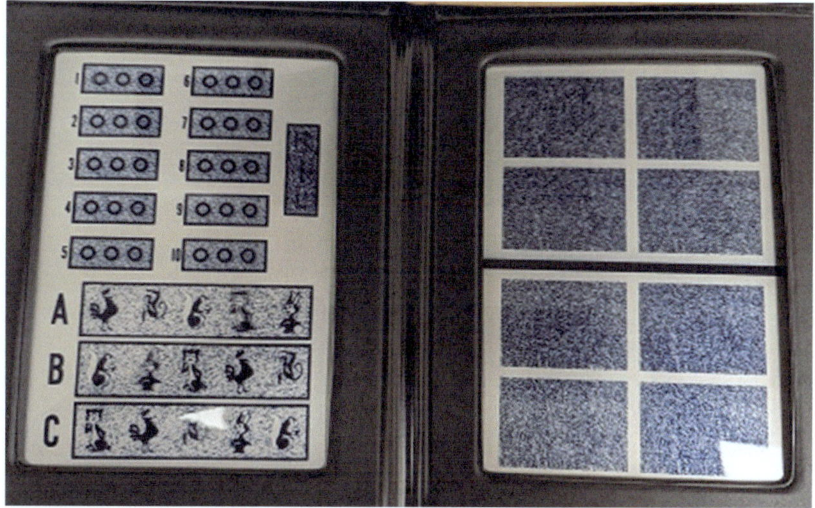

Fig. 8.3 Randot Stereotest

stereograms, although there is some evidence that monocular cues may still be available [10, 11]. Tests of global stereopsis require very accurate oculomotor (vergence) alignment (i.e., bifoveal fixation) to detect the depth of the disparity stimulus [11].

8.4 Neurophysiology of Stereopsis

Many areas of the brain respond to correlated random dot stereograms and can therefore be considered to support stereoscopic depth perception [12]. Both dorsal and ventral portions of the brain are involved in stereopsis, and brain areas V3/V3a are important in processing random dot stereograms. The literature suggests that neural substrates for global and local stereopsis are different. For example, disparity detectors in the primary visual cortex are thought to be important in processing global stereopsis but may not be as significant in processing local stereopsis [13].

8.5 Advantages of Stereopsis

Binocular viewing is advantageous for some tasks compared to monocular tasks. However, these advantages are not necessarily always correlated with stereopsis. Conversely, there is emerging evidence that stereopsis provides specific advantages in tasks such as hand-eye coordination and adapting to terrain changes while walking [14]. O'Connor and colleagues found that individuals with no global stereoacuity performed worse on fine motor tasks compared to peers with normal stereoacuity [15]. Finally, reduced stereopsis may contribute to a greater risk of falls in elderly individuals [16].

Some occupations, such as surgeons, pilots, or architects, may require the applicants to demonstrate a particular level of stereoacuity for licensure. These requirements are supported to some extent by studies such as that of Burgess et al. who found that stereoacuity worse than 120″ was correlated with reduced surgical performance on an ophthalmic surgical simulator [17]. Al-Saud et al. demonstrated that dentists performed better when stereoscopic cues were available [18].

An emerging area of study is dynamic stereopsis. This is the ability of individuals to extract motion-in-depth information from changes in retinal disparity over time and changes in the retinal image velocity between the two eyes of an approaching object. Dynamic stereopsis could be of value, for example, in avoiding or intercepting objects, as in driving or sports. It has been shown that individuals who lack static stereopsis may be able to detect the motion of an object in depth [16].

In summary, studies suggest that stereoscopic depth perception enhances an individual's quality of life and that recovering stereopsis (in the case of stereoblind individuals) and improving stereopsis (in individuals with reduced stereopsis) are, therefore, worthwhile goals. Susan Barry describes a particularly compelling example of the impact of obtaining stereopsis in adulthood in her book entitled "Fixing My Gaze." [12].

8.6 Clinical Usefulness of Stereoacuity Measurements

Performance on clinical tests of stereopsis can be considered the "best indicator" [19] or the "gold standard" for binocular function, as stereoscopic depth discrimination generally requires good vision, good eye movement control, and properly functioning binocular neural processing [20]. Thus, while stereoscopic discrimination thresholds in individuals with a well-functioning visual system are very low (less than 10 s of arc), these thresholds are very sensitive to and can be elevated by a variety of visual issues.

Saladin has summarized the ocular issues that can negatively influence stereopsis [19]. Saladin's list includes reduced contrast sensitivity or blur from uncorrected refractive error or amblyopia, uncompensated horizontal or vertical heterophoria resulting in fixation disparity, suppression, aniseikonia, fatigue, and age.

Given this extensive list of conditions that could potentially impact stereoscopic thresholds, it seems that tests of stereopsis can be used to screen for several visual disorders. However, some studies doubt the usefulness of stereoacuity testing as a screening tool. For example, Ohlsson et al. concluded that commonly used clinical stereoacuity tests (Lang II, Frisby, Randot, Titmus Stereo Fly, TNO) are inadequate in screening for amblyopia and strabismus [21], and Richardson et al. reported that stereoacuity measures in preschool children were not useful in screening for unilateral vision impairment [22]. On the other hand, there is also evidence to support the efficacy of stereoscopic tests in screening for vision disorders [23–25] when performed in combination with other tests [26–28]. Prior to discussing these studies, it should be noted that visual deficits are more likely to negatively affect global stereopsis compared to local stereopsis [7]. Schmidt concluded that the Random Dot E distance stereotest held promise as a (perhaps singular) screening test for detecting vision problems (refractive error, ocular coordination, visual acuity) in preschool children [23]. Later, the Vision in Preschoolers (VIP) study group reported several findings related to screening preschool children for visual abnormalities. In one study, this group concluded that in screening preschool children for targeted disorders, including amblyopia, strabismus, significant refractive error, and unexplained reduced visual acuity, stereopsis tests (Random Dot E and Stereo Smile II) were less sensitive than refractive and acuity measures [27]. In the same study, a direct comparison of the Random Dot E and Stereo Smile II tests showed that the Stereo Smile II test was somewhat more sensitive in detecting vision anomalies. In 2014, the VIP study group demonstrated that preschoolers with no measurable stereoacuity as assessed with the Stereo Smile II stereoacuity test (now termed the PASS or Pediatric Assessment of Stereopsis with a Smile stereoacuity test; range of disparities 480–60 s of arc) were 16.2 times more likely to have a (VIP) targeted vision disorder [26]. In that same study, preschool children who were detected to have a target disorder had a median stereoacuity of 120 s of arc compared to a median value of 60 s of arc in children with no target disorder. In 2015, an expert panel published screening recommendations for children 36–72 months of age [28]. These screening recommendations were directed at detecting amblyopia, strabismus, and significant refractive error. The panel concluded that while tests of monocular visual acuity and instrument-based measures of autorefraction are considered "best practice" screening methods, adding the Stereo Smile II stereotest (i.e., the PASS test) (Fig. 8.4) to these best practice methods may improve the detection of vision anomalies (particularly strabismus).

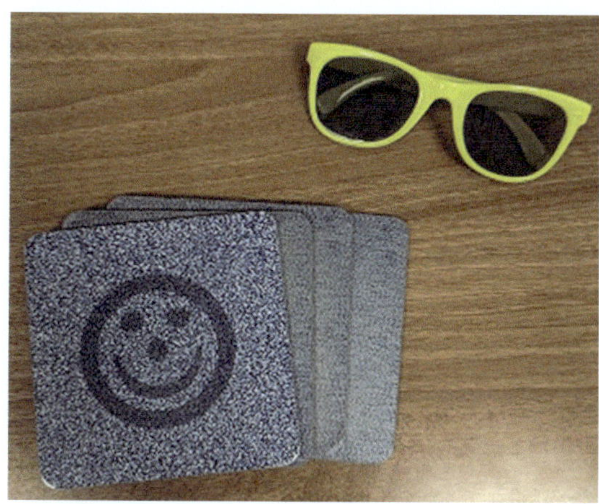

Fig. 8.4 Preschool Assessment of Stereopsis with a Smile 2 (PASS 2 Stereotest)

Lastly, stereopsis is reduced to a greater extent in strabismus than in anisometropic amblyopia [14], and this agrees with some (but not all) experimental results demonstrating that screening for strabismus with stereoscopic tests is more effective than screening for anisometropic amblyopia with these tests [21, 25].

As alluded to previously, stereoacuities obtained by different stereotests generally do not match. These discrepancies can be at least partially attributed to differences in the type of disparity employed (global or local) [29], or differences in the method used to achieve dichoptic separation (anaglyphic versus polarized) [7], or differences in the method by which the stereoscopic thresholds are assessed (e.g., 2 or 4 alternative forced choice) [30]. Measures of stereopsis can be used to assess the outcome of clinical interventions such as refractive correction, orthoptic training [19, 31], and strabismus surgery [16], so it is important that practitioners use the same stereotest in the pretreatment and posttreatment phases. An additional reason for the differences in results between stereotests may relate to the test–retest variability of these tests [11, 12, 32–34]. Values for reliability assessed in this way can be rather low, making it difficult to assess changes in stereopsis brought about by ophthalmic treatment.

8.7 Technique

8.7.1 General Clinical Instructions for Stereoacuity Testing with Common Static Stereotests

The practitioner should follow the manufacturer's instructions for each test. General instructions for practitioners in testing stereoacuity with typical static clinical tests include:

1. Provide proper visual correction for significant refractive error, as blur from uncorrected refractive error influences the testing results. Clinically stereoacuity is often performed before refraction. If stereoacuity is absent or reduced initially and a large change in refractive error is subsequently measured, then the stereoacuity testing should be repeated with the best vision correction. This can often occur during the same appointment for older children and adults. For younger children, where inattentiveness could influence the stereopsis test, stereoscopic testing may occur at another appointment.
2. Provide proper illumination by pointing a stand lamp at the test plates for near stereoacuity tests. Ensure that there are no shadows or glare on the test plates.
3. Hold the test booklets directly before the patient and ensure that the vergence posture is appropriate for the test distance.
4. Hold the test still and instruct the patient not to move their head during testing. Holding the test booklet and the head still helps to avoid monocular parallax.
5. For patients with intermittent strabismus, measure stereoacuity before any dissociating test, such as monocular visual acuities or cover test [35].
6. For patients with strabismus, perform stereoacuity testing at the distance at which the strabismus is manifest [36]. Distance stereopsis, for example, is a more useful measurement in cases of divergence excess exotropia than is near stereopsis [37]. For those with normal

binocular vision, stereoacuity does not tend to vary at different testing distances [38].

7. Because most stereoacuity tests are crossed disparity tests, ask the patient to identify or match the target/figure that is "closer or popping out."
8. For the Titmus Stereo Fly stereotest, to improve confidence that patients are actually seeing the depth from the disparity, consider rotating the test booklet to reverse the direction of the disparity or compare the results with glasses that result in different images for the two eyes with the results with glasses that only allow for the same image in the two eyes [16].

8.7.2 Specific Aspects of Clinical Stereoacuity Testing

Stereopsis develops in children as young as 3 months and can reach adult-like levels between 5 [39] and 12 years of age [40]. Normative stereoacuity data in children can vary according to the clinical stereotest and the patient's age. A larger interpupillary distance may also be correlated with better stereoacuity [2]. For example, a group of age-related values has been reported by Birch et al. for the Randot Preschool Stereoacuity test (Fig. 8.5).

The Randot Preschool Stereoacuity test has a high completion rate in preschool patients [41]. However, Read et al. have reported that about one-half of children with binocular issues could pass the test. The test is no more sensitive in detecting amblyopia than detecting strabismus [42]. The means and lower tolerance limits (defined as the disparity value 2 standard deviations from the mean and above which 95% of the population "would be expected to perform" in a particular age-group), as reported by Birch et al. for the Randot Preschool Stereoacuity test (four-book version), are as follows [43]:

• 3 years:	100″	Lower limit 400″
• 4 years:	100″	Lower limit 200″
• 5 years:	60″	Lower limit 200″
• 7–8 years:	30″	Lower limit 60″
• 11–18 years:	30″	Lower limit 60″

These mean values are similar to the age normative values for stereoacuity summarized by Reading et al. who reported norms of approximately 150″ for ages 3–4 years, 70″ for ages 4–5 years, and 40″ for ages 5–8 years on various stereoacuity tests [3].

Of course, normative stereoacuity values that can be applied across different stereotests are difficult to establish. In addition to the aforementioned differences in test design, tests vary in the maximum and minimum disparities included. Further, differences between children also factor into the choice of stereotest administered to a particular patient. For example, a younger child may resist wearing stereoacuity spectacles; thus,

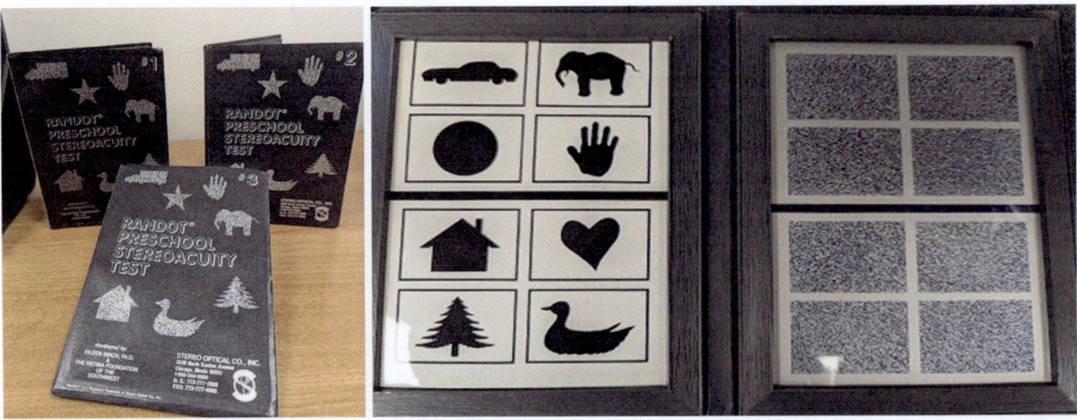

Fig. 8.5 Randot preschool stereoacuity test

a glasses-free test such as the Lang Stereotest (Fig. 8.6) may be preferred, although elimination of monocular cues with spectacle-free tests cannot be guaranteed [11].

For monitoring improvement in binocularity with interventions such as amblyopia treatment, refractive correction, or orthoptic therapy, ideally, a stereotest should contain adequate disparity levels to assess changes resulting from treatment [25]. However, assessing changes in stereopsis that result from interventions in young children can be difficult, at least partially because of issues around testability. Testability is broadly defined as a measure of how readily children can complete a test of stereopsis. In general, testability shows a large range of values (31–81% as calculated by O'Connor and Tidbury) until about 5 years of age [16].

Assuming normal binocular function for older children and adults, stereoacuity can often be measured to near threshold values. Saladin suggests that achieving good scores on stereoacuity testing (15–20″) is indicative of a well-functioning accommodation and disparity vergence system and that threshold values >40″ are suggestive of visual dysfunction [19].

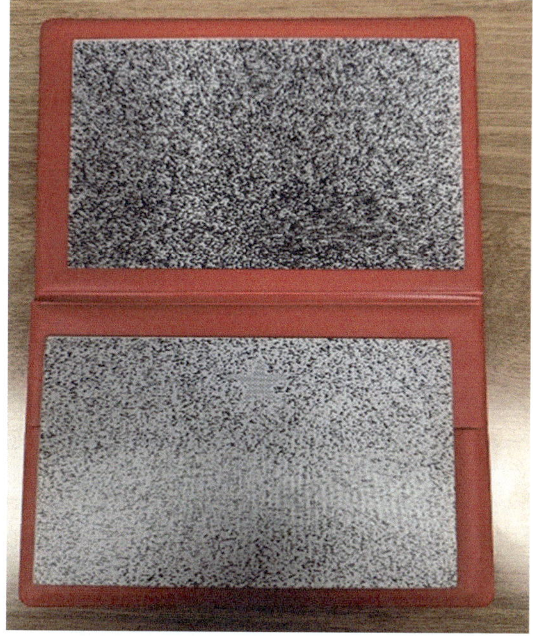

Fig. 8.6 Lang Stereotest I and II

As a guide for stereoacuity in adults, Piano et al. published normative ranges and upper limits of normality for 16–40-year-olds on several stereoacuity tests [44]. These values were as follows:

Test	Median	Upper limit of normality
• Preschool Randot	Median 30″	Upper limit of normality 70″
• Frisby	Median 20″	Upper limit of normality 40″
• Distance Randot	Median 60″	Upper limit of normality 160″
• Frisby-Davis-2	Median 10″	Upper limit of normality 25″
• TNO	Median 60″	Upper limit of normality 120″

While the list of potential stereoacuity tests is extensive (Table 8.1), a practitioner survey addressing those stereotests used in the British Isles and the USA and Canada found the Frisby stereotest is the most used test in the British Isles for both younger and older pediatric cohorts while the Titmus Stereo Fly and Randot circles/animals were more commonly used in the USA and Canada [20]. The difference in preferred stereotests is likely secondary to disparate recommendations from professional organizations in different geographic areas. Global stereopsis indicates that a patient is bifoveally fixating and that constant strabismus is unlikely [11, 45], and local stereoacuity thresholds can be more indicative of peripheral stereopsis or may be subject to measurement artifacts because of monocular cues [8, 11]. In summary, when choosing a stereoacuity test, the clinician must decide which test is appropriate for the situation with regard to patient demographics, the goal of the stereoacuity testing (presence or absence of stereopsis vs. threshold testing), and the distance of testing.

8.8 Advancing Technology

Computerized stereo tests continue to be developed. The Senaptec Sensory Station Depth Perception (https://senaptec.com) and the M&S Smart System Tablet (https://www.mstech-eyes.

com) include stereotests. Other systems that include stereopsis testing are digital visual acuity systems such as M&S technologies SPV (contour, https://www.mstech-eyes.com), Thomson Test Chart (random dot stimulus, https://www.thomson-software-solutions.com), Reichert ClearChart 4P (https://www.reichert.com), and the Hoya EyeGenius (https://eyegeniushoya.com/. Many of these systems have yet to be evaluated for reliability and sensitivity. StereoTAB is a random dot stereo test app for iPad/iPhone to measure stereopsis using anaglyphic glasses (apps.apple.com).

The ASTEROID (Accurate STEReotest On a mobile Device) system from Newcastle University (https://www.ncl.ac.uk/business-and-partnerships/expert-solutions/licensing/asteroid) is in development as a game-based stereoacuity test with a (global) disparity range of 12–1200″ [46]. Other systems in development for measuring stereoscopic depth include the eRDS system, that uses a global target in a two-alternative force choice method, and the Vivid Vision Virtual Reality system, which has a range of 15–2400″ of local stereoacuity [47].

8.9 Summary of Clinical Application and Interpretation

Stereopsis testing is an important part of vision screening in addition to visual acuity and refraction for visual conditions, including uncorrected refractive error, strabismus, and anisometropic amblyopia [28]. Stereoacuity testing is often performed early in the ocular examination. Having a positive stereo response, in particular with global stereopsis testing, suggests that visual acuity is relatively equal (monocular asymmetry in visual acuities affects stereopsis more than bilateral symmetrically reduced acuities), that the vision is reasonably clear, and that bifoveal fixation exists (at least at the time and distance of testing). Strabismic and amblyopic patients have worse thresholds on global stereopsis tests than on local stereopsis tests [11]. Cooper reported that in testing individuals with a random dot stimulus, all patients with constant strabismus (with or without amblyopia) failed, as did all people with microtropia [33]. Some but not all patients with anisometropic amblyopia or intermittent strabismus passed. Characteristics of microtropia can include a strabismic deviation of less than 5°, anomalous retinal correspondence, motor fusion, and foveal suppression [48]. An important advantage of a random dot stereogram over a line (contour) stereogram is that patients with microtropia will not achieve stereopsis using a global (random dot) stereopsis stimulus, but these patients may demonstrate local stereopsis [49] (perhaps worse than 100 s of arc) [48].

In children, once a binocular disorder such as strabismus amblyopia, anisometropic amblyopia, strabismus or significant refractive error is detected, prompt referral to an eye care provider for management of these conditions is required as earlier interventions are associated with better binocular outcomes. Implementing newly developed therapies, such as perceptual learning approaches to improve stereopsis should also be considered. While it has been thought that there is a relatively short critical period for the development of stereopsis that ends at a very young age, recent studies have demonstrated that stereopsis, in some cases, may be developed or improved even in adulthood [14]. Additionally, orthoptic training for vergence disorders in children and adults can reduce fixation disparity, likely leading to improved stereoscopic depth perception [19]. The potential stereopsis that may be attained following strabismus surgery can be estimated using a synoptophore in which the location of the stimuli seen by each eye is placed at the strabismic angle of deviation [16].

Measures of stereopsis can be important in other ways. Birch et al. reported that patients with infantile esotropia who had undergone strabismus surgery but had no stereopsis after surgery were far more likely to need another surgery than those who demonstrated stereopsis postoperatively. In addition, patients who were corrected optically for accommodative esotropia but had no stereopsis after this correction needed surgery to a far greater extent than children who demonstrated stereopsis after correction [50].

Stereoacuity can play a role in the management of an amblyopic patient. For example, during amblyopia treatment in which the patient's visual acuity has stabilized but the stereoacuity is absent or highly deficient, this could result in an extended management period. Because of the variability in stereotesting, it can be difficult to determine the amplitude of changes in stereoacuity that can be considered significant or clinically meaningful. Adams et al. determined that a change of approximately 2 octaves (i.e., a change in the stereopsis threshold by a factor of 4) was necessary to exceed the test–retest variability (Preschool Randot, near Frisby stereotests, Frisby-Davis distance (FD2), distance Randot stereotests) [32].

8.10 Conclusion

The presence and quality of stereoscopic depth perception can significantly impact an individual's quality of life; therefore, assessing stereopsis and applying interventions to improve stereopsis are important in clinical practice. Commonly used clinical stereopsis tests vary in the method by which the disparity is created: global/cyclopean (random dot stereogram) or local/contour, the method by which dichoptic viewing is achieved (e.g., anaglyphic stimuli, polarized stimuli, lenticular technology), the number of choices at each disparity level (e.g., two-alternative forced choice or four alternative forced choice) and the maximum and minimum disparities available. Thus, normative values attained on one stereotest are unlikely to match those of other stereotests. Clinicians should therefore use the same stereotest for initial and post-intervention stereopsis assessments.

In terms of screening patients for visual abnormalities, this is best performed with random dot stimuli (global stereopsis) rather than contour stimuli (local stereopsis). There is no single test of stereopsis to screen for vision disorders such as strabismus and amblyopia adequately, and therefore screenings should include a test of (global) stereopsis along with tests of visual acuity and refraction.

It may be possible to overcome some of the limitations of printed stereoacuity tests with computer-based measurements. These methods may allow for the presentation of disparities at more levels, more opportunities to test depth detection at a particular disparity multiple times (thereby improving test–retest variability), and the ability to apply psychophysical approaches (e.g., the staircase method) that allow for a more accurate estimate of stereoscopic thresholds [11, 16]. Lastly, computer-based techniques may allow for assessing thresholds for motion in depth, a visual characteristic that is potentially important in everyday life.

References

1. von Noorden G, Campos E. Binocular vision and ocular motility: theory and management of strabismus. 6th ed. Mosby Inc.; 2002.
2. Howard I, Rogers B. Binocular vision and stereopsis. New York: Oxford University Press; 1995.
3. Reading R. Binocular vision: foundations and applications. Woburn, MA: Butterworth Publishers; 1983.
4. Yamada T, Scheiman M, Mitchell GL. A comparison of stereopsis testing between red/green targets and polarized targets in children with normal binocular vision. Optometry. 2008;79(3):138–42.
5. Leske DA, Birch EE, Holmes JM. Real depth vs randot stereotests. Am J Ophthalmol. 2006;142(4):699–701.
6. Wu H, Jin H, Sun Y, Wang Y, et al. Evaluating stereoacuity with 3D shutter glasses technology. BMC Ophthalmol. 2016;16(1):45.
7. Vancleef K, Read JCA, Herbert W, et al. Overestimation of stereo thresholds by the TNO stereotest is not due to global stereopsis. Ophthalmic Physiol Opt. 2017;37(4):507–20.
8. Stereopsis CJ. In: Eskridge JB, Amos JF, Bartlett JD, editors. Clinical procedures in optometry. J.B. Lippincott Co: Philadelphia, PA; 1991. p. 121–34.
9. Tyler C. Cyclopean vision. In: Cronly-Dillon J, Regan D, editors. Binocular vision. Boca Raton, FL: CRC Press Inc; 1991. p. 38–74.
10. O'Toole AJ, Kersten DJ. Learning to see random-dot stereograms. Perception. 1992;21(2):227–43.
11. Read JCA. Stereo vision and strabismus. Eye. 2015;29(2):214–24.
12. Levi DM. Learning to see in depth. Vis Res. 2022;200:108082.
13. Ohzawa I. Mechanisms of stereoscopic vision: the disparity energy model. Curr Opin Neurobiol. 1998;8(4):509–15.
14. Levi DM, Knill DC, Bavelier D. Stereopsis and amblyopia: a mini-review. Vis Res. 2015;114:17–30.

15. O'Connor AR, Birch EE, Anderson S, et al. The functional significance of stereopsis. Invest Ophthalmol Vis Sci. 2010;51(4):2019–23.
16. O'Connor AR, Tidbury LP. Stereopsis: are we assessing it in enough depth? Clin Exp Optom. 2018;101(4):485–94.
17. Burgess S, Kousha O, Khalil M, et al. Impact of stereoacuity on simulated cataract surgery ability. Eye (Lond). 2021;35(11):3116–22.
18. Al-Saud LM, Mushtaq F, et al. Drilling into the functional significance of stereopsis: the impact of stereoscopic information on surgical performance. Ophthalmic Physiol Opt. 2017;37(4):498–506.
19. Saladin J. Phorometry and stereopsis. In: Benjamin W, editor. Borish's clinical refraction. 2nd ed. St. Louis, MO: Butterworth Heinemann; 2006. p. 899–960.
20. Vancleef K, Read JCA. Which Stereotest do you use? A survey research study in the British Isles, the United States and Canada. Br Ir Orthopt J. 2019;15(1):15–24.
21. Ohlsson J, Villarreal G, Abrahamsson M, et al. Screening merits of the Lang II, Frisby, Randot, Titmus, and TNO stereo tests. J AAPOS. 2001;5(5):316–22.
22. Richardson SR, Wright CM, Hrisos S, et al. Stereoacuity in unilateral visual impairment detected at preschool screening: outcomes from a randomized controlled trial. Invest Ophthalmol Vis Sci. 2005;46(1):150–4.
23. Schmidt PP. Vision screening with the RDE stereotest in pediatric populations. Optom Vis Sci. 1994;71(4):273–81.
24. Ancona C, Stoppani M, Odazio V, et al. Stereo tests as a screening tool for strabismus: which is the best choice? Clin Ophthalmol. 2014;8:2221–7.
25. Fricke TR, Siderov J. Stereopsis, stereotests, and their relation to vision screening and clinical practice. Clin Exp Optom. 1997;80(5):165–72.
26. Ciner EB, Ying GS, Kulp MT, et al. Stereoacuity of preschool children with and without vision disorders. Optom Vis Sci. 2014;91(3):351–8.
27. Schmidt P, Maguire M, Dobson V, et al. Comparison of preschool vision screening tests as administered by licensed eye care professionals in the Vision In Preschoolers Study. Ophthalmology. 2004;111(4):637–50.
28. Cotter SA, Cyert LA, Miller JM, et al. Vision screening for children 36 to <72 months: recommended practices. Optom Vis Sci. 2015;92(1):6–16.
29. Antona B, Barrio A, Sanchez I, et al. Intraexaminer repeatability and agreement in stereoacuity measurements made in young adults. Int J Ophthalmol. 2015;8(2):374–81.
30. Vancleef K, Read JCA, Herbert W, et al. Two choices good, four choices better: for measuring stereoacuity in children, a four-alternative forced-choice paradigm is more efficient than two. PLoS One. 2018;13(7):e0201366.
31. Poltavski D, Biberdorf D, Praus PC. Which comes first in sports vision training: the software or the hardware update? Utility of electrophysiological measures in monitoring specialized visual training in youth athletes. Front Hum Neurosci. 2021;15:732303.
32. Adams WE, Leske DA, Hatt SR, et al. Defining real change in measures of stereoacuity. Ophthalmology. 2009;116(2):281–5.
33. Cooper J, Feldman J. Random-dot-stereogram performance by strabismic, amblyopic, and ocular-pathology patients in an operant-discrimination task. Am J Optom Physiol Optic. 1978;55(9):599–609.
34. Birch EE, Wang J. Stereoacuity outcomes after treatment of infantile and accommodative esotropia. Optom Vis Sci. 2009;86(6):647–52.
35. Pediatric Eye Disease Investigator Group. Intermittent Exotropia Testing Procedures Manual; 2012, pp. 12–4.
36. Pang Y, Gnanaraj L, Gayleard J, et al. Interventions for intermittent exotropia. Cochrane Database Syst Rev. 2021;9(9):Cd003737.
37. Yildirim C, Mutlu FM, Chen Y, et al. Assessment of central and peripheral fusion and near and distance stereoacuity in intermittent exotropic patients before and after strabismus surgery. Am J Ophthalmol. 1999;128(2):222–30.
38. Wong BP, Woods RL, Peli E. Stereoacuity at distance and near. Optom Vis Sci. 2002;79(12):771–8.
39. Ciner EB, Schanel-Klitsch E, Herzberg C. Stereoacuity development: 6 months to 5 years. A new tool for testing and screening. Optom Vis Sci. 1996;73(1):43–8.
40. Oduntan AO, Al-Ghamdi M, Al-Dosari H. Randot stereoacuity norms in a population of Saudi Arabian children. Clin Exp Optom. 1998;81(5):193–7.
41. Birch E, Williams C, Hunter J, et al. Random dot stereoacuity of preschool children. ALSPAC "Children in Focus" Study Team. J Pediatr Ophthalmol Strabismus. 1997;34(4):217–22.
42. Read JCA, Rafiq S, Hugill J, et al. Characterizing the Randot preschool stereotest: testability, norms, reliability, specificity and sensitivity in children aged 2-11 years. PLoS One. 2019;14(11):e0224402.
43. Birch E, Williams C, Drover J, et al. Randot preschool stereoacuity test: normative data and validity. J AAPOS. 2008;12(1):23–6.
44. Piano ME, Tidbury LP, O'Connor AR. Normative values for near and distance clinical tests of stereoacuity. Strabismus. 2016;24(4):169–72.
45. Fawcett SL, Birch EE. Validity of the Titmus and Randot circles tasks in children with known binocular vision disorders. J AAPOS. 2003;7(5):333–8.
46. McCaslin AG, Vancleef K, Hubert L, et al. Stereotest comparison: efficacy, reliability, and variability of a new glasses-free stereotest. Transl Vision Sci Technol. 2020;9(9):29.
47. Denkinger S, Antoniou M-P, Tarello D, et al. The eRDS v6 stereotest and the vivid vision stereo test: two new tests of stereoscopic vision. Transl Vis Sci Technol. 2023;12(3):1.

48. Houston CA, Cleary M, Dutton GN, et al. Clinical characteristics of microtropia—is microtropia a fixed phenomenon? Br J Ophthalmol. 1998;82(3):219–24.
49. Lang J. Anomalous retinal correspondence update. Graefes Arch Clin Exp Ophthalmol. 1988;226(2):137–40.
50. Birch EE, Stager DR Sr, Berry P, et al. Stereopsis and long-term stability of alignment in esotropia. J AAPOS. 2004;8(2):146–50.

9 Color Vision

Amithavikram R. Hathibelagal

9.1 Introduction

Color vision testing is important and should be done routinely, especially in children, to screen for color vision deficiency (CVD). Most individuals are unaware of this condition, and it is usually detected when they fail occupational-related color vision tests, leading to adverse psychological consequences [1]. Some experience difficulties in day-to-day activities such as driving, identifying a suitable matching pair of clothes, etc. This highlights the importance of assessing color vision regularly and providing suitable career counseling to people with color vision issues. CVD is an X-linked condition [2], and therefore, its prevalence is higher in males (Caucasians [3]: 8% and Indians [4]: 3%). This chapter will focus briefly on the history of the development of color vision tests, the principles of color vision, and their application in the development of color vision tests.

9.2 History

One of the oldest reports on congenital color vision deficiency comes from the famous English chemist John Dalton (1766–1844) [5], who had abnormal color vision (deutan defect). The development of modern color vision tests can be traced back to a train accident (the Lagerlunda collision in Switzerland in 1875); however, it was not conclusively proved that it was caused by the train operator's abnormal red/green CVD [6]. Nevertheless, this incident triggered the need to assess color vision (in different professions as a part of the recruitment process) and led to the subsequent development of color vision tests.

9.3 Principles of Color Vision and Its Testing

In humans, three classes of cone photoreceptors mediate color vision: short-wavelength sensitive cones (S cones; peak sensitivity: 440 nm), medium-wavelength sensitive cones (M cones; peak sensitivity: 530 nm), and long-wavelength sensitive cones (L cones; peak sensitivity: 560 nm) [7, 8].

Color has three attributes: hue, saturation, and value. The interplay of these three factors is used in the design of the color vision testing. The color names we use daily are called hues (e.g., blue, green, or red). The different shades of a given hue are called saturation; for example, dull red (less saturated) vs. bright red (more saturated), etc. Individuals with CVD typically require higher saturation levels to identify the hues and distin-

A. R. Hathibelagal (✉)
Brien Holden Institute of Optometry and Vision Sciences, Prof. Brien Holden Eye Research Centre, L V Prasad Eye Institute, Hyderabad, India

T. Das, P. Satgunam (eds.), *Ophthalmic Diagnostics*, https://doi.org/10.1007/978-981-97-0138-4_9

guish them correctly. The underlying principles of color vision testing are based on color confusion axes—the colors lying on a given color confusion axis are indistinguishable for those with CVD. The orientation of the confusion axes in the color space varies with the type of CVD. Noise (static or dynamic) is introduced in colour vision tests to ensure that the discrimination ability tested is based on chromatic contrast, not luminance contrast.

9.4 Types of Color Vision Deficiencies

Color vision deficiency refers to a condition in which one or more cone class(es) are missing or their function is altered or completely absent. The peak spectral sensitivity of the affected cone class is altered relative to normal trichromats (individuals with normal color vision). Depending on the severity and cone class affected, CVD can be broadly categorized as anomalous trichromacy, dichromacy, or monochromacy (Fig. 9.1).

Anomalous trichromacy is a milder form of CVD in which the peak spectral sensitivity of the L or M cone is abnormal (corresponding to protanomaly or deuteranomaly, respectively). Relative to normal trichromats, there is a reduced wavelength gap between the peak spectral sensitivities of L and M cones, which can adversely affect color discrimination, mostly in the wavelength range between 500 to 700 nm. Tritanomaly is rare, because there is a large gap between the spectral sensitivities of either L or M cones and the S cone spectral sensitivity.

Dichromacy is a relatively severe form than anomalous trichromacy. In dichromats, one type of cone is missing or lacks complete function (protanopia—L cones missing; deuteranopia—M cones; and tritanopia—S cones).

Monochromatism refers to a condition in which only one photoreceptor class is functioning or present (either the rod or cone). Conditions with L- and M-cone monochromacy are much rarer; S - cone monochromatism (also called Blue cone monochromatism; BCM) is a type of cone monochromacy where the L and M cones are missing and functional S-cones are present. Patients with BCM tend to have normal blue-yellow colour vision and absence of red-green colour vision. Rod monochromatism is also called achromatopsia, where only rod function is present. Its symptoms include extremely poor color perception (almost in shades of gray), poor visual acuity, and photophobia.

9.5 Tests for Color Vision Deficiency

Based on the testing design and principles, the tests for CVD can be broadly categorized as follows: (a) pseudoisochromatic tests, (b) color arrangement tests, (c) color-matching tasks, and (d) threshold-based digital color vision tests. The following section will discuss each of the test categories and a few important examples for each of them.

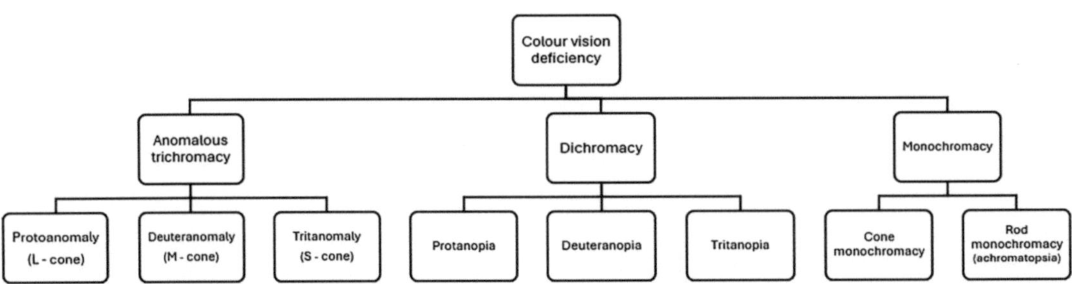

Fig. 9.1 A flowchart showing the different types of color vision deficiencies based on the affected photoreceptor classes

9.5.1 Pseudoisochromatic Test Design Pattern

The plates are called “pseudo” isochromatic because they appear falsely isochromatic (The word ‘Iso’ is derived from the Greek root *isos*, which means equal/same) to an individual with CVD. Such tests can be rapidly administered and are mainly used for screening red-green (R-G) defects. The pseudo isochromatic plates typically incorporate four different test designs, namely transformation, vanishing, hidden-digit design, and classification plates.

9.5.1.1 Ishihara Plates

Ishihara (named after Professor Shinobu Ishihara from Tokyo, Japan) plates are the most used color vision screening test globally. Their popularity as a screener is due to their simplicity and high sensitivity in detecting color vision deficiency. The Ishihara test can perform well even in challenging light environments. Arabic numerals/tracings are used in the foreground, and the background consists of dots of varying shape, chromaticity, and lightness to reduce the role of luminance (brightness changes) in detecting the target. In each version, the Ishihara test uses all four test designs to screen and identify the type of R-G defects (Table 9.1). Colored dots are chosen around the red region where the protan and deutan confusion axes are similar. Thus, isolating protan from deutan using the Ishihara test is challenging compared to other pseudoisochromatic tests.

Table 9.1 Different types of plates in each of the versions of the Ishihara color vision test

Type of plate	38-plate edition	24-plate edition	16-plate edition
Demonstration	1	1	1
Transformation (Screening)	2–9	2–7	2–9
Vanishing (Screening)	10–17	8–13	
Hidden digit (Screening)	18–21	14–15	
Classification	22–25	16–17	10
Tracing	26–38	18–24	11–16

The demonstration plate (Fig. 9.2a) has varying lightness and hence can be seen by anyone whose visual acuity is better than 20/200 (logMAR: 0.0), including a rod monochromat. Transformation plates refer to the plates in which the individual with CVD will misread the numbers as opposed to normal trichromats (Fig. 9.2b). Vanishing test design plates are those in which individuals with CVD cannot read the numbers. Hidden-digit plates can be read by individuals with CVD but not by normal trichromats. The classification plates are built so that the individual numbers are constructed from different color confusion axes, allowing differentiation between protan and deutans (Fig. 9.2c). For example, in the classification plate with the numeral “42” on it, only “4” is seen by the deutans, and only “2” is seen by the protans. This helps in categorizing types of defects. Tracing plates are used for people who cannot read (Fig. 9.2d).

The application of criterion for determining ‘pass/fail’ is important in the usage of Ishihara plates. It is important for clinicians to note that the number of plates read does not indicate the severity of colour vision loss [9]. There are three editions of plates: the 38-, 24-, and 16-plate. Even normal trichromats make a few errors in the Ishihara plates. Therefore, if one keeps a strict criterion of allowing no errors in the first 25 plates in the 38-plate editions, then ~18% of normal trichromats also fail. Typically, 2 or fewer errors in a 24-plate edition are considered normal. A summary of the pass/fail criteria in different versions of the charts [10] is shown in Table 9.2.

There are a few limitations to the Ishihara test. One of the challenges is that it is easy to get a copy, learn and memorize, and pass the test. Using a wrong criterion of pass/fail can lead to misdiagnosis. The ability of the Ishihara plates to differentiate protans from deutans is limited. Also, the tracing plates are not suitable for children.

9.5.1.2 HRR Plates

The HRR plates are a type of pseudoisochromatic plates originally developed by Hardy, Rand, and Rittler [11, 12] and it was named

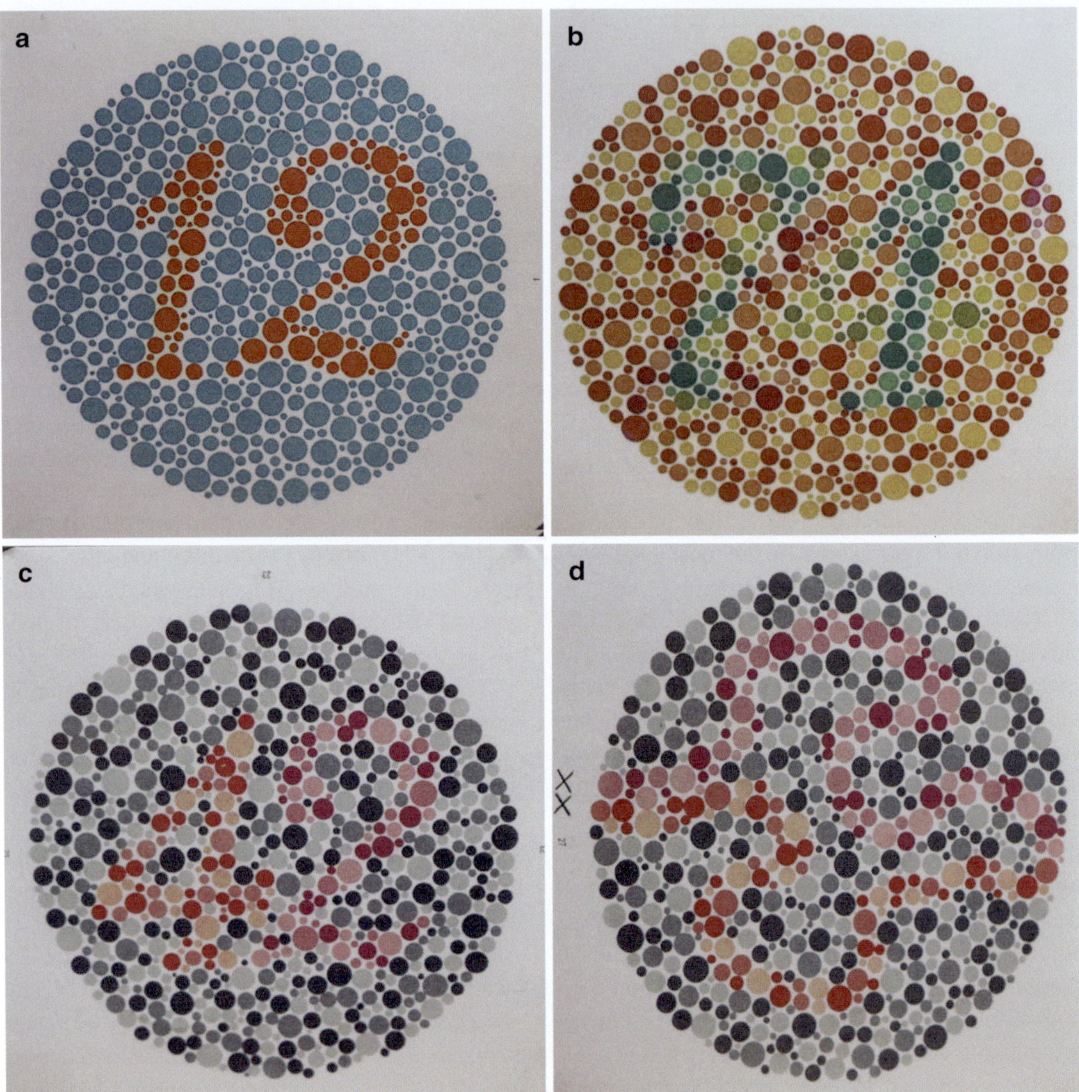

Fig. 9.2 Example of different designs of plates from an Ishihara pseudoisochromatic test. (**a**) Demonstration plate. (**b**) Transformation plate. (**c**) Classification plate. (**d**) Tracing plate

Table 9.2 Criteria for pass and fail for different versions of the Ishihara plate

Criteria for scoring (number of errors)	38-Plate edition	24-Plate edition	16-Plate edition
Pass	4 or less	2 or fewer	2 or fewer
Fail	8 or more	6 or more	4 or more

after them. The first edition of the HRR plates was published in 1955 by the American Optical Company (USA), and the recent editions (third, 1991, and fourth edition, 2002) were developed with Neitz and Bailey, and marketed by Richmond Products (USA) [13]. Unlike the Ishihara plates, the background noise in HRR plates is chosen on either side of the white region (where the confusion axes of protans and deutans are divergent); therefore, these plates can distinguish protans from deutans with more sensitivity. In addition, HRR plates can also differentiate between R-G and blue-yellow (B-Y) defects. The first four are demonstration plates (Fig. 9.3a, b are examples of two demo plates). The minimum acuity required to view a demonstration plate is 20/200. The remaining test can be averted if the patient cannot identify symbols in the demo plates. Three symbols (triangle, circle, and cross) are used as a target in any given plate. The screening plate uses a vanishing design of the pseudoisochromatic plates. The screening plates for B-Y are plates 5–6, and R-G are from plates 7–10. The classification (protan vs. deutan) and grading plates for colour vision severity (Fig. 9.3c, d) are from 11 to 20. Individuals with color vision deficiency would require higher saturation levels to detect the targets reliably. Plates 21–25 are used for grading tritan defects. The correct classification of protan/deutan occurs in 86% of the cases. The HRR test works better in children because they can quickly identify shapes than numerals.

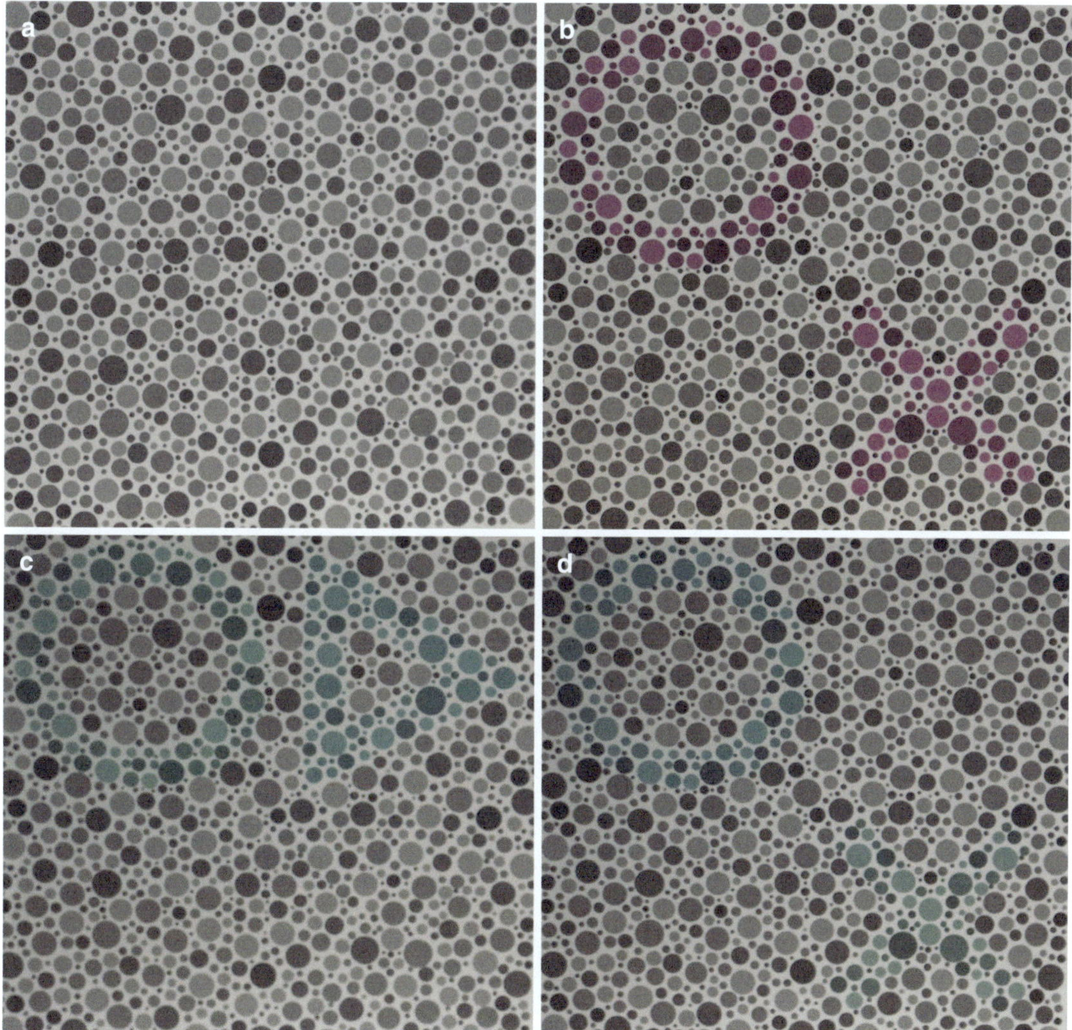

Fig. 9.3 Example of plates from the HRR pseudoisochromatic test. (**a**, **b**) The demonstration plates. Panel (**a**) contains no target. This plate gives a sense of perception to the observer of how the plate appears when there is no target as opposed to one in which a target is present. (**b**) Two targets, the circle and the cross. Panels (**c**, **d**) show the grading plates (the targets in panel (**c**) are more saturated than (**d**)) to categorize the severity of color vision deficiency

9.5.1.3 General instructions for the usage of Pseudoisochromatic plates

The recommended test distance is 75 cm, and each plate is shown perpendicular to the line of sight for not more than 3 seconds. The lighting used for color vision testing should be D65, whose color temperature is about 6500 K. The light source of Illuminant C or similar use should provide illumination in the order of 100–600 lux. Yellow/tungsten light should not be used for testing as it can alter the appearance of the colors. Care should be taken so that the plates are not directly touched with the fingers and exposed to sunlight. The book should be closed when not in use.

9.5.1.4 Patient Instructions and Procedure

Ishihara Plates

The patient is first shown the demonstration plate. If he/she answers correctly, then the test proceeds further. The patient is instructed to read the numbers on the chart, and each plate will be displayed only for 3 seconds.

HRR Plates

The patient is shown some colored symbols and asked to answer the following questions: (a) how many colored symbols are seen? (b) If seen, then what symbols are present, and (c) where are they located? Only when the participant gets the correct answer to all three questions the plate is judged as a "seen," and the patient is given a "pass" response; otherwise, it is recorded as "not seen," and the patient is given a "fail." The severity of HRR does not agree significantly with the anomaloscope classification; however, as a screening tool, it is effective and has a high sensitivity of about ~96% in detecting CVD [13].

The other tests that use the principle of pseudoisochromatic plates are as follows:

- Dvorine test: a combination of pseudoisochromatic plates and naming tests
- Dalton pseudoisochromatic plates [14]: Cost-effective tool for screening for CVD
- City University plates [15]
- CVTME (Color Vision Testing Made Easy): for pediatric subjects [16]

9.5.2 Color Arrangement Tests

The color arrangement task involves arranging colored caps in a sequential manner that represents gradual changes in colors from one to another hue. In this test, individuals with CVD will arrange colors in the palette in a sequence that is perceptually very different from normal trichromats. The errors in a sequence of numbers behind the color caps indicate the magnitude of the defect, and the pattern allows the identification of the defect type. The tests can detect both congenital and acquired CVDs. The most common color arrangement tests are (a) the FM 100 hue test and (b) the D15 test.

9.5.2.1 FM 100 Hue Test

This test consists of 85 caps subdivided into 4 sets of boxes (22 in first box and 21 in next three boxes). In each box, the first color is fixed. The last color of each box and the first subsequent color in the next box have the same chromatic properties to allow continuation. Caps are chosen to have the same brightness and saturation but different hues. Caps are confused by individuals with CVD for those colors that lie on the confusion axis.

Procedure: The participant is first shown how the colors are expected to be arranged. The starting cap is retained; the rest of the caps in the first set are removed from the box and placed loosely in a random manner by the examiner, and the participant is instructed to arrange them in the natural sequence of changing colors, as shown previously. The test is conducted under Macbeth White light conditions (color temperature: 6500 K). Once the given series of caps in one set is arranged, a similar procedure is followed for the subsequent boxes.

Scoring and analysis: The boxes are flipped over to note the sequence of numbers on the back of the color caps. There could be some minor errors even for those with normal color vision. There will be large errors in sequence in people with CVD. The error score for each cap is the absolute sum of differences between adjacent caps. The error score of each color cap can be plotted on a radial line; the subsequent polar plots can reveal the type and severity of the defect. The total score can be calculated by summing up the errors of all caps and subtracting 170 (2 × 85 caps). Quantifying and plotting the score can be expedited by entering the scores in template Excel sheet.

Advantages:

- Quantifies the severity of CVD unlike other screening tools.
- Useful to quantify colour vision deficiency even in acquired retinal diseases

Disadvantages:

- Time-consuming
- Performance is associated with IQ [17]

9.5.2.2 D15 Test

This test is similar to the FM 100 hue test, except that the D15 test is a screening tool. This test involves a color arrangement task in which the patient arranges 15 caps in a natural sequential manner. The step sizes in chromaticity are much larger in the D15 test than in the FM 100 hue test. The number on the back of the color caps can be mapped on a special charting map to identify the type of CVD. In the D15 test, the samples are shown in the color space (Fig. 9.4a). Colors become more desaturated as one moves toward the neutral point. The lines are joined based on the numbers on the color caps, and the resultant lines parallel to the confusion axis yield the type of defect (Fig. 9.4b).

There are other types of color arrangement tasks, such as:

(a) ColorDx D15 test

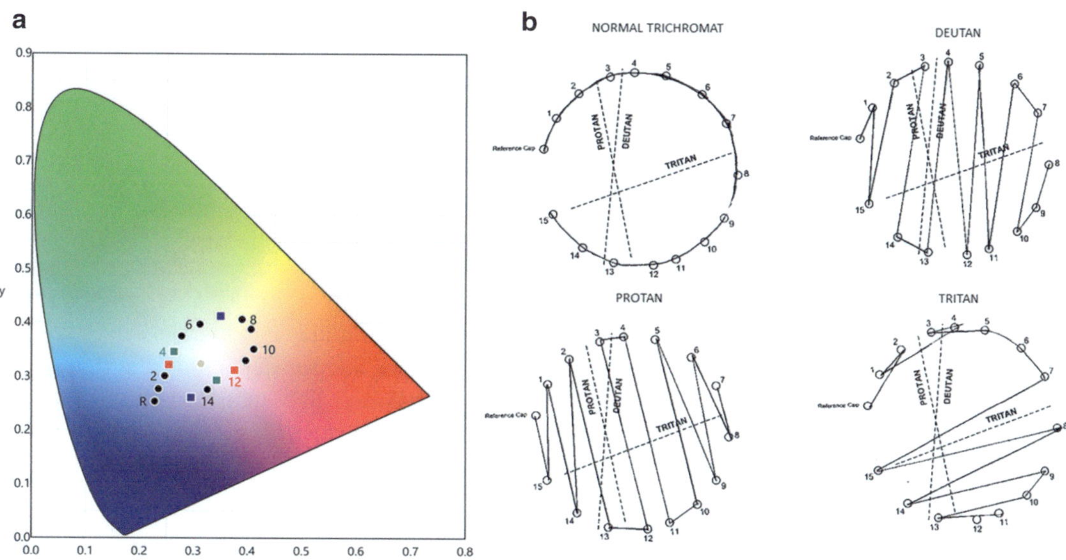

Fig. 9.4 CIE coordinates of D15 caps in the CIE 1931 color space (panel **a**) and interpretation of the results. R refers to the reference cap (panel **a**). A normal trichromat is expected to make no errors (panel **b** - upper left). The lines that emerge parallel to 4 and 13 will likely be deutan defects (panel **b** - upper right). Similarly, patterns of a line parallel to 3 and 12 represent the protan defect (panel **b** - lower left). The lines emerging parallel to 7 and 15 caps represent the tritan defect (panel **b** - lower right). Note that D15 does not distinguish between anomalous trichromats vs. dichromats

(b) Desaturated D15 test
(c) Lanthony D15 test

9.5.3 Color Matching

9.5.3.1 Anomaloscope

The anomaloscope works on the principle of color matching. It allows differentiation between anomalous trichromats and dichromats. The test can also be used to subclassify the type of CVD. In this test, the subject views a 2° circular field. The upper half comprises of a green (549 nm) and red (664 nm) mixture, which the operator controls. The observer controls the lower half field which is a yellow field (589 nm). There is an adapting screen (9 cm) called the Trendelenburg screen below the eyepiece used for preadapting before a color match to obtain stable color-matching results. The outcomes are categorized by the size of the matching range and the midpoint position. The red/green mixture range can vary from 0 (pure green) to 73 (pure red). The R-G setting and wavelength specifications can vary slightly across different instrument manufacturers. The normal midpoint position for trichromats is around 40 units and a matching range of 3–4 units. Matches made by individuals with CVD are not acceptable to normal trichromats. Deuteranomalous individuals require more green, and protanomalous individuals require more red in color matching. One way to differentiate a protanope from a deuteranope is based on the luminance of the yellow (too dark in protanopes vs. normal luminance in deuteranopes). The anomaly quotient is derived using the R/G ratio of the tested individual divided by the R/G ratio of a normal trichromat.

An anomaly quotient >1.33 indicates a protanomaly, and <0.75 indicates a deuteranomaly. One of the disadvantages of an anomaloscope is that it requires the examiner administering the test to be trained. The Pickford-Nicolson anomaloscope is more customizable in terms of field size and the type of defect that can be investigated. One of the general instructions for any anomaloscope testing would be to avoid naming the color and ask the observer what they perceive. Additionally, the establishment of a device-specific, population-specific normative database is recommended.

The other tests based on the color-matching principle are as follows:

(a) The Medmont-C test, which allows one to differentiate protans from deutans.
(b) The Sloan achromatopsia test is used for detecting rod monochromats.
(c) The City University Test is also based on color matching.

9.5.4 Threshold-Based Digital Color Vision Tests

Digital color vision tests are usually threshold-based tests. The most common threshold-based tests are as follows:

(a) CAD (Color Assessment and Diagnosis) test
(b) Cone contrast test
(c) Cambridge color Test

9.5.4.1 CAD Test

The Color Assessment and Diagnosis (CAD) test was developed by Barbur et al. at City, University of London (U.K.) [18, 19]. It consists of a specialized color-calibrated display connected to another computer with a pre-installed CAD program. The saturation threshold is measured in each of the 16 different hues and separate chromatic thresholds, namely R-G and B-Y thresholds are computed. The normative values for the CAD test have been established [19]. Based on comparisons with the age-matched normative values, the severity of color vision is classified as mild, moderate, or severe color vision loss [20].

9.5.4.2 Procedure

The procedure involves identifying the least amount of saturation required for a given hue to detect the direction of the target. In this task, a colored target moves in one of the four diagonal directions (Fig. 9.5a), and the participant's task is

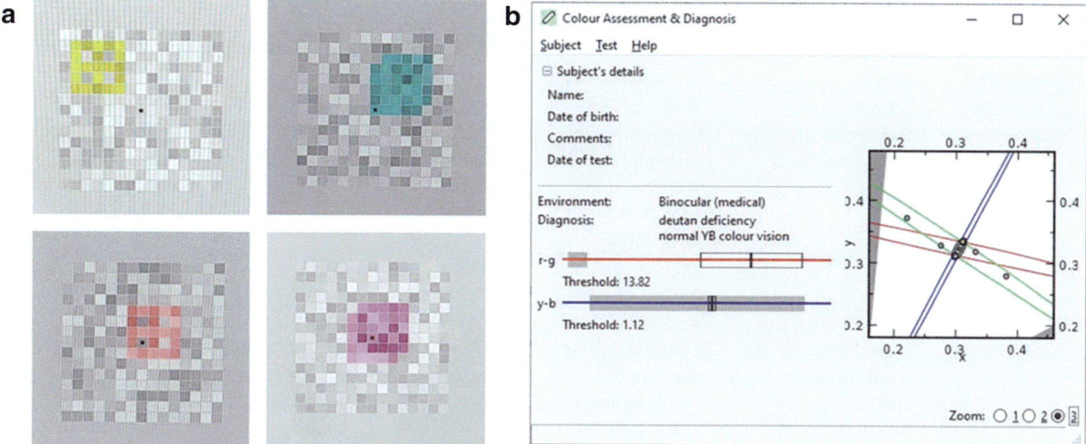

Fig. 9.5 A screengrab of the CAD test stimuli and the summary of the CAD test report. Panel (**a**) shows four different colored targets in a dynamic noise background (note that the noise [black and white squares] appears static in this figure; however, the noise is dynamic during the test). At any point during the test, only one colored stimulus would be presented. Panel (**b**) shows the CAD summary results of an individual with deutan deficiency and normal Y-B color vision. Chromatic thresholds computed for each hue direction are plotted in the color space of the 1931 CIE (Commission Internationale de l'éclairage) on panel (**b**). The small central ellipse indicates the normative values from a large cohort of normal trichromats. The thresholds outside the ellipse are abnormal and aligned with the deutan confusion lines (green)

to identify the location where the targets' end position will be. The difficulty (saturation) of the target is adjusted based on an adaptive staircase procedure. A resultant single outcome variable is obtained separately for R-G and B-Y color vision (Fig. 9.5b). The lower the CAD score, the better the color vision.

The same group that developed the CAD test developed the CAD screener program. This test is aimed at only screening the CVDs. The CAD screener has high sensitivity and specificity and is a 2-alternate forced-choice test. The target moves either in the upper left or upper right direction. Only those who fail the CAD screener test are recommended for complete CAD testing. Currently, the CAD test is used for occupational color vision purposes in aviation and transport industries in the UK.

9.5.4.3 Rabin Cone Contrast Test

Cone contrast is a letter-based digital color vision test [21]. The cone-isolating axis is L, M, or S cone. There are a total of 20 letters. The larger the number of letters read by the person across varying levels of chromatic contrast, the higher the score (indicating normal trichromatic vision). Conversely, lower scores indicate CVD and they can be graded.

9.5.4.4 Cambridge Color Test

The Cambridge Color Test [22] is now part of a suite of tests developed by Cambridge Research Systems (Kent, U.K.). The test works on the principle of pseudoisochromatic plates. There are two different test modes: the Ellipse test and the Trivector test. The participant's task is to identify the opening's direction (1 of 4 options) in the letter C. This procedure is repeated for different hues, and the results are presented as ellipses. The bigger the ellipse, the poorer the color vision. The orientation provides the chromatic axis classifying protans/deutans/tritans.

Besides the above four categories of colour vision tests described, there color-naming tests are typically used for occupational purposes. The important colors for transport and navigation are red, green, orange, and white [20]. In many countries, including India, the lantern test is used to

Table 9.3 Comparison across different color vision tests

Parameters	Pseudoisochromatic plates	Color arrangement tests	Color-matching tests	Color-naming tests	Digital color vision tests
Advantages	Easy to use Relatively cheaper High sensitivity	Both versions (screening and quantification) are available Makes the task interesting	Anomaloscope can distinguish anomalous trichromats from dichromats	Easy to use Practical	Can be used in screening as well as for quantification of the severity of CVD
Disadvantages	Wear and tear of the plates over time Lack of uniform cut-off criteria can result in poor specificity The number of plates read does not indicate the severity of the color vision loss	Monocular cues can affect test results Understanding the task is challenging for some subjects	Extensive training of the operator is required Expensive	Often, the manufacturer does not support repair and spare parts, especially for lantern tests	Expensive and regular calibration Cannot distinguish between anomalous trichromats and dichromats
Examples	Ishihara, HRR plates, Dalton Isochromatic plates, Dvorine plates	D15, FM 100 Hue test, Lanthony desaturated test	Medmont C and Anomaloscope testing	City University Test, Lantern tests	CAD test, Cambridge Color Test, Rabin Cone Contrast Test
Indications	Screening purpose	Screening and quantifying the type of defect and severity	To differentiate the types of CVD (anomalous vs dichromats).	To test the naming of colors for usage in an occupational environment	Can be used to quantify the severity of congenital and acquired conditions Also suitable for setting up occupational safety color vision standards

grade and assess the severity of color vision loss. There are many versions of lantern tests, such as the Holmes Wright, CN Lantern, Edridge-Green lantern, and Farnsworth lantern tests. The Dvorine test also has a color-naming component present in it. The summary of the different types of color vision tests is provided in Table 9.3.

Several commercially available lenses use different wavelength-filtering mechanisms across the visible spectrum to claim that CVD can be 'cured'. The "true improvements" with these filters are typically noticed in individuals with anomalous trichromacy and not with dichromats. The variable results of these filters could be attributed to the lack of a classification of anomalous trichromats from dichromats in many of the studies and the type of task performed by the participants. Therefore, the outcomes of aids for CVD is not straightforward to judge and should be dealt on a case-to-case basis.

9.6 Acquired Color Vision Deficiency

Acquired color vision deficiency is distinct from congenital color vision deficiency in several aspects, such as type of defect, magnitude, and stability (see Table 9.4 for more details). Therefore, it is critical that monocular testing is

Table 9.4 Difference between congenital and acquired color vision deficiency

Congenital color vision deficiency	Acquired color vision deficiency
Mostly R-G defect	Can be either R-G or B-Y defect
Stable throughout the life	Can improve or worsen depending on the magnitude of the disease
Other visual functions, such as acuity and contrast sensitivity are normal	Other visual functions are also affected
Type of defect can be identified	Can be non-specific
Males are more affected	No gender predilection

Table 9.5 Common retinal and optic nerve diseases that show acquired color vision deficiencies

R-G defect	B-Y defect
Optic neuritis	Age-related macular degeneration
Papillitis	Chorioretinitis
Leber's optic atrophy	Central serous retinopathy
Stargardt disease[a]	Glaucoma[a]
Fundus flavimaculatus[a]	Myopic retinal degeneration
Dominant cystoid macular dystrophy[a]	Diabetic retinopathy
Best disease[a]	Retinitis pigmentosa
	Papilledema[a]
	Hereditary autosomal dominant optic atrophy[a]

B-Y Blue-yellow, *R-G* Red-green
[a]Indicate exceptions to Koellner's rule

done in individuals with acquired color vision testing. Retinal or optic nerve diseases are the two most common reasons for acquired color vision deficiency (see Table 9.5 for more details). Koellner's rule states that the inner retina and optic nerve defects cause R-G defects, and the outer retinal and media defects cause B-Y defects. However, there are several exceptions to this rule. Color vision can also be considered a functional biomarker to monitor the efficacy of treatment outcomes in retinal diseases [23, 24]. Color vision can be adversely affected even in systemic conditions, such as prediabetes [25], before ocular involvement. Color vision outcomes can also help in arriving at the correct diagnosis. For example, autosomal dominant tritan (B-Y) defect is specific to autosomal dominant optic atrophy. In addition, the Verriest classification, named after the ophthalmologist Guy Verriest, is the most commonly used classification to categorize acquired R-G and B-Y defects to predict the potential diagnosis [26].

9.7 Conclusions

It is important to test color vision regularly in clinical practice. It is also crucial to decide on the choice of color vision test based on one's understanding of the strengths and limitations of the test and its requirements on an individual basis. Depending on the severity and type of color vision defect, one can be counseled regarding viable career choices and suggest potential aids for helping in everyday life.

Funding Hyderabad Eye Research Foundation.

Disclosure None.

References

1. Hathibelagal AR. Implications of inherited color vision deficiency on occupations: a neglected entity! Indian J Ophthalmol. 2022;70:256–60.
2. Deeb SS. Molecular genetics of color vision deficiencies. Clin Exp Optom. 2004;87:224–9.
3. Birch J. Worldwide prevalence of red-green color deficiency. J Opt Soc Am A. 2012;29:313–320.
4. Krishnamurthy SS, Rangavittal S, Chandrasekar A, Narayanan A. Prevalence of color vision deficiency among school-going boys in South India. Indian J Ophthalmol. 2021;69:2021–5.
5. Hunt DM, Dulai KS, Bowmaker JK, Mollon JD. The chemistry of John Dalton's color blindness. Science. 1995;267:984–8.
6. Mollon JD, Cavonius LR. The Lagerlunda collision and the introduction of color vision testing. Surv Ophthalmol. 2012;57:178–94.
7. Wald G. The receptors of human color vision: action spectra of three visual pigments in human cones account for normal color vision and color-blindness. Science. 1964;145:1007–16.
8. Brown PK, Wald G. Visual pigments in human and monkey retinas. Nature. 1963;200:37–43.
9. Rodriguez-Carmona M, O'Neill-Biba M, Barbur JL. Assessing the severity of color vision loss with

implications for aviation and other occupational environments. Aviat Space Environ Med. 2012;83:19–29.
10. Pokorny J, Collins B, Howett G, Lakowski R, Lewis M. Procedures for testing color vision. National Research Council Washington Committee on Vision; 1981.
11. Hardy LH, Rand G, Rittler MC. H–R–R polychromatic plates. J Opt Soc Am. 1954;44:509–23.
12. Rand G, Rittler MC. An evaluation of the AO HRR pseudoisochromatic plates: a test for detecting, classifying, and estimating the degree of defective color vision. AMA Arch Ophthalmol. 1956;56:736–42.
13. Cole BL, Lian KY, Lakkis C. The New Richmond HRR pseudoisochromatic test for color vision is better than the ishihara test. Clin Exp Optom. 2006;89:73–80.
14. Narayanan A, Venkadesan M, Krishnamurthy SS, Hussaindeen JR, Ramani KK. Dalton's pseudo-isochromatic plates and congenital color vision deficiency. Clin Exp Optom. 2020;103:853–7.
15. Honson VJ, Dain SJ. Analysis of the mark II edition of the City University color vision test. Am J Optom Physiol Optic. 1987;64:277–83.
16. Cotter SA, Lee DY, French AL. Evaluation of a new color vision test:"Color Vision Testing Made Easy®". Optom Vis Sci. 1999;76:631–6.
17. Cranwell MB, Pearce B, Loveridge C, Hurlbert AC. Performance on the Farnsworth-Munsell 100-hue test is significantly related to nonverbal IQ. Invest Ophthalmol Vis Sci. 2015;56:3171–8.
18. Squire TJ, Rodriguez-Carmona M, Evans AD, Barbur JL. Color vision tests for aviation: comparison of the anomaloscope and three lantern types. Aviat Sp Env Med. 2005;76:421–9.
19. Barbur JL, Rodriguez-Carmona M, Harlow AJ (2006). Establishing the statistical limits of "normal" chromatic sensitivity. Ottawa: CIE Publication x030:2006.
20. Barbur JL, Rodriguez-Carmona M. Color vision requirements in visually demanding occupations. Br Med Bull. 2017;122:51–77.
21. Rabin J, Gooch J, Ivan D. Rapid quantification of color vision: the cone contrast test. Invest Ophthalmol Vis Sci. 2011;52:816–20.
22. Mollon JD, Regan JP. Cambridge color test. Handb. [homepage Internet]. Cambridge Cambridge Res. Syst. Ltd; 2000.
23. Abdel-Hay A, Sivaprasad S, Subramanian A, Barbur JL. Acuity and color vision changes post intravitreal dexamethasone implant injection in patients with diabetic macular oedema. PLoS One. 2018;13:e0199693.
24. Yadav G, Narayanan R, Hathibelagal AR. Chromatic and flicker threshold changes in age-related macular degeneration following anti-VEGF treatment. Clin Exp Optom. 2021:1–7.
25. Rodriguez-Carmona M, Bastaki Q, Barbur JL. Loss of color and flicker sensitivity in subjects at risk of developing diabetes. Invest Ophthalmol Vis Sci. 2019;60:1304.
26. Verriest G. Further studies on acquired deficiency of color discrimination. J Opt Soc Am. 1963;53:185–95.

10 Smartphone-Based Ophthalmic Imaging

Anand Sivaraman, Divya Parthasarathy Rao, and Shanmuganathan Nagarajan

10.1 Introduction

Smartphones are ubiquitous assets in medical diagnostics [1]. The VISION 2020 "Right to Sight" Global Initiative, introduced by the World Health Organization (WHO) and the International Association for the Prevention of Blindness (IAPB), aims to eliminate needless visual impairment and maximize the functional potential of those with unavoidable blindness [2, 3]. Conditions needing immediate attention include refractive errors, cataracts, diabetic retinopathy (DR), glaucoma, corneal blindness, and childhood blindness [2, 4].

Smartphones have been the flagbearers of technology and innovation for over two decades. They are the personal digital assistants of healthcare professionals, with more than 87% using either a smartphone or a tablet in their practice [5]. Their ease of use, portability, connectivity, and documentation ability through capturing high-resolution photos and videos at considerable speed with improved camera sensors, fast processors, high storage capacities, and applications have made them excellent choices for point-of-care testing. Ophthalmology relies heavily on investigations, and in this regard, smartphone-based ophthalmic imaging has gained widespread adoption in eye care. It is a versatile tool for patient education, telemedicine-based screening, and diagnosis using AI-based triaging, academic research, and clinical documentation. Additionally, they serve as affordable solutions for resource-constrained settings.

10.2 A Brief History of Smartphone-Based Ophthalmic Devices: Evolution of Technology

Retinal vasculature is the only part of the human circulatory system that can be viewed non-invasively. Hence, fundus photography using smartphone-based devices showed potential in detecting retinal and, subsequently, systemic diseases [6]. Lord et al. were the first to demonstrate the possibility of using a slit lamp and +78D lens in combination to perform indirect ophthalmoscopy with a +20D lens and phone camera, along with a penlight, and showed intra-operative captures on a smartphone using a microscope [7, 8]. Bastawrous et al. modified the design for capturing images from videos wherein one could use the flashlight of the phone itself without a separate penlight [9]. In this design, one could simply hold a +20D/+28D lens in one hand and the

A. Sivaraman (✉) · S. Nagarajan
Remidio Innovative Solutions Pvt,
Bengaluru, India
e-mail: anand@remidio.com; shan@remidio.com

D. P. Rao
Remidio Innovative Solutions Inc., Glen Allen, VA, USA
e-mail: drdivya@remidio.com

T. Das, P. Satgunam (eds.), *Ophthalmic Diagnostics*, https://doi.org/10.1007/978-981-97-0138-4_10

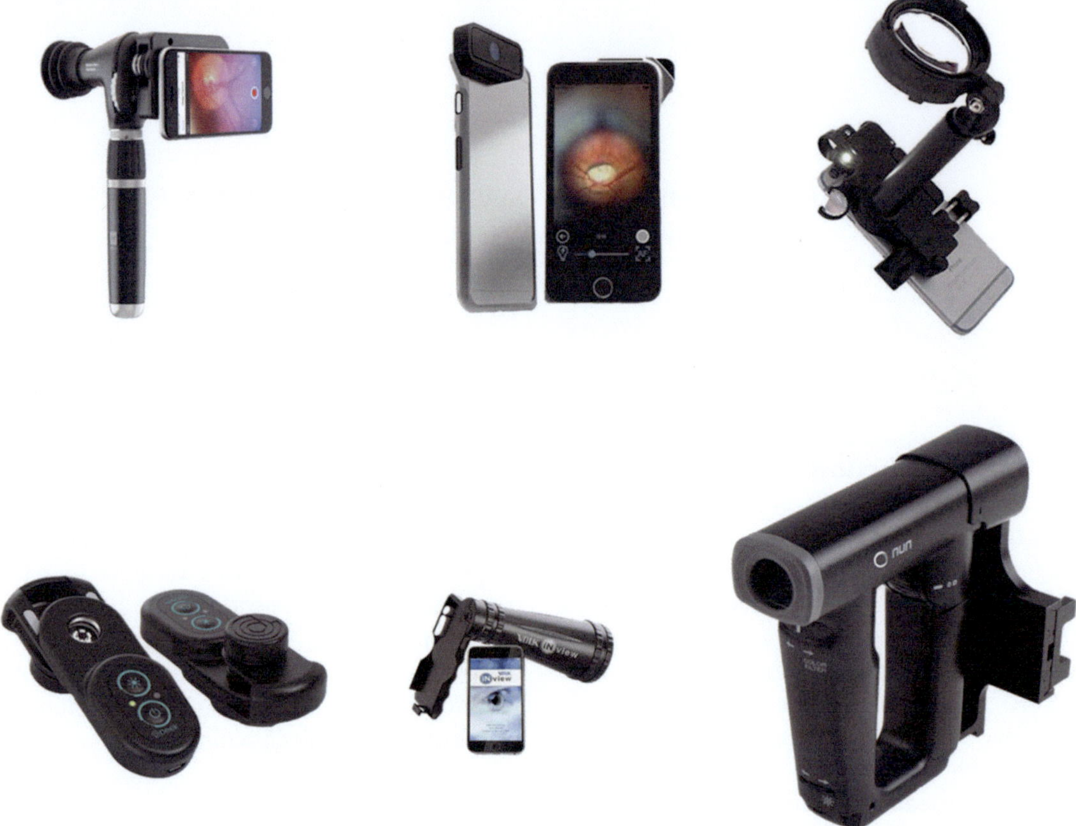

Fig. 10.1 Adapter-based fundus imaging: (from left to right; first row) the iExaminer, D-Eye, and Paxos Scope; (second row) PEEK Retina, Volk iNview, and the oDocs Nun

smartphone in the other. Haddock et al. further improvised on this method by using an application to modify the focus, intensity, and exposure of the camera while capturing the video. In the same device, a Koeppe lens was used in addition to the 20D lens to keep the eyelids open, keep the cornea wet, and get a better field of view under anesthesia [10]. Ryan et al. compared the use of a 20D lens in one hand and an iPhone 5 in the other to capture videos of each eye and compared the screenshots taken from those videos to standard 3-field non-mydriatic and 7-field mydriatic retinal photography on 300 pharmacologically dilated people with diabetes with good sensitivity and specificity [11]. This led to further developments in smartphone-based image acquisition for ophthalmology with improved sensors, image processing, and light sources; these techniques also leveraged the use of 3D printed adapters and eventually developed stand-alone devices integrated with smartphones to capture ophthalmic images [12, 13]. The iExaminer was the first smartphone-based fundus imaging adapter approved by the US FDA in 2013 [12]. Following this, multiple adapter-based fundus imaging modalities like D-Eye, PaxoScope, PEEK Retina, Volk iNView, and ODocsNun (Fig. 10.1) have been validated in various settings primarily for monitoring diabetic retinopathy. These systems relied on applications to adjust light settings or modify the light coming from the camera flash [6, 8]. The systems also used optical designs such as coaxial illumination or cross-polarizer-based designs, often requiring pupillary dilation, and had a field of view (FOV) between 20° and 55° in a single shot [12–14]. Such adapters were major breakthroughs as they could, to some extent, reduce the operational skills needed (due to their ergonomic design) to image the central and peripheral retina through montages [14].

Advantages [15]

- The implementation of point-of-care diagnostics for patients at risk
- Their optical designs come with pre-defined illumination and imaging paths that eliminate the need for manual alignment of the illuminating beam with the optical axis for capturing images

Disadvantages [6, 15, 16]

- The use of coaxial illumination in adapters causes corneal glare and reflex artifacts
- The need for mydriasis for a wider view of the retina
- The cross-polarizers used to eliminate reflection artifacts might lead to non-uniform illumination of the retina causing overexposure of the optic disc and a lack of illumination of the tertiary vessels around the macula
- The distribution of colors is a function of the LED used in smartphones and is not under the control of the photographer
- The ability of the illumination to meet the ISO15004 ophthalmic safety standard needs to be established for every phone used

This chapter will describe some of the smartphone-based imaging modalities currently used and practiced in eye care. In the process, we will also introduce some commercially available and regulatory body-approved devices that the authors are familiar with. This should not be construed as a promotion of these products as describing all devices is out of the scope of this chapter.

10.3 Fundus Imaging

Present-day smartphone-based devices are moving toward high-quality, reflex-free fundus images. Two of these devices are described below.

10.3.1 Fundus on Phone (FOP) and Non-mydriatic Fundus on Phone (FOP NM)

Non-mydriatic fundus on phone (FOP NM-10) (Remidio Bangalore, India) captures ~45° FOV retinal image without dilation (Fig. 10.2) [17]. The device can be used in a desktop or hand-held mode as per the user's needs [18–20].

Technology: The FOP utilizes a patented annular illumination-based optical design, infrared (IR) light, and the voice coil motor of the

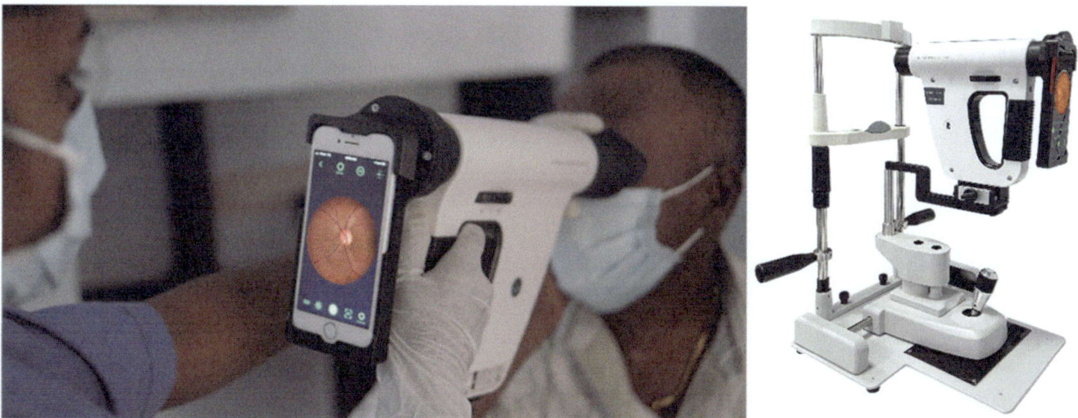

Fig. 10.2 The fundus on phone (FOP) device, Hand-held (left) and desktop (right) modes of use

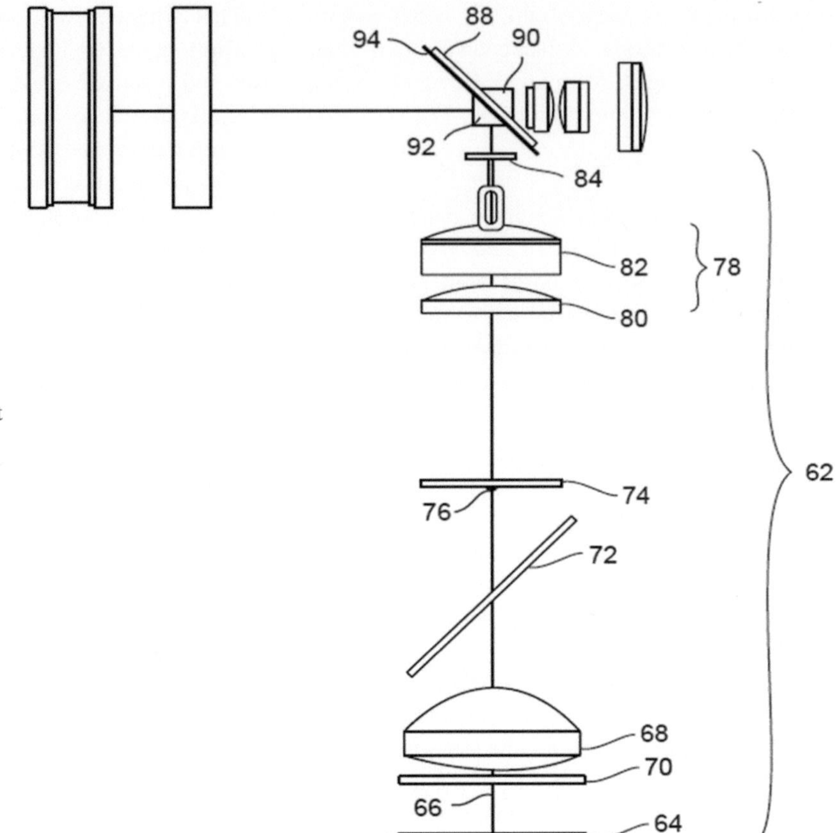

Fig. 10.3 The optical design of the fundus on phone devices (detailed optical design available at reference patent: retinal imaging device: US20140146288A1). Notations: 60—retinal imaging device, 62—illumination module, 64—light source, 66—illumination axis, 68—condenser lens, 70—diffuser, 72—beam splitter, 74—transparent plate, 76—light absorber, 78—projection lens system, 80—plano-convex lens, 82—doublet lens, 84—shield, 86—cornea illumination doughnut, 88—perforated mirror, 90—hollow cylinder 92—projected portion of the hollow cylinder, 94—an elliptical stopper, 96—pupil illumination doughnut

smartphone camera to remove chromatic aberrations, improve image quality, and obtain high-quality images without reflection artifacts. The optical design of the FOP includes an illumination module and an imaging module set perpendicular to each other, with the help of multiple beam splitters, condensing lenses, mirrors, absorbers, and diffusers, devoid of cross-polarizers [16, 21]. An annular illumination-based design provides the camera with a clear central imaging. A porosity mirror, placed between the condensing (Objective) and imaging lens, ensures that all reflections are absorbed, leaving no glare or corneal reflection artifacts (Fig. 10.3) [22].

The FOP and the FOP NM-10 have been validated in multiple settings for detecting different grades and severities of diabetic retinopathy (DR) and in the tele-screening of DR in real-world settings [18–20].

10.3.2 Vistaro

The Vistaro™, a wide-field fundus imaging system, (single shot ~60°) can image an ~90° FOV with two fields, covering more than a standard 7-field ETDRS could visualize [16]. The device, albeit mydriatic, works on a minimum pupil size of 5 mm. It has a unique auto-capture algorithm (Fig. 10.4) to automatically capture images upon reaching the correct working distance. The device captures images of people with refractive errors from −20D to +20D. The Vistaro™ is equipped with a unique patient-management software to capture and store images at all times. When there is internet connection available, the device also backs up the images to a Health Insurance Portability and Accountability Act (HIPAA)-compliant cloud server. The stored images can be sent to specialists over third-party applications, in real time, or on a feed-forward basis using telemedicine [16].

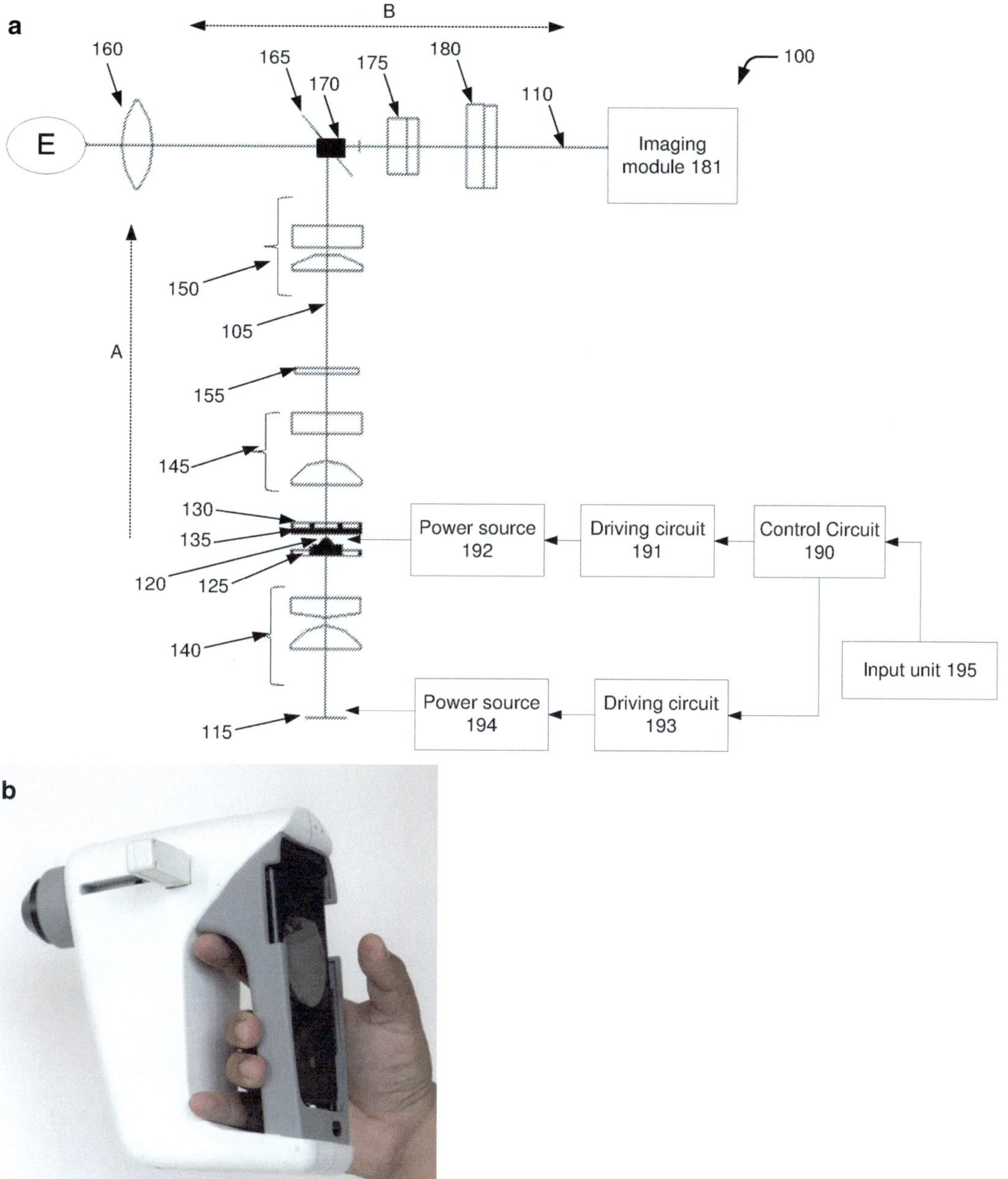

Fig. 10.4 The schematic diagram of the optical design of the hardware (**a**) and a photograph of the Vistaro handheld device (**b**) [16]. Detailed optical design and description available at reference patent: EP3379994A4). Notations: 100—retinal imaging apparatus, E—subject's eye, 105—illumination axis, 110—imaging axis, 115, 120—light sources arranged on the illumination axis, 160—objective lens, 165—porosity mirror, 170—porosity tube, 175—a collimating lens, 180—a converging lens, 181—an imaging module placed along the imaging axis (110), 125, 130—two ring-shaped shields, 135—a diffuser, 140—first condenser lens, 145—second condenser lens, 150—one projection lens, 155—a transparent plate placed along the illumination axis (105). The first shield (125) has a central opaque portion on which an observation light source (120) is mounted and an outer pair of coaxial annular transparent regions. The diffuser (135) is placed before the observation light source (120). The second shield (130) has a central opening portion and is mounted on the diffuser (135), which is adapted to receive the illumination light beam emitted from the observation light source (light-emitting diode [LED]; 120) mounted on the first shield (125)

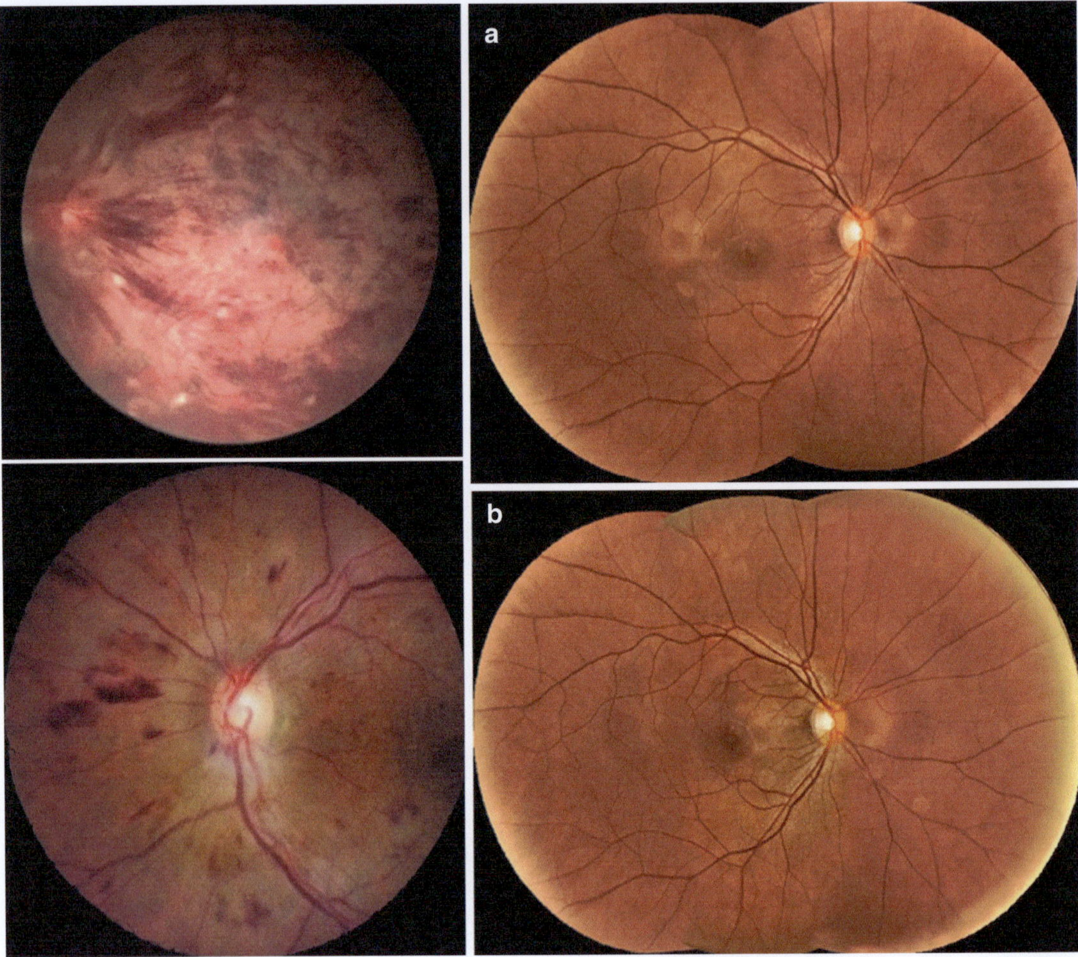

Fig. 10.5 Smartphone-based camera fundus photograph. Left top: central retinal vein occlusion on FOP NM 10; Left bottom: retinal hemorrhage on FOP NM 10. Right top: a two-field montage; Right bottom: a three-field montage captured on the Vistaro™. (All images have been reproduced under the Creative Commons Non-commercial License)

Clinical Applications: State-of-the-art smartphone-based imaging devices like the FOP and the Vistaro™ offer multiple benefits [16, 18–20, 23], such as reflection artifacts-free retinal images (Fig. 10.5), wireless connectivity, secure cloud storage, and artificial intelligence. The limitations include the need for mydriasis (in those with small pupils for FOP) and the non-availability of essential in-clinic features such as autofluorescence and fluorescein angiography [7].

10.4 Anterior Segment Imaging

The early possibility of imaging the anterior segment using smartphones was demonstrated by Barsam et al. [24]. They used the iPhone 3G with a standard Haag-Streit BM 900 slit lamp (Koniz, Switzerland) under different diffuse illumination settings [25]. It required holding the iPhone with the one hand vertically and aligning the camera lens closely with one of the viewing eyepieces from the slit lamp biomicroscope while viewing

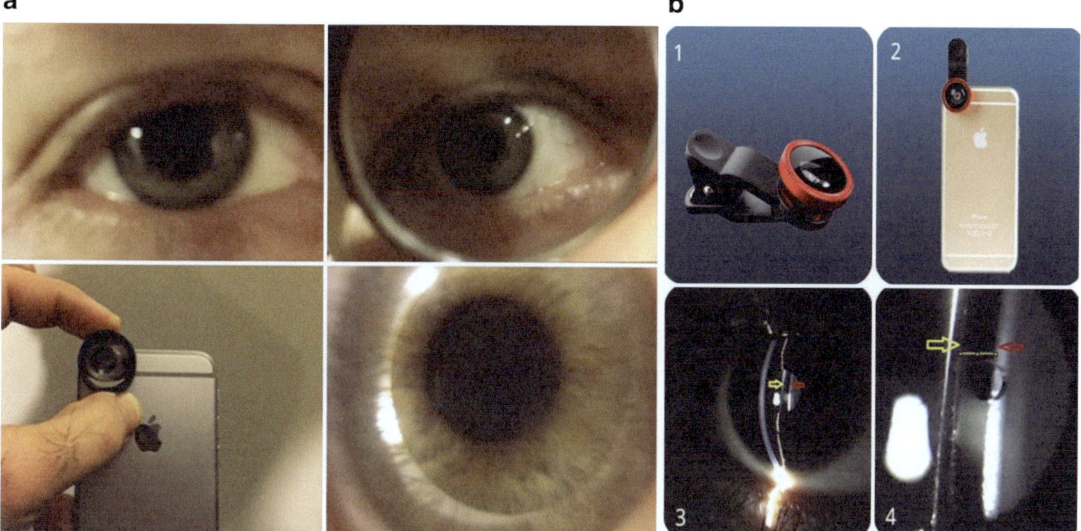

Fig. 10.6 (**a**) A prototype showing the use of a macro lens with smartphones to view the anterior segment [26]. (**b**) A prototype to show ICL measurement using macro lenses clipped to a smartphone [27]. (All images have been reproduced under the Creative Commons Non-commercial License)

the image on the iPhone [24]. Although this was tedious for the operator, it paved the way for many possibilities in imaging different parts of the anterior segment using different attachments to the smartphone like a macro lens, gonio lens, etc. [25] (Fig. 10.6). This advancement enabled various clinical applications, including but not limited to measuring the Implantable Collamer Lens (ICL) vault, imaging the iridocorneal angle, positioning toric intraocular lens (IOL) with a protractor, and quantifying corneal endothelial cells [24–28].

Using smartphones with adapters or lenses requires patients to remain seated to obtain well-focused images, which can be particularly challenging when dealing with elderly patients.

10.4.1 Digitizing Analog Slit Lamps

10.4.1.1 Anterior Imaging Module (AIM)

The AIM (Remidio, Bangalore, India) digitizes a slit lamp.

Technology: AIM uses high-quality anti-reflection (AR) coated binocular optics combined with a 70/30 beam splitter design, to match the magnification drum optics of slit lamps with 3-step or higher magnification. It is designed to fit snugly into the smartphone sensor at its lowest magnification, requiring no additional adjustments between the eyepiece and the slit lamp (Fig. 10.7) [29]. The depth of focus can be adjusted to visualize different anterior structures of the eye and adnexa. The plane of focus on the phone can be adjusted according to the structure imaged (Figs. 10.7 and 10.8). When adjusting the slice of focus toward the desired structure, a shallow focus effect is created in front of and behind the focal point, resulting in a layered appearance. By ensuring that the autofocus of the smartphone app is disabled, the optical assembly ensures that the position of the joystick of the slit lamp determines the focus (Fig. 10.8) [29].

Clinical Applications: The smartphone-based design ensures instant photo documentation. This process helps avoid errors associated with manual documentation and reduces the time required for diagnosis (Figs. 10.9 and 10.10). Additionally, the photographer can click an image while still seeing through the eyepiece, as the design ensures that what the photographer sees through the eyepiece gets documented, following the equivalence of foci in the design.

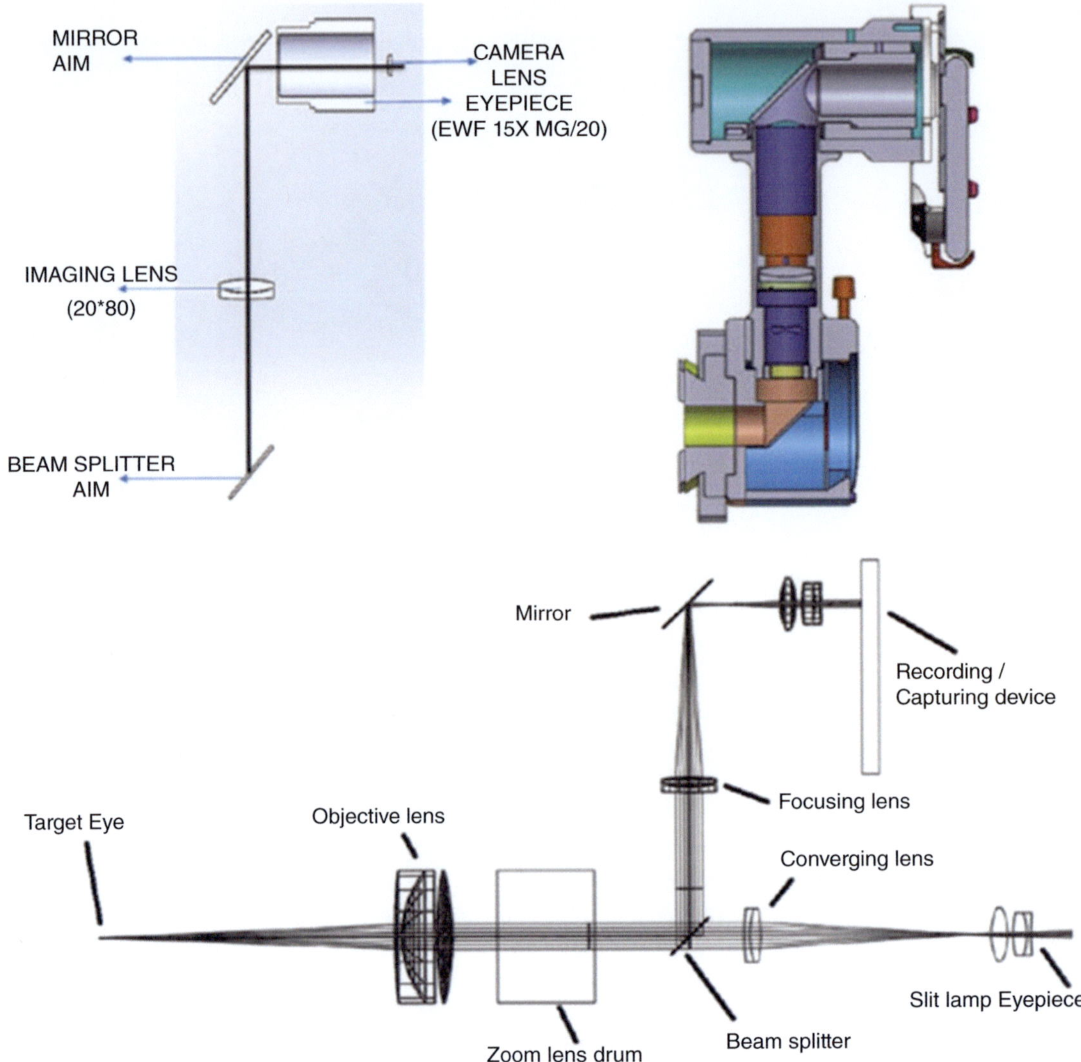

Fig. 10.7 Optical design of the anterior imaging module. (Image reproduced under the Creative Commons Non-commercial License)

10.4.2 Portable Slit Lamps Based on Smartphones

Smartphones can make slit lamps portable and accessible for larger audiences, especially in remote, resource-constrained settings. Several adapter-based systems that utilize 3D printed technology have been primarily used and validated for detecting and grading lens pathologies [30]. Stand-alone systems with separate, standardized light sources have also been developed. We describe one such device here: the PSL D20 [31]. Another hand-held slit lamp device is briefly described in Chap. 35.

10.4.2.1 PSL D20

The PSL D20 (Remidio, Bangalore, India) is a novel, smartphone-based, portable digital slit lamp with separate paths for illumination and imaging to obtain high-quality, artifact-free anterior segment images (Fig. 10.11) [31].

Technology: Light from the LED source passes through the condenser lens as a single convergent beam and then through the illumination lens. It is then reflected via an anti-reflection-

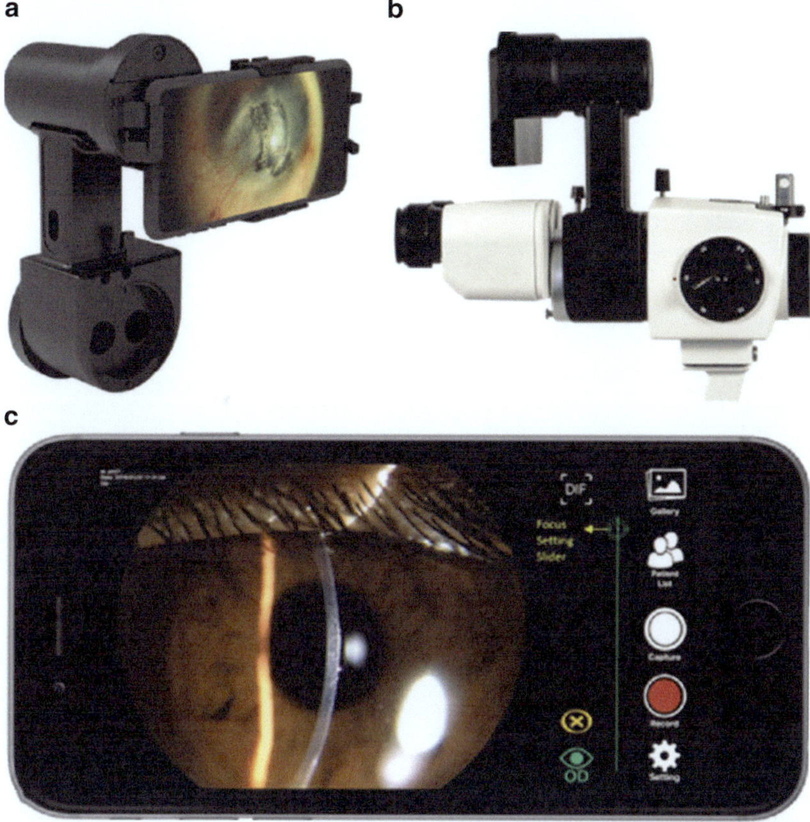

Fig. 10.8 (**a**) Hardware design of the anterior imaging module (AIM). (**b**) The AIM mounted on a conventional slit lamp. (**c**) Anterior segment imaging on AIM [29]. (All images have been reproduced under the Creative Commons Non-commercial License)

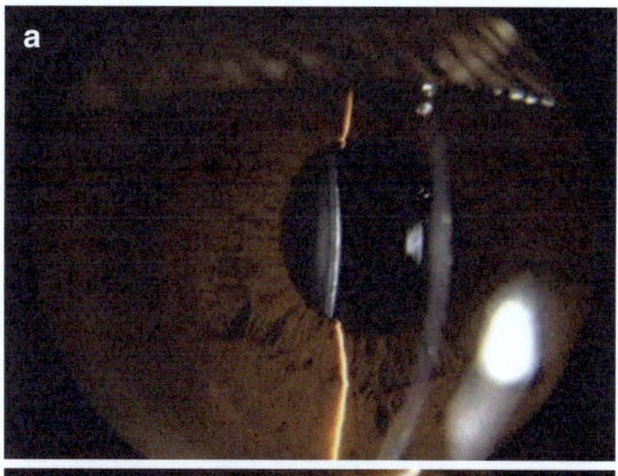

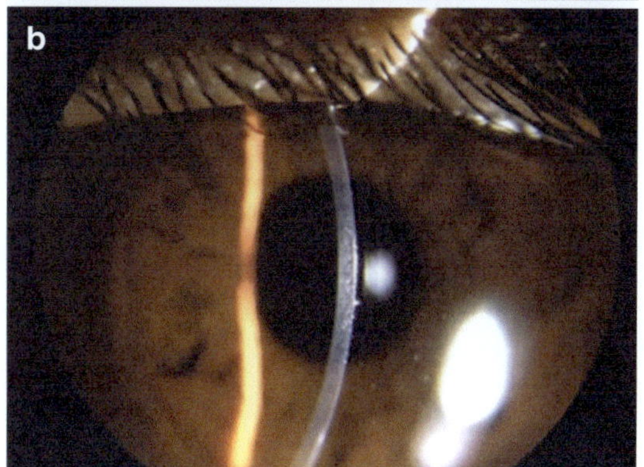

Fig. 10.9 (**a**) An anterior segment image shows the iris plane and lens in focus. (**b**) An anterior segment image showing the plane of the cornea in focus. (All images have been reproduced under the Creative Commons Non-commercial License)

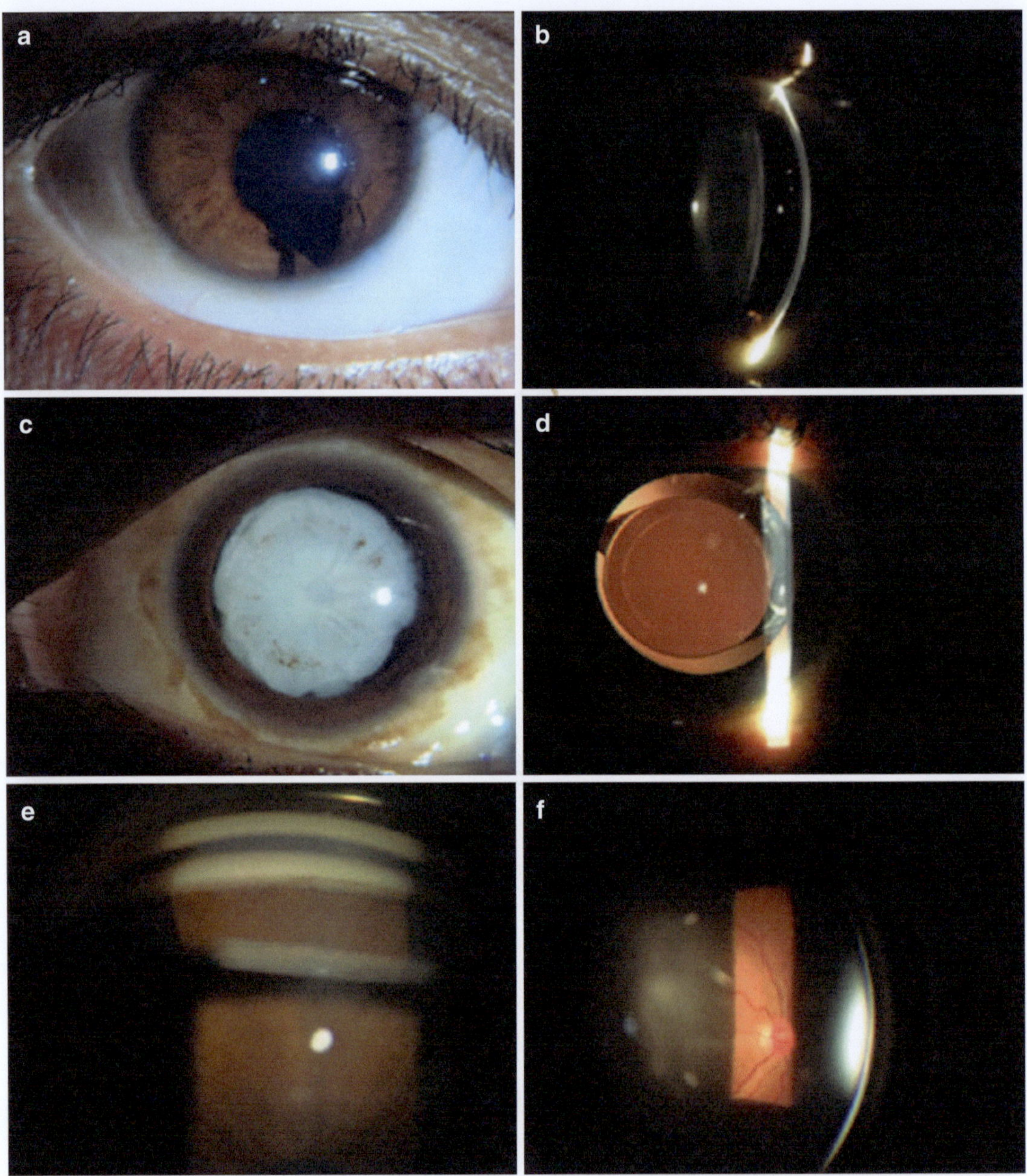

Fig. 10.10 Quality of images and range of pathologies covered by the AIM. (**a**) Diffuse illumination showing a congenital inferonasal coloboma (25×). (**b**) Optical section showing a clear lens (25×). (**c**) Diffuse illumination depicting a hyper mature cataract with iris pigments on the anterior lens surface (25×). (**d**) Retro illumination shows a well-centered capsulorhexis with a single-piece posterior chamber IOL in the capsular bag (16×). (**e**) Gonioscopy showing an open inferior angle up to the ciliary body band with possible neovascularization of the angle (25×). (**f**) Slit lamp biomicroscopy with a 90D volk lens showing a healthy optic disc (25×). (All images have been reproduced under the Creative Commons Non-commercial License)

coated right-angled prism to illuminate the eye. Depending on the physician's requirement, the entire illumination set-up is mounted on a slit swiveling system that can be rotated to 45° on both sides. The reflected ray then passes along the imaging plane, crossing two sets of imaging lenses, that the smartphone captures after an optical magnification. The slit width can be controlled between 0 and 12 mm. The length of the slit is fixed at 12 mm (Fig. 10.11) [31].

The device features an adjustable headrest for convenient manual focusing, ensuring that the object of focus is visible on the phone screen. This stability enables easy image capture by simply looking at the phone screen. The PSL D20 can be efficiently operated using four controls: a button to toggle between background illumination lights (blue, green, and white LEDs) and, one to capture the image, a knob to adjust the slit beam intensity, all easily accessible within the grasp of the thumb. The knob to adjust the variable slit width is located on the swiveling optomechanical unit underneath the prism. The controls offer user convenience in adjusting to ambient light conditions while imaging a patient's eye. To maintain consistent angles during an examination, the optomechanical illumination unit is supported by a pair of ball spring plungers, providing the necessary friction (Fig. 10.12) [31].

Clinical Applications: A pilot study demonstrated the PSL D20's performance in photo documentation and its feasibility in teleophthalmology practice [31]. Optical sections across the lens (Fig. 10.13a, e, and f) and retro illumination (Fig. 10.13h) allow for objective cataract grading (as per the Lens Opacities Classification System (LOCS) III scale). The optic disc evaluation (Fig. 10.13i) was done using a 90D lens, and the green filter enhances the delineation of conjunctival blood vessels (Fig. 10.13d). Fluorescent dye with a blue filter can evaluate the tear film break-up time (TBUT). Additionally, the PSL-D20 has been validated for asynchronous and synchronous teleconsultation [31].

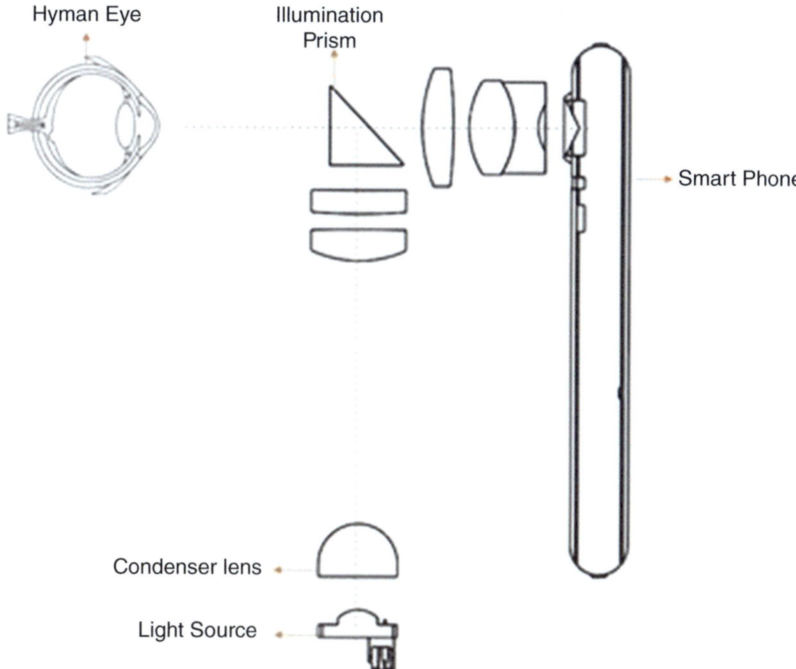

Fig. 10.11 The optical design of the PSL D20 (Image has been reproduced under the Creative Commons Non-commercial License)

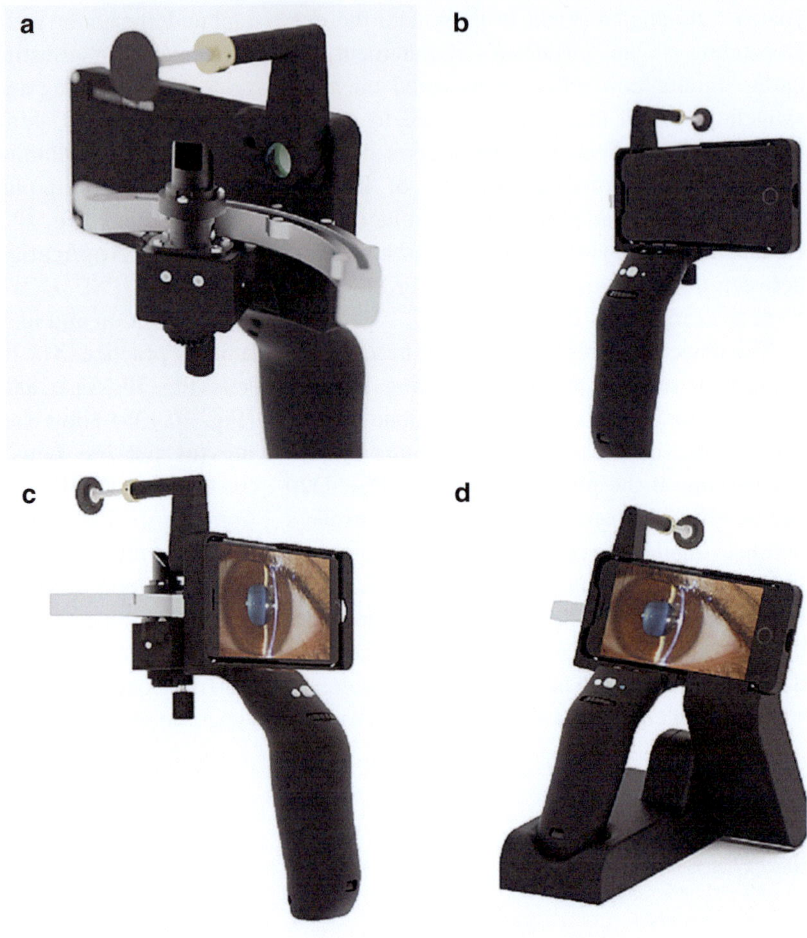

Fig. 10.12 The PSL D20 hardware along a swiveling optomechanical unit (All images have been reproduced under the Creative Commons Non-commercial License)

While we await large-scale, real-world studies to further validate the clinical impact of smartphone-based anterior segment devices like the AIM and PSL D20, they hold promise with their unique set of advantages (portability, unique design, connectivity, dedicated patient-management software, HIPAA-compliant storage servers), [29, 31] and shortcomings (concomitant use of gonioscope lenses and applanation tonometry is not possible, difficult retroillumination, limited smartphone sensor resolution, and limitations in magnification for viewing corneal endothelium and for estimating anterior chamber flare).

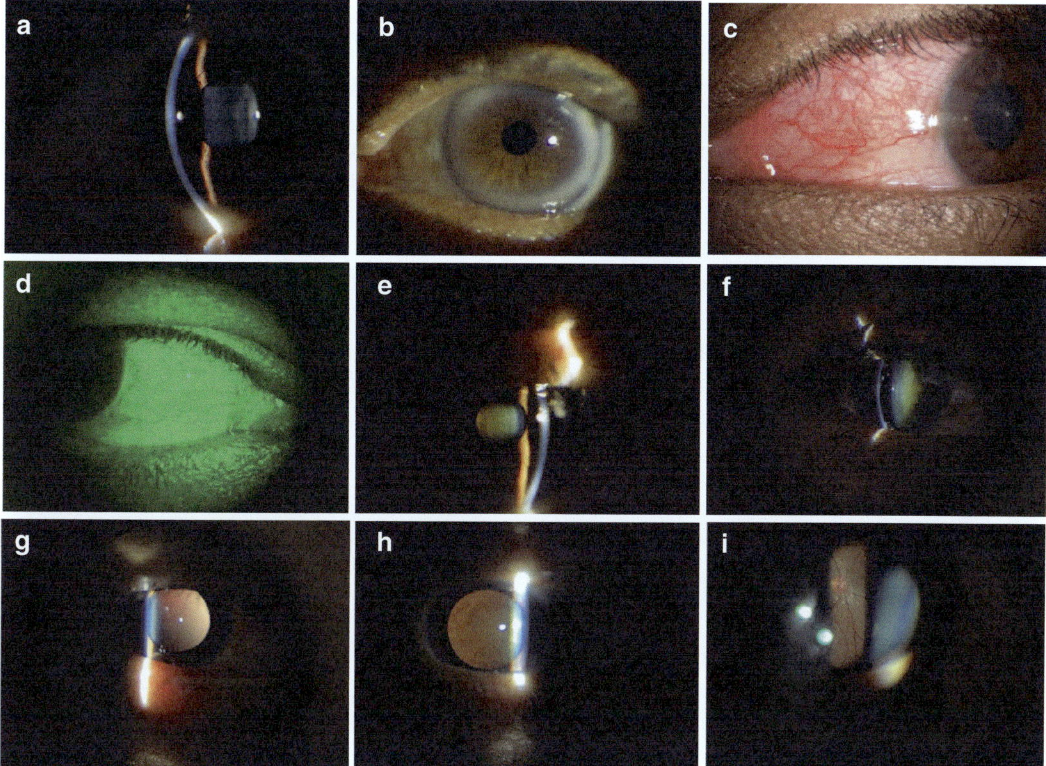

Fig. 10.13 The quality of images captured by the PSL D20 [31]. (**a**) A narrow slit beam is projected at an angle of 45°. It cuts an optical section through the clear lens obtained at a magnification equivalent to 16× on standard slit lamp. (**b**) Diffuse illumination provides evenly balanced lighting. This image shows a dense arcus senilis in a pseudophakic eye captured at a magnification equivalent of 10× on standard slit lamp. (**c**) Diffuse illumination showing diffuse conjunctival hyperemia captured at a magnification equivalent of 10× on standard slit lamps. (**d**) Conjunctival vessels are better visualized in green filters (captured at a magnification equivalent of 10× on standard slit lamps). (**e**) A narrow slit beam cuts an optical section through the lens with a nuclear cataract (LOCS III grade NO 4 and NC 4; captured at a magnification equivalent of 16× on standard slit lamps). (**f**) A narrow slit beam cuts an optical section through the lens with a nuclear cataract (LOCS III grade NO 3 and NC 3; captured at a magnification equivalent of 10× on standard slit lamps). (**g**) Retroillumination technique showing a good fundal glow with no peripheral cortical or posterior subcapsular opacities (captured at a magnification equivalent of 10× on standard slit lamps). (**h**) Retroillumination imaging showing posterior subcapsular cataract (LOCS grade P5; captured at a magnification equivalent to 10×). (**i**) PSL biomicroscopy with a 90D lens shows clear media with a normal optic disc in a view captured at a magnification equivalent of 10× on standard slit lamps. (All images have been reproduced under the Creative Commons Noncommercial License)

10.5 Artificial Intelligence in Smartphone-Based Ophthalmic Imaging Devices

Artificial intelligence (AI) is a cutting-edge technology capable of handling and analyzing large amounts of data. Since smartphones are extensively used to capture image-based data; integrating AI can aid in analyzing and processing this data to generate point-of-care diagnostic support output. In ophthalmology, AI has shown promising results over the past decade in detecting various conditions like DR, age-related macular degeneration (AMD), retinopathy of prematurity (ROP), glaucoma, cataracts, and other anterior segment diseases [32].

Most AI algorithms used for ophthalmic diagnosis have been cloud-based (for example, Google

AI, EyeArt, IDx-DR), requiring a working internet connection, which can be challenging in remote areas with limited internet access [33]. To address this, integrating AI algorithms into smartphone-based devices can make ophthalmic diagnosis more accessible to a larger population. Initially intended for screening and triaging patients for specialist referrals, AI algorithms on smartphones can also facilitate autonomous decisions in the absence of ophthalmic professionals, improving eyecare equity [34, 35]. This requires robust development with diverse datasets, no inherent bias, and real-world testing in the population for which it is intended to be used. Several AI algorithms have been validated on smartphone-based devices (either with adapters or on a standalone basis) for screening DR and glaucoma; these have demonstrated high diagnostic accuracies and have the potential to bridge gaps in eyecare access for a broader population [32–41].

An offline AI algorithm can overcome the limitation of the availability of an internet connection. The Medios AI algorithm is one such innovation implemented after real-world studies to detect referable DR and glaucoma (Fig. 10.14) [20, 33, 34, 36, 37].

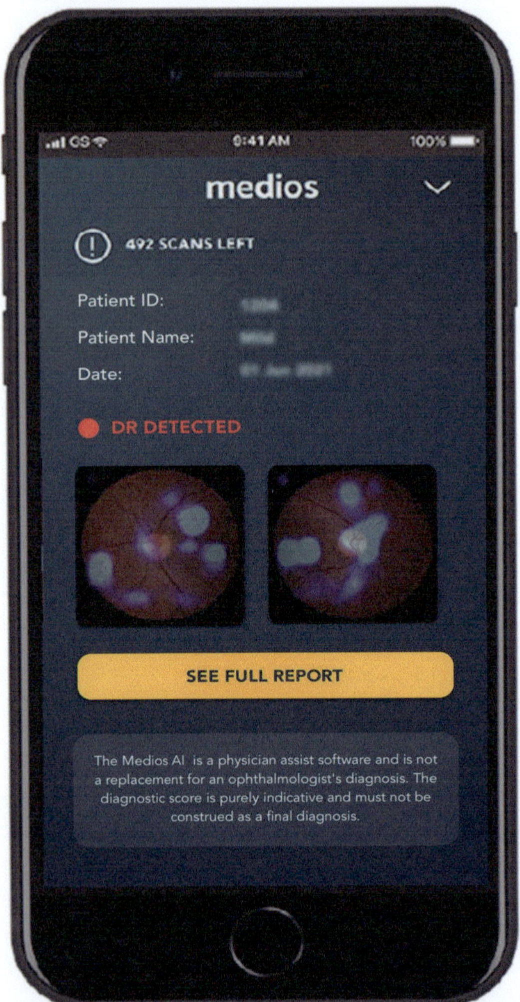

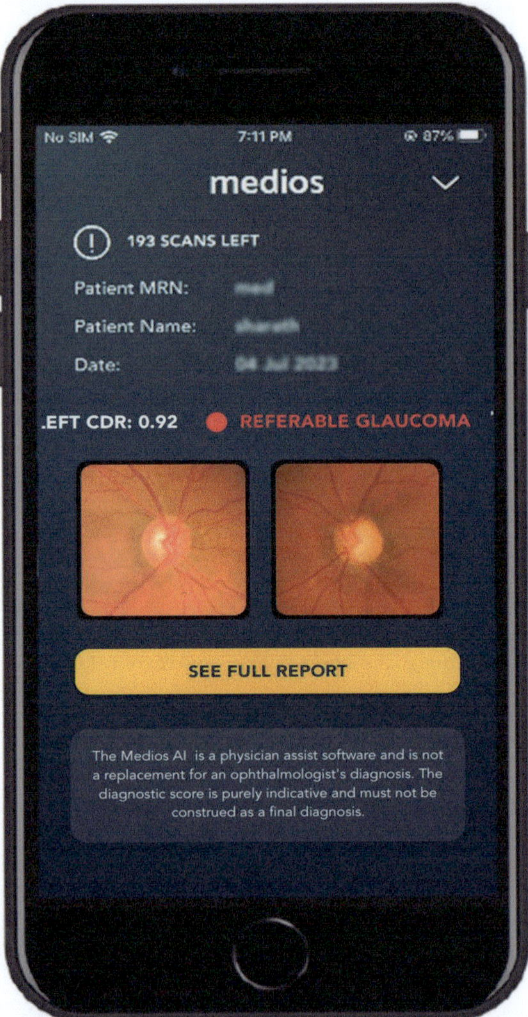

Fig. 10.14 The user Interface of Medios AI, an offline AI algorithm that can generate a report within seconds of image capture highlighting the lesions (left) for referable DR and for referable glaucoma (right)

The technology utilizes shallow architectures to optimize operational efficiency while maintaining high accuracy.

10.6 Smartphone-Based Microscope Video Recording

Intra-operative video recording benefits surgical education, helping patients understand surgical processes and improving overall surgical outcomes. There is a growing demand for high-quality video recordings over verbal feedback, drawings, or images [42]. Smartphones offer a portable and cost-efficient tele-surgical solution for objective, point of view (POV) video recording with good resolution and wireless connectivity [42–44]. Stereoscopic videos captured on smartphones have also been used to create 3D models of body parts, providing enhanced visualization through both anaglyph glasses and head-mounted displays [43, 44].

History: Early examples of using smartphones for surgical video recording were provided by Kimyon et al. and Nair et al. who demonstrated the use of selfie-sticks to record surgical videos [45, 46]. Ho et al. demonstrated the feasibility of smartphone-delivered stereoscopic vision for microsurgical use [47]. Hickman et al. provided a qualitative and quantitative evaluation of the potential of surgical videos captured on smartphones for surgical education and learning via self-recording and self-review across two training facilities in Nepal [48]. The same system was used to transmit 15 different surgeries live via Skype from Nepal to a surgical ophthalmology trainer in South Africa to evaluate the feasibility of live consultation. The overall video quality was high in 65% of the cases for self-review and in 92.9% of live-streamed cases via Skype.

One such device, which was developed in India (Remidio, Bangalore) is described below.

10.6.1 Microscope Recording Device (MRD)

This is a smartphone-based surgical video recording device (Fig. 10.15). It works on an intelligent acquisition software that allows for customized FOV selection, ISO control, and selection of depth of focus during recording, enabling the user to create professional videos [49]. The videos are shared to a local storage wirelessly and seamlessly using proprietary technology. The device can also be used to stream surgeries live on third-party applications. MRD has been compared to current state-of-the-art cameras and has been used to document multiple ophthalmic surgeries [49].

The limitations of the MRD are as follows: (A) it requires custom-designed holders for different smartphone models and (B) it may not be ideal for vitreoretinal surgeries due to low intra-operating light conditions.

10.7 Virtual Reality (VR)-Based Visual Field Perimeter

VR-based perimeters use a VR headset to perform a visual field test. The VR headset contains a display screen and two high-power aspheric lenses to magnify the screen and create a virtual image. The images on the screen are displayed in a side-by-side format, such that after magnification via lenses, the eyes will fuse the two images into one and create depth perception. Though this depth perception is not of much use in VR-based perimeters, the ability to simulate each eye individually offers a big advantage as the visual field is evaluated monocularly and the eye patch is not required in VR-based perimeters. Test programs (24-2, 30-2, 10-2), strategies (thresholding eg. full threshold, Zest, SITA-like; suprathreshold, TOP), and other parameters (reliability and global indices, stimulus presentation, stimulus response window controls) as used in conventional perim-

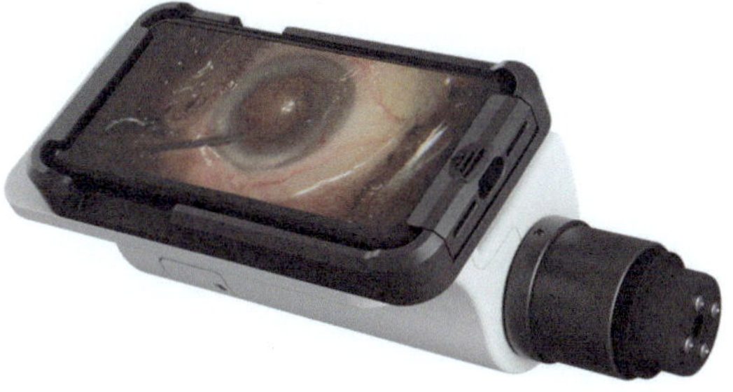

Fig. 10.15 The microscope recording device

eters are made available. In addition, the final report formats remain similar to conventional perimeters; however, they differ in the principle of the projecting stimulus. Such a device is described in Chap. 35.

10.8 Conclusion

Smartphone-based ophthalmic diagnostics have emerged as game-changing technologies in eye care. These devices offer unparalleled convenience, portability, and telemedicine capabilities, enabling enhanced patient triaging, photo documentation, and objective assessments. From the early adapter-based designs to the present-day high-quality devices algorithms, the evolution of smartphone-based ophthalmic diagnostics has witnessed significant advancements. The utilization of AI-based algorithms has further propelled the effectiveness of these devices by automating referrals and reducing dependency on internet connectivity or skilled personnel. As a result, smartphone-based ophthalmic diagnostics hold the potential to bridge gaps in healthcare accessibility, especially in remote and underserved areas, while providing cost-efficient and scalable solutions. With continuous technical advancements and ethical, responsible integration of AI, these devices are set to revolutionize eye care. This may ultimately lead to improved patient outcomes and a significant reduction in preventable eye diseases globally.

Funding Anand Sivaraman: None; Divya Parthasarathy Rao: None; Shanmuganathan Nagarajan: None.

Disclosure Anand Sivaraman: Co-founder, and Shareholder, Remidio Employee; Divya Parthasarathy Rao: Medical Director, Remidio employee; Shanmuganathan Nagarajan: Head of Optics R&D; Remidio Employee.

References

1. Hernández-Neuta I, Neumann F, Brightmeyer J, Ba Tis T, Madaboosi N, Wei Q, et al. Smartphone-based clinical diagnostics: towards democratization of evidence-based health care. J Intern Med. 2019;285(1):19–39.
2. Ramke J, Evans JR, Habtamu E, Mwangi N, Silva JC, Swenor BK, et al. Grand challenges in global eye health: a global prioritisation process using Delphi method. Lancet Healthy Longev. 2022;3(1):e31–41.
3. Kumar A, Vashist P. Indian community eye care in 2020: achievements and challenges. Indian J Ophthalmol. 2020;68(2):291–3.
4. Deshpande M. Vision 2020: right to sight—India. Med J Armed Forces India. 2008;64(4):302–3.
5. Ventola CL. Mobile devices and apps for health care professionals: uses and benefits. Pharm Ther. 2014;39(5):356–64.
6. Iqbal U. Smartphone fundus photography: a narrative review. Int J Retina Vitr. 2021;7:44.
7. Lord RK, Shah VA, San Filippo AN, Krishna R. Novel uses of smartphones in ophthalmology. Ophthalmology. 2010;117(6):1274–1274.e3.
8. Pujari A, Saluja G, Agarwal D, Selvan H, Sharma N. Clinically useful smartphone ophthalmic imaging techniques. Graefes Arch Clin Exp Ophthalmol. 2021;259(2):279–87.
9. Bastawrous A. Smartphone Fundoscopy. Ophthalmology. 2012;119(2):432–433.e2.
10. Haddock LJ, Kim DY, Mukai S. Simple, inexpensive technique for high-quality smartphone fundus photography in human and animal eyes. J Ophthalmol. 2013;2013:e518479.
11. Ryan ME, Rajalakshmi R, Prathiba V, Anjana RM, Ranjani H, Narayan KMV, et al. Comparison among methods of retinopathy assessment (CAMRA) study: smartphone, nonmydriatic, and mydriatic photography. Ophthalmology. 2015;122(10):2038–43.
12. Myung D, Jais A, He L, Blumenkranz MS, Chang RT. 3D printed smartphone indirect lens adapter for rapid, high quality retinal imaging. J Mob Technol Med. 2014;3(1):9–15.
13. Russo A, Morescalchi F, Costagliola C, Delcassi L, Semeraro F. A novel device to exploit the smartphone camera for fundus photography. J Ophthalmol. 2015;2015:e823139.
14. Karakaya M, Hacisoftaoglu RE. Comparison of smartphone-based retinal imaging systems for diabetic retinopathy detection using deep learning. BMC Bioinform. 2020;21(Suppl 4):259.
15. Panwar N, Huang P, Lee J, Keane PA, Chuan TS, Richhariya A, et al. Fundus photography in the 21st century—a review of recent technological advances and their implications for worldwide healthcare. Telemed J E Health. 2016;22(3):198–208.
16. Sivaraman A, Nagarajan S, Vadivel S, Dutt S, Tiwari P, Narayana S, et al. A novel, smartphone-based, teleophthalmology-enabled, Widefield fundus imaging device with an autocapture algorithm. Transl Vis Sci Technol. 2021;10(12):21.
17. Remidio FOP NM-10 | Non Mydriatic Hand Held Fundus Camera [Internet]. [cited 2023 May 16]. https://www.remidio.com/products/fop
18. Rajalakshmi R, Arulmalar S, Usha M, Prathiba V, Kareemuddin KS, Anjana RM, et al. Validation of

smartphone based retinal photography for diabetic retinopathy screening. Merigan WH, editor. PLoS One. 2015;10(9):e0138285.
19. Sengupta S, Sindal MD, Baskaran P, Pan U, Venkatesh R. Sensitivity and specificity of smartphone-based retinal imaging for diabetic retinopathy: a comparative study. Ophthalmol Retina. 2019;3(2):146–53.
20. Natarajan S, Jain A, Krishnan R, Rogye A, Sivaprasad S. Diagnostic accuracy of community-based diabetic retinopathy screening with an offline artificial intelligence system on a smartphone. JAMA Ophthalmol. 2019;137(10):1182–8.
21. Anand S, Pramod K, Shanmuganathan N. Retinal imaging device [internet]. US9398851B2, 2016 [cited 2023 May 16]. https://patents.google.com/patent/US9398851B2/en#citedBy
22. Tran K, Mendel TA, Holbrook KL, Yates PA. Construction of an inexpensive, hand-held fundus camera through modification of a consumer "point-and-shoot" camera. Invest Ophthalmol Vis Sci. 2012;53(12):7600–7.
23. Sivaprasad S, Sahasranamam VI, George S, Sadanandan R, Gopal B, Premnazir L, et al. Burden of diabetic retinopathy amongst people with diabetes attending primary care in Kerala: Nayanamritham Project. J Clin Med. 2021;10(24):5903.
24. Barsam A, Bhogal M, Morris S, Little B. Anterior segment slitlamp photography using the iPhone. J Cataract Refract Surg. 2010;36(7):1240–1.
25. Bolster NM, Giardini ME, Livingstone IA, Bastawrous A. How the smartphone is driving the eye-health imaging revolution. Expert Rev Ophthalmol. 2014;9(6):475–85.
26. Mohammadpour M, Mohammadpour L, Hassanzad M. Smartphone assisted slit lamp free anterior segment imaging: a novel technique in teleophthalmology. Contact Lens Anterior Eye. 2016;39(1):80–1.
27. Pujari A, Kishore A, Makwana T, Sharma N. A simple tool to assess an implantable collamer lens vault. J Cataract Refract Surg. 2019;45(6):883–4.
28. Toslak D, Thapa D, Erol MK, Chen Y, Yao X. Smartphone-based imaging of the corneal endothelium at sub-cellular resolution. J Mod Opt. 2017;64(12):1229–32.
29. Dutt S, Vadivel SS, Nagarajan S, Galagali A, Christy JS, Sivaraman A, et al. A novel approach to anterior segment imaging with smartphones in the COVID-19 era. Indian J Ophthalmol. 2021;69(5):1257–62.
30. Hu S, Wu H, Luan X, Wang Z, Adu M, Wang X, et al. Portable hand-held slit-lamp based on a smartphone camera for cataract screening. J Ophthalmol. 2020;2020:1037689.
31. Dutt S, Nagarajan S, Vadivel SS, Baig AU, Savoy FM, Ganapathy VM, et al. Design and performance characterization of a novel, smartphone-based, portable digital slit lamp for anterior segment screening using telemedicine. Transl Vis Sci Technol. 2021;10(8):29.
32. Dutt S, Sivaraman A, Savoy F, Rajalakshmi R. Insights into the growing popularity of artificial intelligence in ophthalmology. Indian J Ophthalmol. 2020;68(7):1339–46.
33. Sosale B, Aravind SR, Murthy H, Narayana S, Sharma U, Gowda SGV, et al. Simple, mobile-based artificial intelligence algorithm in the detection of diabetic retinopathy (SMART) study. BMJ Open Diabetes Res Care. 2020;8(1):e000892.
34. Sosale B, Sosale A, Murthy H, Sengupta S, Naveenam M. Medios– an offline, smartphone-based artificial intelligence algorithm for the diagnosis of diabetic retinopathy. Indian J Ophthalmol. 2020;68(2):391.
35. Sheikh A, Bhatti A, Adeyemi O, Raja M, Sheikh I. The utility of smartphone-based artificial intelligence approaches for diabetic retinopathy: a literature review and meta-analysis. J Curr Ophthalmol. 2021;33(3):219–26.
36. Varshney T, Parthasarathy DR, Gupta V. Artificial intelligence integrated smartphone fundus camera for screening the glaucomatous optic disc. Indian J Ophthalmol. 2021;69(12):3787.
37. Shroff S, Rao DP, Savoy FM, Shruthi S, Hsu CK, Pradhan ZS, et al. Agreement of a novel artificial intelligence software with optical coherence tomography and manual grading of the optic disc in glaucoma. J Glaucoma. 2023;32(4):280.
38. Li F, Song D, Chen H, Xiong J, Li X, Zhong H, et al. Development and clinical deployment of a smartphone-based visual field deep learning system for glaucoma detection. Npj Digit Med. 2020;3(1):1–8.
39. Nakahara K, Asaoka R, Tanito M, Shibata N, Mitsuhashi K, Fujino Y, et al. Deep learning-assisted (automatic) diagnosis of glaucoma using a smartphone. Br J Ophthalmol. 2022;106(4):587–92.
40. Mrad Y, Elloumi Y, Akil M, Bedoui MH. A fast and accurate method for glaucoma screening from smartphone-captured fundus images. IRBM. 2021;43:279.
41. Chen D, Ho Y, Sasa Y, Lee J, Yen CC, Tan C. Machine learning-guided prediction of central anterior chamber depth using slit lamp images from a portable smartphone device. Biosensors. 2021;11(6):182.
42. Hakimi AA, Hu AC, Pham TT, Wong BJF. High-definition point-of-view intraoperative recording using a smartphone: a hands-free approach: POV surgical recording using a smartphone. Laryngoscope. 2019;129(3):578–81.
43. Barbero-García I, Lerma JL, Marqués-Mateu Á, Miranda P. Low-cost smartphone-based photogrammetry for the analysis of cranial deformation in infants. World Neurosurg. 2017;102:545–54.
44. Philbrick SM, Baskin DE. Recording and viewing stereoscopic ophthalmic surgical videos with smartphones. Can J Ophthalmol. 2018;53(3):222–8.
45. Kimyon S, Pamukcu C, Mete A, Saygılı O. A novel technique for surgical video recording and imaging: smartphone and selfie stick. Surg Innov. 2016;23(6):620–2.
46. Nair AG, Kamal S, Singh S. A "flexible tripod" mounted videocamera: an economical and effective method to record

oculoplastic surgeries. Indian J Ophthalmol. 2019;67(9): 1460–2.

47. Ho DK, hong. Using smartphone-delivered stereoscopic vision in microsurgery: a feasibility study. Eye. 2019;33(6):953–6.
48. Hickman MS, Dean WH, Puri L, Singh S, Siegel R, Patel D. Ophthalmic Telesurgery with a low-cost smartphone video system for surgeon self-reflection and remote synchronous consultation: a qualitative and quantitative study. Telemed Rep. 2022;3(1):30–7.
49. Remidio MRD: How to [Internet]. 2021 [cited 2023 Jun 22]. https://www.youtube.com/watch?v=UPm4pdYKEuM

11 Cataract Grading Systems

Maneck Nicholson, Swapnali Sabhapandit, Mekhla Naik, and Somasheila I. Murthy

11.1 Introduction

The cornerstone of cataract diagnosis is slit lamp biomicroscopic examination. The surgeon needs to determine whether the density of the cataract accounts for the reduction in vision and, therefore, warrants surgery. For such an evaluation to be consistent, it is pertinent to have a standardized system for the grading and classification of cataracts, which would help not only in the accurate diagnosis, grading, and assessment of progression, but also in clinical research and documentation. With the advent of newer technologies, the grading of cataracts has shifted from a subjective to a more objective assessment.

11.2 History

The evolution of cataract surgery over the last quarter of a century has resulted in many iterations in the grading of cataracts. Till the mid-1970s, when intracapsular cataract extraction (ICCE) was the standard of care, qualitative grading systems largely emphasized nuclear color as the index of the severity of cataract formation [1, 2]. Before 1976, animal lenses were erroneously believed to be adequate models of the human lens, and descriptive terms and organizational guidelines varied among clinicians and countries. A summary of these historical classifications is provided in Table 11.1.

M. Nicholson (✉) · M. Naik · S. I. Murthy
Shantilal Shanghvi Eye Institute, Mumbai, India
e-mail: smurthy@lvpei.org

S. Sabhapandit
Institute of Ophthalmic Sciences, AIG Hospitals, Hyderabad, India

T. Das, P. Satgunam (eds.), *Ophthalmic Diagnostics*, https://doi.org/10.1007/978-981-97-0138-4_11

Table 11.1 Historical lens classification system

Classification system	Main features	Advantages	Disadvantages
American Cooperative Cataract Research Group (CCRG)	Divides lens into nucleus and cortex, and further subdivides the cortex into 6 zones: subcapsular anterior (SCA), subcapsular posterior (SCP), anterior cortical (CXA), equatorial cortical (CXE), posterior cortical (CXP), and supranuclear (SN, a zone found between the cortical and the nuclear zones)	Comprehensive system Identifies different zones of opacification	Designed primarily for ex vivo use Photography is tedious
Oxford Clinical Grading System	Uses target projection ophthalmoscopy to generate photographs and assess cataracts, graded on a scale from 0 to 5	In vivo grading system Uses readily available equipment	Variable in inter-observer agreement Mixed results among physicians
Wilmer System	Uses 4 standard photographs for grading nuclear opacity based on visual acuity, density, and extent	High intra- and inter-observer agreement Examines posterior subcapsular and cortical opacities using retroillumination	Inter-observer agreement poor for posterior subcapsular cataracts
Wisconsin Grading System	A semi-quantitative grading system based on a large population-based study, with nuclear sclerosis graded on a scale of 0 to 5 and cortical cataracts in nine separate lens segments	Reproducible	Limited features assessed
Japanese Cooperative Cataract Epidemiological Study Group (JAPCCESG)	Utilizes a set of standard photographs, with cataracts graded as early (I), moderate (II), or advanced (III) and subdivided into cortical, nuclear, and subcapsular opacities	Simple grading system Correlates well with the patient's visual experience of a cataract	Limited features assessed Less comprehensive than other systems

11.3 Lens Opacification Classification System

The lens opacification classification system (LOCS) system was developed in the NEI (National Eye Institute, USA)-sponsored Lens Opacities Case-Control Study [3]. It is a widely used system for classifying and grading lens opacities or cataracts. It helps in assessing the severity and type of cataract present in an individual's eye. It has gone through multiple revisions over the years, with LOCS I and LOCS II being earlier versions and the most recent and widely adopted version LOCS III.

The aim was to provide a simple, highly reproducible system of in vivo cataract classification. This classification uses a set of standard photographs which define the extent of opacification in two major lens zones—cortical and posterior subcapsular—and the intensity of opalescence in the third major zone, the nucleus. Nuclear color and opalescence were evaluated separately, as it was found that the color had less to do with cataract severity than previously thought.

11.3.1 Development of LOCS

The Lens Opacities Classification System I (LOCS I) was developed in 1988 and provided a simpler but reproducible way to classify nuclear, cortical, and posterior subcapsular opacities. It used a combination of subjective grading by ophthalmologists and slit-lamp biomicroscopy to assess cataract severity. It also found for the first time that visual acuity was not a useful criterion, citing that equatorial and anterior cortical opacification could be quite advanced without reducing a patient's visual acuity. This led to the adoption of using a set of standard retroilluminated black-and-white photographs for the classification of cortical and posterior subcapsular cataracts and a single-color slit-lamp photograph for the classification of nuclear color and opalescence. The adoption of this system marked a pivotal shift in cataract assessment by emphasizing morphology over visual acuity. Unaggregated cortical changes played a minor role in visual acuity, prompting LOCS I to prioritize clustered aggregation as an early indicator of cataract.

The Lens Opacities Classification System II (LOCS II) was introduced in 1989 to address some of the shortcomings of LOCS I. It refined the grading scales for nuclear, cortical, and posterior subcapsular opacities, and included additional descriptions for different types of cataracts. LOCS II aimed to reduce subjectivity in grading and improve the consistency of cataract grading among different observers. Although LOCS II was an improvement over LOCS I, some limitations and challenges in accurately classifying and quantifying cataracts remained. Vision was again left out of the grading system, because of the inconsistent relationship between loss of visual acuity and extent of lens abnormality. Instead, colored standards were used, and the number of reference standards was increased. LOCS II uses 4 standards for nuclear opalescence, 5 cortical standards, and 4 subcapsular standards. Good inter-observer and intra-observer agreement in cataract grading made this classification useful for longitudinal as well as cross-sectional cataract studies.

The Lens Opacities Classification System III (LOCS III) is the most recent and widely accepted version of the LOCS system. It was developed in 1993 and introduced an objective grading system that uses standardized photographs of the lens to assess cataract severity. It incorporates five standardized photographs, each representing a specific degree of nuclear opalescence, nuclear color, and cortical and posterior subcapsular cataract. By comparing the patient's lens with the reference photographs, ophthalmologists can assign numerical grades to each component of the cataract, allowing for better quantification and comparison of cataract severity. It was developed by Chylack et al. (1993) [4] and adapted from the LOCS II. Nuclear opalescence (NO) and nuclear color (NC) are graded on a scale of 1–6, cortical cataracts (C) on a scale of 1–5, and posterior subcapsular cataracts on a scale of 1–5. LOCS III grading introduced a paradigm shift in using photographs of the crystalline lens rather than slit-lamp examination in providing a more objective measure of cataract. The decimalized grading and expanded sets of reference photographs provide a more sensitive grading system than LOCS II (Table 11.2).

11.3.2 LOCS III in Clinical Practice (Fig. 11.1)

LOCS III has been used in several cross-section and population studies. It is also important in clinical practice. The essential requirement to effectively use the LOCS III scale for grading cataracts include prior training of the graders (including ophthalmologists), slit lamps with standardized illumination, and availability of colored photographs of the LOCS III scale for quick reference. A Singapore study tested the reliability of LOCS III grading between observers at different levels of ophthalmology experience and inferred that familiarity with the manual and discussion between the graders increased the interobserver agreement [5].

11.3.3 Surgical Implications of LOCS III

One study found a linear correlation between LOCS III features for nuclear color and opalescence and average phacoemulsification power and time [6]. An increase in the nuclear density of cataract was found to increase the phacoemulsification energy exponentially. LOCS III is, therefore, a useful tool in creating a surgical plan for nuclear cataract procedures [7–9]. The relation of the lens density (measured by IOL-Master 700

Table 11.2 Comparison of LOCS I, II, and III

Classification method	LOCS I	LOCS II	LOCS III
Nuclear Opalescence (NO)	0–2	0–4	1–6
Nuclear Color (NC)	0–2	0–2	1–6
Posterior Subcapsular Cataract (PSC)	0–2	0–4	1–5
Cortical Cataract (CC)	0–2	0–5	1–5
Methodology	Set of standard photographs, consisting of one slit-lamp color photograph used to grade nuclear opalescence and nuclear color and three black-and-white retroillumination photographs used for posterior subcapsular and cortical classifications. The standard photographs are reproduced on an 8.5 × 11 inch transparency and placed on a light box located at eye level behind the patient's right shoulder when the patient is seated at the slit lamp. The classifier can easily refer to the standards during the examination, which is done with the patient's pupils maximally dilated.	Nuclear color (NC) is graded by comparing the color of the posterior cortical–posterior subcapsular reflex to the nuclear I (NI) standard (the same standard used in LOCS I). The examiner uses the low-magnification view of the slit lamp with the slit beam oriented approximately 45° to the patient's visual axis, and the slit height and brightness are set to equal those in the standard photograph. The classifier envisions an aggregate opacity by aggregating all contiguous and non-contiguous opacities into one zone. The size of the opaque zone relative to the size of the opaque zone in the standards determines the class chosen to grade the cataract. In the LOCS classification, the cortical and posterior subcapsular zones are graded individually as C and P.	

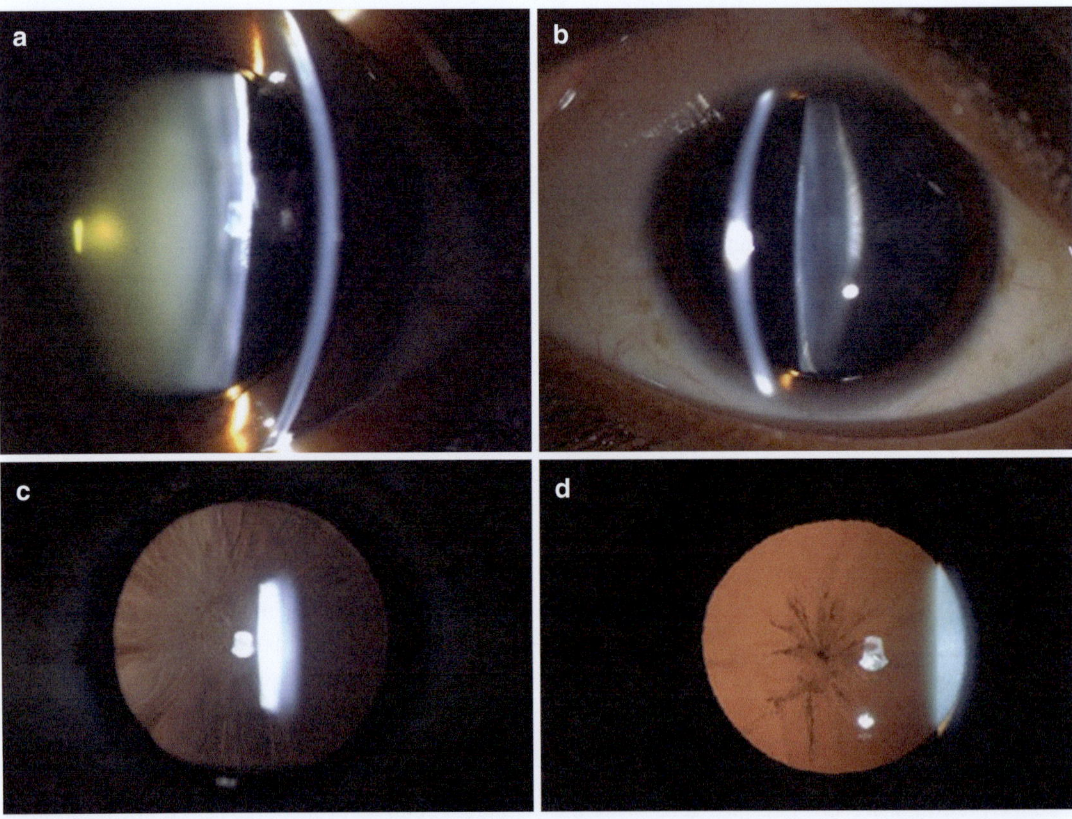

Fig. 11.1 LOCS III grading system. (**a**) Cross-sectional view of nuclear opalescence (**NO4, NC4**). (**b**) Cross-sectional view of nuclear opalescence of grade (**NO1, NC1**). (**c**) Cortical cataract with a central posterior subcapsular cataract in retroillumination (**C4P1**). (**d**) Posterior subcapsular cataract (**P3**)

(Carl Zeiss, Germany), using Swept source-optical coherence tomography, SS-OCT, technology) and phacodynamic parameters has also shown a significant correlation [10].

11.3.4 Limitations of LOCS III

Despite being a widely used system in crystalline lens classification, LOCS III is not without limitations [4]. First, the system relies on subjective assessments by clinicians, introducing variability and inconsistencies in grading. Second, it may not adequately capture important aspects of cataracts beyond lens opacity, such as their impact on vision quality or specific opacities. Third, the grading scale's ordinal categories may lack the necessary granularity to accurately represent the full range of cataract severity. Four, there is no categorization for anterior subcapsular or polar cataracts. LOCS III was primarily developed using data from older populations and may be subject to age-related biases. Regular maintenance of slit lamps and bulbs is necessary to prevent grading errors caused by inadequate illumination. Lastly, while LOCS III is commonly used in research, its clinical relevance and predictive ability for visual outcomes are limited.

11.4 Other Methods of Classification

11.4.1 Slit Lamp Based

1. Duncan et al. (1997) [11] proposed an objective classification system for nuclear opacification based on computer analysis of slit-lamp images of human lenses. They used a digital camera to capture the images of the lenses and then applied image processing techniques to analyze opacification patterns in the images. The image analysis included different levels of nuclear opacity and identified various characteristics of the opacity, such as the location and size of the opacity, its color, and its texture. Based on these characteristics, nuclear opacities were categorized into five grades, from grade 0 (no visible opacity) to grade 4 (severe opacity that obscures the underlying structures of the lens). This system is also reported to have good agreement between observers.
2. Hall et al. (1999) [12] proposed a novel method to assess the severity of nuclear cataracts by developing a laser slit-lamp. This device comprises an illumination arm that generates a slit of laser light, a viewing arm with an attached beam splitter, and a high-sensitivity charge-coupled device (CCD) camera. A video image of the laser-illuminated anterior segment is sent to a computer, and the amount of light backscattered from the lens nucleus is used to grade the cataract. Image analysis software is used to calculate the measure of lens opacity for each laser slit-lamp image. The study found a linear relationship and good correlation between LOCS III scores and laser slit-lamp grading.
3. Babizhayev et al. (2003) [13] used intraocular light scattering to grade cataracts. An increase in the light scattering due to random fluctuations in the refractive index of cataractous eyes contributes to the impairment of the retinal image. This degradation is due to the forward scattering of the light. However, for a clinician using the slit-lamp, only the backscatter of light is available to diagnose cataract severity. Babizhayev et al. (2003) designed a diagnostic instrument, the Halometer, to measure intraocular light scattering. They introduced a new method of computer-generated analysis of lens images to measure the severity of cataracts. The researchers used the grading methods of Taylor and West (1989) [3] to objectively document and grade the lens opacities seen on a slit-lamp image. They generated 3D topography images of the lens to provide a better understanding of lens characteristics.
4. Li et al. (2009) [14] described a technique that addressed the disadvantage of the system proposed by Duncan et al. (1997) [11] (the John Hopkins group). Given that Duncan et al.

(1997) used features along the visual axis ignoring the rest of the lens, the model was based solely on anatomical landmarks. In this study, anatomical structure in the lens image was detected using a modified active shape model (ASM) which was described by the authors in earlier work [15]. Based on the anatomical landmark, local features were extracted. Support vector machine regression was employed to train a grading model for grade prediction. The success rate of this feature extraction was 95%.

5. Srivastava et al. (2014) [16] built the lens classification system as an extension of their earlier work of an automatic grading system for nuclear cataracts, the Automatic Cataract Screening from Image Analysis Nuclear Cataract (Version 0.10). In a healthy eye, clear visibility of the lens parts leads to distinct edges in the lens region, but these edges become less distinct with increasing severity of cataracts. At higher grades of nuclear cataract, these landmarks are less distinct. This indicates the utility of gradient information for the NC grading task. Their classification focuses on the automatic grading of nuclear cataract (NC) from slit-lamp images, aiming to reduce the labor-intensive process of manual grading. The authors incorporated visibility cues by introducing gray-level image gradient-based features for the automatic grading of NC.

11.4.2 Using Retinal Images

1. Abdul Rahman et al. (2008) [17] used Discrete Fourier Transforms (DFT) to quantify the optical degradation of a retinal image of a cataractous eye.
2. Xiong et al. (2017) [18] developed a method independent of slit-lamp images using blurriness in retinal images with vitreous opacity. They analyzed the three types of data: the pixel number of visible structures, mean contrast between vessels and background, and local standard deviation. Based on the extracted features, a decision tree was trained to classify retinal images into five grades of blurriness. This system graded cataracts with an 81.1% accuracy and a kappa value of 0.7435, compared to clinical grading.

11.4.3 Using Other Imaging Modalities

1. Wong et al. (2015) [19] compared the reliability of lens density measurements with anterior segment optical coherence tomography (AS-OCT) and its association with LOCS III grading. Significant correlations were found between LOCS III NO and NC scores and the AS-OCT nuclear cataract density measurements. The association score was slightly higher than LOCS III and had high repeatability; thus, the AS-OCT provides a better surrogate of lens density than the colors of the LOCS III scoring system. Unlike Scheimpflug photography, AS-OCT provides a clear visualization of the posterior cortex and capsule of the lens. However, this study only evaluated lens nucleus density and ignored the anterior and posterior cortex.
2. Pei et al. (2008) [20] aimed to investigate the relationship between lens density measured with the Pentacam (Oculus GmbH, Germany) Scheimpflug System and the LOCS III scoring system. A positive linear relationship between the lens density measured by the Pentacam and the LOCS III grading score was observed, with a stronger correlation with the nuclear opacity (NO) score than nuclear color (NC) score. The study concluded that lens density as a quantitative and objective parameter can represent the degree of nuclear opacity and associated visual impairment due to nuclear cataract.

11.4.4 Deep Learning Artificial Intelligence in Cataract Classification

In recent years, deep learning (DL) has emerged as a promising tool for the automatic detection

Table 11.3 Overview of deep learning artificial intelligence in cataract classification systems

Study	AI method	Image analysis	Result
Xu et al. (2013) [21]	Group Sparsity Regression (GSR)	Slit-lamp images	Mean absolute error of 0.336 and 69.0% integral agreement ratio with clinical grading
Gao et al. (2015) [22]	Convolutional-Recursive Neural Networks (CRNN)	Medical images	70.7% exact agreement ratio against clinical integral grading
Wu et al. (2019) [23]	Residual Neural Network (ResNet)	Eye images	Established a 3-step sequential AI algorithm for the diagnosis and referral of cataracts
Zhang et al. (2017) [24]	Deep Convolutional Neural Network	Fundus images, pre-processed with a G-channel filter	Achieved an AUC of 93.52% for cataract detection and 86.69% for severity grading
Dong et al. (2017) [24]	Combination of machine learning and deep learning	Fundus images	Reported high levels of accuracy for cataract detection and severity grading
Li et al. (2018) [24]	Deep learning with ResNet-18 and ResNet-50	Fundus images, pre-processed with a G-channel filter	Achieved an AUC of 87.7% for severity grading and 97.2% for cataract detection
Ran et al. (2018) [24]	Combination of deep convolutional neural network and random forest	Slit-lamp images	Achieved high levels of accuracy for cataract detection and grading, outperforming other state-of-the-art methods

and grading of cataracts from various types of medical images. Several studies have explored different DL techniques and algorithms for achieving accurate and reliable diagnoses (Table 11.3).

11.5 Conclusion

The progress made in grading systems over the years indicates the continued research toward improving the diagnosis and management of cataract. Integrating digital imaging technology and artificial intelligence algorithms has further enhanced the accuracy and efficiency of cataract grading systems, assisting clinicians with a more comprehensive and reliable diagnosis. With the increasing prevalence of cataracts and an aging population, the need for accurate and efficient grading systems is more crucial than before.

Funding None.

Disclosure None.

References

1. Pirie A. Color and solubility of the proteins of human cataracts. Investig Ophthalmol. 1968;7(6):634–50.
2. Truscott RJ, Augusteyn RC. Changes in human lens proteins during nuclear cataract formation. Exp Eye Res. 1977;24(2):159–70.
3. Taylor HR, West SK. The clinical grading of lens opacities. Aust N Z J Ophthalmol. 1989;17(1):81–6.
4. Chylack LT Jr, Wolfe JK, Singer DM, et al. The lens opacities classification system III. The Longitudinal Study of Cataract Study Group. Arch Ophthalmol. 1993;111(6):831–6.
5. Tan AC, Loon SC, Choi H, Thean L. Lens opacities classification system III: cataract grading variability between junior and senior staff at a Singapore hospital. J Cataract Refract Surg. 2008;34(11):1948–52.
6. Bencic G, Zoric-Geber M, Saric D, Corak M, Mandic Z. Clinical importance of the lens opacities classification system III (LOCS III) in phacoemulsification. Coll Antropol. 2005;29(Suppl 1):91–4.
7. Davison JA, Chylack LT. Clinical application of the lens opacities classification system III in the performance of phacoemulsification. J Cataract Refract Surg. 2003;29(1):138–45.
8. Makhotkina NY, Berendschot T, van den Biggelaar F, Weik ARH, Nuijts R. Comparability of subjective and objective measurements of nuclear density in cataract patients. Acta Ophthalmol. 2018;96(4):356–63.

9. Lim SA, Hwang J, Hwang KY, Chung SH. Objective assessment of nuclear cataract: comparison of double-pass and Scheimpflug systems. J Cataract Refract Surg. 2014;40(5):716–21.
10. Wu X, Chen L, Li Z, Zhao YE. Correlation between lens density measured by swept-source optical coherence tomography and phacodynamic parameters of centurion phacoemulsification. Curr Eye Res. 2023;48:1–9.
11. Duncan DD, Shukla OB, West SK, Schein OD. New objective classification system for nuclear opacification. J Opt Soc Am A Opt Image Sci Vis. 1997;14(6):1197–204.
12. Hall NF, Lempert P, Shier RP, Zakir R, Phillips D. Grading nuclear cataract: reproducibility and validity of a new method. Br J Ophthalmol. 1999;83(10):1159–63.
13. Babizhayev MA, Deyev AI, Yermakova VN, et al. Image analysis and glare sensitivity in human age-related cataracts. Clin Exp Optom. 2003;86(3):157–72.
14. Li H, Lim JH, Liu J, et al. An automatic diagnosis system of nuclear cataract using slit-lamp images. Annu Int Conf IEEE Eng Med Biol Soc. 2009;2009:3693–6.
15. Li H, Lim JH, Liu J, Wong TY. Towards automatic grading of nuclear cataract. Annu Int Conf IEEE Eng Med Biol Soc. 2007;2007:4961–4.
16. Srivastava R, Gao X, Yin F, et al. Automatic nuclear cataract grading using image gradients. J Med Imaging (Bellingham). 2014;1(1):014502.
17. Abdul-Rahman AM, Molteno T, Molteno AC. Fourier analysis of digital retinal images in estimation of cataract severity. Clin Experiment Ophthalmol. 2008;36(7):637–45.
18. Xiong L, Li H, Xu L. An approach to evaluate blurriness in retinal images with vitreous opacity for cataract diagnosis. J Healthc Eng. 2017;2017:5645498.
19. Wong AL, Leung CK, Weinreb RN, et al. Quantitative assessment of lens opacities with anterior segment optical coherence tomography. Br J Ophthalmol. 2009;93(1):61–5.
20. Pei X, Bao Y, Chen Y, Li X. Correlation of lens density measured using the Pentacam Scheimpflug system with the Lens Opacities Classification System III grading score and visual acuity in age-related nuclear cataract. Br J Ophthalmol. 2008;92(11):1471–5.
21. Xu Y, Gao X, Lin S, et al. Automatic grading of nuclear cataracts from slit-lamp lens images using group sparsity regression. Med Image Comput Comput Assist Interv. 2013;16(Pt 2):468–75.
22. Gao X, Lin S, Wong TY. Automatic feature learning to grade nuclear cataracts based on deep learning. IEEE Trans Biomed Eng. 2015;62(11):2693–701.
23. Wu X, Huang Y, Liu Z, et al. Universal artificial intelligence platform for collaborative management of cataracts. Br J Ophthalmol. 2019;103(11):1553–60.
24. Goh JHL, Lim ZW, Fang X, et al. Artificial intelligence for cataract detection and management. Asia Pac J Ophthalmol (Phila). 2020;9(2):88–95.

12 Biometry and Intraocular Lens Power Calculation

Swapnali Sabhapandit, Srinivas K. Rao, Dennis S. C. Lam, Afra Abdussamad, Mounica Sai Konda, and Sanjeev P. Srinivas

12.1 Introduction

Cataract surgery is one of the most common surgical procedures performed worldwide [1]. Along with removing the cataractous lens, cataract surgery aims to provide clear vision to the patient with or without glasses. Therefore, accurate intraocular lens (IOL) power calculation is essential. The refractive power of the eye primarily depends on the cornea, the lens, the ocular media, and the axial length (AL) of the eye. Hence, the corneal curvature, the anterior chamber depth, and the AL should be accurately measured to precisely calculate the power of the IOL to be implanted and its final position in the eye. The power of the IOL is calculated from these parameters.

12.2 Biometry

The calculations for determining the power of IOLs have undergone several generations of changes. Monofocal IOLs, which provide good uncorrected distance vision after surgery, continue to be the most popular choice of IOLs even today. Precision biometry is essential for implanting premium IOLs, such as multifocal and toric IOLs.

Steps in the calculation of IOL power include [2]:

1. Measuring the corneal power (keratometry) and AL of the eye.
2. Using the appropriate IOL calculation formula.

The decision to use emmetropia for distance versus mono vision is discussed with the patient, and IOL power is decided based on these parameters.

12.2.1 Types of Biometry

12.2.1.1 Ultrasound Biometry

Technology: In ultrasound biometry, the time taken for the ultrasound waves to travel through

S. Sabhapandit (✉) · M. S. Konda
Institute of Ophthalmic Sciences, AIG Hospitals, Hyderabad, India

S. K. Rao · S. P. Srinivas
Darshan Eye Care and Surgical Centre, Chennai, India

D. S. C. Lam
International Eye Research Institute of The Chinese University of Hong Kong, Shenzhen, China

C-Mer International Eyecare Group, Hong Kong, China
e-mail: dennislam@hkcmer.com

A. Abdussamad
GMR Varalakshmi Campus, L V Prasad Eye Institute, Vishakhapatnam, India

T. Das, P. Satgunam (eds.), *Ophthalmic Diagnostics*, https://doi.org/10.1007/978-981-97-0138-4_12

Table 12.1 Comparison of ultrasound and optical biometry

Ultrasound biometry	Optical biometry
Measures along the anatomical axis	Measures along the visual axis
Measures AL from the corneal epithelium to the internal limiting membrane of retina	Measures AL from the corneal epithelium to the Bruch's membrane
Uses ultrasound waves (10 MHz)	Uses infrared light waves (780–820 nm; 8× resolution of UV rays)
AL accuracy: 0.10–0.12 mm	AL accuracy: 0.012 mm
Corneal contact required	No corneal contact
Operator variations: Significant	Operator variations: Negligible
Cost-effective	Expensive

AL Axial length, *UV* Ultraviolet

the eye is used to estimate the AL of the eye. However, this step has the maximum chances of errors as contact with the applanation probe can indent the cornea, resulting in an underestimation of the AL. The immersion method of ultrasound biometry avoids compression of the cornea [2].

Clinical application: Although ultrasound biometry can measure the anterior chamber depth and the lens thickness in addition to the AL, it does not provide keratometry values; hence, the corneal power must be measured with a keratometer or topographer.

12.2.1.2 Optical Biometry

Recently, optical biometry methods have been used to calculate AL and corneal power more accurately (Table 12.1) [2].

Technology: Optical biometry is a non-contact automated method. Three models are widely available and employ different techniques, such as laser partial coherence interferometry (PCI), optical low-coherence reflectometry (OLCR), and swept-source optical coherence tomography (SS-OCT). They offer the advantage of performing both keratometry and AL measurements. The comparison between the three technologies is shown in Table 12.2.

12.2.1.3 Newer Technologies in Biometry

The recently evolved biometry technologies are listed in Table 12.3.

12.2.1.3.1 IOL Master 500 (Carl Zeiss Meditec AG, Jena, Germany)

This PCI-based optical biometer was launched in 2000.

Technology: The IOL Master 500 uses an infrared light wave (780 nm)-emitting semiconductor laser diode. It measures optical AL instead of anatomical AL, which results in better refractive outcomes after cataract surgery.

Clinical Application: It performs keratometry, measures AL and other ocular parameters, and calculates IOL power. Its main limitations are its inability to measure AL in opaque media like dense cataracts and patients with low visual acuity because of fixation difficulties [3].

12.2.1.3.2 IOL Master 700 (Carl Zeiss Meditec AG, Jena, Germany)

This is the first swept-source OCT-based optical biometer device.

Technology: It uses 1050 nm wavelength lasers to create OCT images of the entire eye and helps the surgeon to visualize entire longitudinal sections of the eye. The device performs 2000 scans/second. Compared to the IOL master 500, this device has a higher acquisition rate for measuring AL in eyes with dense and posterior subcapsular cataracts.

Clinical Application: It can calculate AL precisely in poorly fixating eyes with the help of foveal images. This fixation check can also help find macular pathologies like macular holes, which can be verified with retina OCT. Additionally, it can identify unusual ocular geometries like lens tilt or decentration [4].

12.2.1.3.3 AL-Scan (Nidek, Gamagori, Japan)

Technology: The PCI-based biometer uses an 830 nm infrared laser diode for AL measurement

Table 12.2 Comparison of IOL Master 500, IOL Master 700, and Lenstar biometry

Parameters	IOL Master 500 (Carl Zeiss Meditec AG, Jena, Germany)	LENSTAR (Haag Streit, Koeniz, Switzerland)	IOL Master 700
Technology	Partial coherence interferometry (PCI)	Optical low-coherence reflectometry (OLCR)	Swept-source optical coherence tomography (SS-OCT)
Light source	Semiconductor diode laser (780 nm)	Superluminescent diode laser (820 nm)	Rapid-cycle tunable wavelength laser Source (1050 nm)
Principle	Laser interferometry; dual-beam setup, reflection from the cornea and reflection from retina assessed in parallel	Laser interferometry; Standard Michelson interferometer setup, a patented rotating glass cube system is used to change the optical path length in the reference arm	SS-OCT technology; Length measurement is based on swept-source frequency-domain OCT enabling a 44 mm scan depth with 22 μ resolution in tissue.
White to white diameter	Range: 8–16 mm; Resolution: 0.1 mm	Range: 7–16 mm; Resolution: 0.01 mm	Range: 8–16 mm Resolution: 0.1 mm
Keratometry	Range: 5–10 mm Resolution: 0.01 mm Measured at 6 points	Range: 5–10.5 mm Resolution: 0.01 mm Measured at 32 points	Range: 5–11 mm Resolution: 0.01 mm Measured at 18 points
Anterior chamber depth	Not measured directly; it uses an image-based slit lamp system for ACD measurements, measured from the front of the cornea to the front of the lens Range: 1.5–6.5 mm Resolution: 0.01 mm	Measures ACD directly; measures aqueous depth from the back of the cornea to the front of the lens Range: 1.5–6.5 mm Resolution: 0.01 mm	Measured from the front of the cornea to the front of the lens Range: 0.7–8 mm Resolution: 0.01 mm
Axial length	Range: 14–38 mm Resholution: 0.01 mm	Range: 14–32 mm Resolution: 0.01 mm	Range: 14–38 mm Resolution: 0.01 mm
Corneal thickness	Not measured	Measured Range: 0.3–0.8 mm	Measured Range: 0.2–1.2 mm
Lens thickness	Not measured	Measured Range: 0.5–6.5 mm	1–10 mm (phakic eye), 0.13–2.5 mm (pseudophakic eye)
Retinal thickness	Not measured	Measured	Measured
Ability to perform biometry through dense cataracts	Poor	Better	Better penetration rates even in dense cataracts

ACD Anterior chamber depth, *OCT* Optical coherence tomography

[5]. In 10 s, the machine can measure AL, the radius of the corneal curvature, anterior chamber depth, central corneal thickness, white-to-white distance (WWD), and pupil size. Anterior segment observation is done with Scheimpflug imaging and double mire ring keratometry. It has three-dimensional auto-tracking technology to follow eye movements along the *X*–*Y*–*Z* directions to ensure accurate eye alignment. Once the appropriate alignment is completed, the automated scanner immediately captures the image and data. It also has an in-built ultrasound biometer.

12.2.1.3.4 Aladdin Ocular Biometer (Topcon, Tokyo, Japan)

Technology. It combines OLCR biometry (using an 820 nm superluminescent diode) with anterior topography, Zernike corneal wavefront analysis, and pupillometry [6]. It provides information about corneal asphericity by mapping 24 Placido ring reflections and analyzing 1024 data points

Table 12.3 Newer biometry machines

Name	Launch year	Technology	Advantages
Al-scan (Nidek)	2012	Partial coherence interferometry	1. Rapid assessment 2. 3D auto-tracking 3. In-built ultrasound biometer
Aladdin (Topcon)	2012	OLCR biometry	1. Extensive corneal topography 2. Keratoconus screening 3. Onboard toric IOL calculators: Barrett IOL suite and Abulafia–Koch regression formula 4. Post-refractive IOL calculations 5. Aberrometry analysis (Zernike)
Galilei G6 (Ziemer)	2019	OCT-based	1. High-definition topography, anterior segment tomography, and optical biometry 2. Designed for femto cataracts 3. Patented iris-based motion compensation 4. Artificial intelligence-based programs for screening ectasia-susceptible corneas
Eyestar 900 (Haag Streit)	2017	SS-OCT	1. Built-in tear film quality assessment leads to highly precise keratometry, complemented by swept-source OCT-based laser precision biometry, topography, pachymetry, and tonometry of the entire eye. 2. Anterior chamber B-scan imaging, including the lens, helps in the identification of lens tilt and decentration 3. All data needed can be collected in less than 40 s
Argos (Movu)	2020	SS-OCT	1. Image acquisition for biometry and keratometry takes less than 1 s 1. High accuracy even in densest cataracts through enhanced retinal visualization mode 1. Equipped with video keratometry
OA 2000 (Tomey)	2014	Fourier domain OCT	1. High tissue penetration capability, which enables high-speed scans even through dense cataracts 2. Integrates topography, AL, lens thickness, and pachymetry which yields the perfect data set for ray tracing

AL Axial length, *IOL* Intraocular lens, *OCT* Optical coherence tomography, *OLCR* Optical low-coherence reflectometry, SS-OCT Swept-source optical coherence tomography;

using its real corneal radii technology. The images are captured at a working distance of around 8 cm.

Clinical Application: It also provides extensive information on the status of the anterior surface of the cornea, including the presence of corneal irregularities, keratoconus, and higher order aberrations. Pupillometry uses infrared and white laser emission diodes (LEDs) to assess photopic and mesopic pupil sizes.

12.2.1.3.5 Galilei G6 Dual Scheimpflug Analyzer (Ziemer, Port, Switzerland)

Technology: The Galilei G6 combines OCT-based scanning for optical biometry, dual-Scheimpflug imaging, and Placido-disc topography [7]. The topography provides data on anterior corneal curvature, surface irregularities, and tear film quality. The Scheimpflug tomography provides corneal pachymetry and elevation data, 3-D anterior chamber analysis, and ray tracing capabilities. Optical biometry allows the determination of AL, lens thickness (LT), and other intraocular distances for planning the construction of premium IOLs. The repeatability and reproducibility of the scanning results from the Galilei G6 device have a high level of agreement with those from the Pentacam.

12.2.1.3.6 Eyestar 900 (Haag Streit, Koeniz, Switzerland)

This launched in 2017.

Technology: The SS-OCT technology provides precise measurements, comprehensive topography (elevation map of the front and back of the cornea) and pachymetry maps, complete cornea-to-retina biometry, keratometry, and high-quality, detailed cross-sectional eye images [8]. The SS-OCT also improves the signal-to-noise ratio because the narrow-bandwidth wavelength light source has high tissue penetration and image quality.

12.2.1.3.7 Argos Advanced Optical Biometer (Movu, Santa Clara, CA)

Technology: This biometer uses the 1060 nm and 20 nm bandwidth SS-OCT technology to obtain two-dimensional OCT images of the entire eye [3]. The AL is measured from the corneal surface to the retinal pigment epithelium using refractive indexes that correspond to each tissue; this ensures that the AL is the sum of four lengths from four segments, namely corneal thickness, anterior chamber depth, lens thickness, and the thickness of the vitreous humor. Keratometry is obtained from OCT information in combination with a 2.1 mm diameter ring made up of 16 infrared LEDs. The unit displays the anterior corneal radius of curvature (R), the average value (RAV), and the K readings using a 1.3375 corneal index of refraction.

12.2.1.3.8 OA-2000 (Tomey, GmbH, Nurnberg, Germany)

Technology: This Fourier domain OCT combines optical biometry, corneal topography, and keratometry values to provide anterior chamber depth, AL, and central corneal thickness [3]. It measures corneal curvature using a Placido disc-based topography technique and has nine rings, each with 256 points, in a 5.5 mm zone projected onto the cornea. The latter helps create a topography map to detect irregular astigmatism and compare the pre-and post-surgery shape of the cornea. It is also helpful for analyzing eyes after laser-assisted in situ keratomileusis (LASIK) and other refractive procedures and for implantation of toric IOLs (to identify the axis of orientation of the toric IOL).

12.3 IOL Power Calculation Formulae

The formulae for calculating power for IOLs have evolved through several iterations; these are discussed below.

1. *Theoretical*: The first-generation formulae were based on mathematical and geometric principles used in the optics of the eye and theoretical constants [9]. They used a fixed power based on the patient's refraction and the optics of the eye.
2. *Regression:* These are the second-generation formulae. These were calculated by analyzing postoperative outcomes and using this data retrospectively, by regression analysis, to arrive at the desired IOL power [10].
3. *Vergence:* The third and fourth-generation formulae incorporate theoretical (geometric optics) and regression formulae. These are used to accurately estimate the effective lens position, i.e., the distance from the cornea to the principal plane of the IOL [9].
4. *Ray tracing*: In this method, the biometer uses individual rays that refract light on all surfaces of the lens and cornea [9]. It calculates the postoperative lens position as a fraction of the crystalline lens thickness and the anterior chamber depth (ACD). This approach allows accurate calculation of the lens position independent of the corneal status.
5. Deep learning and artificial intelligence (AI): Recently, to overcome the difficulties in predicting refractive outcomes of different IOLs, deep learning of large datasets and AI networks has been used to fine-tune such outcomes [9]. The Hill-RBF (Radial Basis Function) calculator, Ladas Superformula, Kane formula, FullMonte IOL software, Multilayer Perceptron (MLP), and Support Vector Machine Regression model are some of the newer AI-powered software where the refractive outcome for a particular IOL is

Table 12.4 Classification of IOL power calculation methods

Method	Formula
Historical/ refraction based	IOL power = (1.25 × pre-op spherical equivalent
Regression analysis based	SRK I, SRK II
Vergence formulae based	Two variables: SRK-T; Holladay 1; Hoffer Q Three variables: Haigis, Ladas Five variables: Barrett Universal II Seven variables: Holladay 2
Artificial intelligence based	Hill-RBF Clarke neural network
Ray tracing based	Oculix PhacoOptics Olsen

IOL Intraocular lens

predicated on the input of variables like the K value, ACD, AL, surgeon factor, and desired refraction. For example, studies have shown that Hill-RBF 2.0 online software is highly reliable as the post-surgery refractive error after using this software is less than 0.5D.

12.3.1 Classification of Different Formulae for Calculating the Power for IOLs

In 2017, Koch et al. introduced a classification for the formulae used to calculate the power of IOLs to celebrate the 50th anniversary of Fyodorov's sentinel article on a formula for calculating the power of an IOL [11]. The classification, the method of calculation, and the data used for these formulae are shown in Table 12.4.

12.4 Newer Formulae

The newer generation formulae include the Holladay 2, Barrett Universal II, and the Hill-RBF [9, 12]. The common factor in all these formulae (except the Hill-RBF) is the need to predict the effective lens position (ELP).

The **Holladay I** is a third-generation regression formula based on AL. The outcomes for eyes with ALs between 22.00 mm and 26.00 mm are comparable to other third-generation formulae, such as the SRK/T [9].

The **Hoffer Q** is a third-generation formula useful for eyes with AL <22.00 mm as it performs better than other third-generation formulae for these conditions [12].

The **SRK/T:** This popular third-generation formula is more accurate for long eyeballs (with AL >26.00 mm) as compared to other third-generation formulae [13].

The **Holladay 2:** This is a fourth-generation formula [9]. It uses keratometry values, AL, ACD, lens thickness, horizontal white-to-white diameter (WTW), patient age, and preoperative refraction to calculate ELP and appropriate IOL power. However, no one has reported if its use is more advantageous than appropriately selected third-generation formulae.

The **Olsen:** This is a fourth-generation formula using keratometry, AL, ACD, lens thickness, and horizontal WTW values [9]. This formula performs better than third-generation formulae for eyes with ALs between 20.00 mm and 26.00 mm.

The **Haigis:** This is a fifth-generation formula. Very good outcomes have been reported for eyes across the AL range using this formula [9]. The accuracy is maintained for eyes >28.00 mm. For best results, three IOL constants are needed, and the normative data of at least 500 eyes must be optimized to arrive at the accurate IOL power.

The **Barrett Universal II (Barrett U2):** This formula is suitable for all types of eyes regardless of the AL. It also predicts the power for all types of IOL designs available today [9]. The AL, keratometry values, optical ACD, desired postoperative refraction, and optional variables of lens thickness and horizontal WTW are required for IOL power calculation. This method is advantageous because it can predict the powers of IOLs for highly myopic eyes and negative-powered IOLs without requiring specialized constants or AL modification.

The **Hill-Radial Basis Activation Function:** This is an online AI-powered formula calculator which shows great promise in optimizing refractive outcomes in the future for any type of IOL [9]. It is not dependent on the ELP and uses normative data from 12,400 eyes to predict the refractive success of a particular IOL. This calculator is available on the Lenstar suite biometer.

The **Okulix:** This newer IOL formula calculation program is based on the "ray tracing" principle. It introduces the concept of the "true geometrical position" of the IOL. It uses the anterior and posterior central curvature radii, asphericity of IOL surfaces, central IOL thickness, and index of refraction to describe the IOL position. It may find particular use for the positioning of toric and phakic IOLs and calculating the powers for IOLs in post-keratorefractive surgery eyes [14].

Intraoperative wavefront aberrometry: This topographer can perform aphakic and pseudophakic refractive measurements in the operating room during surgery. This allows the surgeon to confirm or revise the power of the IOL during surgery, optimize the IOL location, and plan arcuate corneal incisions based on the requirements for astigmatic corneas [15].

Clarke's neural network: This is a computer-based neural network that mimics biological neurons to predict a mathematical correlation with the multiple inputs received by the network. The advantage of such a network is that it can predict a single outcome from multiple variables, including discontinuous predictions, and is unbiased with initial data. Clarke et al. used such a network with inputs on preoperative AL, K values, ACD, and lens thickness [16]. They trained the network using a personalized Holladay program to predict the power of the IOL for patients operated on by a single surgeon. The prediction error was +0.27 D.

Several other neural networks have been tested for the prediction of refractive power in cataract surgery with satisfyingly high accuracy [17]. However, the system has not been tested with heterogeneous data, and no randomized trials have validated them.

12.5 Special Circumstances

12.5.1 Aphakia

Newer devices have modes specially programmed for aphakia. Options are available for aphakic modes in the current biometers, wherein the calculation compensates for the change in the speed of the sound waves travelling through the aqueous or vitreous humor. Most values remain similar in the theoretical equations, except for the manufacturer's ACD and the measured K reading. As the manufacturer's ACD is intended for in-the-bag placement, unless special lenses are utilized, the value should be reduced by 0.25 mm for sulcus placement [18].

12.5.2 Pseudophakia

Optical biometry is preferred in such cases as it offers a more accurate correction of the AL by a correction factor, which varies according to the type and thickness of the lens used [19]. For example, in polymethylmethacrylate (PMMA) lenses, the conversion factor is +0.45; for silicone lenses, it is either −0.56 or −0.41 (depending on the style and the manufacturer); for acrylic lenses, it is +0.30.

These conversion factors must be applied to the formulae.

In newer devices, prefilled data is available as per the implant type.

$$\text{TAL} = \text{AAL}1532 \pm (\text{cf} \times t)$$

The lens thickness (t) is obtained from the manufacturer.

12.5.3 Keratoconus

Patients with keratoconus have unusually steep corneas with higher keratometry and ACD values; thus, the ELP would differ. In such situations, the IOL power is calculated in the following manner:

1. The posterior corneal power is calculated, and the total power of the cornea that uses true refractive indices is then incorporated into the formula used to calculate the power of the IOL.
2. Specifically, customized formulae for calculating the power of the IOL for keratoconus patients, such as the Kane keratoconus

or Barrett true K for keratoconus, must be used [20].
3. The corneal power map from the topography data is assessed to understand the suitability of toric IOLs for such patients.

Kane and Barrett True K formulae are the two most frequently used formulae in people with keratoconus.-.

12.5.3.1 The Kane Formula [21]

- It minimizes the effect of corneal power on the ELP prediction and enables better accuracy in calculating the IOL power.
- The target refraction is kept unchanged for corneas with the keratometry up to 48.00 D, aiming for mild myopic refraction of −0.50 to −1.00 D in eyes with average corneal power between 48.00 and 59.00 D. In eyes with keratometry >59 D, the aim is for −1.50 to−2.50 D.

12.5.3.2 The Barrett True K Formula for Keratoconus [22]

- The keratoconus option from the drop-down menu in the Barrett True K formula is available on the Asia Pacific Association of Cataract and Refractive Surgeons (APACRS) (https://www.apacrs.org/#).
- There is an option to input anterior corneal values, thereby letting the Barrett True K formula predict the total corneal values; however, the input may also be measured from posterior corneal values if available.
- If a measured posterior corneal value is available either from the IOL Master or Pentacam, then either of these can be selected from the drop-down menu in the calculator.

12.5.4 Pediatric Cataracts

In children, the currently available data are sufficient to build a consensus formula for accurate IOL power calculation. Some studies state that it is preferable to use theoretical formulae because they are generally more precise for small eyes. In pediatric studies, these formulae appear slightly more accurate than regression formulae [23].

Table 12.5 Rule of thumb for IOL power calculation in children pediatric eyes

Age of patient	Percentage of IOL power planned for emmetropia (%)
0–2 months	Controversial
>2 months to 2 years	80
>2 years to 8 years	90
>8 years	100

IOL Intraocular lens

While errors in AL measurement, K measurement, and IOL power calculation show up immediately in postoperative refraction, these errors are not the main source of unexpected refractive outcomes. Growth of the eye, which is generally not very predictable, is responsible for these "refractive surprises." [9]

In the Aphakia Treatment Study, different formulae were compared for minimum prediction error [9]. The results showed that among the Hoffer Q, Holladay1, Holladay 2, SRK II, and SRK/T formulae, SRK/T had the lowest mean prediction error. On the other hand, both the Holladay 1 (44%) and SRK/T (46%) had the highest percentage of outcomes within 1D of the predicted power.

In the case of children who require long-term care, an additional focus should be on the permissible extent of under-correction (based on the likely growth of the eye in a specific child) (Table 12.5) [24].

12.5.5 Eyes with Silicone Oil

Oil has a high refractive index, which alters its refraction; therefore, calculating the IOL power in silicon oil-filled eyes is challenging. Hence, predicting the ELP and obtaining accurate IOL power and residual refractive power are difficult [25]. Numerous studies have shown that the fourth-generation IOL power assessment formulae (Holladay 2, Barrett Universal II, Olsen, and Haigis) have high accuracy in adult patients [26]. Also, the Haigis, Barrett Universal II, and SRK/T formulae are superior to the Holladay 1, Holladay 2, and Hoffer Q formulae in longer eyes with silicon oil [26, 27].

Among the biometry machines, the IOL Master 700 measures all biometric indices (ACD, K values, and AL) and has specific formulas for IOL power assessment [28]. In the third-generation formulae, including the Holladay 1, SRK/T, and Hoffer Q formulae, postsurgical ACD depends on the AL of the eye and corneal curvature [26].

12.5.6 Calculation of the IOL Power After Refractive Surgery

The advent of corneal refractive surgery in the 1990s and its increasing popularity have resulted in those patients now presenting for cataract surgery. The altered corneal profile adds further complexity to accurately estimating the power of the IOLs for these eyes. This has been largely overcome by multiple new-generation calculation formulae. These formulae mainly depend on the net corneal power based on the direct anterior and posterior corneal curvature measurement by advanced topography techniques [29, 30]. This overcomes the difficulty of calculating the keratometric index of the cornea due to changes in the anterior corneal shape. Some formulae use the pre- and post-LASIK corneal measurements for calculating the correct IOL power [9].

The challenge of accurately determining the IOL power is increased in radial keratotomy patients due to the unpredictable biomechanical properties of the cornea. The consensus is to use the central 3 mm corneal power in such eyes. Studies have shown that using the Barrett True K formula produces minimum postoperative refractive surprises in people with radial keratotomy [9].

12.5.6.1 Clinical History Method

- Holladay first introduced this method; it is theoretically easy but unreliable when relevant data cannot be provided [31].
- The formula for calculating the power for the IOL is $K = \text{KPRE} - \text{RCC}$.

  where *K* Calculated corneal power, *KPRE* Corneal power before refractive surgery, *RCC* Change in manifest refraction at the corneal plane

12.5.6.2 Contact Lens Over-Refraction Method

- This method, introduced by Riddley, is practical and inexpensive [32]. However, this method did not gain popularity as it was inaccurate in eyes with poor visual acuity, such as in dense cataracts.
- The formula used is $K = \text{BCL} + \text{PCL} + \text{RCL} - \text{RNoCL}$.

  where *BCL* Contact lens base curve, *PCL* Contact lens power, *RCL* Contact lens over-refraction, *RnoCL* The spherical equivalent of the manifest refraction without a contact lens

12.5.6.3 Topography-Based Post-LASIK Adjusted Keratometry

These regression formulae are based on the analysis of post-LASIK corneal topography central K values (TK) in LASIK eyes. The true corneal power is predicted using only the single central postoperative TK. A few popular formulae used are the Wang Koch Maloney, adjusted Atlas, Double K, Masket, Shammas, Haigis-L, Hoffer Q, and Galilei formulae.

The **Wang Koch Maloney** method uses the pre- and post-LASIK/PRK anterior and posterior corneal power to predict post-refractive corneal power. If pre-surgery corneal power is not available, then a mean posterior corneal power is used for the calculation [33].

The **Shammas formula** uses post-refractive surgery keratometry values for power calculation [9]. This reduces the dependency on pre-surgery measurements for calculations.

The **Masket formula** determines the surgically induced refractive power along with SRK/T or Hoffer Q for myopic or hyperopic patients, respectively. This enables the adjustment of the predicted IOL power [34].

The **Haigis-L formula** utilizes the ACD which does not change with refractive surgery and corrects for myopic or hyperopic eyes during IOL power calculation [13]. This formula is incorporated into the IOL Master 700 platform.

The **Double K formula** uses the pre-refractive surgery corneal power estimate for predicting the ELP, while the post-refractive power is used for vergence calculation. This helps in the better prediction of ELP after cataract surgery. This formula is incorporated in the SRK/T, Holladay II, and Hofer Q online calculations [35].

The **Barrett True K formula** holds promise for accurate calculation of IOL power in post-LASIK eyes [9].

The American Society of Cataract and Refractive Surgery (ASCRS) website has an online calculator incorporating all these formulae for IOL power calculation in post-refractive surgery eyes [9].

The net corneal power for all these newer formulae can be measured using the Pentacam, Orbscan, or anterior segment OCT.

12.5.7 Piggyback IOLs

Piggyback IOLs are necessary due to residual high refractive errors caused by inaccurate biometry, errors in IOL power calculation, and placement of incorrectly powered IOLs. While lower residual powers can be corrected by refractive surgery, larger errors will need either an IOL exchange or the placement of an additional IOL in the ciliary sulcus to obtain refractive neutrality [19, 36]. The adjustments required for this secondary IOL placement in the ciliary sulcus include calculations for:

- Myopic correction: $P = 1.0 \times \text{Error}$
- Hyperopic correction: $P = 1.5 \times \text{Error}$

  where P The needed power in the piggyback lens, *Error* The residual refractive error that needs to be corrected

The implantation of piggyback IOLs may lead to intralenticular opacification, iris chafing with pigment release, and a higher risk of glaucoma.

12.5.8 High Myopia

A study by MacLaren et al. showed that postoperative refraction is overestimated when the SRK/T formula was used for IOL power calculation with estimates of the AL in extreme myopia with both ultrasound and optical biometry [37].

Wang et al. evaluated the accuracy of refractive prediction of four IOL power calculation formulae in eyes with ALs >25.0 mm and proposed a method to optimize AL measurements to improve the accuracy of such calculations. According to this study, the proposed method significantly reduced the percentage of long eyes with a hyperopic outcome [38].

Holladay1 2-center optimized AL = 0:8814 × IOLMaster AL + 2:8701
Haigis 2-center optimized AL = 0:9621 × IOLMaster AL + 0:6763
SRK/T 2-center optimized AL = 0:8981 × IOLMaster AL + 2:5637
Hoffer Q 2-center optimized AL = 0:8776 × IOLMaster AL + 2:9269

In another study, Wang et al. proposed the Holladay Nonlinear AL adjustment method to optimize AL calculations in long eyes (AL >24.00 mm) with the Holladay 2 formula [39].

12.5.9 Toric IOL

Toric IOL is a technology that meets the increasing expectations of spectacle-free vision after cataract surgery in people with astigmatism. However, refractive surprises can sometimes happen even after the implantation of toric IOLs. Repositioning or rotating the IOL is indicated when the IOL is placed in an incorrect position during surgery but not when the rotation occurs in the postoperative period. The Toric Results Analyzer (https://www.astigmatismfix.com), developed by Berdahl and Hardten, helps analyze the alignment of an already placed toric IOL. This toric analyzer helps determine if the refractive surprise can be decreased by rotating the IOL by comparing the current location of the toric IOL and a patient's refraction. It simultaneously helps calculate the required IOL rotation and the expected residual refraction [40].

12.6 Errors in Iol Power Calculation

Errors in IOL power calculations have three sources: operator-induced, machine-induced, or surgeon-induced.

- *Operator-induced:* This may include biometry on the wrong patient, incorrect calculation formulae or IOL selection, or inaccurate IOL labelling. In ultrasound biometry, an excessive indentation of the cornea or improper alignment of the probe may cause wrong IOL power calculation. The operator may also miss noting dryness in the eyes during the recording, which may contribute to errors. Manual entries also are prone to error.
- *Machine-induced*: Improper calibration of the machine can cause errors in the IOL power calculation.
- *Surgeon-induced*: Incorrect selection of an IOL and/or improper placement of the IOL during surgery can lead to postoperative refractive surprises.

12.7 Techniques Used in IOL Power Measurement

The pre-operative workup for cataract surgery includes biometry to obtain measurements for calculating the most accurate intraocular lens power for each patient.

12.7.1 Ultrasound Biometry Must Be Performed by Following These Steps

- Ask the patient to sit comfortably and look straight at a fixation point to measure the AL along the visual axis.
- Select the appropriate mode based on the patient's eye status, such as cataract, aphakia, pseudophakia, or silicone oil-filled globe, as the velocity of ultrasound waves varies in each medium.
- For contact ultrasound biometry, instill a topical anesthetic drop in the eye, place the ultrasound probe over the cornea without compression, and align it along the visual axis. The probe should be sterilized before use.
- A scleral shell filled with saline is placed between the eye and the probe for immersion ultrasound biometry. Proper alignment of the probe is necessary for accurate AL measurement.
- The AL value and keratometry readings (measured using a keratometer) must be used in an appropriate IOL power calculation formula to calculate the power of the IOL to be implanted.

12.7.2 Optical Biometry Must Be Performed by Following These Steps

- Ask the patient to sit in front of the machine with their chin resting comfortably on the chin rest.
- Ask the patient to blink their eyes to ensure the even spreading of the tear film on the cornea and look at the internal fixation target in the machine.
- The instrument will automatically track the test eye, and the scanner will move.
- The machine will scan the eyes and retrieve the data needed for IOL power calculation, including corneal curvature measurements, anterior chamber depth, WTW diameter, and AL.
- IOL power will be calculated and displayed according to different lens-specific constants and the formulae selected. Other data, like astigmatism measurements, will also help the surgeon plan the surgery.

Different modes are available in eyes with previous cataract or retinal surgeries, such as aphakic, pseudophakic, silicone oil-filled phakic/aphakic/pseudophakic eye, phakic IOL, and piggyback lens.

12.8 Conclusion

The accuracy of IOL power selection for cataract surgery has advanced significantly in the past decade. With the increasing expectations of patients and constantly evolving IOL designs, accurate biometry measurements and calculation of IOL power using appropriate formulae are crucial for successful surgeries with the desired refractive outcomes and patient satisfaction. Newer IOL formulae have been created to generate a single algorithm that can accurately determine the appropriate IOL power for a wide range of eye dimensions. The Barrett Universal II formula has achieved consistently accurate results across a large range of ALs. The current biometers and formulae have made it possible to achieve outcomes within the range of ±0.50 D with minimum astigmatism for most patients. However, achieving the target postoperative refraction is still challenging in silicone oil-filled eyes, irregular corneas, and post-refractive surgery eyes.

Disclosure None.

References

1. Rossi T, Romano MR, Iannetta D, et al. Cataract surgery practice patterns worldwide: a survey. BMJ Open Ophthalmol. 2021;6(1):e000464. https://doi.org/10.1136/bmjophth-2020-000464.
2. Nemeth J, Fekete O, Pesztenlehrer N. Optical and ultrasound measurement of axial length and anterior chamber depth for intraocular lens power calculation. J Cataract Refract Surg. 2003;29:85–8.
3. Borgia A, Raimondi R, Sorrentino T, et al. Swept-source optical coherence tomography-cased biometry: a comprehensive overview. Photo-Dermatology. 2022;9(12):951. https://doi.org/10.3390/photonics9120951.
4. Akman A, Asena L, Güngör SG. Evaluation and comparison of the new swept source OCT-based IOLMaster 700 with the IOLMaster 500. Br J Ophthalmol. 2016;100:1201–5.
5. Hoffer KJ, Savini G. Comparison of AL-Scan and IOL Master 500 partial coherence interferometry optical biometers. J Refract Surg. 2016;32:694–8.
6. Mandal P, Berrow EJ, Naroo SA, et al. Validity and repeatability of the Aladdin ocular biometer. Br J Ophthalmol. 2014;98:256–8.
7. Moshirfar M, Tenney S, McCabe S, Schmid G. Repeatability and reproducibility of the galilei G6 and its agreement with the pentacam® AXL in optical biometry and corneal tomography. Expert Rev Med Devices. 2022;19:375–83.
8. Higashiyama T, Mori H, Nakajima F, Ohji M. Comparison of a new biometer using swept-source optical coherence tomography and a conventional biometer using partial coherence interferometry. PLoS One. 2018;13(4):e0196401. https://doi.org/10.1371/journal.pone.0196401.
9. Xia T, Martinez CE, Tsai LM. Update on intraocular lens formulas and calculations. Asia Pac J Ophthalmol. 2020;9:186–93.
10. Menezo JL, Chaques V, Harto M. The SRK regression formula in calculating the dioptric power of intraocular lenses. Br J Ophthalmol. 1984;68:235–7.
11. Koch DD, Hill W, Abulafia A, Wang L. Pursuing perfection in intraocular lens calculations: I. Logical approach for classifying IOL calculation formulas. J Cataract Refract Surg. 2017;43:717–8.
12. Hoffer KJ. The Hoffer Q formula: a comparison of theoretic and regression formulas. J Cataract Refract Surg. 1993;19:700–12.
13. Retzlaff J, Sanders DR, Kraff MC. Development of the SRK/T intraocular lens implantation power calculation formula. J Cataract Refract Surg. 1990;16:333–40.
14. Saiki M, Negishi K, Kato N, et al. Ray tracing software for intraocular lens power calculation after corneal excimer laser surgery. Jpn J Ophthalmol. 2014;58:276–81.
15. Ianchulev T, Salz J, Hoffer K, et al. Intraoperative optical refractive biometry for intraocular lens power estimation without axial length and keratometry measurements. J Cataract Refract Surg. 2005;31:1530–6.
16. Clarke GP, Burmeister J. Comparison of intraocular lens computations using a neural network versus the Holladay formula. J Cataract Refract Surg. 1997;23:1585–9.
17. Sramka M, Slovak M, Tuckova J, Stodulka P. Improving clinical refractive results of cataract surgery by machine learning. PeerJ. 2019;7:e7202. https://doi.org/10.7717/peerj.7202.
18. Nakhli FR, Emarah K, Jeddawi L. Accuracy of formulae for secondary intraocular lens power calculations in pediatric aphakia. J Curr Ophthalmol. 2017;29:199–203.
19. Karjou Z, Jafarinasab MR, Seifi MH, et al. Secondary piggyback intraocular lens for management of residual ametropia after cataract surgery. J Ophthalmic Vis Res. 2021;16:12–20.

20. Vandevenne M, Webers V, Segers M, et al. Accuracy of intraocular lens calculations in eyes with keratoconus. J Cataract Refract Surg. 2023;49:229–33.
21. Connell BJ, Kane JX. Comparison of the Kane formula with existing formulas for intraocular lens power selection. BMJ Open Ophthalmol. 2019;4:e000251. https://doi.org/10.1136/bmjophth-2018-000251.
22. Savini G, Abbate R, Hoffer KJ, et al. Intraocular lens power calculation in eyes with keratoconus. J Cataract Refract Surg. 2019;45:576–81.
23. O'Gallagher MK, Lagan MA, Mulholland CP, et al. Paediatric intraocular lens implants: accuracy of lens power calculations. Eye (Lond). 2016;30: 1215–20.
24. Dahan E, Drusedau MUH. Choice of lens and dioptric power in pediatric pseudophakia. J Cataract Refract Surg. 1997;23(Suppl 1):618–23.
25. El-Baha SM, Hemeida TS. Comparison of refractive outcome using intraoperative biometry and partial coherence interferometry in silicone oil-filled eyes. Retina (Philadelphia). 2009;29:64–8.
26. Hou Y, Liu L, Wang G, et al. Different lens power calculation formulas for the prediction of refractive outcome after phacoemulsification with silicone oil removal. BMC Ophthalmol. 2022;22:74. https://doi.org/10.1186/s12886-022-02304-2.
27. Wang JK, Hu CY, Chang SW. Intraocular lens power calculation using the IOLMaster and various formulas in eyes with long axial length. J Cataract Refract Surg. 2008;34:262–7.
28. Kunavisarut P, Poopattanakul P, Intarated C, Pathanapitoon K. Accuracy and reliability of IOL master and A-scan immersion biometry in silicone oil-filled eyes. Eye. 2012;26:1344–8.
29. Savini G, Hoffer KJ. Intraocular lens power calculation in eyes with previous corneal refractive surgery. Eye Vis (Lond). 2018;5:18. https://doi.org/10.1186/s40662-018-0110-5.
30. Langenbucher A, Haigis W, Seitz B. Difficult lens power calculations. Curr Opin Ophthalmol. 2004;15:1–9.
31. Holladay JT. Consultations in refractive surgery. Refract Corneal Surg. 1989;5:203.
32. Ridley F. Development in contact lens theory–moulding, computation, and veiling. Trans Ophthalmol Soc. 1948;68:385–401.
33. Wang L, Booth MA, Koch DD. Comparison of intraocular lens power calculation methods in eyes that have undergone LASIK. Ophthalmology. 2004;111:1825–31.
34. Masket S, Masket SE. Simple regression formula for intraocular lens power adjustment in eyes requiring cataract surgery after excimer laser photoablation. J Cataract Refract Surg. 2006;32:430–4.
35. Aramberri J. Intraocular lens power calculation after corneal refractive surgery: double-K method. J Cataract Refract Surg. 2003;29:2063–8.
36. Mehta R, Aref AA. Intraocular lens implantation in the ciliary sulcus: challenges and risks. Clin Ophthalmol. 2019;13:2317–23. https://doi.org/10.2147/OPTH.S205148.
37. MacLaren RE, Sagoo MS, Restori M, Allan BD. Biometry accuracy using zero- and negative-powered intraocular lenses. J Cataract Refract Surg. 2005;31:280–90.
38. Wang L, Shirayama M, Ma XJ, Kohnen T, Koch DD. Optimizing intraocular lens power calculations in eyes with axial lengths above 25.0 mm. J Cataract Refract Surg. 2011;37:2018–27.
39. Wang L, Holladay JT, Koch DD. Wang-Koch axial length adjustment for the Holladay 2 formula in long eyes. J Cataract Refract Surg. 2018;44(10):1291–2.
40. Berdahl, J. and Hardten, D. Toric results analyzer, Berdahl & Hardten Astigmatism Fix Calculator. https://www.astigmatismfix.com/. Accessed: 16 May 2023.

13 Imaging in Cataract

Supriya Sharma, Maneck Nicholson, Prashant Gupta, Prajakta Dandekar, and Somasheila I. Murthy

13.1 Introduction

In the quest for improved quality of vision and to match the increasing expectations of people, cataract surgical techniques and designs for intraocular lenses (IOLs) have undergone a remarkable evolution in the past decade. Improvement in the quality of vision has been possible through our improved understanding of optical aberrations, which can often cause post-operative dissatisfaction. While the introduction of aspheric IOLs addresses this problem, assessment of pre-operative aberrations is necessary and is made possible by aberrometry-measuring devices. Imaging the lens using Scheimpflug technology objectively documents the changes in the lens and detects various types of cataracts, which helps in surgical planning. The anterior segment optical coherence tomography (AS-OCT) and ultrasound brightness scan (B scan) have added new dimensions to managing complex cases. Over the past two decades, IOL power calculations have been modified using data from corneal topography, resulting in increased precision in achieving the targeted refraction [1, 2]. Common sources of error in calculating refraction include imprecise axial length measurements and incorrect keratometry [3]. Many keratometry devices do not measure posterior corneal astigmatism, often resulting in under or over-estimating the total corneal astigmatism, particularly in eyes where toric IOL implantation is indicated. Obtaining accurate biometric data is one of the major challenges in the preoperative planning of cataract surgery.

Of the various preoperative imaging modalities explored in the past to improve surgical outcomes, in this chapter we have highlighted four imaging modalities that help the surgeon anticipate intraoperative complications and achieve better postoperative results and patient satisfaction.

13.2 Aberrometry (iTRACE, Tracey Technologies, Houston, TX)

Aberrations occur when light from a point source does not converge to or diverges from a single point after transmission through an optical system [4]. Aberrations are a major cause of poor quality of vision. The various refracting surfaces like the tear film, cornea, and lens are primarily responsible for inducing ocular aberrations in the

S. Sharma (✉) · M. Nicholson · P. Dandekar · S. I. Murthy
Shantilal Shanghvi Eye Institute, Mumbai, India
e-mail: supriya.sharma@ssei.ind.in; maneck.nicholson@ssei.ind.in; prajakta.dandekar@ssei.ind.in; somasheila.murthy@ssei.ind.in

P. Gupta
Kallam Anji Reddy Campus, L V Prasad Eye Institute, Hyderabad, India
e-mail: prashant.gupta@lvpei.org

T. Das, P. Satgunam (eds.), *Ophthalmic Diagnostics*, https://doi.org/10.1007/978-981-97-0138-4_13

eye [5]. Several factors affect the quality of vision, such as refractive/wavefront error, light scatter, binocular summation, illumination (pupillary size), and neuro adaptation [6]. The commonly performed diagnostic procedures to evaluate the quality of vision include contrast sensitivity and vision testing in different illumination levels by glare test and aberrometry. Different aberrometers work on various principles such as Hartmann-Shack (outgoing reflection aberrometry), Tscherning, Ray tracing (retinal imaging aberrometry), and automatic retinoscopy (slit sciascopy). Aberration-correcting IOLs have largely replaced traditional IOLs, which has helped select the appropriate IOL for customized cataract surgery.

13.2.1 Principle of the iTrace

The iTrace uses ray-tracing aberrometry to dynamically measure and analyze wavefront aberrometry while also analyzing corneal topography, allowing the surgeon to separate visual function into a corneal component and an internal optic component to calculate higher order aberrations and refractive data [7]. This system combines ray tracing aberrometry wavefront analysis, advanced corneal topography, autorefraction, pupillometry, and auto keratometry in a single device. In an emmetropic eye, the 64 laser beams would focus on the fovea, but due to ocular aberrations at the level of the cornea and lens, these points shift to other retinal areas with respect to the reference. This deviation of the emergent wavefront from the original wavefront, which entered the eye, is measured as an ocular aberration.

13.2.2 Image Acquisition Technique

This is a non-contact test. Once the patient is seated comfortably, the machine takes an image in about 30 s (Fig. 13.1). It sends 64 laser beams four times sequentially, making 256 individual rays enter through the pupil. The aberrations in the path of the laser beam (cornea and internal structures) cause a shift in the location of the laser beam when it reaches the retina. These laser beams pass through multiple points on the pupil. By analysing the process of using the entry and exit of laser beams, a real wavefront (WF) error is obtained. This method obtains the forward aberrations of light that go through the pupil.

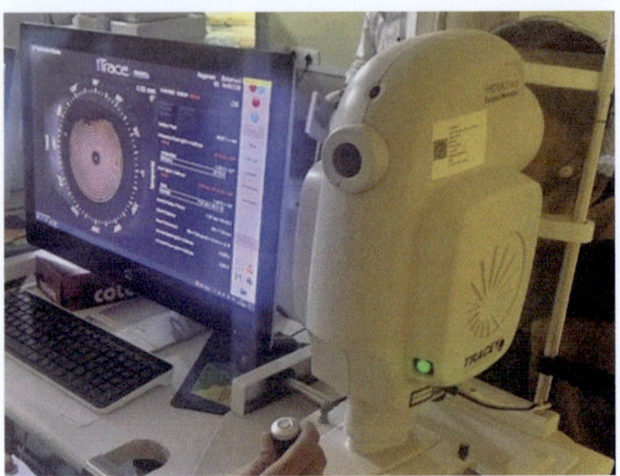

Fig. 13.1 Aberrometry using iTrace testing

13.2.3 Clinical Applications

13.2.3.1 Localization of the Origin of the Aberration

The "wavefront and corneal topography" display on the iTrace help localize the origin of the aberrations [6, 8]. The aberration may originate from the lens (depicted by the internal optics map), cornea, or the entire eye. Localizing the exact source helps in targeted treatment, thus eliminating the aberrations from that source and contributing to better post-operative quality of vision (Fig. 13.2).

13.2.3.2 Selecting Spherical vs. Aspherical IOL [3, 9]

Asphericity (Q value) is a geometric measure of ellipsoid surfaces, with a change in curvature from the center toward the edge. A normal cornea is prolate with negative asphericity (−0.23 μm), as the center is more curved than the periphery, inducing a positive spherical aberration of +0.28 μm. However, in young adults, the negative spherical aberration of the crystalline lens

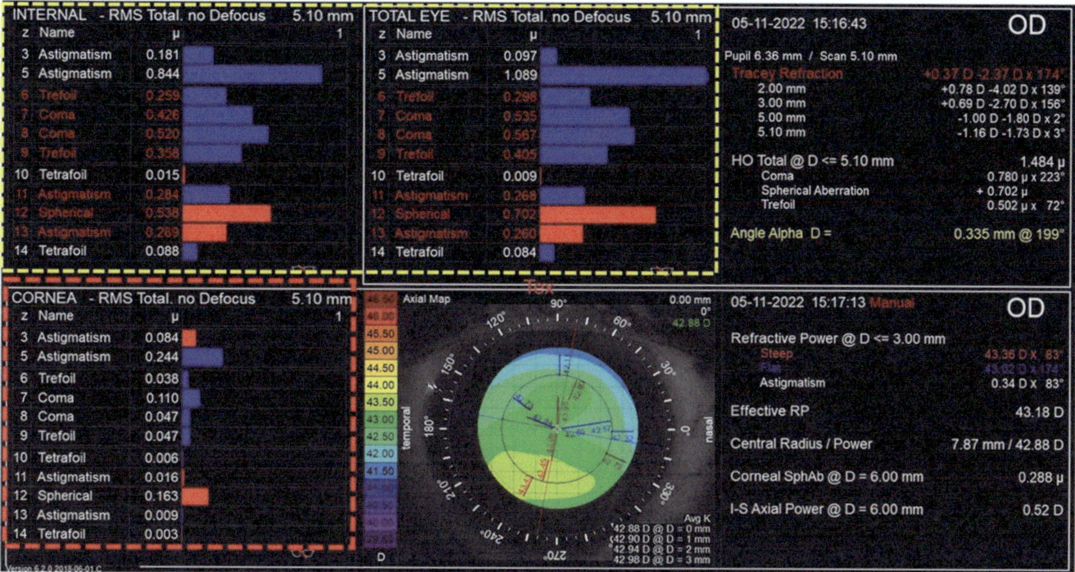

Fig. 13.2 Chang analysis display map on iTrace. These maps show color-coded wavefront aberrations of the eye (internal aberrations [lenticular and retinal] of the eye—top left corner, yellow dotted box; corneal aberrations—lower left corner, red dotted box; and total eye aberrations—top middle, yellow dotted box) measured in microns of error. The error can be positive or negative (the red color indicates that the wavefront is in front of the reference plane, and the blue color indicates that the wavefront is retarded in relation to this plane). Decomposition in each of the Zernike polynomials is represented in red and blue bars depending on the value of the sign. The map in this figure represents the Chang analysis display of the right eye showing minimal corneal aberrations (red dotted box); thus, the cause of the higher order aberrations is likely to be lenticular

compensates for the corneal aberration, thereby maintaining a good quality of vision. This changes with age and cataract formation. The residual aberration of the eye after cataract surgery is planned by the visual need of the patient and preoperative aberration of the cornea. The figure represents Dr. Devgan's decision-making tree for selecting aspheric lenses (Fig. 13.3) [10].

13.2.3.3 Preoperative Assessments for Premium IOLs [11, 12]

13.2.3.3.1 Measurement of Higher Order Aberrations (HOAs)

Addressing the HOAs before surgery is required to prevent post-operative dysphotopsia, glare, and haloes. These phenomena occur due to the splitting of the image, resulting in loss of contrast sensitivity, regardless of the type of multifocal IOL (diffractive or refractive) implanted. Among the HOAs, coma (asymmetrical aberration) is commonly associated with these ocular symptoms, and a value of more than 0.32 μm is considered a contraindication for multifocal IOL implantation. The iTrace helps to separate aberrations from the anterior cornea from those in the entire eye. If there are minimal HOAs in the cornea, and the overall optical quality of the cornea is good, the patient will likely benefit from a premium IOL (assuming optical alignment, as discussed subsequently, is not an issue). Conversely, if the cornea shows significant HOAs and poor optical quality, the patient may not achieve the best vision after implanting a premium IOL.

13.2.3.3.2 Measurement of Angle Kappa and Angle Alpha

Angle kappa is the angle between the visual and pupillary axis. Angle alpha is the angle between the visual axis and the center of the limbus or the optical axis (Fig. 13.4). If the multifocal IOL is significantly decentered in the eye due to a large angle alpha or angle kappa (>0.5 mm), the patient may look through the diffractive rings

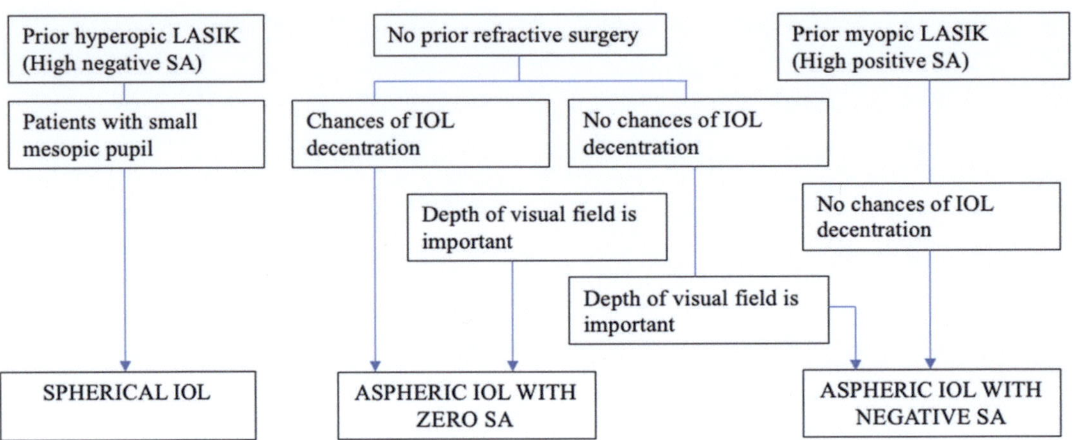

Fig. 13.3 Dr. Devgan's decision-making tree for selecting an aspheric intraocular lens based on the patient's ocular characteristics and visual requirements. *IOL* Intraocular lens, *LASIK* Laser-assisted in situ keratomileusis, *SA* Spherical aberration

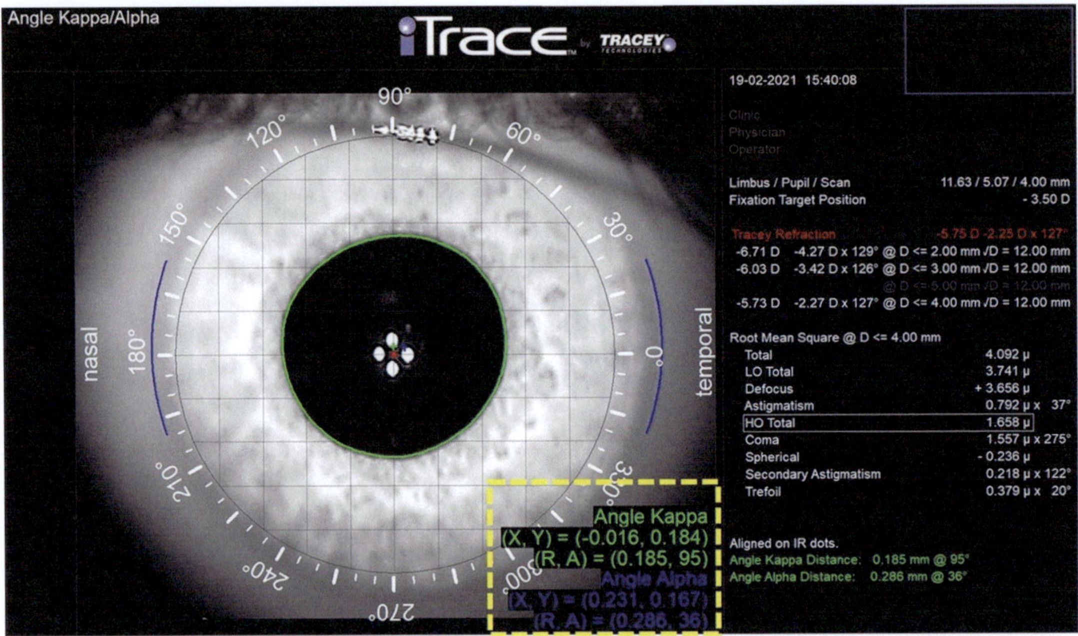

Fig. 13.4 The angle kappa and alpha display of the iTrace. The visual axis is marked with the red cross; the center of the pupil (green circle) is marked with the green cross; the center of the limbus (blue circle) is marked with the blue cross. The screen displays the measurements of these distances in both polar and rectilinear coordinates in the bottom right of the eye image (yellow dotted box)

rather than the central optical zone as intended; this induces higher order aberrations and decreases postoperative visual function. For similar reasons, these angles are also important while planning a toric IOL, particularly in eyes with against-the-rule astigmatism. Hence, preoperative assessment of the angle alpha and angle kappa is important, and a value of >0.5 mm is considered a contraindication for multifocal IOL placement (Fig. 13.5).

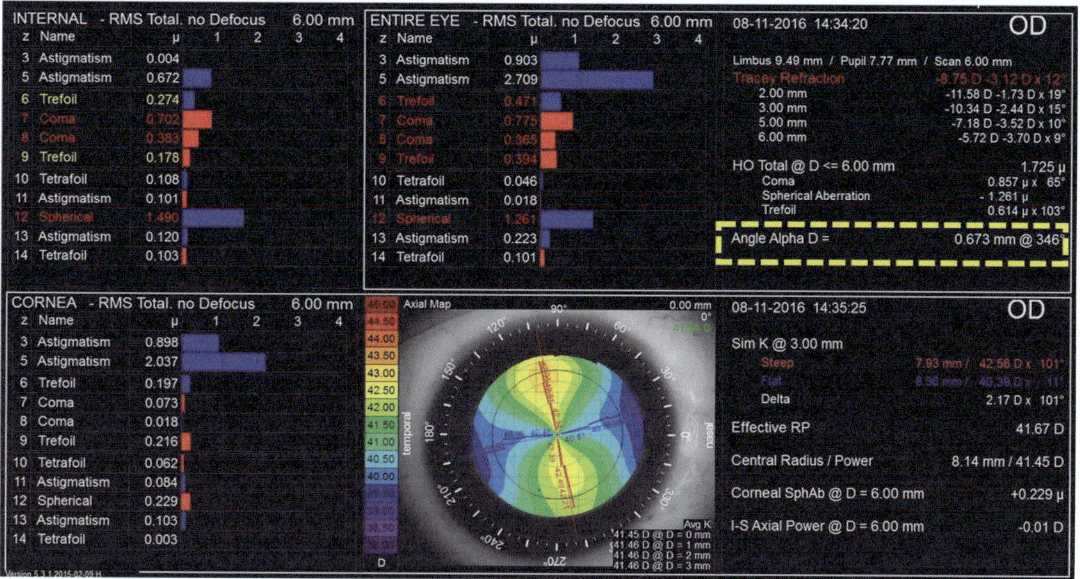

Fig. 13.5 The Chang analysis display map on the iTrace depicting a high angle alpha (0.67 mm @ 346°, yellow dotted box) in the right eye. This patient may not be an ideal candidate for multifocal IOL implantation

13.2.3.3.3 Planning for Toric IOLs [13]

The iTrace helps one to decide if the patient's internal optics compensates for any corneal astigmatism and accordingly decide the need for a toric IOL. Implantation of toric IOLs should be preferred in people with high corneal astigmatism but who never required astigmatism correction previously due to the compensation of their natural lens. The iTrace also offers integrated tools, allowing surgeons to increase the precision with which the characteristics of the toric IOLs are planned. The Hoya Toric Calculator, surgically induced astigmatism analysis, and the Zaldivar Toric Caliper help to enhance the accuracy of power selection, placement, and postoperative assessment of toric IOLs. The toric calculator provides several power alternatives and expected residual cylinder outcomes to help surgeons choose the appropriate toric power for the intended result. The precise location of the placement axis with reference to the usual surgical markings is determined as the last step.

13.2.3.4 Dysfunctional Lens Index (DLI)

The iTrace visual function analyzer provides objective lens outcomes such as the dysfunctional lens index (DLI) and opacity grade to measure crystalline lens degeneration (Fig. 13.6) [14]. DLI values vary from 0 to 10, with a lower value associated with a more dysfunctional lens suggestive of cataract, while a higher number is associated with improved lens performance or optically clear crystalline lens. The opacity grade metric assesses how much energy reaches the retina from 128 sequential and independent beams that enter the pupil. The device reads the variance and intensity of the energy reaching the retina generating a map of the opacity or scatter graded from 0 to 5. This grading is similar to the lens opacification classification system (LOCS) cataract grading. Thus, DLI and opacity grade are parameters which assist in the diagnosis and the optimal timing of cataract surgery.

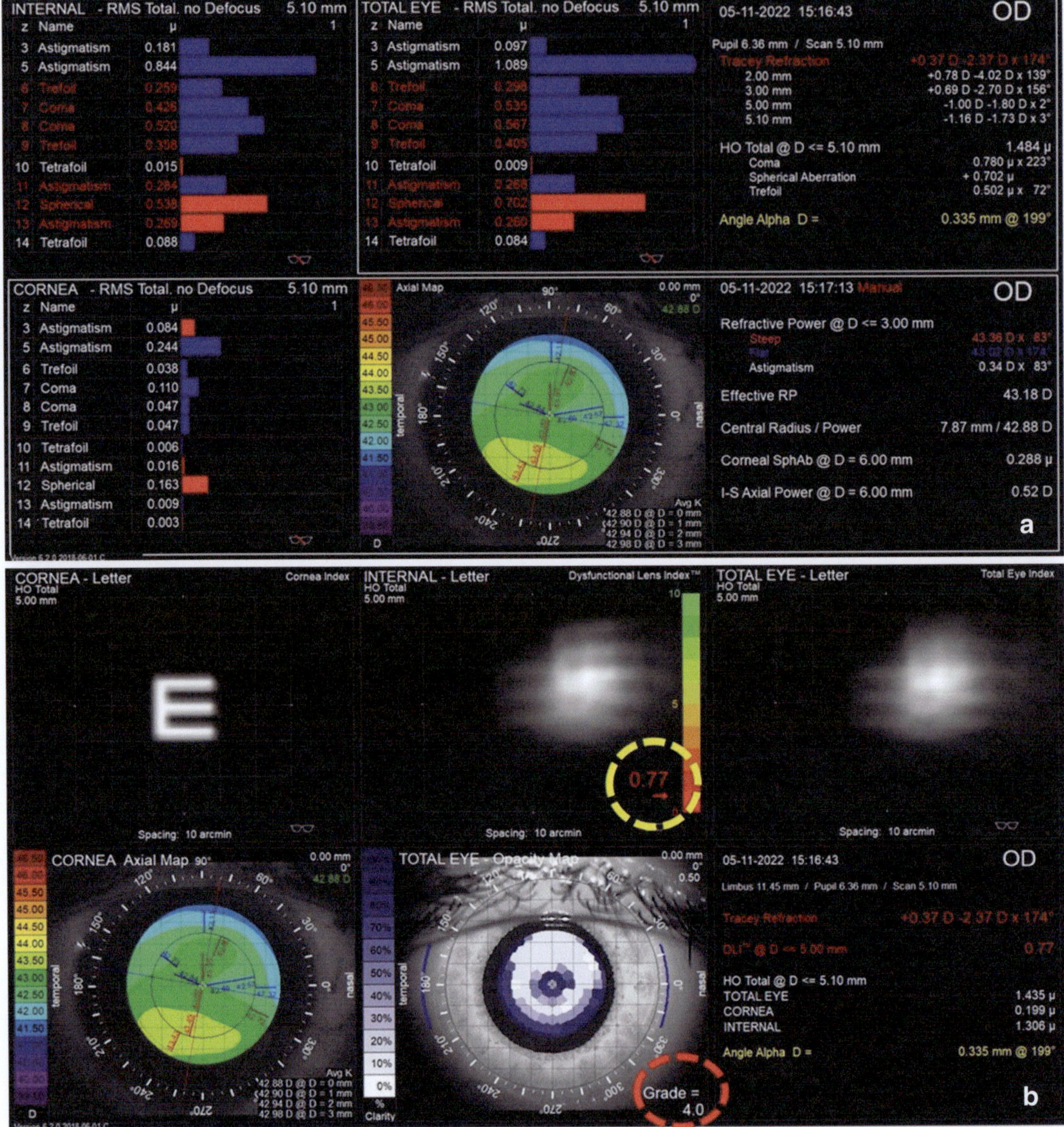

Fig. 13.6 The Chang analysis display map of the right eye of a 64-year-old man shows high internal and total higher order aberrations contributed mainly by the mature cataract (**a**). The dysfunctional lens index (DLI) map shows a DLI value of 0.77 (dotted yellow circle), and the opacity map depicted a cataract of grade 4 (red dotted circle) (**b**). These two parameters suggest a dysfunctional lens due to a mature cataract

13.3 Scheimpflug Imaging (OCULUS Pentacam®)

A standardized and objective cataract grading is required from clinical and research perspectives [15]. The current literature has described several classification systems, such as the LOCS III, age-related eye disease study, and laser slit-lamp evaluation [16–18]. Of these, the LOCS III is the most popular. The grading quality depends on slit-lamp examination, lens photography, patient age, and best-corrected visual acuity (BCVA); thus, it is fundamentally a subjective technique that often depends on the examiner's experience [18, 19]. Scheimpflug imaging has overcome these limitations.

13.3.1 Principle of Scheimpflug Imaging

The Scheimpflug imaging system is credited to Theodor Scheimpflug [18]. It captures an obliquely inclined object with a maximum depth of focus and minimal image distortion. This is accomplished by shifting the plane of the film (sensor) in relation to the camera lens. In a conventional camera, the film plane and lens plane stay parallel, resulting in a plane of focus that is also parallel to these planes. The slit-lamp imaging device can only concentrate on a portion of the crystalline lens at a given time (the anterior capsule, nucleus, or posterior capsule) [19]. Other parts remain out of focus and cannot be accurately analyzed to assess the lens density. The lens plane is inclined to the film plane in the Scheimpflug imaging system, causing the focus plane to shift along the line of intersection (Scheimpflug line). All the points on this line will remain focused and can be analyzed simultaneously.

The first Scheimpflug imagining system used to evaluate the crystalline lens in vivo was developed by N Brown and subsequently by Hockwin et al. [20–22]. Since then, an array of imaging systems have been developed, including the Oxford Scheimpflug System, Topcon SL-45 (Topcon, Tokyo, Japan), Zeiss Scheimpflug video camera (Carl Zeiss Meditec, Dublin CA), and Nidek EAS-1000 (Nidek, Japan) [23–26]. The rotating Scheimpflug allows a 360-degree examination of lens density, eliminating the need for multiple scans across multiple meridians. The Scheimpflug densitometry software analyzes the cataract or loss of lens transparency based on the principle of reflectometry (measuring the reflected light) [27]. The lens density on a scale of 0–100 (0 = no cloudiness to 100 = completely opaque lens) is calculated using individual photographs. The peak value at a specific location within the nucleus is measured and combined with the mean and maximum nucleus density [28].

13.3.2 Image Acquisition

The patients are positioned comfortably before the Pentacam® device. They are asked to rest their chin on the chin rest and focus on a target within the device. The OCULUS Pentacam® consists of a rotating Scheimpflug camera. The rotational measuring procedure generates Scheimpflug images in three dimensions, with the dot matrix fine-meshed in the center due to the rotation. The pupil's size, direction, and fixation are recorded by a second camera positioned in the center of the eye. It takes 2 s to generate a complete image of the anterior eye segment. Any eye movement is detected by a second camera and corrected in the process. The Pentacam® calculates a 3D model of the anterior eye segment from as many as 25.000 distinct elevation points.

The topography and pachymetry of the entire anterior and posterior surfaces of the cornea from limbus to limbus are calculated and depicted. The analysis of the anterior eye segment includes a calculation of the chamber angle, volume, and height and a manual measuring function that can be applied to any location in the anterior chamber of the eye. Images of the anterior and posterior surfaces of the cornea, the iris, and the anterior and posterior surfaces of the lens are generated in a moveable virtual eye. The densitometry of the lens and cornea is automatically quantified. The Scheimpflug images taken during the examination are digitalized in the main unit, and all image data are transferred to the computer unit. When the test is finished, the computer unit calculates a 3D virtual model of the anterior eye segment, from which all additional information is derived.

Pentacam Nuclear Staging (PNS) is a built-in lens densitometry program that delivers average and maximum lens density and a cataract grading score ranging from 0 to 5 [29]. The surgeon can create a more specialized preoperative plan for the cataract surgery with an objective evaluation of cataract density and volume.

13.3.3 Clinical Applications

13.3.3.1 Preoperative Adjustment of Phacoemulsification Parameters

A preoperative assessment of the cataract density helps to customize the operative planning for every individual [28]. Intraoperative phacoemul-

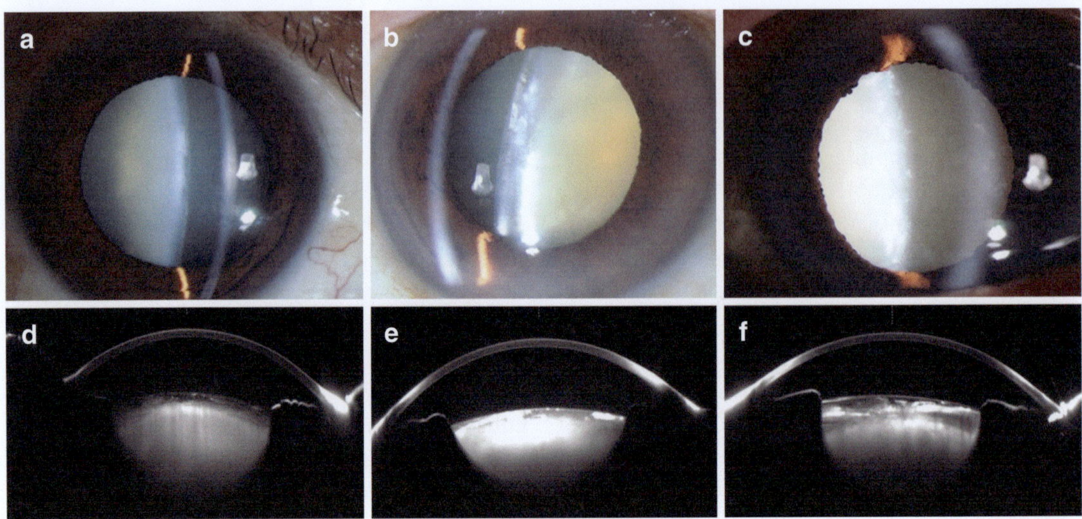

Fig. 13.7 Slit-lamp image of a mature cataract (white and brunescent) and hyper mature cataract (**a–c**) with corresponding Scheimpflug images on the Oculus Pentacam® (**d–f**). A mature nuclear cataract with anterior subcapsular cataract (**a**) is seen as a uniform increase in opalescence of the nucleus, with a band of increased density observed in the deep anterior cortex, while the cortex anterior to it appears clear (**d**). A mature brunescent cataract (**b**) is seen as an increase in density involving the anterior subcapsular, cortical, and nuclear regions (**e**). A hypermature cataract (**c**) shows hypodensity in the anterior subcapsular area corresponding with the liquified lens matter and hyperdense areas in the anterior cortex corresponding to the calcific plaques. The central hyperdense nucleus is surrounded by a liquified cortex seen as a hypodense area around the central nucleus (**f**)

sification energy depends on the nuclear density of the cataract (Fig. 13.7). The Scheimpflug imaging may help the surgeon to plan phacoemulsification, using the lowest power of ultrasound energy required to extract the cataract with a specific density profile, thereby minimizing endothelial cell damage and postoperative inflammation [30].

In the technique described by Nixon, cataracts are graded using the software on the Oculus Pentacam® to develop a three-dimensional (3D) image of the cataract through a dilated pupil [31]. The PNS software does not grade the cortical portion of a cataract or posterior subcapsular cataract (PSC). Instead, a 3D template is placed posterior to the anterior cortex and anterior to the posterior cortex, measuring only the optical density of the nucleus. For the first time, this study compared the effect of modified phaco-setting after Scheimpflug imaging cataract grading with standardized phaco-settings in eyes with uneventful cataract surgery. This difference was most significant for patients with the lowest and the highest cataract grades (Grade 1 or Grades 4 and 5), with no significant difference between the adjusted and standardized parameters in eyes with Grade 2 or 3 nuclear cataracts.

For grading of lens opacities, the Scheimpflug imaging depends on the morphological lens changes, which is more precise than the LOCS III system of cataract grading [27]. Additionally, it allows detecting even minute changes in the cataract progression. There is enough literature supporting a stronger correlation between Scheimpflug imaging grading and phacoemulsification parameters than LOCS III grading.

13.3.3.2 Traumatic Cataract

Cataracts may be an early or late complication of ocular trauma.

The role of Scheimpflug imaging in assessing the status of the posterior capsule was first described in an isolated case report by Grewal et al. in 2007 [29]. They showed that the posterior capsule rupture (PCR) with the lens matter escaping into the vitreous cavity (named it "pseudo-posterior lenticonus"). Sen et al. reported the sensitivity and specificity of this technique in eyes with traumatic cataracts as 70% and 85%, respectively [32]. However, Scheimpflug imaging is an optical method, and hence it is prone to poor image quality due to media opacity caused by corneal scars, very dense cataracts, and hyphema.

13.4 Anterior Segment Optical Coherence Tomography (AS-OCT)

Over the past three decades, optical coherence tomography (OCT) has evolved from time-domain OCT (TD-OCT), through spectral-domain OCT (SD-OCT), to the most current swept-source OCT (SS-OCT). The SS-OCT (tunable swept laser, 1050 nm) is superior to the SD-OCT (diode laser, 840 nm) due to increased scanning speed, number, and area [32]. Pujari et al. described the utility of the Fourier-domain AS-OCT CASIA-2 (Tomey Corp.) for preoperative evaluation of the posterior capsule integrity in patients with posterior polar cataracts [33]. This imaging modality is a non-invasive and non-contact in vivo imaging system for the ocular tissues that provide cross-sectional images from the corneal surface to the anterior hyaloid face, with a detailed assessment of the lens morphology. With AS-OCT, ocular biometry and morphological evaluation of the ocular structures are possible in a short period and with good clinical reproducibility. Currently, two anterior segment OCT (AS-OCT) models are commercially available, the Visante OCT (Carl Zeiss Meditec, Dublin, CA, USA) and the slit-lamp OCT (SLOCT) (Heidelberg Engineering, GmbH, Dossenheim, Germany) [34].

In the following sections, we describe the role of AS-OCT in objectively assessing cataract grades, intralenticular changes in white/mature cataracts, and posterior capsular changes in posterior polar and traumatic cataracts.

13.4.1 Principle of the AS-OCT

The AS-OCT technique creates high-resolution cross-sectional images of the anterior segment of the eye using the principle of low-coherence interferometry. The method compares the light reflected by the tissue structure being studied to the light reflected by a reference mirror and evaluates the delay and intensity of that light. The combination of these two signals results in an interference phenomenon. The device uses these signals to create a sagittal cross-section image of the studied structure. The signal intensity is dependent on the optical characteristics of the tissues. The posterior region of the eye was first visualized using OCT technology utilizing a wavelength of 820 nm. The newer models employ a super luminescent diode (SLD) of a longer wavelength (1310 nm) to allow better penetration through light-retaining tissues like the sclera and the limbus to improve visualization of the anterior segment.

13.4.2 Image Acquisition

The patient is seated comfortably before the machine. The patient's chin is placed on a support, and the patient is advised to focus on a fixation target to keep the eye steady during image capture. A near-infrared light source is directed into the eye, and the reflected light is used to create detailed images. The AS-OCT technique generates a series of A-scans (axial scans) representing the reflections of the near-infrared light from different tissue layers in the anterior segment. These A-scans are combined to create a 2D cross-sectional image of the examined structures. The captured A-scan data is processed to create detailed cross-sectional images. The software performs mathematical analyses to determine the thickness, depth, and shape of the cornea, iris, anterior chamber, and lens.

13.4.3 Clinical Applications

13.4.3.1 Early Cataract

Automated grading systems for cataracts on the AS-OCT technique have been constantly explored to overcome the inter-observer variability and bias of the LOCS III system [35]. Investigators have measured and correlated lens density on AS-OCT with cataract severity; an average lens density of 73.8-pixel units was suggestive of cataract with more than 95% sensitivity and 90% specificity [36, 37]. Often, the

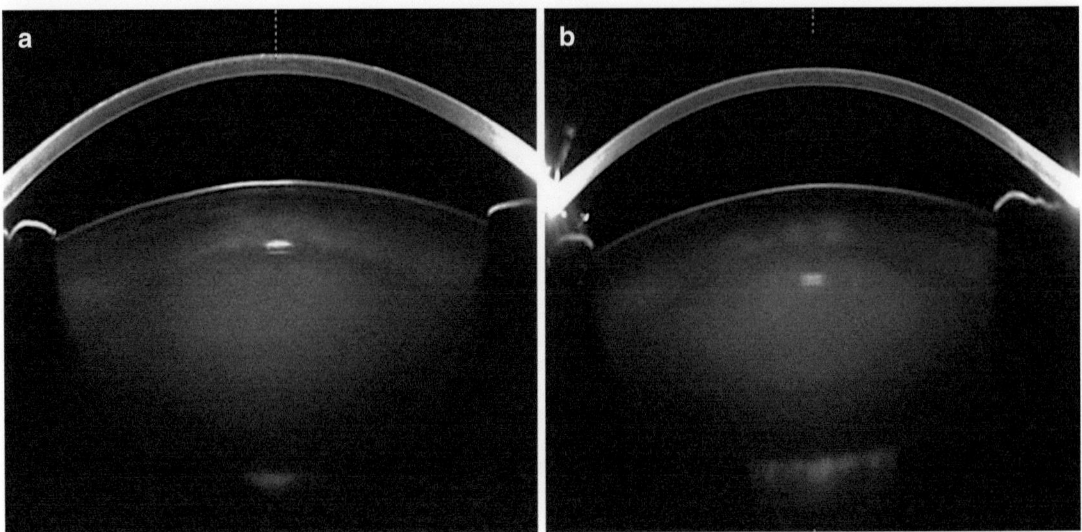

Fig. 13.8 The AS-OCT image showing hyperintensity along the posterior capsule suggests a posterior polar cataract (**a**). The posterior capsule appears intact as it can be traced continuously from the posterior paracentral region to the most dependent part of the lens under the opacity. Conversely, the hyperintensity is poorly defined with active herniation of the lens matter into the vitreous cavity, suggestive of a defect in the posterior capsule in the area of the posterior polar cataract (**b**)

patient's visual acuity alone may not be sufficient to assess the severity of the cataract. In these events, AS-OCT-based nuclear density data can serve as an additional guide to surgical planning.

13.4.3.2 Posterior Sub-capsular Cataract (PSC)

The AS-OCT technique demonstrates vacuolar changes along the posterior sub-capsular region [38].

13.4.3.3 Mature/Hypermature/White Cataracts

Intralenticular and posterior sub-capsular and capsular changes are difficult to detect clinically in denser cataracts. As the lens matures, the lens fibers undergo liquefaction with an accumulation of fluid within the bag, characterized as hypoechoic areas detected on the AS-OCT images. In such eyes, targeted needle aspirations may be performed intraoperatively to reduce the lenticular bag pressure, thus preventing rhexis-related complications, such as an uncontrolled extension of the rhexis [39]. Pujari et al. used AS-OCT images to understand the natural progression of mature cataracts measuring the intralenticular and anterior lens curvature changes, which [40] they graded into three stages as follows: Stage 1: "vacuolation" or "early lamellar separation" was characterized by tiny hypoechoic areas within the anterior lens substance, indicating early separation of the lens fibers. These cases carried the minimum risk of rhexis-related intraoperative complications. Stage 2: "advanced stage of lamellar separation" characterized by advanced lens fiber liquefaction causing wider hypoechoic areas within the anterior lens substance, with minimal bulge along the anterior lens surface with no liquefied lens material. These eyes carry fewer risks of rhexis-related complications. Stage 3: extensive lysis with excessive accumulation of liquefied material characterized by large hypoechoic areas and marked anterior lens bulge. These eyes carry the maximum risk of rhexis-related complications.

13.4.3.4 Posterior Polar Cataract (PPC)

In eyes with PPC, dysplastic lens fibers form a discoid plaque-like opacity at the posterior pole, interfering with the assessment of the underlying capsular integrity during a clinical examination [33] (Fig. 13.8a). The incidence of posterior capsular rupture (PCR) in PPC ranges from 7.1% to 36% [41]. Preoperative knowledge of the integrity of the posterior capsule (PC) can provide insight into improving surgical outcomes (Fig. 13.8b).

Several studies attempted preoperative identification of posterior capsular defects in eyes with PPC using cross-sectional images of the lens [42]. However, limitations like image resolution and magnification resulted in discrepancies between AS-OCT predictions and intraoperative findings. Pujari et al. used a modified posterior segment OCT (with a +20D lens) to predict posterior capsule integrity in eyes with PPC [33]. Two important parameters are the "contour" and "capsule." They proposed that the PC be traced from the adjacent paracentral region to the posterior-most dependent part of the lens from either side. The PC can be labelled "intact" if the continuity is maintained throughout. The posterior "contour" can have 3 possibilities: (1) conical sign: "active herniation" of the lens matter into the anterior vitreous cavity; (2) "moth-eaten appearance": the lens excavates into the posterior lens substance; (3) "zigzag ectatic appearance": inherent weakness of the posterior capsule. Concerns such as the quality of the scan and magnification should be addressed before any conclusions are made. Better-quality images were obtained using the swept source AS-OCT. This device provides images from the anterior to the posterior lens capsule in a single frame, with better resolution and magnification of up to 200 times, with minimal degradation of the image quality.

13.4.3.5 Traumatic Cataracts

In traumatic cataracts, accurate assessment of the cataract is often hampered due to coexisting complications like corneal laceration, severe inflammatory reactions in the anterior chamber, swollen cortical matter, and hyphema. A thorough preoperative knowledge of posterior capsule integrity is important to prevent unintentional extension of the PCR and loss of lens material into the vitreous cavity [43]. Preoperative AS-OCT helps identify any traumatic damage to the lens capsule, cortex, zonules, and vitreous prolapse. Kuriyan et al. reported AS-OCT-based vacuolar changes representing intracellular spaces in the anterior subcapsular region in an eye with a traumatic subluxated cataract [43]. The lens capsule and zonular integrity dictate the placement of the IOL; the ASOCT can detect and prepare the surgeon accordingly.

13.5 Ultrasound B-Scan

In people with mature and total cataracts, the fundus view is obscured. In such cases, B-scan ultrasonography is an indispensable tool that helps in surgical planning. Ultrasound is safe, inexpensive, and readily available than other imaging techniques, such as computed tomography (CT) and magnetic resonance imaging (MRI) [44].

13.5.1 Principle

Acoustic waves in ultrasound are produced by particle consistency oscillation within the medium. The B-scan gives vital information about the vitreous, retina, choroid, and sclera. The B (brightness) mode demonstrates the shape and topographic relationship of lesions in the posterior segment. A high-frequency (8–10 MHz) probe is used in ocular echography because it provides a more detailed picture than the low-frequency probes.

13.5.2 Image Acquisition [45]

Ultrasound can be performed through the patient's eyelids or by placing the probe directly on the surface of the eye with adequate topical anesthesia. The patient is advised to look in the direction of the quadrant to be examined, with the probe marker pointing superiorly or nasally. Initially, the gain is set high. From the limbus to the fornix, rocking and rotational movements are performed so that the probe tip moves a smaller distance than the base of the probe, which moves significantly. The probe is rotated around the globe in different quadrants so that the sound waves pass through the center of the eye. Since anterior segment structures require a standoff couplant, the immersion B-scan uses a water bath over the eyes. This method allows the probe to be offset from the eye sufficiently to place the anterior segment in the focal plane to observe the anterior segment, including the entire lens.

13.5.3 Clinical Applications

13.5.3.1 Detection of Posterior Segment Pathology

Several studies have reported the usefulness of B-scan ultrasonography in identifying posterior segment pathologies in eyes with mature and traumatic cataracts [46, 47]. The reported incidence of posterior segment pathology in eyes with opaque media is up to 66% [47]. Posterior vitreous detachment is the most common finding, with a sensitivity of 64.2% and specificity of 100%. Parchand et al. reported the sensitivity and specificity of this technique in identifying rhegmatogenous retinal detachment (92.31% and 98.31%, respectively), posterior vitreous separation (96.2% and 100%, respectively), and vitreous hemorrhage (100% for both) [48].

13.5.3.2 Detection of Zonular Weakness and Posterior Capsule Breach

In traumatic cataract, or where the view of the lens is obscured either due to corneal pathologies such as edema, scars, or anterior chamber hyphema, immersion or contact B-scan can detect gross zonular dehiscence, lens subluxation or dislocations, and larger posterior capture ruptures.

13.5.3.3 Intralenticular Foreign Bodies

In rare cases, the presence of an intra-ocular foreign body due to penetrating trauma (such as those occurring during a road traffic accident, blast injury, or hammer/chisel injury), when a foreign body is suspected but not immediately visible due to swollen cortical matter, poor patient cooperation, or anterior chamber inflammation, the precise anatomical location of the intralenticular foreign body can be obtained using the immersion B-scan [49] (Fig. 13.9).

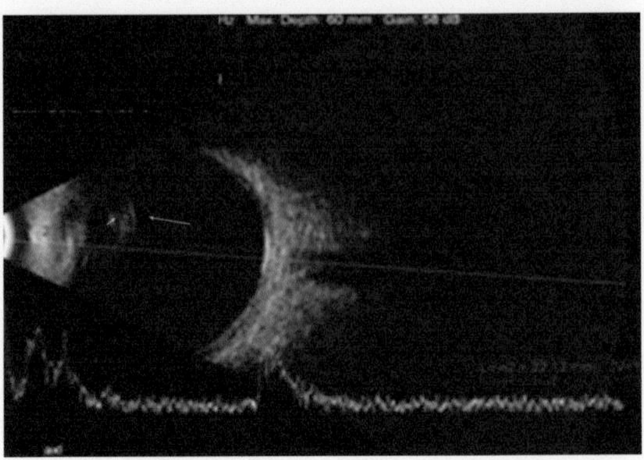

Fig. 13.9 Ultrasound B-scan immersion technique photograph showing high reflective dot echo (yellow arrowhead) within the lens matter with an intact posterior capsule (green arrow) confirming the diagnosis of an intralenticular foreign body

13.6 Conclusion

Preoperative imaging modalities are relatively simple and rapid, with a fairly easy learning curve. Anatomical details of the crystalline lens, such as the lens density, integrity of the posterior capsule, type of cataract, and existing comorbidities, can be assessed quickly and objectively with good repeatability. Aberrometry guides the surgeon in selecting an appropriate IOL and helps diagnose the cause of post-operative distressing symptoms. These techniques also have great potential in documenting cataract progression in longitudinal studies and clinical trials. Scheimpflug imaging is a rapid and simple-to-perform diagnostic procedure. It is extremely useful in children whose cooperation is usually poor. The lens densitometry measurements are easy, quick, repeatable, and objective methods to assess lens changes over time. The versatility of the Scheimpflug imaging technique is useful in diagnosing various degrees of cataract, posterior-capsule rupture, and traumatic cataracts; this makes it an invaluable but neglected tool for modern cataract surgeons. The AS-OCT technique is helpful in complex lenticular pathologies. Finally, the immersion mode of B-scan ultrasound is useful in uncooperative patients and open globe injuries.

Over the years, people's expectations have increased with the evolution of cataract surgery techniques and technologies. Consequently, the preoperative assessment has expanded to include discussions of the patient's visual expectations and various surgical options, each of which may have its own medical and financial considerations. Various diagnostic tests performed at the preoperative visit enable the surgeon to anticipate and address these to achieve optimal functional outcomes.

Funding None.

Disclosure None.

References

1. Lee AC, Qazi MA, Pepose JS. Biometry and intraocular lens power calculation. Curr Opin Ophthalmol. 2008;19:13–7.
2. Sahin A, Hamrah P. Clinically relevant biometry. Curr Opin Ophthalmol. 2012;23:47–53.
3. Davison JA, Potvin R. Preoperative measurement vs. intraoperative aberrometry for the selection of intraocular lens sphere power in normal eyes. Clin Ophthalmol Auckl NZ. 2017;11: 923–9.
4. Marcos S. Aberrometry: basic science and clinical applications. Bull Soc Belge Ophtalmol. 2006;302:197–213.
5. Salmon TO, van de Pol C. Evaluation of a clinical aberrometer for lower-order accuracy and repeatability, higher-order repeatability, and instrument myopia. Optom St Louis MO. 2005;76:461–72.
6. Parede TRR, Torricelli AAM, Mukai A, et al. Quality of vision in refractive and cataract surgery, indirect measurers: review article. Arq Bras Oftalmol. 2013;76:386–90.
7. Molebny VV, Panagopoulou SI, Molebny SV, et al. Principles of ray tracing aberrometry. J Refract Surg Thorofare NJ. 1995;2000(16):S572–5.
8. Pallikaris IG, Panagopoulou SI, Molebny VV. Clinical experience with the Tracey technology wavefront device. J Refract Surg Thorofare NJ. 1995;2000(16):S588–91.
9. Beiko GHH. Personalized correction of spherical aberration in cataract surgery. J Cataract Refract Surg. 2007;33:1455–60.
10. Khanna A. Role of asphericity in choice of IOLs for cataract surgery. Delhi J Ophthalmol. 2015;25:185–9.
11. Miháltz K, Vécsei-Marlovits P. The impact of visual axis position on the optical quality after implantation of multifocal intraocular lenses with different asphericity values. Graefes Arch Clin Exp Ophthalmol. 2021;259:673–83.
12. Jun I, Choi YJ, Kim EK, et al. Internal spherical aberration by ray tracing-type aberrometry in multifocal pseudophakic eyes. Eye. 2012;26:1243–8.
13. Niu Y, Lin H, Qin Y, et al. Three-random-point marking method for toric intraocular lens alignment using the iTrace aberrometer. J Ophthalmol. 2021;2021:6695454. https://doi.org/10.1155/2021/6695454.
14. Martínez-Plaza E, Ruiz-Fortes P, Soto-Negro R, et al. Characterization of dysfunctional lens index and opacity grade in a healthy population. Diagn Basel Switz. 2022;12:1167. https://doi.org/10.3390/diagnostics12051167.
15. Chylack LT, Wolfe JK, Singer DM, et al. The lens opacities classification system III. The Longitudinal Study of Cataract Study Group. Arch Ophthalmol Chic Ill. 1960;1993(111):831–6.
16. Age-Related Eye Disease Study Research Group. The age-related eye disease study (AREDS) system for classifying cataracts from photographs: AREDS report no. 4. Am J Ophthalmol. 2001;131:167–75.
17. Hall NF, Lempert P, Shier RP, et al. Grading nuclear cataract: reproducibility and validity of a new method. Br J Ophthalmol. 1999;83:1159–63.
18. Grewal DS, Grewal SPS. Clinical applications of Scheimpflug imaging in cataract surgery. Saudi J Ophthalmol. 2012;26:25–32.
19. West SK, Rosenthal F, Newland HS, Taylor HR. Use of photographic techniques to grade nuclear cataracts. Invest Ophthalmol Vis Sci. 1988;29:73–7.
20. Brown N. An advanced slit-image camera. Br J Ophthalmol. 1972;56:624–31.
21. Brown SI, Bloomfield SE, Pearce DB. A follow-up report on transplantation of the alkali-burned cornea. Am J Ophthalmol. 1974;77:538–42.
22. Hockwin O, Dragomirescu V, Laser H. Measurements of lens transparency or its disturbances by densitometric image analysis of Scheimpflug photographs. Graefes Arch Clin Exp Ophthalmol Albrecht Von Graefes Arch Klin Exp Ophthalmol. 1982;219:255–62.
23. Brown NA, Bron AJ, Sparrow JM. Methods for evaluation of lens changes. Int Ophthalmol. 1988;12:229–35.
24. Kashima K, Trus BL, Unser M, Edwards PA, Datiles MB. Aging studies on normal lens using the Scheimpflug slit-lamp camera. Invest Ophthalmol Vis Sci. 1993;34:263–9.
25. Magno BV, Freidlin V, Datiles MB. Reproducibility of the NEI Scheimpflug cataract imaging system. Invest Ophthalmol Vis Sci. 1994;35:3078–84.
26. Foo KP, Maclean H. Measured changes in cataract over six months: sensitivity of the Nidek EAS-1000. Ophthalmic Res. 1996;28(2):32–6.

27. Pei X, Bao Y, Chen Y, Li X. Correlation of lens density measured using the Pentacam Scheimpflug system with the lens opacities classification system III grading score and visual acuity in age-related nuclear cataract. Br J Ophthalmol. 2008;92:1471–5.
28. Jeria S, Aggarwal A, Singh K, et al. Assessment of age-related cataract using scheimpflug imaging system and its correlation with phacoemulsification parameters. J Clin Diagn Res [Internet]. 2020; [cited 2023 Jun 3]. https://jcdr.net/article_fulltext.asp
29. Grewal DS, Brar GS, Grewal SPS. Correlation of nuclear cataract lens density using Scheimpflug images with Lens Opacities Classification System III and visual function. Ophthalmology. 2009;116:1436–43.
30. Baradaran-Rafii A, Rahmati-Kamel M, Eslani M, et al. Effect of hydrodynamic parameters on corneal endothelial cell loss after phacoemulsification. J Cataract Refract Surg. 2009;35:732–7.
31. Nixon DR. Preoperative cataract grading by Scheimpflug imaging and effect on operative fluidics and phacoemulsification energy. J Cataract Refract Surg. 2010;36:242–6.
32. Gabriele ML, Wollstein G, Ishikawa H, et al. Optical coherence tomography: history, current status, and laboratory work. Invest Ophthalmol Vis Sci. 2011;52:2425–36.
33. Pujari A, Yadav S, Sharma N, et al. Study 1: evaluation of the signs of deficient posterior capsule in posterior polar cataracts using anterior segment optical coherence tomography. J Cataract Refract Surg. 2020;46:1260–5.
34. Ramos JLB, Li Y, Huang D. Clinical and research applications of anterior segment optical coherence tomography—a review. Clin Exp Ophthalmol. 2009;37:81–9.
35. Wong AL, Leung CKS, Weinreb RN, et al. Quantitative assessment of lens opacities with anterior segment optical coherence tomography. Br J Ophthalmol. 2009;93:61–5.
36. Panthier C, Burgos J, Rouger H, et al. New objective lens density quantification method using swept-source optical coherence tomography technology: comparison with existing methods. J Cataract Refract Surg. 2017;43:1575–81.
37. Panthier C, de Wazieres A, Rouger H, et al. Average lens density quantification with swept-source optical coherence tomography: optimized, automated cataract grading technique. J Cataract Refract Surg. 2019;45:1746–52.
38. Enaida H, Nakao I, Ishikawa S, et al. Optical coherence tomography imaging for gas-induced posterior subcapsular cataract after lens-sparing vitrectomy. Can J Ophthalmol. 2020;55:e178–80.
39. Dhami A, Dhami AS, Singh H, Dhami GS. Role of anterior segment optical coherence tomography for safer management of mature white cataracts. J Cataract Refract Surg. 2019;45:480–4.
40. Pujari A, Sharma N. The emerging role of anterior segment optical coherence tomography in cataract surgery: current role and future perspectives. Clin Ophthalmol Auckl NZ. 2021;15:389–401.
41. Hayashi K, Hayashi H, Nakao F, Hayashi F. Outcomes of surgery for posterior polar cataract. J Cataract Refract Surg. 2003;29:45–9.
42. Chan TCY, Li EYM, Yau JCY. Application of anterior segment optical coherence tomography to identify eyes with posterior polar cataract at high risk for posterior capsule rupture. J Cataract Refract Surg. 2014;40:2076–81.
43. Kuriyan AE, Flynn HW Jr, Yoo SH. Subluxed traumatic cataract: optical coherence tomography findings and clinical management. Clin Ophthalmol. 2012;6:1997–9. https://doi.org/10.2147/OPTH.S37393.
44. Qureshi MA, Laghari K. Role of B-scan ultrasonography in pre-operative cataract patients. Int J Health Sci. 2010;4:31–7.
45. Coleman DJ, Dallow RL, Smith ME. Immersion ultrasonography: simultaneous A-scan and B-scan. Int Ophthalmol Clin. 1979;19:67–102.
46. Salman A, Parmar P, Vanila CG, et al. Is ultrasonography essential before surgery in eyes with advanced cataracts? J Postgrad Med. 2006;52:19–22.
47. Anteby II, Blumenthal EZ, Zamir E, Waindim P. The role of preoperative ultrasonography for patients with dense cataract: a retrospective study of 509 cases. Ophthalmic Surg Lasers. 1998;29:114–8.
48. Parchand S, Singh R, Bhalekar S. Reliability of ocular ultrasonography findings for pre-surgical evaluation in various vitreo-retinal disorders. Semin Ophthalmol. 2014;29:236–41.
49. Thapa BB, Singh S, Basnet R, Lamichhane G. Ultrasound immersion technique in the management of intra-lenticular foreign body in low resource setting: a case series. Nepal J Ophthalmol. 2022;14:183–90.

14 Slit Lamp Biomicroscopy

Anahita Kate and Sayan Basu

14.1 Introduction

Ophthalmology distinguishes itself from other medical disciplines by the unique advantage of directly examining the organ it focuses on. The most important instrument that facilitates this is the slit lamp biomicroscope. This indispensable tool provides a gamut of information on the various parts of the eye, from the external ocular surface and adnexa to the lens and posterior segment structures. These can be viewed at different magnifications and with additional filters. The binocularity of this compound microscope augments ocular evaluation and elicits subtle signs [1]. The versatility and precision of the slit lamp have made it an indispensable device for diagnosing and monitoring various ocular conditions, empowering eye care professionals to provide targeted treatments. While there is a general familiarity with the basic functioning of this device, an in-depth understanding can allow ophthalmologists to maximize the potential of a slit lamp in their daily practice. In this chapter, we will explore the different components and applications of the slit lamp, highlighting its invaluable role in ophthalmic practice.

14.2 History

The unique feature of a slit lamp is the alterable slit beam for illumination and the fact that the focal planes of the illuminating and the observer arm coincide to give a binocular, well-illuminated field. The development of the slit lamp has spanned more than two centuries; it can be understood in terms of each of these sections. Historically, the observer arm was put through several innovations while keeping the illumination uniform. In 1823, Purkinje was the first to examine the iris with a microscope and a fixed source of illumination [2]. Nealy, 40 years later, Louis de Wecker used an objective, eyepiece, and a condensing lens to develop the first uniocular slit lamp [3]. Siegfried Czapski subsequently introduced binocularity; it provided the examiner with a stereoscopic view of the ocular structures

A. Kate
Kode Venkatadri Chowdary Campus, L V Prasad Eye Institute, Vijayawada, India
e-mail: dranahitakate@lvpei.org

S. Basu (✉)
Shantilal Shanghvi Cornea Institute, Kallam Anji Reddy Campus, L V Prasad Eye Institute, Hyderabad, India

Prof. Brien Holden Eye Research Centre, Champalimaud Translational Centre for Eye Research, L V Prasad Eye Institute, Hyderabad, India
e-mail: sayanbasu@lvpei.org

T. Das, P. Satgunam (eds.), *Ophthalmic Diagnostics*, https://doi.org/10.1007/978-981-97-0138-4_14

[4]. This eventually paved the way for Allvar Gullstrand to use the concept of a focused slit to illuminate the eye and observe its structures [5]. The source of light was a Nernst lamp with an adjustable slit at the other end. In 1915–16, this illumination system was combined with Czapski's binocular device by Otto Henker, and thus, the slit lamp was invented [3]. In the following years, further improvements were made to the slit lamp, including a swivel design to allow movement of the illuminating arm and different light sources. Hans Goldmann coupled the focal planes of these two arms and engineered a joystick that could control the movement of the entire unit [6]. The introduction of the rotatory magnifying system by Hans Littman enabled a comprehensive examination of the ocular structures [7]. Alfred Vogt played a pivotal role in advancing our understanding of slit lamp examinations through his innovative and meticulous utilization of this tool [8]. His pioneering work, documented in his atlas, helped establish the slit lamp as a crucial instrument in ophthalmology. Over the next few decades, various modifications and advancements were made, including adding filters to enhance contrast and visualization of specific structures within the eye. Additionally, introducing different types of lenses allowed for better magnification and focused examination of different eye regions. With the rapid advancements in technology, modern slit lamps have become even more sophisticated and now feature the ability to capture high-resolution images and videos of the eye.

14.3 Parts of a Slit Lamp

The slit lamp consists of three parts: the illumination system, the observer system, and the mechanical unit coupling these two. Figure 14.1 depicts the different parts of the slit lamp.

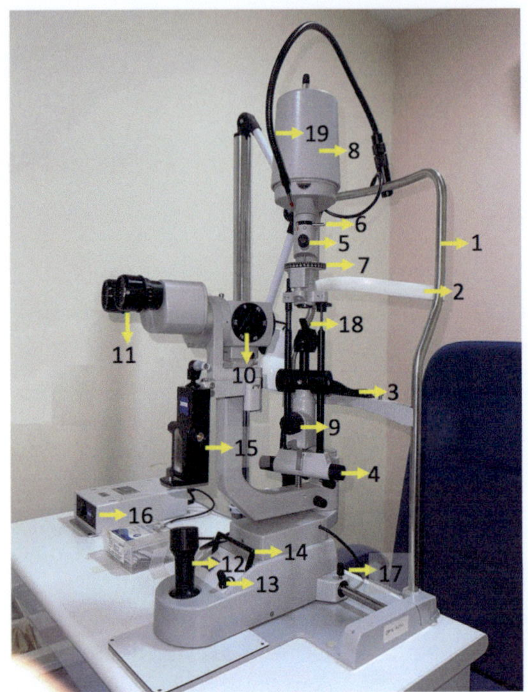

Fig. 14.1 Image of a slit lamp with marked parts. (1) patient frame, (2) forehead band, (3) chin rest, (4) slit width control, (5) slit height control, (6) filters, (7) slit angle indicator, (8) illumination tower, (9) decoupling control, (10) magnification, (11) eyepiece, (12) joystick, (13) illumination knob, (14) base lock, (15) applanation tonometer, (16) power switch, (17) screw lock, (18) reflecting mirror, (19) fixation target

14.3.1 The Illumination Unit

The illumination unit produces a precise slit beam of light of variable length, breadth, and brightness based on the examination area. The light source can be situated above or below the observer unit, as seen in the Haag-Streit (Koniz, Switzerland) and Zeiss (Jena, Germany) slit lamps, respectively. Additionally, prisms and mirrors are used to manipulate the beam of light within the small confines of the illumination unit. The sources of light include halogen lamps, low-voltage incandescent lamps, and light-emitting diodes (LED). The choice of the light source is balanced between its durability and the color temperature. With respect to the latter, light with a greater degree of blue within it is preferred since it scatters easily, thus making detecting pathologies easier [3]. Köhler's principle of illumination is used to produce a homogeneous beam of light wherein the light from the source is transmitted through a collector system of plano-convex lenses and then passed through a slit aperture [9]. This aperture acts as a new light source, emitting rays that pass through the objective lens to generate an image of the slit onto the area under examination. The height and width of the slit beam can be altered by opening the vertical and horizontal shutters of the light aperture. It can also be swiveled across the horizontal plane to pass this light beam through different eye structures. The slit beam can also be rotated through different angles and made completely horizontal. This is particularly useful when measuring different structures and anomalies. It is typically carried out by reducing the slit beam width to 0.5–1 mm and altering the height until it matches the structure being evaluated.

Different filters add perspective to the various pathologies viewed through a slit lamp biomicroscope. These filters are located between the slit aperture and the objective lens. The cobalt blue filter (Wratten 47/47A) is employed with the fluorescein dye and aids in identifying areas where the corneal or conjunctival epithelial layer has been compromised [10]. It also helps evaluate the health of the tear film, perform Seidel's test, and assess the fit of contact lenses. Optionally, a yellow barrier filter that blocks the incoming blue light and improves contrast can also be used. Although the Zeiss slit lamps have an inbuilt filter, models that do not have this feature can have the filter added as an attachment [10]. The red-free filter enhances the evaluation of any area of inflammation, and this is particularly useful in localizing the depth of inflammation in episcleritis and scleritis. A neutral density filter decreases the intensity of the light and enables visualization in symptomatic/photophobic patients. A diffuser is also present external to the illumination arm which can be manually brought into place to illuminate the examined area evenly.

14.3.2 Observer System

This consists of a collation of lenses that help assess the observed area with sufficient magnification to allow the required examination details. This includes two telescopic systems, one at each end of the observer system. A Galilean telescope is present at the objective end of the slit lamp and is formed by a combination of a convex and a concave lens with a total power of +22D [3, 11]. Similarly, a Keplerian/astronomical lens is situated within the eyepiece and is fashioned with two convex lenses with a combined power of 10D [3, 11]. Since the latter produces an inverted image, a Porro prism is placed between the two telescopic systems to correct the same [3, 11]. These telescopes function on the principle that the image formed by one lens falls on the principal focus of the second lens.

Additionally, a graded magnification change is possible either by changing the eyepieces or using an incorporated changer. The latter comprises two Galilean telescopes, which can be rotated to accommodate different orders of magnification. The degree of magnification varies among the slit lamps and can range from 6.3× to 40×. Each eye of the examiner has an independent path between the source and the image formed, thus allowing good stereopsis. The eyepieces converge at an angle of 10–15° to facilitate the same. The eyepieces also feature lenses that can be set to plano or adjusted according to the examiner's refractive error, eliminating the need for them to wear glasses.

14.3.3 The Mechanical System

The illumination and observer systems are connected through a base mechanical unit which not only facilitates the coupling of the two systems but also allows a three-dimensional movement of the entire complex. This is enabled with a joystick that can move forward, backward, and along an up-down axis as well. This is usually accompanied by a lock system that can fix the unit in a desired location. The control of illumination with an intensity rheostat and a power switch is also located within the base of the mechanical unit. The slit lamp has a motorized system that enables vertical movement of the entire unit with a control.

The patient frame consists of a forehead band against which the patient rests the head and an adjustable chin rest beneath this. This frame also has a canthus height marker that indicates the level to which the lateral canthus should be aligned. Ensuring proper alignment of the patient to these three landmarks will ensure that the patient's eyeball falls within the focal plane of the slit lamp system. Two handles extend laterally from this frame over which the patients can rest their hands during examination. A mobile blinking light is also incorporated into the slit lamp to serve as a fixation target for patients in various gaze positions to ensure consistent eye alignment.

14.4 Machine Specifications

The growth and development of the slit lamp have been greatly facilitated by two prominent companies, namely Zeiss and Haag-Streit. These companies have played a pivotal role in advancing the field of ophthalmology by continuously innovating and producing high-quality slit lamps that have become integral tools for eye care professionals worldwide. Today several ophthalmological diagnostics companies manufacture slit lamps, and within each company, the specifications vary based on different models. As describing all these modifications is beyond the scope of this chapter, the salient points of some of these devices are summarized in Table 14.1.

14.5 Examination Techniques

The various methods of examination employed in slit lamp examination are derived from different variations of brightness, height, breadth, and position of the illumination arm. Broadly this can be divided into direct and indirect forms of illumination. In the former, the area of interest is directly illuminated by the light source. In indirect illumination, the examined area is illuminated by the light reflected from a structure posterior to it. These techniques are discussed in detail below.

14.5.1 Direct Illumination

This includes diffuse illumination, focal illumination, and specular reflection.

(i) *Diffuse illumination:* In diffuse illumination, the width of the slit is broad, or a diffuser is used, and a low magnification is preferred. This is typically employed when an even illumination is desired while the initial gross examination is done. It is also used for slit lamp photographs for documentation, in conjunction with a slit beam, to provide context to the structures within the slit (Fig. 14.2).

(ii) *Focal illumination:* This uses the scattering of light within the area of interest to highlight abnormalities (Fig. 14.2). The dimly lit sur-

Table 14.1 Comparison of the commonly used slit lamp platforms

Slit lamp company	Design[a]	Magnification	Light source	Filters
Haag-Streit Slit lamps (Haag-Streit, AG Koniz, Switzerland)	Tower	6.3/10/16/25/40× 10/16/25× 10/16×	LED	Gray, red-free, blue
Zeiss slit lamps (Carl Zeiss AG, Jena, Germany)	Tower/integrated	6/10/16/25/40× 5/8/12/20/32× 10/16/25×	LED/Halogen	Blue, red-free, yellow (optional)
Appasamy (Appasamy Associates, Chennai, India)	Tower	6/10/16/25/40× 10/16/24× 10/16×	LED	Heat-absorbing, red-free, blue
Nidek (Nidek, Gamagori, Aichi, Japan)	Integrated	5/8/12.5/20/32×	LED	Gray, red-free, blue
Topcon (Topcon Medical Systems, Tokyo, Japan)	Tower/integrated	10/16/25× 6/10/16/25/40×	LED/Halogen	Blue, red-free, gray

LED Light emitting diode

[a]Tower: light source from above, integrated: light source from below

rounding area offers a high degree of contrast and makes it easy to detect subtle changes. It provides three-dimensional information, which allows us to understand the profile and thickness of the structure being examined and its position with respect to the source of the light. Within the section of light, structures that are present closer to the source are anterior and vice versa. This is perhaps the most commonly used mode of slit lamp examination and yields a plethora of information depending on the height, width, and angle of the slit. Based on these parameters, focal illumination can further be divided into a parallelopiped and an optical section.

(a) *Parallelopiped*: Here, the width of the slit is between 1 and 2 mm and is placed at an angle of 35°–45°. This provides a three-dimensional block view of different ocular structures and enables localization of the same. Since the field of view is greater than the optical section, it is more sensitive at picking up findings.

(b) *Optical section*: Here, the term "section" is used because the beam of light provides a slit image of a semi-transparent structure which is analogous to a histopathological section of tissue. In an optical section, the width of the slit is extremely narrow and ranges between 0.1 and 0.3 mm, and the angle of illumination can be varied between 30°–50°. The magnification depends on whether the lesion location or thickness is measured. For the former, a higher magnification of 16–25x is preferred, while a magnification of 10–16x can be used for the latter since a decent field of view is also required. The light intensity is another key factor that can improve the sensitivity of slit lamp examination and has to be titrated based on the opacity of

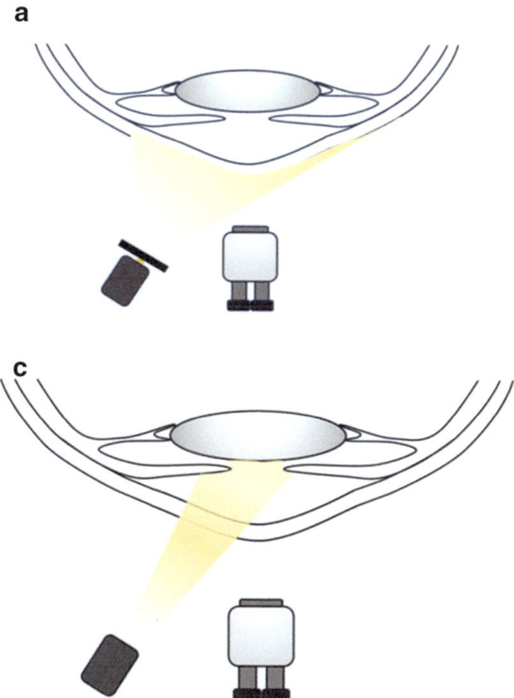

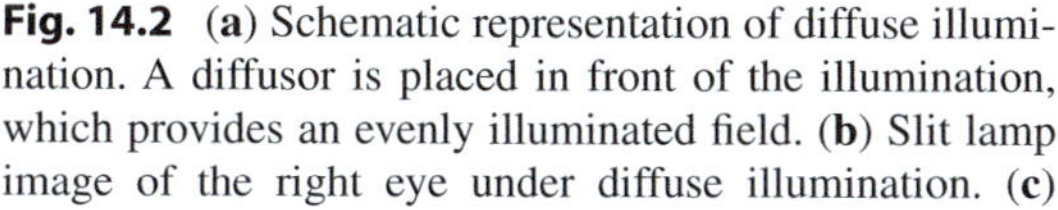

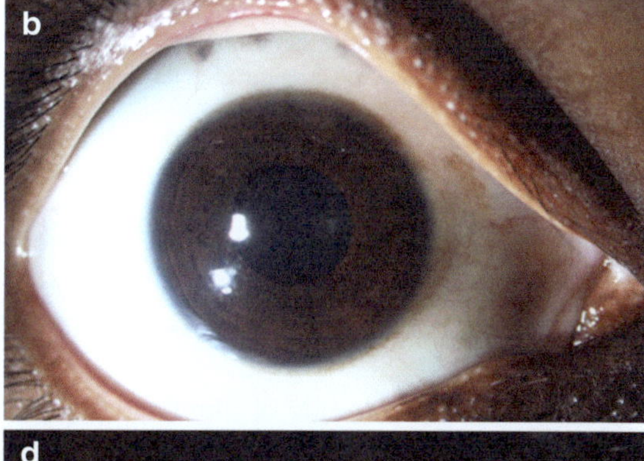

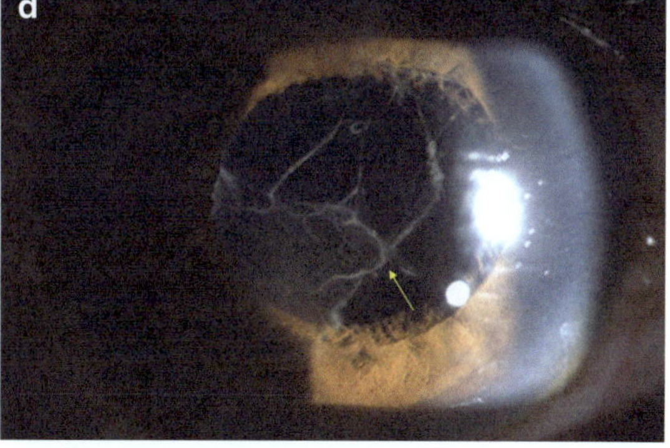

Fig. 14.2 (**a**) Schematic representation of diffuse illumination. A diffusor is placed in front of the illumination, which provides an evenly illuminated field. (**b**) Slit lamp image of the right eye under diffuse illumination. (**c**) Schematic representation of focal illumination with a moderate slit. (**d**) Slit lamp image of a moderate slit with focal illumination depicting fibrin strands in the pupillary plane (yellow arrows)

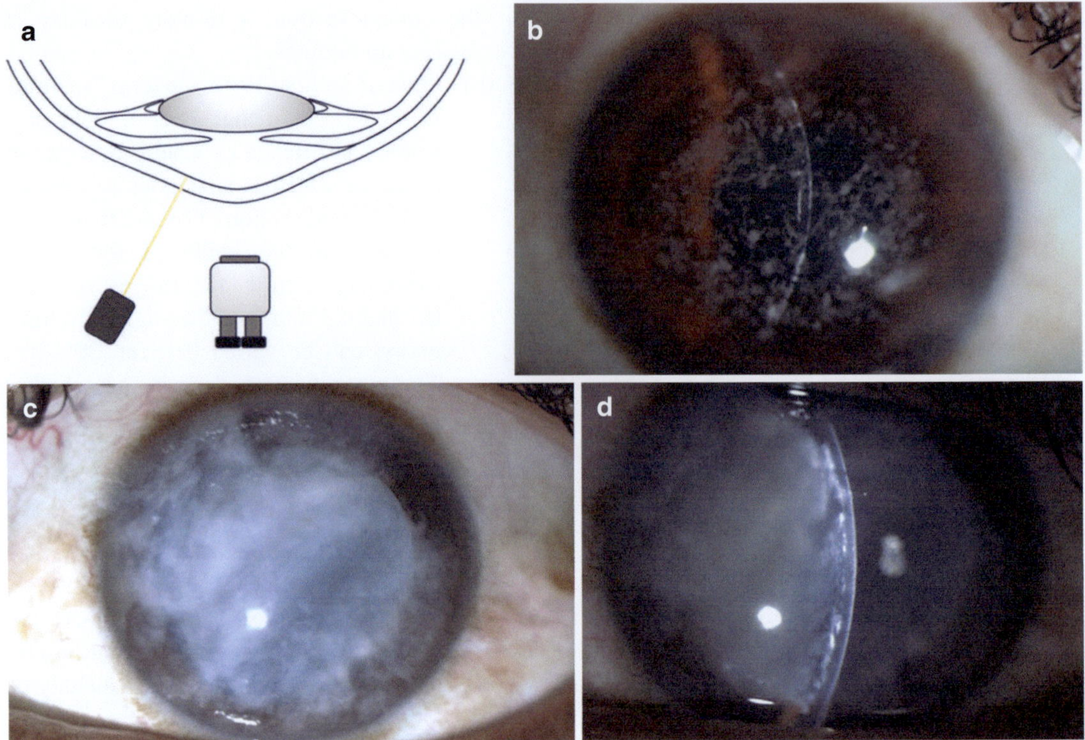

Fig. 14.3 (**a**) Schematic representation of an optical section. (**b**) Slit lamp image of corneal granular dystrophy examined with an optical section which reveals the exact depth of different deposits. (**c**) Diffuse illumination image of an eye with a white media opacity. (**d**) An optical section shows a relatively clear and compact cornea with dispersed loose cortical matter in the anterior chamber and a traumatic cataract. Thus, the optical section helps us understand the structures involved

the structure being examined. Very high or low intensities may mask important findings and should be avoided. Increasing the angle of illumination will increase the width of the optical section and thus enhance the details of the image (Fig. 14.3).

(iii) *Specular reflection:* It uses the principle of specular reflection where the angle of incident light is equal to the angle of the reflected light [12]. To achieve this with a slit lamp, the observer and illuminating arm are placed at an angle of approximately 60° to each other. To begin with, the slit height is reduced to 2–3 mm, and the width is kept around 1 mm with a low-moderate intensity of light. Once the slit is brought into focus, the illuminating arm is moved until the reflection of light is sighted, which is the first Purkinje image. Posterior to this on the corneal endothelium will lie the second Purkinje image, which is usually dimmer. The corneal endothelial cells can be examined within this area (Fig. 14.4). This examination technique can also be used on the conjunctival surface and for the tear film.

14.5.2 Indirect Illumination

This includes proximal illumination, sclerotic scatter, and retro-illumination. The properties of refraction and absorption are used to emphasize subtle changes.

(i) *Proximal illumination:* In this type of illumination, the two arms of the slit lamp are placed in such a way that the examined tissue acts as a light source, and the structures within it are backlit. To achieve this, the illu-

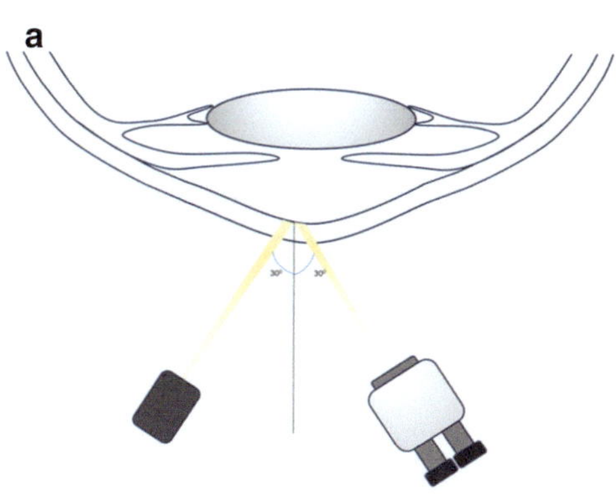

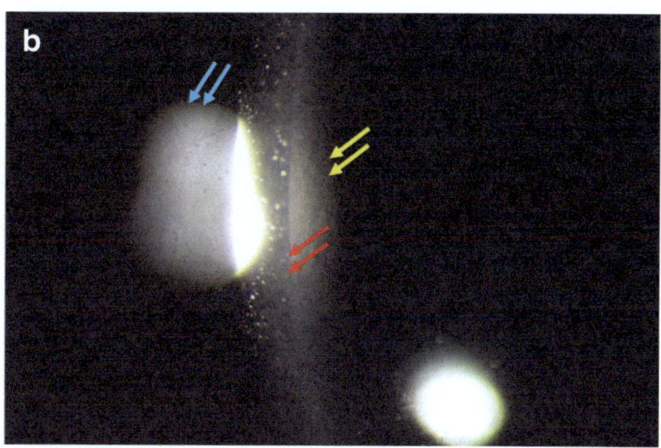

Fig. 14.4 (**a**) Schematic representation of specular reflection, with the incident light angle being equal to that of the reflected light. (**b**) Slit lamp image, which has captured the specular light reflection (blue arrows). The vertical slit must coincide with this image. In this image, the anterior slit image is from the corneal epithelium, and this is the first Purkinje image (red arrows). The second Purkinje image behind it is from the corneal endothelium (yellow arrows)

mination beam is placed tangential to the area of interest such that the light is directed toward its base and gets reflected from it. This is particularly useful to highlight details of semi-transparent structures based on how the light gets refracted or absorbed within them (Fig. 14.5; top row).

(ii) *Sclerotic scatter:* This employs the principle of total internal reflection of light and creates this phenomenon within the cornea. Any structural abnormalities will produce a scattering of light, thus highlighting these areas. However, this technique will not give information on the depth of these irregularities. The illumination arm is first decoupled from the observer arm to perform a sclerotic scatter. A 4–5 mm slit beam is focused on the limbus with a high intensity of light, and the magnification is set so that the entire cornea falls within the field of view. The position of the observer arm is adjusted until a brilliant circle of light is visible, encircling the cornea. This is the point where a total internal reflection of light occurs within the stromal layers. A normal cornea appears dark, which allows the examiner to detect very subtle changes. A limitation of this technique is that it may be challenging to perform on a photophobic patient since it involves a very bright beam of light (Fig. 14.5; bottom row).

(iii) *Retro-illumination:* Here, a posterior structure is used to reflect the light from the source. This can further be divided into direct and indirect retro-illumination based on the position of the area of interest.

(a) *Direct retro-illumination*: In direct retro-illumination, the area of interest is directly illuminated by the light reflected off the iris, lens, or fundus. The angle of the illuminating arm can vary based on the structure that the light has to reflect. In the case of retro-illumination from the iris or the lens, the angle of illumination is kept between 30° and 50°, with a moderate to high light intensity and a slit width of 1.5–2 mm. When retro-illumination from the fundus is desired, the illuminating arm is kept coaxially with a low to moderate light intensity (Fig. 14.6).

(b) *Indirect Retro-illumination* involves placing the area of interest between the slits formed on the cornea and the posterior structure, be it the iris or the lens. The observed area is examined against a dark background which offers a contrast. Increasing the illumination angle creates greater space between the two slits and allows better viewing of the in-between structures (Fig. 14.7). Minimal decentration of the observer arm may be required to visualize the pathologies.

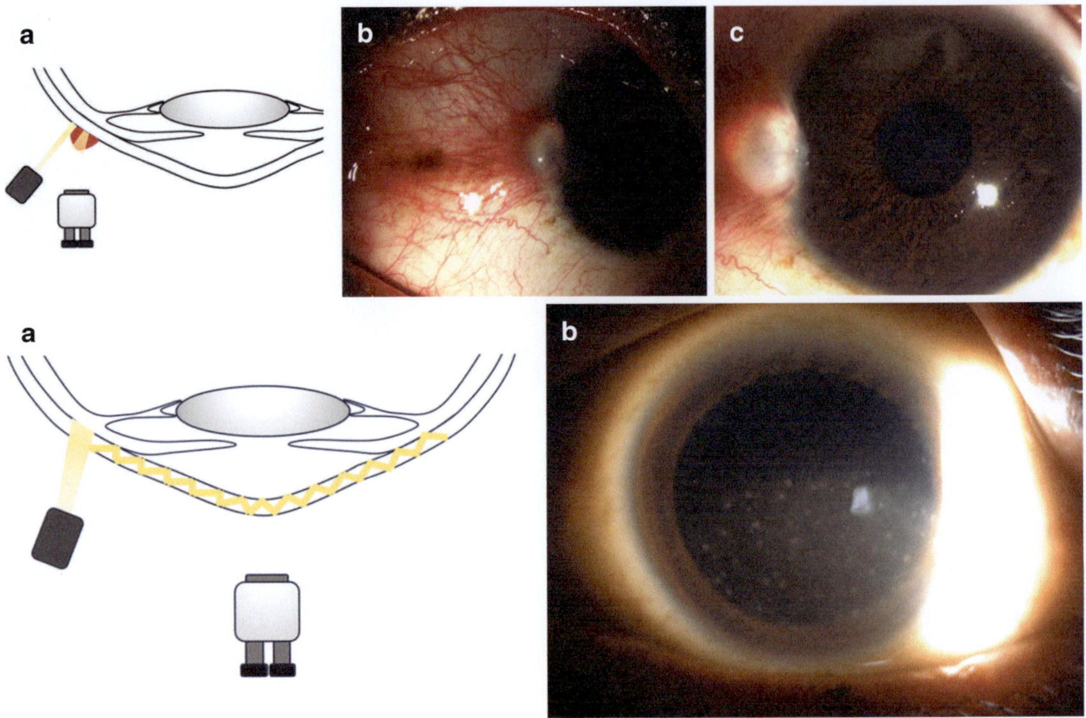

Fig. 14.5 Top Row: (**a**) Schematic representation of proximal illumination wherein light tangential to a mass lesion strikes its bases and acts as a new source of light from within the lesion. (**b**) Slit lamp photograph of a cyst within the head of a pterygium under diffuse illumination. (**c**) The proximal illumination depicts the cystic nature of the lesion. **Bottom Row:** (**a**) Schematic representation of sclerotic scatter. (**b**) Slit lamp image of sclerotic scatter depicting keratic precipitates in the inferior half of the cornea with surrounding corneal haze. The superior half of the cornea, which is relatively uninvolved, appears dark

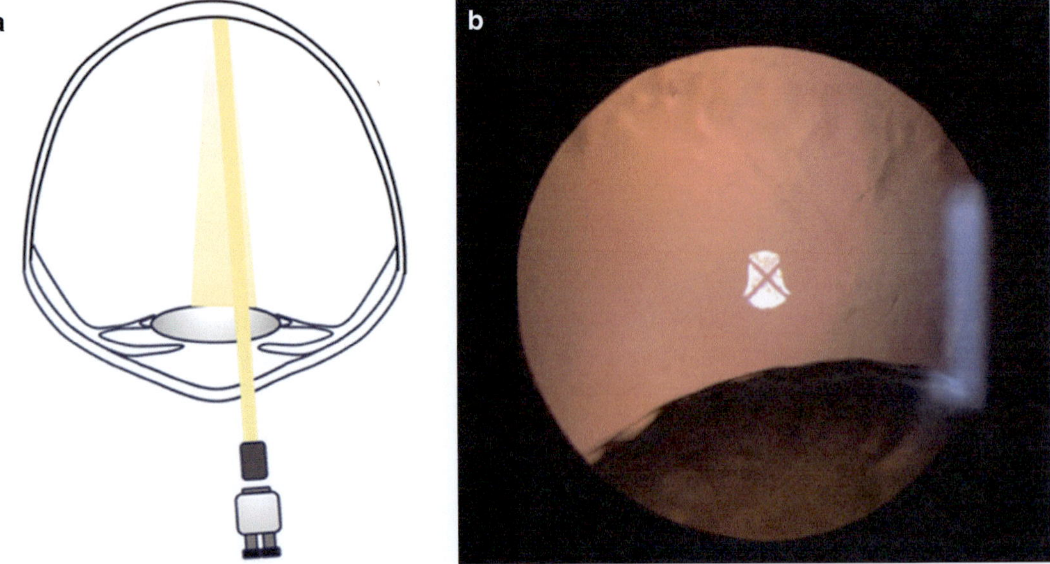

Fig. 14.6 (**a**) Schematic representation of retro-illumination from the fundus. Slit lamp photographs of fundus retro-illumination illustrating. (**b**) A subluxated lens in the inferior half of the pupillary area. (**c**) A lamellar cataract. (**d**) Markings in a toric intraocular lens along with the margins of the capsular bag

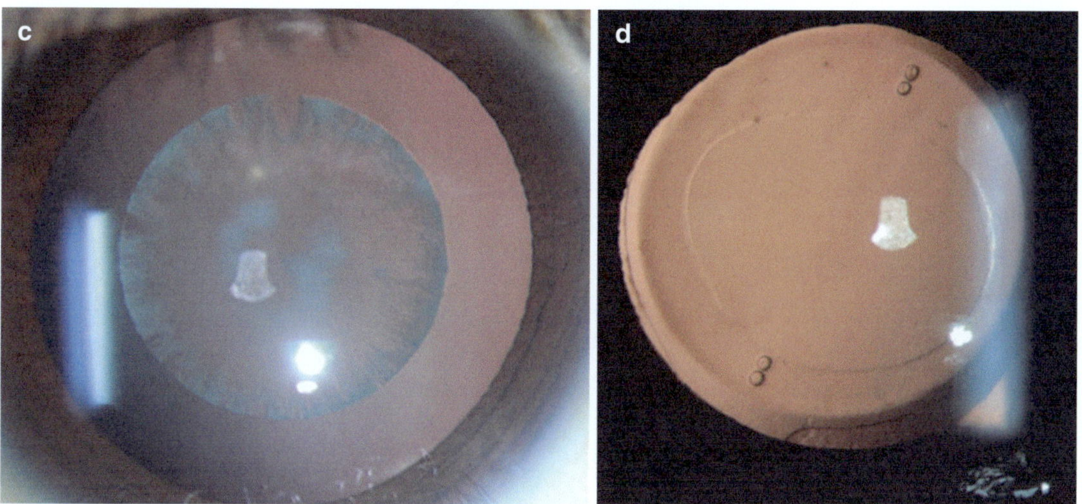

Fig. 14.6 (continued)

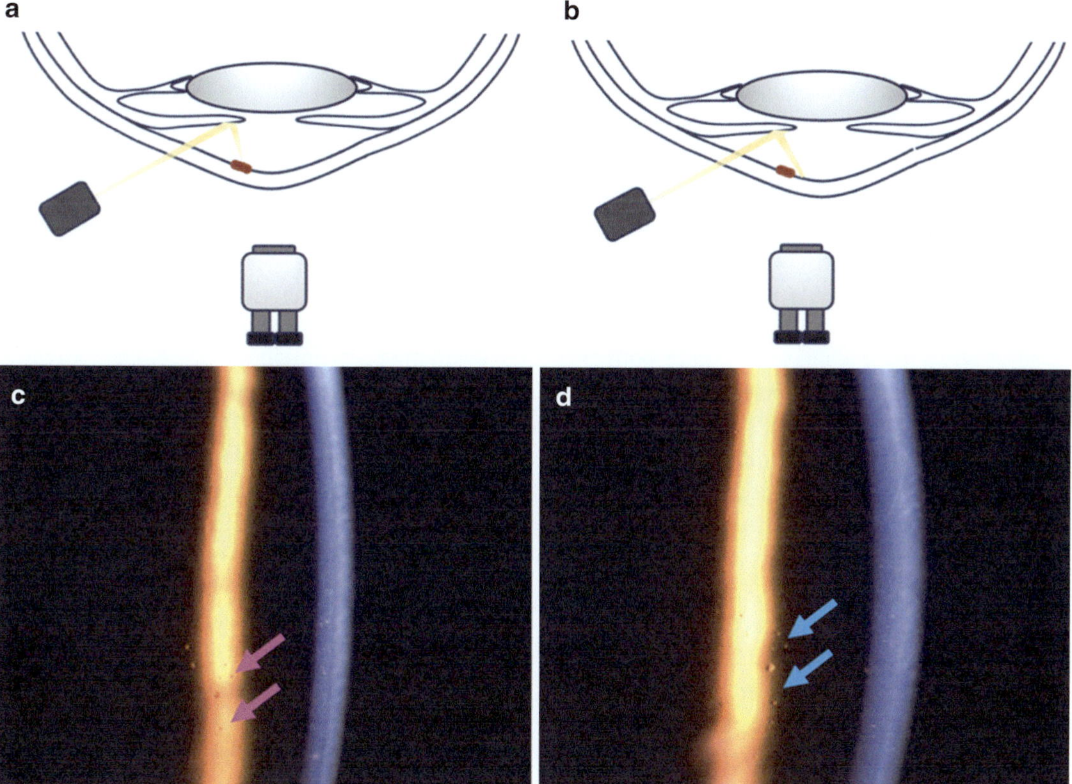

Fig. 14.7 (**a**) Schematic representation of direct retro-illumination wherein the reflected light from the iris falls on the corneal endothelial pigments. (**b**) Schematic representation of indirect retro-illumination wherein the corneal endothelial pigments are visualized between the corneal and the iris slits. (**c, d**) Slit lamp image of corneal endothelial pigments visualized under direct (against a well-lit background, pink arrows) and indirect illumination (against a dark background, blue arrows), (**e**) Diffuse slit lamp photograph depicting temporal corneal edema. Further details are difficult to discern. (**f**) However, on retro-illumination off the iris, the folded Descemet's membrane is visualized under direct retro-illumination (against a lit background, black arrow) and indirect retro-illumination (against a dark background, red arrow)

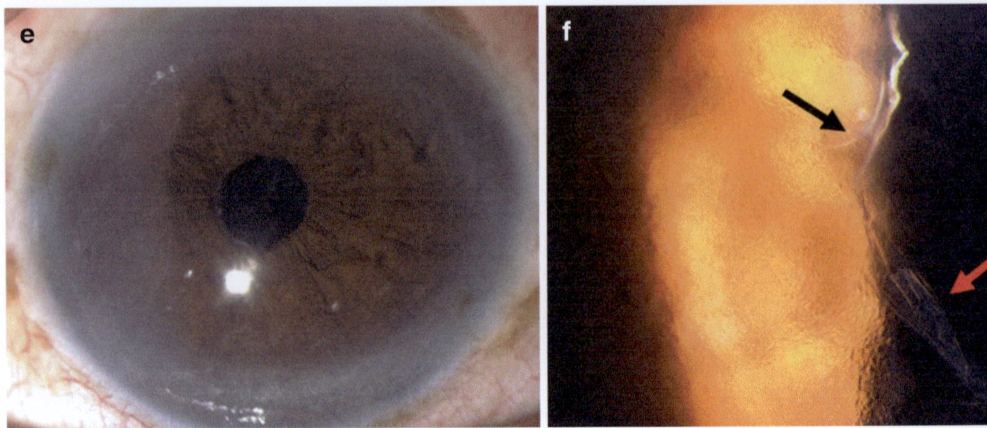

Fig. 14.7 (continued)

14.6 Stepwise Procedure of Examination

1. *Setting up the slit lamp:* A methodical approach to slit lamp examination can ensure that all structures are observed appropriately. Firstly, it is essential to ensure the comfort of the examiner and the patient. It is necessary to sanitize the patient frame and handles with 70% ethanol disinfectant before each examination [13]. The patient's chair is adjusted to the appropriate height, and the chin rest is adjusted so that the lateral canthi of both eyes align with the canthal marker on the patient frame. The eyepiece of the slit lamp is adjusted to the examiner's interpupillary distance and typically set to plano or corrected to accommodate their refractive error. The examiner chair is also adjusted for comfortable sitting with both arms on the table frame. The illumination is then switched on at the lowest setting and gradually increased until the ocular structures are visible. The joystick is moved forward until the structures are clear and focused. Once the area of interest is in the field of view, the slit lamp can be locked into place, and a detailed examination can be carried out. Focusing on the structures such as the cornea, lens, and tear film can be challenging because of their semi-transparent nature. The use of adjacent opaque structures can aid in this process, where the examiner first focuses on them and then slowly shifts both the field and the focus to the desired area of examination. For example, the iris can first be focused on using a moderate slit beam which is then shifted and then moved slightly posteriorly to bring the lens into focus.
2. *Ocular examination:* Before utilizing the slit lamp to examine each eye, it is crucial to assess both eyes under natural light without any aids. This preliminary step is essential for evaluating symmetry, detecting potential issues, and obtaining an overview of any inflammation or mass lesion. The slit lamp examination of each eye typically begins at a low magnification and diffuse illumination. Due to the convex nature of the external surface of the eyeball, the slit lamp unit has to be moved back and forth to bring different structures into focus. A sequential approach for ocular examination will ensure all structures from outwards in are examined meticulously, as described below. Detailed examination techniques of the different structures of the eye have been addressed in the other chapters. This chapter will focus on the different slit lamp techniques and their modifications required based on the structure being examined.

(a) *Lids:* Examination of the lids should include their apposition, lid margin abnormalities or inflammation, and lash abnormalities. Eversion of the lids should be routinely carried out in all cases to detect any foreign bodies, follicles, papillae, etc. This technique can also detect subtle cicatricial changes. Concurrent assessment of puncta will help identify abnormalities of the same.

(b) *Tear film, sclera, and conjunctiva:* The next structure to be examined is the tear film. It is assessed for the presence of any debris, its height, and distribution. This is a dynamic assessment that occurs with each blink. The movement of the debris can be used as a marker to focus on the tear film, typically examined under direct illumination with a moderately wide slit beam. The specular reflection is also used to assess the movement of the lipid layer and to measure the height of the tear film meniscus. This is followed by concurrent examination of the sclera and the conjunctiva-the bulbar and the palpebral. In addition to any mass lesions or signs of inflammation, it is also important to assess any abnormality in the folds, such as excessive laxity or irregularity. The conjunctival examination can be carried out with a combination of an optical section and a moderately wide slit beam to assess the profile of the surface. It is advisable to refrain from using high light intensities as they have the potential to obscure findings due to overexposure. Proximal illumination can reveal the cystic nature of a mass lesion, while specular reflection can be used to detect surface irregularities. The red-free filters are particularly useful while discerning scleral inflammation and should be routinely employed to differentiate between episcleral and scleral inflammation. Scleral nodules or thinning can be best detected using an optical section.

(c) *Limbus and cornea:* The next examination is of the limbal palisades and the cornea. The limbus can be viewed with direct diffuse and focal examination techniques. The use of focal illumination can help understand the profile of the palisades, especially in eyes with lesser degrees of pigmentation. Examination of the cornea uses a combination of different examination techniques. It is important to meticulously examine every layer individually. A lower magnification is required to assess changes such as ectasia, corneal thinning, or edema. Determining the relative depths of different pathologies will require a higher magnification. The illumination angle can be increased to widen the width of the optical section and better understand the exact depth of scars, infiltrates, or foreign bodies. It is recommended to perform the parallelopiped examination before the optical section to detect subtle changes which can be easily missed because of the smaller field of view in the latter. Both direct and indirect retro-illumination can be used to assess the presence of vascularization within the cornea. Similarly, sclerotic scatter is a sensitive technique for evaluating irregularities within the corneal layers. The specular reflection assesses the endothelial layer and detects any guttae or drop-out areas within the cells.

(d) *Anterior chamber:* Since a normal anterior chamber is typically optically clear, subtle changes can get missed even in minor defocus. It is also necessary to use a higher magnification of 16×–25×. For the same reason, it is important to decrease the slit beam height within the pupillary margin to prevent obscuration of the field of view from the backscattering of light from the opaque iris. This conical light beam allows the optics to pick up the scattered light from floating particles within the aqueous humor and elicit Tyndall effect [14]. Reducing the illumination of the examination room can facilitate this process by providing higher contrast. Grading the depth of the anterior chamber using the van Herick grading system can help screen patients with angle closure disease [15].

(e) *Iris:* Focal illumination using a slit beam of varying width helps evaluate the iris pattern and color. Changes in the contour may indicate a local mass lesion, which will not be visible unless a thin slit is used. Similarly, a very high magnification is needed to rule out the presence of neovascularization around the pupillary area. Retro-illumination can identify focal areas of thinning of the iris tissue, which will transmit the reflected light.

(f) *Lens* examination uses an optical section where the illumination angle is usually greater than the one used for examining the cornea. Similar to the examination of the cornea, it is imperative to first examine with a wider slit to detect the presence of small alterations such as glaucomflecken, early posterior subcapsular cataracts, etc. Retro-illumination is perhaps a more sensitive technique for detecting early focal lenticular changes; it must be employed during routine lens examination with the pupil dilated.

(g) *Anterior vitreous:* Examination of the anterior vitreous is similar to the examination of the anterior chamber. It is done using direct illumination with a moderately wide slit beam. Unlike the anterior chamber, the vitreous cavity is not optically clear and has a strand-like appearance that moves with the eyeball's movement. Using a conical light beam helps identify the presence of floating cells, dispersed vitreous hemorrhage, etc.

14.7 Slit Lamps Accessories

This section will discuss different accessories. When used, the utility of the slit lamp can extend beyond the examination of the anterior segment and the vitreous cavity.

1. *Goldmann applanation tonometer:* This instrument is attached either on the side of the slit lamp or superiorly and is swiveled into place when required. It consists of a prism-holding unit, a sensor arm, and a metal house for weights [16, 17]. The prism-holding unit is shaped as a truncated cone with a surface area of 7.35 mm^2 and a diameter of 3.06 mm [16, 17]. It houses a doubling prism which breaks the circular meniscus and needs realignment to measure the intraocular pressure (IOP). The Goldmann applanation tonometer is the current gold standard for measuring IOP (see Chap. 17 for further details).
2. *Lenses:* Several handheld contact and non-contact lenses can augment slit lamp examination. These include lenses for viewing angles, such as the Goldman, Posner, and Sussman lenses. Fundus evaluation with a slit lamp biomicroscope requires a +90D or +78D lens. The distance between the lens and the eye is indirectly proportional to the lens power; thus, a greater distance is required for lenses with lower powers [18]. Ensuring proper cleaning of these lenses is vital to prevent contamination and cross infections [19].
3. *Photography and videography*: This is done using cameras mounted on the slit lamp or with digital compact cameras [20]. The following adjustments are made in the slit lamp to permit photo-videography:
   (a) A beam splitter is required to divide the light traversing back from the patient's eye so that half of it travels to the examiner’s viewing system and the other half is captured by the photography system. Alternatively, a reflex mirror system can divert all the light to the system.
   (b) A crosshair graticule is incorporated in one of the eyepieces, which allows proper centration of the area of photographic interest.
   (c) Alongside the slit beam, a diffuse light source is also necessary during slit lamp examinations. This additional light source

should have an intensity approximately 2–3 times dimmer than the slit beam. This diffuse light provides a softer illumination that complements the focused slit beam, aiding in the observation of subtle details and enhancing the overall visibility of ocular structures.

(d) The camera should be mounted in a manner that it does not interfere with the optics, the observer's movement, or the illumination arm.

(e) The slit lamp is also equipped with an electronic flash feature, specifically designed with minimal exposure unaffected by eye movement. This feature ensures that the flash duration is extremely short, minimizing the risk of motion artifacts and allowing for precise and accurate imaging of the ocular structures.

(f) With the advent of smartphones, it may now be possible to do away with these elaborate systems, which are difficult to maintain and are expensive. Various adapters designed for smartphones enable obtaining high-resolution photographs conveniently during slit lamp examinations [21, 22].

4. *Lasers:* The integration of lasers into slit lamps expands the scope of these instruments from diagnostics to therapeutics. Discussing the indications, techniques, and uses of slit lamp lasers is beyond the scope of this chapter. Briefly, these can be used for treating several conditions, including posterior capsule opacification through capsulotomy, angle closure disease through iridotomy, macular edema, and neovascularization through retinal laser procedures, among others [23–26].

14.8 Recent Advances and Future Directions

There are several new developments in slit lamps. Some of these are as follows:

(i) *Compact and portable*: By reducing the size and weight of the instrument, it becomes more convenient for clinicians to transport and maneuver the slit lamp within clinical settings [27, 28]. It is also advantageous in operating rooms to examine patients under anesthesia and people in the supine position or immobile for various reasons. A handheld slit lamp proves particularly valuable when evaluating children who may not cooperate with a standard slit lamp examination. Additionally, its portability facilitates eye examinations in mass eye screenings, such as in school screenings [27].

(ii) *Incorporation of software within the photography systems* has resulted in "functional slit lamp examination." This technique offers an in vivo method of assessing the hemodynamics of the conjunctiva by providing the blood flow rate, velocity, vessel size, etc. [29] These parameters currently provide an insight into contact lens fitting and dry eye disease, and this may soon expand to include other diseases as well.

(iii) Slit lamps have also been adapted to optical coherence tomography (OCT) machines to enable instant OCT imaging of different ocular structures [30]. Quantitative assessment of the meibomian glands can also be performed with slit lamp adaptors [31].

Similar integration of additional diagnostic modalities, such as automated refractometry, pachymetry, tomography, or optical biometry into the slit lamp platform, holds the promise of comprehensive evaluations within a compact setup. The ability to conduct these investigations with a single instrument permits a more seamless workflow and facilitates rapid decision-making in clinical practice.

14.9 Conclusion

The usefulness of the slit lamp for obtaining high-resolution images and adjustable illumination and magnification has revolutionized the evaluation of the anterior structures of the eye. It allows for identifying subtle abnormalities, precisely measuring structures, and monitoring changes over time. Incorporating handheld lenses further enhance these capabilities, enabling detailed viewing of angle structures and the posterior segment. This aids in identifying pathologies, contributing to better treatment decisions and improved patient outcomes. With newer innovations, the instrument is becoming more compact, allowing a comprehensive range of functionality. Eventually, performing all basic diagnostic investigations with one multipurpose instrument may become possible. By expanding its utility to encompass areas beyond diagnostics, the slit lamp continues to be a cornerstone instrument in ophthalmology, empowering practitioners to provide comprehensive care and deliver improved ocular health outcomes for their patients.

Acknowledgments The authors are grateful to Drs. Simmy Chaudhary, Anasua Kapoor, Shilpa Tarani, and Rashmi Deshmukh for sharing their clinical photographs for publication.

Funding Hyderabad Eye Research Foundation, Hyderabad, India.

Disclosure None.

References

1. Yuan J, Jiang H, Mao X, et al. Slit-lamp photography and videography with high magnifications. Eye Contact Lens. 2015;41(6):391–7.
2. Mazurak M, Kusa J. Jan Evangelista Purkinje: a passion for discovery. Tex Heart Inst J. 2018;45(1):23–6.
3. Gellrich M. The slit lamp. 3rd ed. Berlin: Springer; 2013.
4. Muirhead JF. Adolph Barkan (1845-1935), European ophthalmologist in San Francisco. JAMA Ophthalmol. 2014;132(3):346–9.
5. Ehinger B, Grzybowski A. Allvar Gullstrand (1862–1930)—the gentleman with the lamp. Acta Ophthalmol. 2011;89(8):701–8.
6. Gloor BRP. Hans Goldmann (1899-1991). Eur J Ophthalmol. 2010;20(1):1–11.
7. Littmann H. A new slit lamp apparatus. Am J Ophthalmol. 1950;33(12):1863–70.
8. Vogt A. Atlas of the slitlamp-microscopy of the living eye. Surv Ophthalmol. 1962;7:316–21.
9. Sanderson J. Fundamentals of microscopy. Curr Protoc Mouse Biol. 2020;10(2):e76.
10. Srinivas SP, Rao SK. Ocular surface staining: current concepts and techniques. Indian J Ophthalmol. 2023;71(4):1080–9.
11. Kaur K, Gurnani B. Slit-lamp biomicroscope. In: StatPearls [Internet]. Treasure Island (FL): StatPearls Publishing; 2023. [cited 2023 Jul 1]. http://www.ncbi.nlm.nih.gov/books/NBK587440/.
12. Martin R. Cornea and anterior eye assessment with slit lamp biomicroscopy, specular microscopy, confocal microscopy, and ultrasound biomicroscopy. Indian J Ophthalmol. 2018;66(2):195–201.
13. Fritz B, Paschko E, Young W, et al. Comprehensive compositional analysis of the slit lamp bacteriota. Front Cell Infect Microbiol. 2021;11:745653.
14. Oshika T, Mori M, Araie M. A new approach to the study of aqueous humor dynamics by measuring the intensity of Tyndall's effect. J Fr Ophtalmol. 1990;13(10):471–80.
15. Baskaran M, Oen FTS, Chan YH, et al. Comparison of the scanning peripheral anterior chamber depth analyzer and the modified van Herick grading system in the assessment of angle closure. Ophthalmology. 2007;114(3):501–6.
16. Zeppieri M, Gurnani B. Applanation tonometry. In: StatPearls [Internet]. Treasure Island (FL): StatPearls Publishing; 2023. [cited 2023 Jun 30]. http://www.ncbi.nlm.nih.gov/books/NBK582132/.
17. Brusini P, Salvetat ML, Zeppieri M. How to measure intraocular pressure: an updated review of various tonometers. J Clin Med. 2021;10(17):3860.
18. Gellrich MM. The fundus slit lamp. Springerplus. 2015;4:56.
19. Sobolewska B, Buhl M, Liese J, Ziemssen F. Slit lamps and lenses: a potential source of nosocomial infections? Eye (Lond). 2018;32(6):1021–7.
20. Honavar S, Sen M. Beauty and the beam: Slit-lamp photography essentials [Internet] [cited 2023 Jun 30]. https://ijoreports.in/article.asp?issn=2772-3070;year=2022;volume=2;issue=3;spage=643;epage=646;aulast=Honavar
21. Ludwig CA, Murthy SI, Pappuru RR, et al. A novel smartphone ophthalmic imaging adapter: user feasibility studies in Hyderabad, India. Indian J Ophthalmol. 2016;64(3):191–200.
22. Muth DR, Blaser F, Foa N, et al. Smartphone slit lamp imaging-usability and quality assessment. Diagnostics (Basel). 2023;13(3):423.
23. Modena DAO, Miranda ACG, Grecco C, et al. Efficacy and safety of ND:YAG 1064 nm lasers for photoepilation: a systematic review. Lasers Med Sci. 2020;35(4):797–806.
24. He M, Jiang Y, Huang S, et al. Laser peripheral iridotomy for the prevention of angle closure: a single-Centre, randomised controlled trial. Lancet. 2019;393(10181):1609–18.
25. Saha BC, Kumari R, Sinha BP, et al. Lasers in glaucoma: an overview. Int Ophthalmol. 2021;41(3):1111–28.

26. Yadav NK, Jayadev C, Rajendran A, Nagpal M. Recent developments in retinal lasers and delivery systems. Indian J Ophthalmol. 2014;62(1):50–4.
27. Hu S, Wu H, Luan X, et al. Portable handheld slit-lamp based on a smartphone camera for cataract screening. J Ophthalmol. 2020;2020:1037689.
28. Yazu H, Shimizu E, Sato S, et al. Clinical observation of allergic conjunctival diseases with portable and recordable slit-lamp device. Diagnostics (Basel). 2021;11(3):535.
29. Shu X, Wang J, Hu L. A review of functional slit lamp biomicroscopy. Eye Vis (Lond). 2019; 6:15.
30. Mueller M, Schulz-Wackerbarth C, Steven P, et al. Slit-lamp-adapted fourier-domain OCT for anterior and posterior segments: preliminary results and comparison to time-domain OCT. Curr Eye Res. 2010;35(8):722–32.
31. Arita R, Itoh K, Maeda S, et al. A newly developed noninvasive and mobile pen-shaped meibography system. Cornea. 2013;32(3):242–7.

Corneal Topography 15

Rashmi Deshmukh and Sayan Basu

15.1 Introduction

The cornea is the anterior transparent optical element of the eye. It plays a vital role in focusing the rays of light on the retina. It contributes to two-thirds of the total refractive power of the eye. In Greek, "*topos*" means "place" and "*graphien*" means "to write." Topography relates to studying a surface. Corneal topography was developed as a technique to analyze the anterior surface of the cornea. Traditionally, topography refers to a two-dimensional representation of the corneal surface. In contrast, "*tomos*" means "section"; corneal tomography is a three-dimensional representation of the cornea derived from the anterior and the posterior surfaces of the cornea [1]. A good understanding of the principles of corneal topography and tomography and the ability to interpret these images accurately is crucial to diagnose corneal disorders such as keratoconus, pellucid marginal degeneration, keratoglobus, regular or irregular astigmatism, or corneal ectasia following refractive surgery. With the recent increase in the number of people opting for refractive surgery, corneal topography has become an indispensable tool for screening them for their eligibility and determining the procedure of choice.

15.2 History

The first measurements of the corneal shape were reported by Scheiner in 1619. He used convex mirrors of different curvatures next to the eye to see the reflections of window panes until he found a mirror reflecting an image of the same size as the cornea [2]. Cuignet developed the first keratoscope to see the reflected image from the cornea, and the first keratometer was developed by Helmholtz in 1854. Using a keratometer made it possible to measure the curvature of the central 3 mm of the cornea by assessing the distance between two pairs of reflected points. In 1882, Placido developed a disc with alternating black and white concentric rings with a convex lens at the center of the disc to view the reflected image. This disc named after him (Placido disc) is still widely used by reflection-based topographers. Using the Placido disc in keratometers made it possible to analyze data from a large surface area of the cornea. The following century did not see much progress until the developments of contact

R. Deshmukh (✉) · S. Basu
Shantilal Shanghvi Cornea Institute, Kallam Anji Reddy Campus, L V Prasad Eye Institute, Hyderabad, India
e-mail: sayanbasu@lvpei.org

T. Das, P. Satgunam (eds.), *Ophthalmic Diagnostics*, https://doi.org/10.1007/978-981-97-0138-4_15

lens fitting techniques made it necessary to get information about the mid-peripheral curvature of the cornea. Further developments in cataract surgeries, keratoplasties, and corneal refractive surgeries necessitated the measurements of the curvature of a large area of the cornea. Developments in videokeratoscopy made these measurements possible. Further development of the Scheimpflug principle used the principle of projection rather than reflection to generate true elevation data.

15.3 Principles and Technology

15.3.1 Reflection-Based Systems

Many topography systems use the principle of reflection-based imaging. The principle is to direct the reflected light from the corneal surface onto a two-dimensional image capture system. A reflection-based topographer typically has a Placido disc; it is illuminated and projected onto the cornea. The reflected image from the cornea is captured and analyzed to determine the shape of the cornea. Keratoscopes and videokeratoscopes are examples of topographers based on this principle. The NIDEK-OPD (Nidek Technologies, Gamagori, Japan) scan combines a Placido disc with ray tracing aberrometry and measures anterior corneal curvature, refraction, and pupil size [3]. Most Placido-based topographers use 22 rings with an angular resolution of 2° and can be divided into small and large cone topographers. Small cone systems image more data points and are hence more accurate, but it might be challenging to image deep-set eyes with these systems [4].

There are some limitations to this technology. The posterior cornea cannot be measured. Anterior corneal measurements with the help of reflected mires might miss minor abnormalities. A healthy ocular surface is a prerequisite for a good image; hence, using this technology on people with ocular surface disorders is difficult. Another major limitation is limited corneal coverage, as it obviates measurements from the paracentral and peripheral cornea (Fig. 15.1).

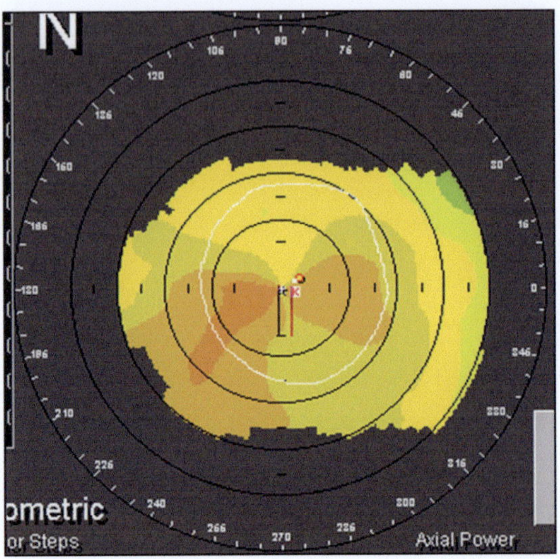

Fig. 15.1 Corneal topography using Placido disc technology shows poor peripheral cornea coverage

15.3.2 Slit Scanning System

Slit scanning topography combines the reflection of a Placido disc with the projection of a slit beam, similar to a slit lamp biomicroscope [5]. The slit beam is moved across the cornea, getting refracted at the anterior and posterior corneal surfaces. Ray tracing triangulation allows the mathematical analysis of the reflected and refracted rays of light to analyze the anterior and posterior surfaces of the cornea. Simultaneous measurements of the anterior and posterior corneal surface enable global pachymetry measurement. Orbscan I (Orbscan, Inc., Salt Lake City, UT, USA) was the first attempt at imaging the posterior corneal surface using a slit scanning system. A Placido disc was incorporated in the Orbscan II (Bausch & Lomb, Rochester, NY), and the latest version, Orbscan IIz (Bausch & Lomb, Rochester, NY), has an integrated Hartmann-Shack aberrometer [6].

15.3.3 Scheimpflug Imaging

The Scheimpflug principle describes the optical imaging condition when the plane of an object is not parallel to the film of the camera; it has the advantage of achieving a wide depth of focus. It was described by Theodor Scheimpflug, an Austrian navy officer who noticed this phenomenon could correct the perspective distortion of aerially acquired photographs. The Pentacam (Oculus, Inc., Lynnwood, WA), Galilei (Ziemer, Port, Switzerland), and Sirius (CSO, Italy) imaging devices use this principle for corneal tomography [7]. The devices use sub-pixel edge detectors to precisely detect corneal and anterior chamber edges. This technology allows the measurements of anterior and posterior cornea, anterior chamber angle and depth, and corneal and lenticular densitometry measurements (Fig. 15.2) [8].

The Pentacam is the most popularly used Schiempflug system. It has a static camera in the center to image the pupil center and control fixation. A second rotating camera with a slit light source obtains slit images from 0° to 180°. The analysis is then converted into detailed topography and thickness maps.

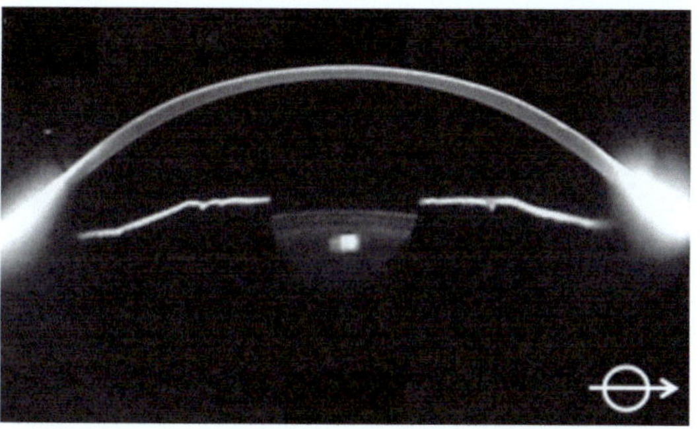

Fig. 15.2 A Scheimpflug image showing the cornea, anterior chamber, and lens imaging

15.4 Color Coding Systems

The analyzed measurements represent keratometry, pachymetry, and elevation maps. These maps show individual data points and are represented using the Louisiana State University Color Coded maps. In this scale, the warmer colors (orange and red) represent steeper corneas, thinner areas, and areas with a higher elevation than the reference surface. The cooler colors (violet and blue) represent flatter curvatures, thicker corneas, and areas that are depressed compared to the reference surface. The greens and the yellows are seen in normal corneas.

The color scale can further be absolute or normalized. An absolute scale has a fixed color coding system with the same colors representing the same dioptric steps for a particular instrument. However, subtle changes are easily missed since the dioptric steps are large. In contrast, in a normalized scale, the system identifies the minimum and maximum values for each map and automatically distributes the colors in a gradient manner. Since the increment step assigned to each color is smaller, this scale gives more topographic details (Fig. 15.3).

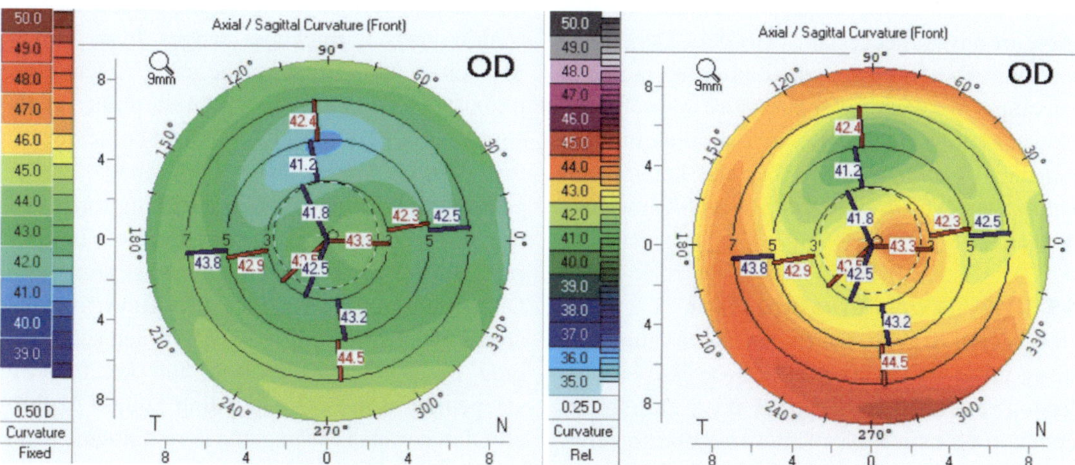

Fig. 15.3 Absolute (right) and normalized (left) scale of the same keratometry map

15.5 Concept of Best-Fit Sphere

The concept of the best-fit sphere is a fundamental principle in corneal topography aimed at understanding the baseline curvature of the cornea. The corneal surface is prolate, and its shape is complex, varying across different regions. The best-fit sphere represents a smooth, symmetrical sphere that minimizes the deviations or differences between the two when superimposed onto the irregular corneal surface. It is a reference point to analyze and quantify corneal curvature changes accurately [9].

Elevation-based topography uses the best-fit sphere as a reference surface and plots the points above or below the reference surface [10]. The areas below the reference surface are represented in cool colors, and the areas above the reference surface are represented in warm colors.

15.6 Topography Maps

15.6.1 Keratometry Maps

Keratometry is the measurement of the corneal radius of curvature. It is defined as the curvature of the circle that touches the cornea at a given point of interest. Keratometry maps essentially provide details of the curvature of the cornea at a given point. Consequently, these maps help assess whether the cornea is regular or irregular (as in corneal scars), steep or flat and whether there are any corneal ectatic disorders. Depending on the method used for calculating the radius of curvature, keratometry or curvature maps are displayed as either sagittal (axial) curvature maps or tangential curvature maps. Normal keratometry values range from 41D to 46D with a mean of 43D [11].

15.6.1.1 Axial Curvature Maps

In this type of map, the radius of curvature at a given point on the corneal surface is measured from a reference axis (optical axis). Due to this common reference axis, small irregularities may not be visible or "smoothened out" as they are much smaller than the large corneal diameter. These maps are calculated assuming that all the rays of light striking the corneal surface are refracted, forcing a focal point through the optical axis as a reference axis and assuming that the center of rotation of the best-fit sphere center lies on the optical axis. It gives a good global view of the cornea averaging out the values and reducing noise. Axial curvature maps are particularly useful in classifying the corneal shape and determining the base curve of the contact lenses for fitting. However, details of minor irregularities may be missed [12].

15.6.1.2 Tangential Maps

These maps more closely represent the actual curvature of the cornea over the axial map. The tangential radius of curvature is calculated at each point with respect to its neighboring points by fitting the best-fit sphere. It means that the tangents are projected at each point, and curvature is measured along the tangent. This type of map recognizes sharp power transitions more easily than the axial map and is more sensitive to irregularities on the corneal surface. It is useful for evaluating corneal shape, assessing refractive surgery candidates, surgically induced changes, and fitting contact lenses [13].

15.6.2 Pachymetry Maps

These maps show the distribution of corneal thickness at various points on the cornea. Normal central corneal thickness ranges from 500 to 550 μm and gradually increases toward the limbus. Most often, the thinnest point on the cornea would be close to or almost coincide with the corneal apex. Pachymetry maps are of particular importance while screening for refractive surgery. A normal corneal thickness is a prerequisite for performing laser vision correction. Displacement of the thinnest location from the apex indicates ectasia, especially when accompanied by posterior elevation and keratometric steepening at the corresponding points. A globally thin cornea is seen in the keratoglobus, while a thick cornea might indicate endothelial dysfunction.

15.6.3 Elevation Maps

The anterior and posterior elevation maps display the areas in the anterior and posterior corneal surface above and below the reference surface. The most used reference surface is the best-fit sphere. However, best-fit ellipse and best-fit toric ellipsoid can also be used. During screening for refractive surgery, a best-fit sphere to the central 8 mm zone provides adequate data points to recognize subtle ectasias and astigmatism [14].

15.7 Interpretation of Maps

A typical quad map consists of 4 maps: the keratometry map (usually axial keratometry), pachymetry map, anterior elevation map, and posterior elevation map. However, since the displays might differ between each machine, one must read a map and look for the red flag signs pointing toward ectasias.

15.7.1 Orbscan

A normal Orbscan quad map includes a keratometry map, pachymetry map, and anterior and posterior elevation maps with measurements displayed at the center (Fig. 15.4).

The Rousch and Efkarpides criteria give the typical red flag signs on an Orbscan map.

15.7.1.1 Rousch Criteria [15]

(a) A thinnest pachymetry of <470 μm.

(b) A difference of >100 μm from the thinnest point to the values of the 7 mm optic zone implies a steep gradient of thinning from mid-periphery to the thinnest point.

(c) The thinnest point on the cornea should correspond with the highest point of elevation of the posterior corneal surface. A posterior high point should be >50 μm above the best-fit sphere on posterior elevation maps. A best-fit sphere of power >55D on the posterior profile is required.

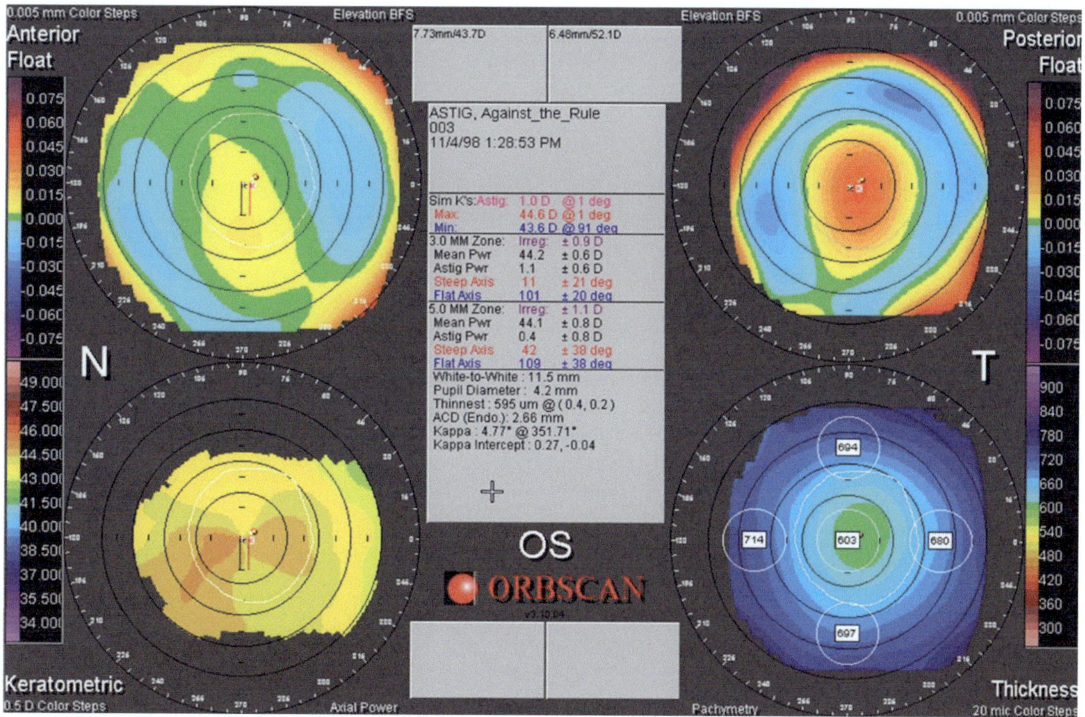

Fig. 15.4 An Orbscan quad map with anterior elevation map (top left), posterior elevation map (top right), keratometry map (bottom left), and pachymetry map (bottom right). The central box displays measurements of various parameters

(d) A relative difference of >100 μm between the highest and lowest point on the posterior elevation map must be seen.

(e) Keratometric mean power map readings of >46D and a lazy C on the axial power map are suspect when the astigmatism shifts >20° from a straight line.

(f) A change within the central 3 mm optic zone of the cornea of more than 3D from superior to inferior can be correlated to the presence of vertical coma (the commonest aberration in keratoconus).

(g) Composite integrated information, which includes the highest point on the posterior elevation, coincides with the highest point on the anterior elevation, the thinnest point on pachymetry, and the point of steepest curvature on the power map, can be acquired.

Additionally, the Efkarpides criteria suggest that ratio of the radii of the anterior and posterior best-fit spheres of the cornea should be >1.21. An astigmatic discrepancy of >1.5D in the 3 mm zone and a discrepancy of >2D in the 5 mm zone should be an alert sign.

15.7.2 Pentacam

A standard Pentacam map (Fig. 15.5) displays certain numerical values on the left-hand side of the map.

- **Quality specification (QS):** Specifies the quality of the topographic capture and should be displayed as "OK." Otherwise, the Pentacam software tends to extrapolate the missing information leading to false readings in the missed areas.
- **K-readings:** K1 indicates flat keratometry, K2 indicates steep keratometry. Consider flat K while treating myopia (should not be <34D

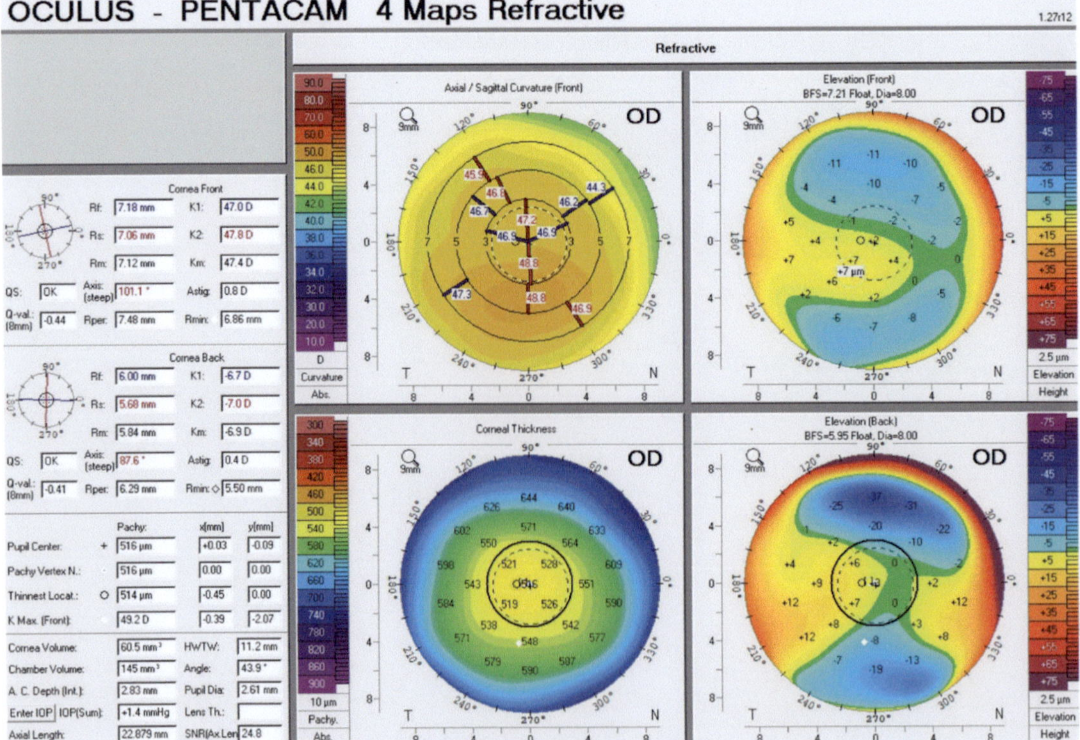

Fig. 15.5 Normal Pentacam display of a quad map with axial keratometry map (top left), pachymetry map (bottom left), anterior elevation map (top right), and posterior elevation map (bottom right). The rectangular display on the left shows various parameters

post-treatment) and steep K while treating hyperopia (should not be >48D post-treatment). Ectatic corneas tend to have higher steep K values.

- **Corneal astigmatism:** The total corneal astigmatism after considering posterior corneal astigmatism should be compared with the manifest refraction to exclude causes of incongruence, such as lenticular astigmatism, posterior subcapsular cataract, tear film disturbance, etc. The axes of astigmatism are also displayed.
- ***Q* value:** This value describes the shape of the cornea, which is typically aspheric. The normal corneal asphericity ranges from −0.2 to −0.3. A positive *Q* value indicates oblate cornea, and a more negative value indicates increased prolate shape.
- **Thinnest location:** This category gives an idea about corneal thickness, but one should refer to the thickness map to have a complete picture of the case. It is very important to study the relationship between the thinnest location and the pachymetric apex according to the thickness and location.
- **Pupil center location:** This is important when carrying out decentration of the ablation profile, especially when treating hyperopia.

15.7.2.1 Red Flag Signs of Ectasia on Pentacam Map

(a) The elevation values on the front surface map should not exceed 12 μm. Values between +13 μm and +15 μm are suspicious, and any value >+15 μm is considered a risk factor.

(b) The elevation values on the back surface map should not exceed +17 μm. Values between +18 μm and +20 μm are suspicious, and any value >+20 μm is considered a risk factor.

(c) The difference between the back and front surfaces (back–front) should not exceed +5 μm at the same point. For example: if the back is +12 μm and the front is +4 μm at the same point, it is suspicious, although both values are within the normal limits.

(d) If there is any isolated island on either front or back surfaces, it would be suspected, even with values within the normal limits.

(e) In the pattern on the keratometric map, as shown with Placido images, any inferior–superior asymmetry arouses suspicion. Compare the thickness at the apex with the thickness at the thinnest location. A difference of >10 μm that increases during follow-ups is suspicious.

(f) An inferior–superior difference in the central 4 mm zone of >30 μm is abnormal.

(g) The difference between the examined cornea and its fellow eye at the same point should be <30 μm.

15.8 Applications of Corneal Topography

(a) As a screening tool to identify regular and irregular corneas and astigmatism.

(b) To identify corneas suitable for laser vision correction and to determine the corneal shape and thickness for planning the surgery.

(c) Identify corneal ectatic disorders such as keratoconus, pellucid marginal degeneration, and keratoglobus.

(d) Planning intracorneal ring segments requires adequate pachymetry in the mid-peripheral cornea, measured on corneal topography systems.

(e) Contact lens fitting is based on the corneal curvature and best-fit sphere measurements.

(f) Comparison of corneal topography scans over time indicates progression of corneal ectasias.

15.9 Conclusion

Topography is an excellent tool to screen potentially borderline cases in clinical practice. Placido disc-based devices are very useful tools; however, they are less sensitive to changes on the posterior surface of the cornea. Newer diagnostic devices like elevation-based topographers, single and dual Scheimpflug imaging, and LED technology help one better understand the posterior surface of the cornea and pachymetry. These newer modalities can help diagnose ectatic disease in the preclinical stage, thus allowing early treatment.

Funding Hyderabad Eye Research Foundation (HERF), Hyderabad, India.

Disclosure None.

References

1. Ambrósio R, Belin MW. Imaging of the cornea: topography vs tomography. J Refract Surg. 2010;26(11):847–9.
2. Scheiner C. Oculus, Hoc Est: Fundamentum Opticum. Innsbruck, Austria: Daniel Agricola; 1619.
3. Gatinel D, Hoang-Xuan T. Measurement of combined corneal, internal, and total ocular optical quality analysis in anterior segment pathology with the OPD-scan and OPD-station. J Refract Surg. 2006;22(9 Suppl):S1014–20.
4. Ventura BV, Al-Mohtaseb Z, Wang L, Koch DD, Weikert MP. Repeatability and comparability of corneal power and corneal astigmatism obtained from a point-source color light-emitting diode topographer, a Placido-based corneal topographer, and a low-coherence reflectometer. J Cataract Refract Surg. 2015;41(10):2242–50.
5. Liu Z, Huang AJ, Pflugfelder SC. Evaluation of corneal thickness and topography in normal eyes using the Orbscan corneal topography system. Br J Ophthalmol. 1999;83(7):774–8.
6. Oliveira CM, Ribeiro C, Franco S. Corneal imaging with slit-scanning and Scheimpflug imaging techniques. Clin Exp Optom. 2011;94(1):33–42.
7. Kanclerz P, Khoramnia R, Wang X. Current developments in corneal topography and tomography. Diagnostics (Basel). 2021;11(8):1466.
8. Motlagh MN, Moshirfar M, Murri MS, Skanchy DF, Momeni-Moghaddam H, Ronquillo YC, et al. Pentacam® corneal tomography for screening of refractive surgery candidates: a review of the literature, part I. Med Hypothesis Discov Innov Ophthalmol. 2019;8(3):177–203.
9. Gatinel D, Malet J, Hoang-Xuan T, Azar DT. Corneal elevation topography: best fit sphere, elevation distance, asphericity, toricity, and clinical implications. Cornea. 2011;30(5):508–15.
10. Belin MW, Khachikian SS. An introduction to understanding elevation-based topography: how elevation data are displayed—a review. Clin Experiment Ophthalmol. 2009;37(1):14–29.
11. Ghemame M, Charpentier P, Mouriaux F. Corneal topography in practice. J Fr Ophtalmol. 2020;43(1):67–79.
12. Rasheed K, Rabinowitz YS, Remba D, Remba MJ. Interobserver and intraobserver reliability of a classification scheme for corneal topographic patterns. Br J Ophthalmol. 1998;82(12):1401–6.
13. Shah RS, Khandelwal SS, Goshe JM, Haberman ID, Randleman JB. Comparative postoperative topography pattern recognition analysis using axial vs tangential curvature maps. J Cataract Refract Surg. 2020;46(10):1368–73.
14. Smadja D, Santhiago MR, Mello GR, Krueger RR, Colin J, Touboul D. Influence of the reference surface shape for discriminating between normal corneas, subclinical keratoconus, and keratoconus. J Refract Surg. 2013;29(4):274–81.
15. Rousch C. Orbscan II Manual (Salt Lake City, Utha. Orbtek).

Ocular Surface Examination 16

Swati Singh and Sayan Basu

16.1 Introduction

The ocular surface comprises the cornea, limbus, conjunctiva, eyelids, tear film, and lacrimal gland [1, 2]. The ocular surface examination should be performed using the slit lamp and requires vital dyes like Sodium fluorescein and Lissamine green. Different techniques for using a slit lamp have been discussed in Chap. 14. This chapter describes the examination techniques used to arrive at a clinical diagnosis using devices readily available in eye clinics.

S. Singh (✉)
Kallam Anji Reddy Campus, LV Prasad Eye Institute, Hyderabad, India
e-mail: swatisingh@lvpei.org

S. Basu
Shantilal Shanghvi Cornea Institute, Kallam Anji Reddy Campus, LV Prasad Eye Institute, Hyderabad, India
e-mail: sayanbasu@lvpei.org

16.2 Cornea and Conjunctiva

16.2.1 Cornea

The normal cornea is transparent and has a smooth, clear optical surface. The cornea measures 11–12 mm horizontally and 9–11 mm vertically [1]. One should examine the cornea under white light and fluorescein staining. Slit-lamp evaluation of the cornea shows the five layers individually and allows pathology detection at high magnification. Any epithelial irregularities like defects and erosions would take up fluorescein stain (Fig. 16.1) [3]. Different grading systems are used for corneal fluorescein staining, like the National Eye Institute Scoring System and the Oxford Ocular Surface Staining Score [3]. Corneal scarring with an irregular surface will show pooling of the dye and should be differentiated from staining. A high-resolution anterior segment optical coherence tomography (AS-OCT) of the cornea can depict the abnormalities involving the individual layers of the cornea and stromal thickness and provide an infrared photograph of the cornea for better appreciation of the stromal opacification [4, 5] (Fig. 16.2).

16.2.2 Limbus

The limbus is the transition zone between the cornea and the sclera. It contains radially running

T. Das, P. Satgunam (eds.), *Ophthalmic Diagnostics*, https://doi.org/10.1007/978-981-97-0138-4_16

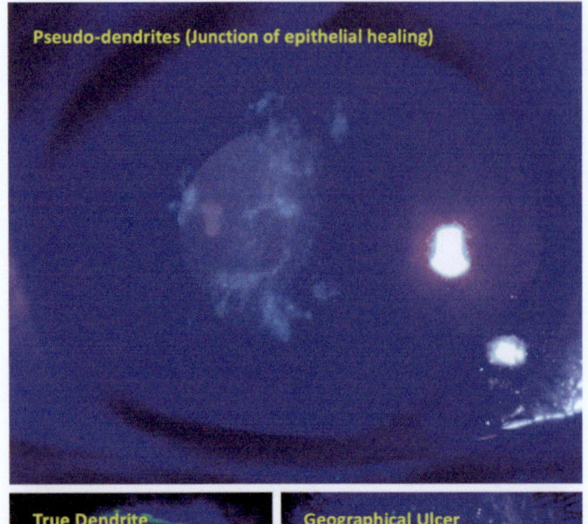

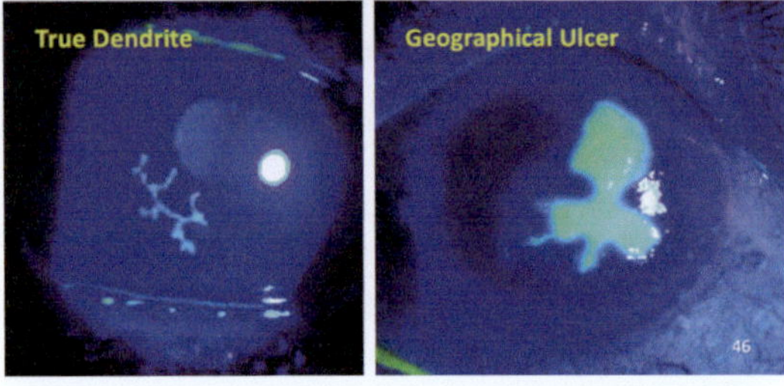

Fig. 16.1 Sodium fluorescein-stained images of the cornea showing stain uptake patterns in pseudo-dendrites, true dendrites, and corneal ulceration

fibrovascular ridges known as the palisades of Vogt that contain limbal stem cells (Fig. 16.3) [5]. The palisades of Vogt are more common in the superior and inferior quadrants and better appreciated in pigmented races. Limbal stem cell deficiency seen in chemical injury results in the loss of the palisades of Vogt (Fig. 16.4). The surface abnormalities that occur at the limbus are pterygium, Horner-Trantas dots, hypertrophied epithelium, and ocular surface malignancy [5].

16.2.3 Conjunctiva

Both the bulbar and palpebral conjunctiva should be examined for any congestion, especially perilimbal congestion, and the presence of symblepharon. Everted upper and lower eyelid examination exposes the lid margin and palpebral conjunctiva better (Fig. 16.5). Presence of follicles suggests conjunctivitis, whereas papillae suggest allergic conjunctivitis. For ocular surface diseases, conjunctival signs like congestion, scarring, symblepharon, and keratinization can suggest chronic

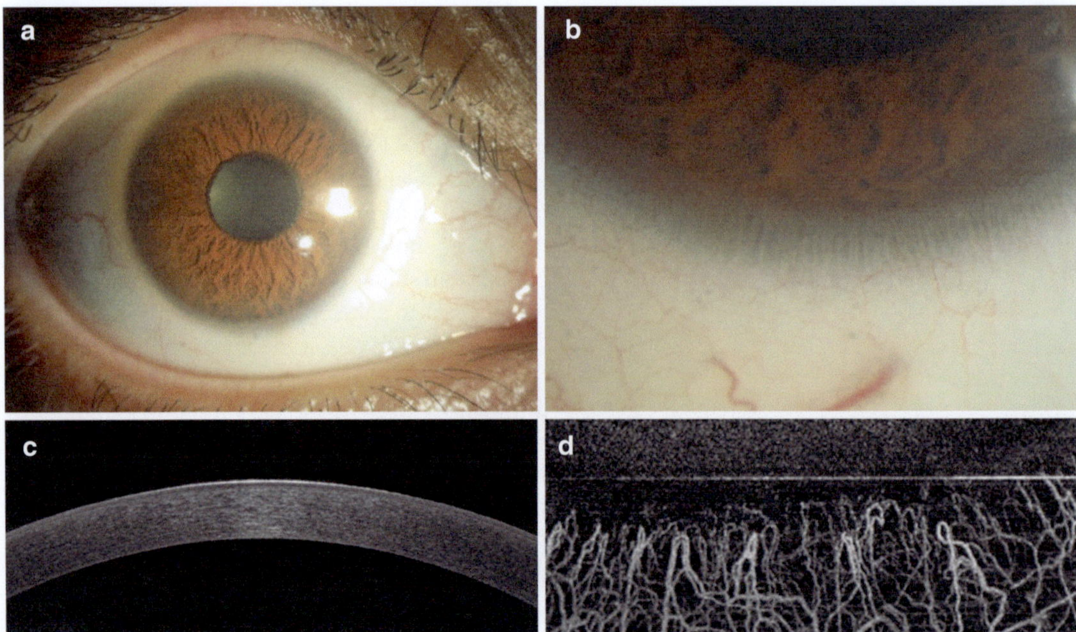

Fig. 16.2 Normal appearance of the cornea and limbus. The healthy cornea is optically transparent (**a**) and surrounded by the annular limbus, which separates it from the opaque sclera. The limbus contains the palisades of Vogt (**b**), which are finger-like projections of the stroma. The optical coherence tomography (OCT) image of the normal cornea shows a smooth, uniform stratified epithelium (**c**) with underlying compact stroma. The OCT angiography image of the normal limbus shows linear anastomosing hairpin loops of the limbal capillaries (**d**) with adjacent avascular corneal stroma

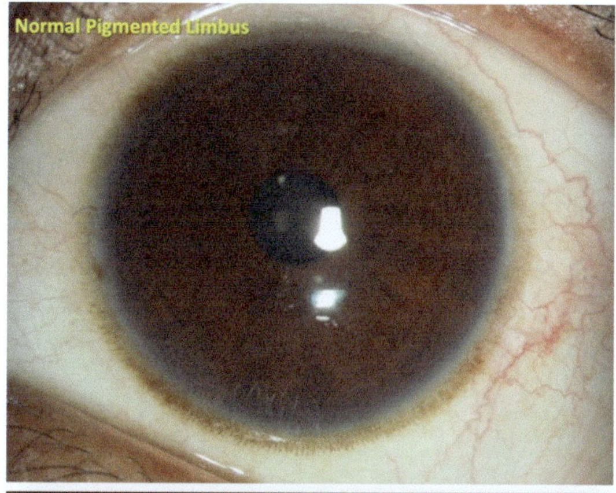

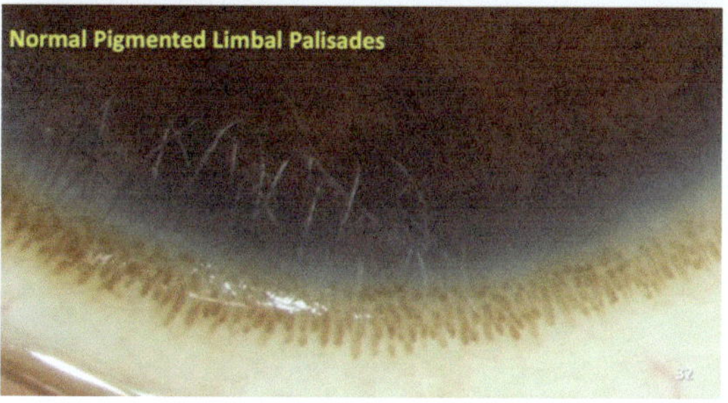

Fig. 16.3 Top and bottom. Pigmented palisades of Vogt in a healthy corneal limbus

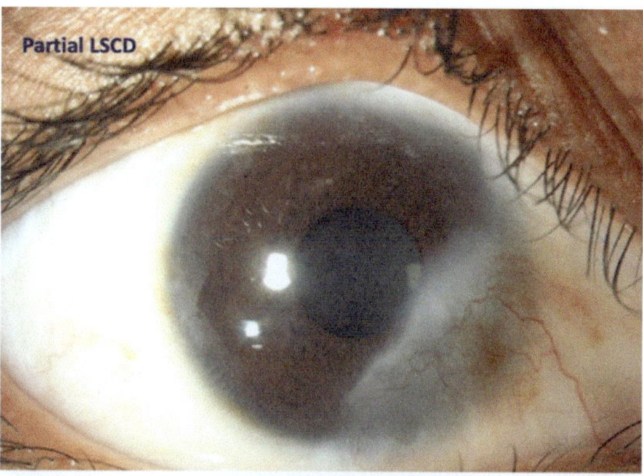

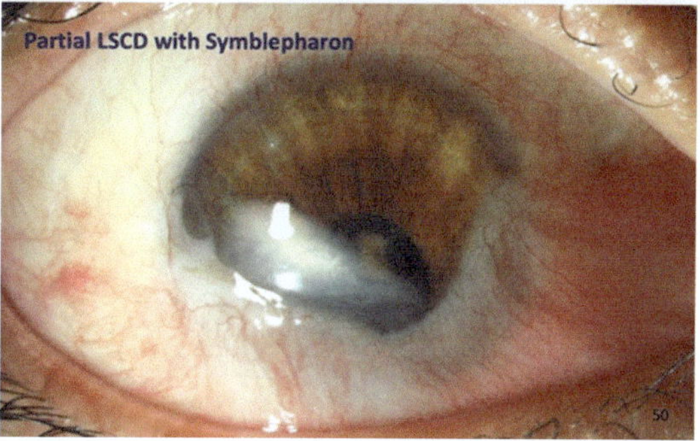

Fig. 16.4 Limbal stem cell deficiency after chemical injury that resulted in conjunctivalization of the cornea is seen in the inferonasal cornea (top) and symblepharon formation with adherence between the palpebral conjunctiva and the cornea (bottom)

cicatrizing conjunctivitis [6]. Subtle symblepharon are picked up by retracting the lower eyelid and instructing the patient to look upward, which better exposes forniceal, nasal symblepharon. The upper and lower fornices must be examined for foreign bodies and scarring, especially in eyes with mucous membrane pemphigoid with otherwise quiet eye. Lid margin conjunctival folds suggest conjunctivochalasis.

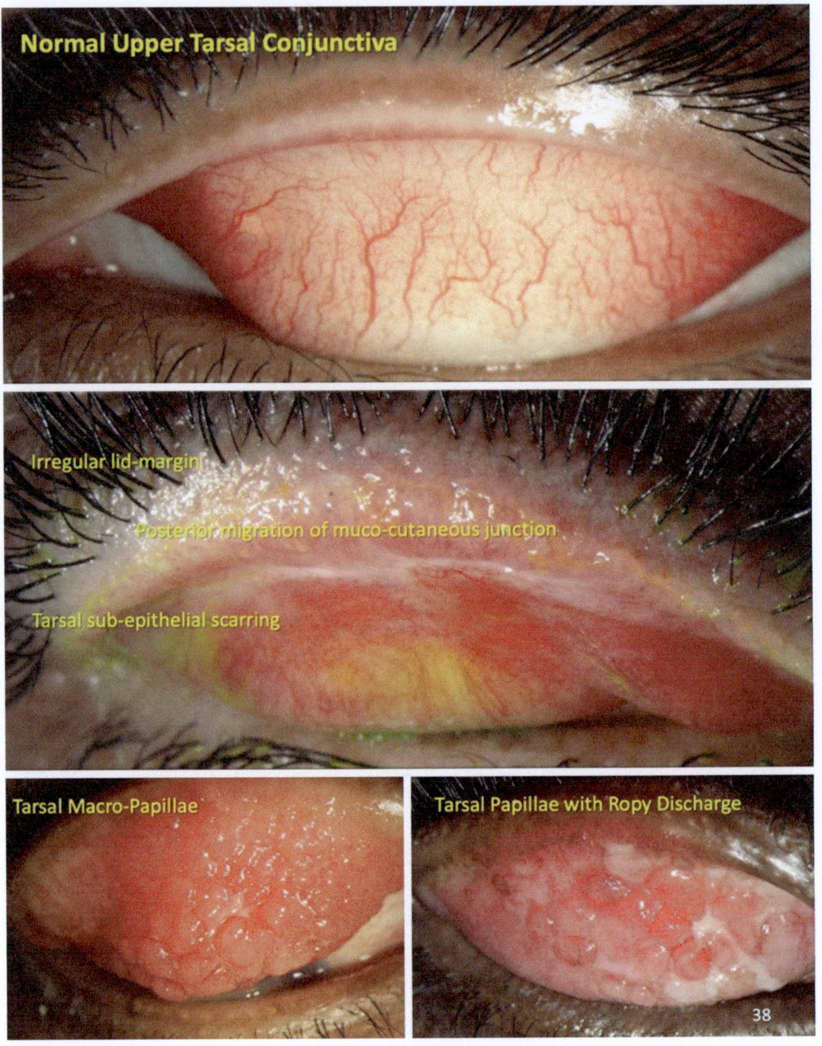

Fig. 16.5 Everted upper eyelid showing normal (upper panel) and scarred tarsal conjunctiva. In the middle panel, the lid margin can be seen as distorted, scarred, and having occluded meibomian gland openings. The lower panel shows giant tarsal papillae with a cobblestone appearance and ropy discharge

16.3 Ocular Adnexa

16.3.1 Eyelid and Eyelid Margin

The eyelids should be examined in a closed and open state for proper apposition evaluation. These must be examined for any signs of lagophthalmos, ectropion, entropion, blepharitis, and any signs of trauma. The entire eyelid margin must be examined for evidence of edema, hordeolum, or chalazion.

The eyelid margin is inspected for three parameters, namely apposition to the globe, mucocutaneous junction, and appearance. The normal lid sits apposed to the globe, where its sharp inner border lies over the bulbar surface where the tear lake resides as a reservoir. These positions are altered in eyelid ectropion or entropion, and the tear lake reservoir is disturbed. The mucocutaneous junction (MCJ) is the area where the free lid epidermis meets the conjunctival epithelium (Fig. 16.6) [7, 8]. This transition is situated at the posterior border of the meibomian gland orifices from where the lid wiper begins. The lid wiper region is part of the eyelid margin in contact with the globe and extends superiorly from the MCJ to the sub-tarsal fold. Any disturbances in the lid wiper region can cause corneal epitheliopathy, termed lid wiper epitheliopathy (LWE; Fig. 16.7) [8]. LWE is observed in lid

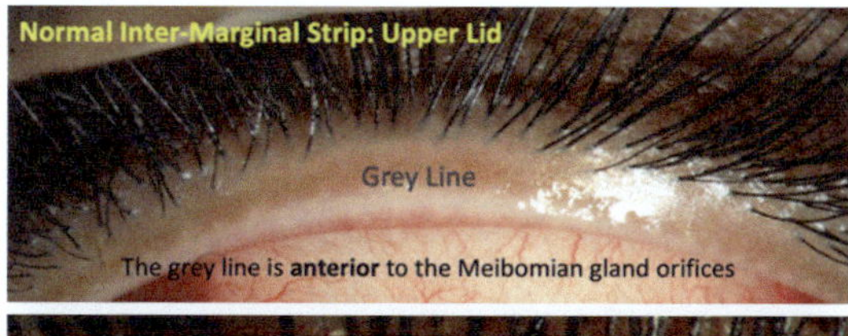

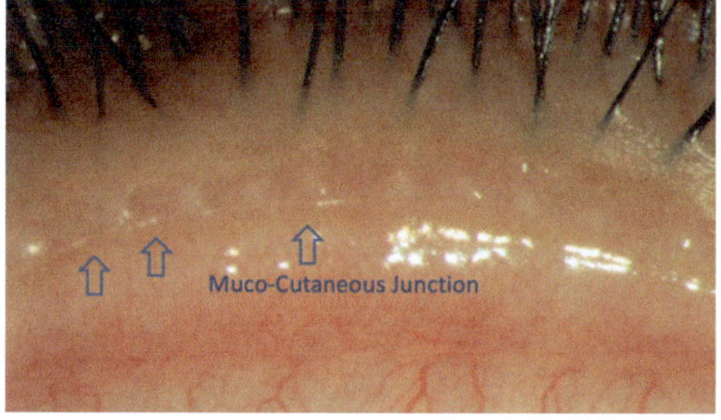

Fig. 16.6 Normal appearance of posterior lid margin showing a gray line and the mucocutaneous junction (MCJ) at the posterior border of the meibomian gland openings

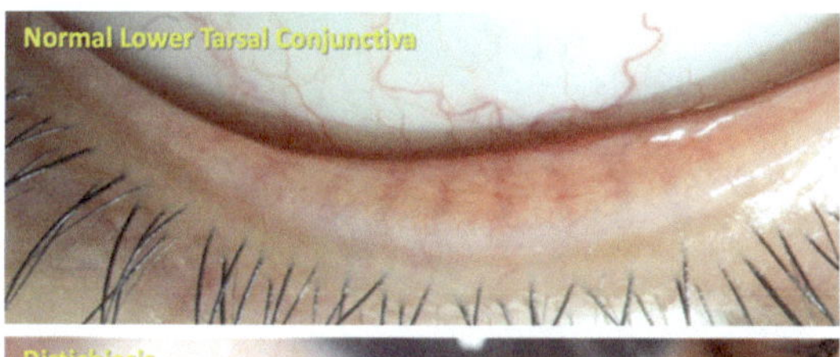

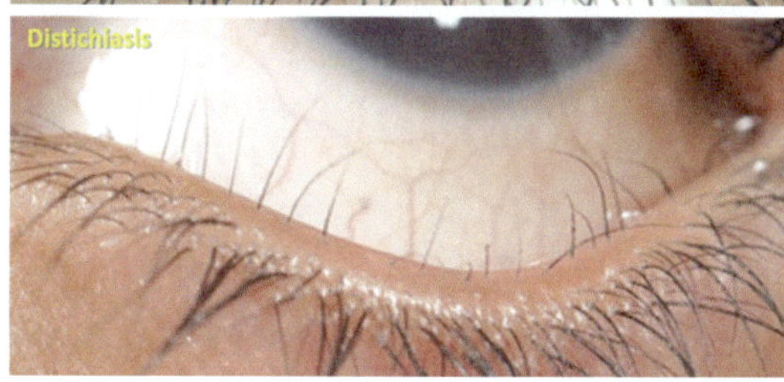

Fig. 16.7 Normal lower eyelid with eyelashes arising from the skin and oriented outwards (upper panel). The lower panel shows aberrant distichiatic eyelashes located at the meibomian gland openings as an extra row other than normal eyelashes

margin keratinization (LMK), contact lens users, and dry eye disease. The MCJ and lid wiper region are examined using fluorescein staining under a cobalt blue filter where the conjunctival epithelium has pooling of the dye (Fig. 16.7). In eyes with LMK, posterior migration of the MCJ occurs and the keratinized epithelium encroaches over the lid wiper region [8]. Also, sometimes, there can be conjunctivalization of the meibomian gland orifices with associated gland blockade as a sign of meibomian gland dysfunction.

Any lid margin notching or thinning, especially in eyes with chemical injury, should also be looked at. An inflamed lid margin would have a congested look with fine telangiectatic vessels around the meibomian gland openings seen in posterior blepharitis. The inferior lid margin should be reflected using a cotton-tipped applicator to better visualize the lower lid margin, lower lash follicles, inferior punctum, and meibomian glands.

16.3.2 Eyelashes

Examine the eyelashes for debris, flakes, crusting, or collarettes. The normal orientation of the eyelash is upwards and outwards. Misdirected eyelashes like those in trichiasis or aberrant eyelashes like those in distichiatic can cause ocular surface staining due to rubbing over the surface epithelium (Fig. 16.8) [9]. Distichiatic lashes can be fine and light-colored and are best examined using the slit lamp.

16.3.3 Periocular Skin

The periocular skin should be examined for any hypo or hyperpigmentation, edema, or signs of inflammation. Contact dermatitis, especially in patients using antiglaucoma medications, would show edematous skin with or without erosion in the medial compartment of the eyelids [6, 10].

16.3.4 Lacrimal Gland

The lacrimal gland contributes to the aqueous component of the tear film via secretory ductules opening into the conjunctiva overlying the palpebral lobe. Traditionally, Schirmer's test and tear film height or area measurement are considered indicators for lacrimal gland function [11]. These techniques give an indirect assessment of the lac-

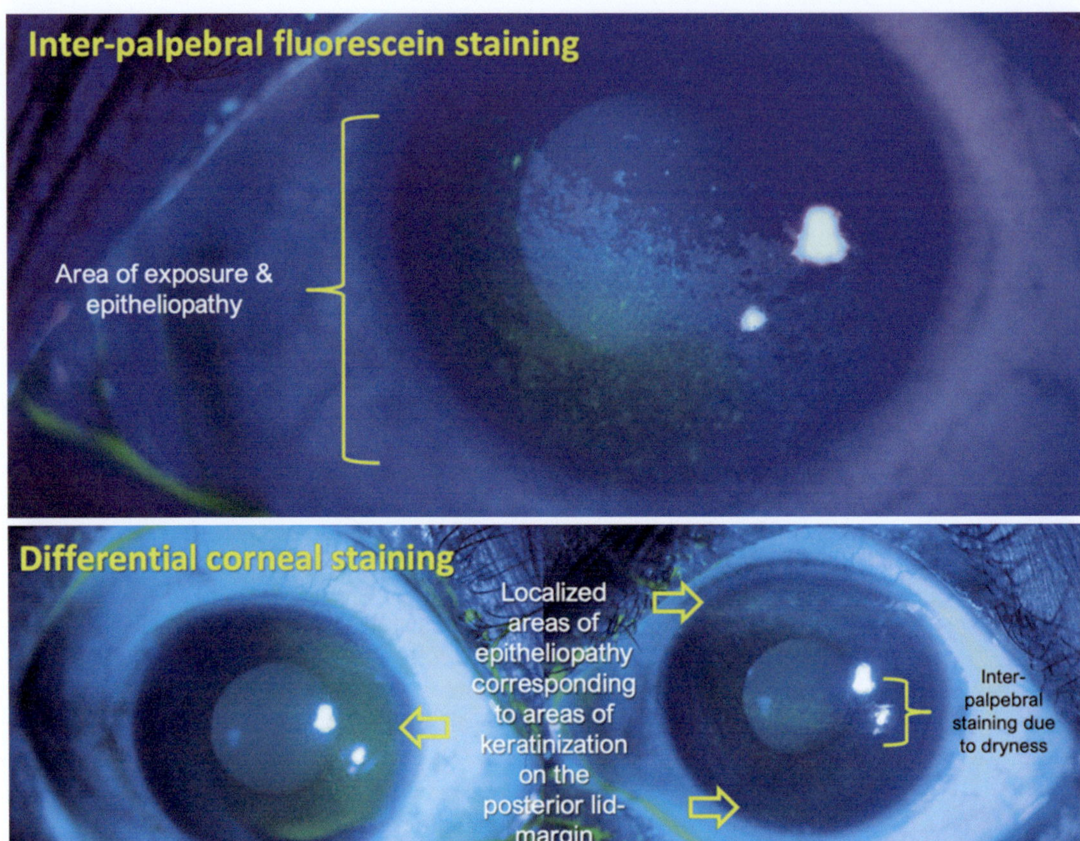

Fig. 16.8 Corneal staining in different ocular conditions. The upper panel shows diffuse inferior corneal staining in the area of exposure in a patient with lagophthalmos. The lower panel shows interpalpebral staining seen in aqueous deficient dry eye disease, whereas sectoral temporal staining is seen in areas of contact with the keratinized lid margin, which is suggestive of lid wiper epitheliopathy

rimal gland activity. The palpebral lobes of the lacrimal gland can be directly visualized during a routine slit-lamp biomicroscopy session by asking the patient to look inferonasal. At the same time, the upper eyelid is lifted superotemporally [12]. The morphology can be divided into size (exposed area), shape (convex or flat), and overlying conjunctival appearance (engorged vessels, whitish areas of subepithelial scarring, or symblepharon). The normal palpebral lobe is a convex-shaped, raised pinkish lobular structure with overlying normal conjunctiva (Fig. 16.9). The lobe lies in the superotemporal fornix extending to or beyond the lateral canthus. The lobe is visibly smaller in patients with Sjogren's Syndrome (SS), whereas cicatrization over the lobe is seen in patients with Stevens-Johnson syndrome (SJS). Under a slit-lamp biomicroscope, a dry 2% sodium fluorescein ophthalmic strip is applied onto the exposed palpebral lobe. The washout of fluorescein stain across the applied area is recorded till secretions start appearing. Normally, 3–5 secretory ductules can be observed in healthy individuals, whereas the number of openings is reduced in individuals with aqueous deficient dry eye [13].

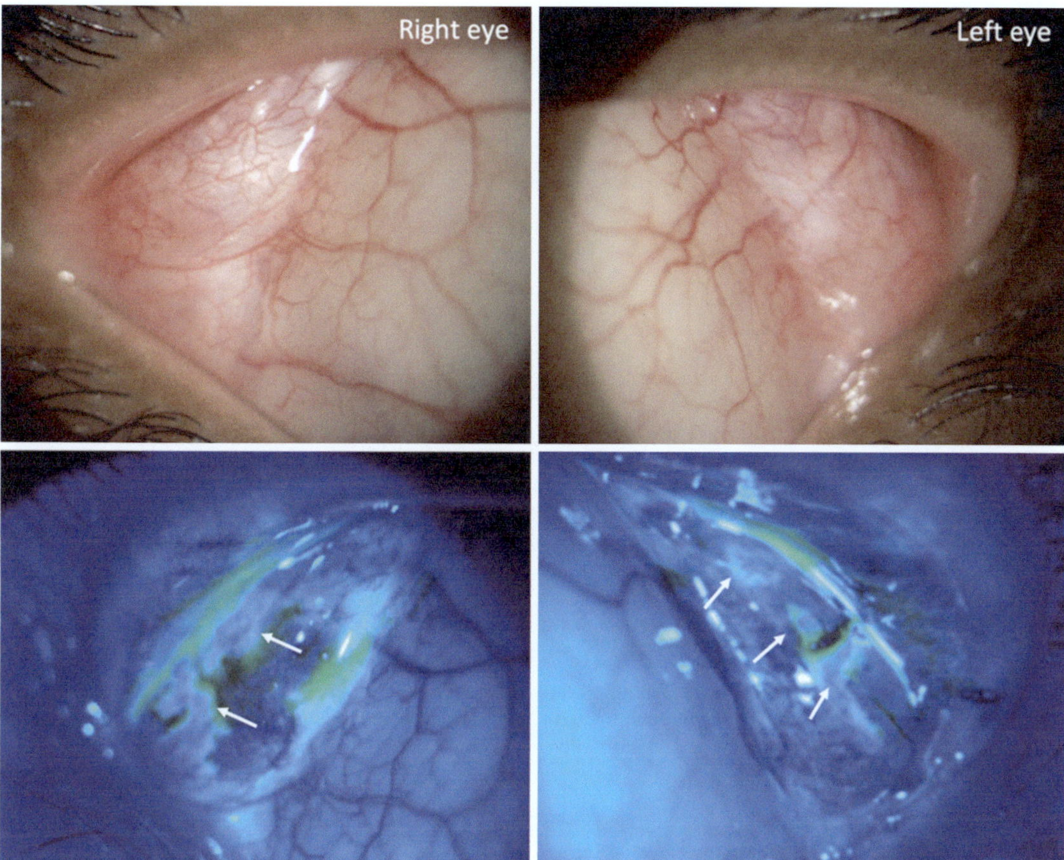

Fig. 16.9 Right and left palpebral lobes of the lacrimal gland in normal individuals. The lobes are convex-shaped and have smooth overlying conjunctiva. The lower panel shows the secretory openings seen as fluorescein washout areas—two on the right side and three on the left side (marked with arrows)

16.3.5 Meibomian Gland

Meibomian glands are lipid-producing glands that secrete a mixture of lipids and some proteins onto the ocular surface. The structure of the meibomian glands can be evaluated using transillumination infrared imaging, such as infrared meibography, and their function can be measured using lipid layer thickness (LLT) and meibum quality or expressibility tests [11]. Normal meibomian glands are seen as whitish vertically running glands within the tarsal plate. Gland dropout and short glands suggest meibomian gland dysfunction [14, 15]. Meibum quality is graded as 0 (clear fluid), 1 (cloudy fluid), 2 (cloudy particulate), or 3 (toothpaste-like). The expressibility of meibum from the central eight glands of the upper and lower eyelids is graded as 0 (all glands expressible), 1 (3 to 4 glands expressible), 2 (1 to 2 glands expressible), and 3 (no glands expressible). The meibographic appearance of normal glands is shown in Fig. 16.10. The normal lipid layer thickness (LLT) varies from 70 to 100 nm [16]. Values <60 nm are considered signs of lipid deficiency. However, the repeatability coefficient of the dry eye diagnostic devices should be kept in mind while interpreting LLT values [17].

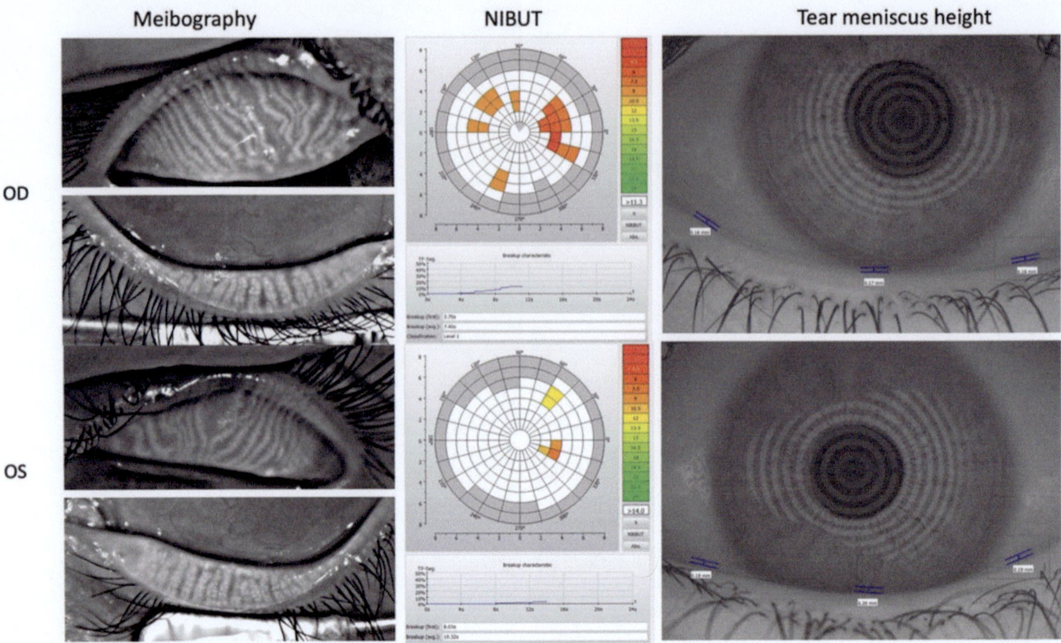

Fig. 16.10 Infrared meibography of the upper and lower eyelids of a normal adult showing vertically running meibomian glands reaching up to the convex tarsal border. Non-invasive tear break-up time (NIBUT; OD = 7.4 s; OS = 10 s) and tear meniscus height were captured in the oculus keratograph of the same individual

16.4 Tear Film Assessment

Tear film tests are crucial in identifying dry eye disease and surface irregularities in ocular surface disorders. The tear film break-up time (TBUT) measures tear stability and can be evaluated in an invasive and non-invasive manner [18]. TBUT is the time taken for the precorneal tear film to break after one blink and is affected in dry eye disease (both aqueous deficient and evaporative types), corneal epithelial irregularities, and surface inflammation with diminished mucus layer attachment to corneal microplicae. A drop of fluorescein is instilled in the conjunctival cul-de-sac, and the patient is instructed not to blink afterward. The time taken for the appearance of the first dry spot is taken as TBUT. The reported mean fluorescein-TBUT values in normal subjects are 7.6 ± 10.4 s [11, 18]. One should repeat the test if the values are <10 s before labelling it pathological. With the advent of non-invasive tests, the accuracy of TBUT is better when tested two or more times. Non-invasive TBUT (NIBUT) measures changes in the reflected videokeratographic mires using topographic systems (Fig. 16.10). The Placido disc projects the mires onto the cornea, and any changes in the mires' regularity are taken as the onset of tear break-up. In one study, the values of NIBUT for 236 healthy individuals of South Indian origin were between 7 s and 10 s in 33% of individuals, and 7% had NIBUT values <7 s [19].

Tear volume is measured using the Schirmer test (invasive) and tear meniscus height (TMH, non-invasive) [20]. A commercially available Whatman 41 filter paper strip is used for the Schirmer test. The proximal part of the strip sits in the conjunctival-cul-de-sac and is inserted in the lateral one-third of the lower eyelid. Both eyes are tested simultaneously, and the moistened segment is measured at the end of 5 min. The strip should not touch the cornea to avoid reflex tear activity. The Schirmer test can be performed with open or closed eyes; however, there is less variation with closed eyes [21]. The different types of Schirmer tests are the Schirmer I (without anesthesia and with open eyes), Schirmer II (after nasal stimulation), and Schirmer III (reflex-stimulated secretion by looking into the sun) [11]. To avoid confusion, defining the Schirmer test with or without anesthesia is better than using I or II [21]. Schirmer test values <10 mm indicate dry eye disease; however, values <5 mm are pathological, and between 5 and 10 mm should be interpreted carefully [22].

For measuring TMH, slit-lamp-based meniscometry and non-invasive optical coherence tomography (OCT) can be used [20]. Due to its non-invasive nature and less chances of reflex tearing, OCT-based TMH is more repeatable and reproducible than the Schirmer test. Time- and spectral-domain OCT can be used for calculating TMH, but they are not interchangeable. The reported normal mean TMH values are 0.29 mm (SD = 0.13 mm, slit lamp), 0.27–0.29 mm (SD = 0.05–0.12 mm, keratograph), and 0.19–0.34 mm (SD = 0.02–0.15 mm, SD-OCT) [23].

16.5 Conclusion

The ocular surface examination should be comprehensive and inclusive of all components of the surface, i.e., cornea, conjunctiva, eyelids, and eyelashes. Fluorescein stain for ocular surface evaluation is crucial and should be performed for every case. Diagnostic devices like ASOCT, ocular surface analyzer, and keratograph for non-invasive tear film assessment are adjunctive tools that help in diagnosis and follow-up evaluations.

Funding Hyderabad Eye Research Foundation, Hyderabad, India.

Disclosure None.

References

1. Kenyon KR. Anatomy and pathology of the ocular surface. Int Ophthalmol Clin. 1979;19(2):3–35.
2. Cher I. Ocular surface concepts: development and citation. Ocul Surf. 2014;12:10–3.
3. Srinivas SP, Rao SK. Ocular surface staining: current concepts and techniques. Indian J Ophthalmol. 2023;71(4):1080–9.
4. Han SB, Liu YC, Noriega KM, Mehta JS. Applications of anterior segment optical coherence tomography in cornea and ocular surface diseases. J Ophthalmol. 2016;2016:4971572.
5. Kate A, Basu S. A review of the diagnosis and treatment of limbal stem cell deficiency. Front Med (Lausanne). 2022;9:836009.
6. Vazirani J, Donthineni PR, Goel S, et al. Chronic cicatrizing conjunctivitis: a review of the differential diagnosis and an algorithmic approach to management. Indian J Ophthalmol. 2020;68(11):2349–55.
7. Knop E, Knop N, Zhivov A, et al. The lid wiper and muco-cutaneous junction anatomy of the human eyelid margins: an in vivo confocal and histological study. J Anat. 2011;218(4):449–61.
8. Shanbhag SS, Singh S, Koshy PG, et al. A beginner's guide to mucous membrane grafting for lid margin keratinization: review of indications, surgical technique and clinical outcomes. Indian J Ophthalmol. 2021;69(4):794–805.
9. Singh S. Distichiasis: an update on etiology, treatment and outcomes. Indian J Ophthalmol. 2022;70(4):1100–6.
10. Adewara B, Singh S. Ocular adnexa and antiglaucoma medications. Int Oph Clin. 2023;63:47.
11. Singh S, Srivastav S, Donthineni PR, et al. Lacrimal and meibomian gland evaluation in dry eye disease: a mini-review. Indian J Ophthalmol. 2023;71:1090.
12. Singh S, Shanbhag SS, Basu S. Palpebral lobe of human lacrimal gland: morphometric analysis in normal versus dry eyes. Br J Ophthalmol. 2021. [Epub].;105:1352. https://doi.org/10.1136/bjophthalmol-2020-316929.
13. Singh S, Shanbhag SS, Basu S. Tear secretion from the lacrimal gland: variations in normal versus dry eyes. Br J Ophthalmol. 2022;106(6):772–6.
14. Singh S, Vemuganti GK, Basu S. Morphological variants of meibomian glands: correlation of meibography features with histopathology findings. Br J Ophthalmol. 2021. [Epub].;107:195. https://doi.org/10.1136/bjophthalmol-2021-318876.
15. Swiderska K, Read ML, Blackie CA, et al. Latest developments in meibography: a review. Ocul Surf. 2022;25:119–28.
16. Finis D, Pischel N, Schrader S, Geerling G. Evaluation of lipid layer thickness measurement of the tear film as a diagnostic tool for Meibomian gland dysfunction. Cornea. 2013;32:1549–53.
17. Singh S, Srivastav S, Modiwala Z, et al. Repeatability, reproducibility and agreement between three different diagnostic imaging platforms for tear film evaluation of normal and dry eye disease. Eye. 2023;37:2042–7.
18. Cox SM, Nichols KK, Nichols JJ. Agreement between automated and traditional measures of tear film breakup. Optom Vis Sci. 2015;92(9):257–e263.
19. Singh S, Srivastav S, Mohamed A, Basu S. Non-invasive tear film assessment in normal population: effect of age, sex, and interparametric relationship. Front Med (Lausanne). 2022;9:894184.

20. Niedernolte B, Trunk L, Wolffsohn JS, et al. Evaluation of tear meniscus height using different clinical methods. Clin Exp Optom. 2021;104(5): 583–8.
21. Serin D, Karsloğlu S, Kyan A, Alagöz G. A simple approach to the repeatability of the Schirmer test without anesthesia: eyes open or closed? Cornea. 2007;26(8):903–6.
22. Singh S, Basu S. Effect of topical anesthesia on the secretory activity of the main lacrimal gland. Cornea. 2020;39(10):e24–5.
23. Donthineni PR, Doctor M, Kate A, et al. Aqueous-deficient dry eye disease: preferred practice pattern guidelines on clinical approach, diagnosis, and management. Indian J Ophthalmol. 2023;71:1332. https://doi.org/10.4103/IJO.IJO_2808_22.

17 Intraocular Pressure

Ramyashri S, Aparna Rao, and Sardar M. Khan

17.1 Introduction

Intraocular pressure (IOP) measurement is essential for diagnosing and managing glaucoma. The Goldmann applanation tonometer (GAT) is the current gold standard for measuring IOP, although several newer technologies are currently available for IOP measurement [1–4]. Some new IOP measurement technologies and devices include dynamic contour tonometry (DCT), ocular response analyzer (ORA), Pascal dynamic contour tonometer (DCT-Pascal), rebound tonometry, Tono-Pen Avia, and the Bioresonator applanation resonance tonometer (ART). This chapter will describe the GAT and the newer devices used for IOP measurement.

R. S
Kallam Anji Reddy Campus, L V Prasad Eye Institute, Hyderabad, India

Drishti Eye Centre, Hyderabad, India

A. Rao (✉)
Kallam Anji Reddy Campus, L V Prasad Eye Institute, Hyderabad, India

L V Prasad Eye Institute, Bhubaneshwar, India
e-mail: aparna@lvpei.org

S. M. Khan
Gullapalli Pratibha Rao International Centre for Advancement of Rural Eye Care, L V Prasad Eye Institute, Siddipet, India

17.2 Goldmann Applanation Tonometry (GAT)

The technique is named after its inventor, Hans Goldmann, who discovered it in 1948 [5].

Technology—By applying a known force to the cornea and measuring the area of applanation (the flattened area), the Goldmann applanation tonometer (GAT) calculates the IOP based on Imbert Fick's law. The device uses a truncated cone with a surface area of 7.35 mm^2 and a diameter of 3.06 mm mounted on a slit lamp. It is lit with a blue filter, and the doubling prism embedded in the cone divides the circular tear meniscus into two equal semicircular halves, which are aligned at their inner edges (Fig. 17.1) to obtain precise applanation of the cornea. The force required to flatten the corresponding surface of the cornea is directly proportional to the IOP in mmHg from the scale of the measuring drum [6].

Technique—The patient is made to sit with his/her forehead firmly placed against the headband and the chin comfortably placed on the chinrest of the device. After adequate anesthesia, the fluorescein dye is added to each eye. The patient's lateral canthus should align at the mark on the headrest column, and the patient is instructed to look straight ahead with eyes wide open. The clean tip of the tonometer biprism with the cobalt blue filter is moved toward the eye to be examined; the filter helps visualize the bright yellow-green fluorescence of the dye. The tip of the biprism is illuminated at a wide angle, and the

T. Das, P. Satgunam (eds.), *Ophthalmic Diagnostics*, https://doi.org/10.1007/978-981-97-0138-4_17

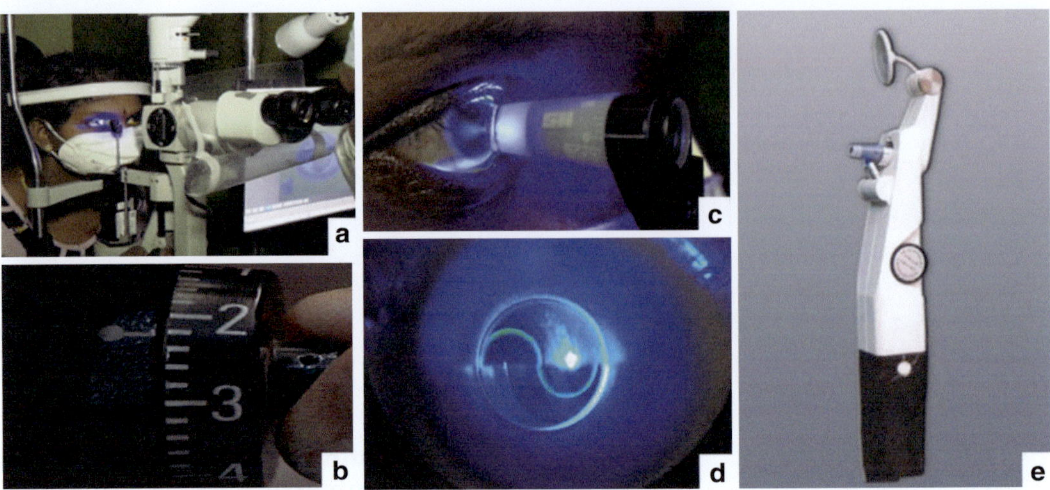

Fig. 17.1 (**a**) Slit-lamp mounted Goldmann applanation tonometer; (**b**) the measuring dial; (**c**) the biprism illuminated with a blue filter; (**d**) the mires of the biprism; and (**e**) the Perkins tonometer

instrument is set at low magnification and highest illumination. The examiner should look monocularly through the oculus to identify the spot of fluorescein on the cornea that has just been applanated (converted into two semicircular halves). The height of the slit lamp is adjusted such that the two halves of the applanated cornea are equal. The force adjustment knob or measuring dial is moved in the appropriate direction such that the inner edges of the two semicircles touch each other but do not overlap. The number on the measuring dial multiplied by 10 gives the IOP in mmHg (Fig. 17.1).

Clinical Application—Goldmann applanation tonometry provides accurate and reproducible IOP measurements; nevertheless, this depends on the physician's (user's) experience. Interobserver variability of ±2 mmHg may be observed [7]. The measurement of IOP using GAT, however, is not without limitations. Since the technique requires the device to contact the cornea, it is a potential source of corneal abrasion and infection. The device is slit-lamp mounted and requires that the patient is in an upright position. Additionally, the IOP value obtained by GAT can be affected by corneal parameters like corneal thickness, curvature, and other biomechanical properties [8]. Any abnormalities such as scarring or other irregularities can result in inaccurate IOP measurements. The technique may also underestimate IOP in thin corneas and overestimate IOP in thick corneas [7, 8]. Other drawbacks of using GAT include interference in IOP measurement due to tear films with too little or too much fluorescein dye, quenching of the dye, and other calibration errors [9].

Recent advancements in technology and design have improved the accuracy and reproducibility of GAT. Newer models use a digital display to provide more precise IOP measurements, and some integrate with electronic medical records for easier tracking and analysis of collected data. A portable version of GAT is the Perkins tonometer, which works on the same principle as the Goldmann applanation tonometer but is useful for people lying supine.

17.3 Dynamic Contour Tonometry

Dynamic contour tonometry (DCT) is a low-contact method of measuring IOP. The technique uses a small probe gently placed near the eye to measure the eye pressure.

Technology—DCT uses a small, sensor-equipped probe that lightly touches the surface of the eye and records the changes in the pressure as the eye is deformed. The sensor of the probe has a flexible and curved surface that conforms to the shape of the cornea, allowing it to measure the pressure accurately [10, 11].

Clinical Application—DCT is more accurate than applanation tonometry, especially in patients with corneal abnormalities, such as scarring or irregular curvature. In addition, DCT is easy to use and requires no special skills or training. However, DCT is affected by eye movements and can result in inaccurate readings, and the devices used are associated with high costs. The comparison of DCT and GAT, and other tonometers is shown in Table 17.1.

New developments and versions of DCT technology [12] include:

- Corvis ST: This is a new generation DCT device developed by Oculus (Switzerland). The Corvis ST measures corneal deformation responses and IOP using a high-speed Scheimpflug camera that captures images of the cornea when a puff of air deforms it. It also provides biomechanical information on the cornea, such as corneal hysteresis.
- DCT Pro: This is an upgraded version of the Pascal DCT tonometer developed by Zeimer (Switzerland). The DCT Pro uses a smaller and more ergonomic probe, which improves patient comfort and ease of use for the operator. It also features enhanced measurement stability, thus improving the accuracy and reproducibility of IOP measurements.
- Bidirectional DCT: This is a new DCT technology developed by Nidek (Japan). The bidirectional DCT uses a two-way air jet to measure IOP, improving accuracy and reducing corneal biomechanics' effect on IOP measurements.
- DCT with Ocular Pulse Amplitude (OPA): This is a new feature added to some DCT devices, such as the Reichert ORA. The OPA measures the pulsatile component of IOP, which reflects changes in blood flow and ocular perfusion [13, 14]. Adding OPA to DCT measurements provides additional information about ocular health and can help diagnose and manage glaucoma and hypertension.

Despite the advantages of other IOP measurement systems, GAT is more widely used and remains the standard of care.

Table 17.1 Comparisons of different tonometers

Schiotz tonometer	Working principle	Indentation
	Relation with cornea	Contact
	Corneal biomechanics	Not considered, but affects the measurements
	Clinical application	Useful in low-resource countries IOP in post-Kpro eyes with scleral indentation
	Availability/cost	Available easily Inexpensive
Goldmann Applanation tonometer	Working principle	Applanation
	Relation with cornea	Contact
	Corneal biomechanics	Affected by corneal biomechanics and corneal thickness
	Clinical application	In all cases, but not accurate when corneal scarring is present
	Availability/cost	Easily available and routinely used by all Current gold standard
Perkins tonometer	Working principle	Indentation
	Relation with cornea	Contact
	Corneal biomechanics	Same as GAT
	Clinical application	Can be used in supine position
	Availability/cost	Can be used as a replacement for GAT

(continued)

Table 17.1 (continued)

Tono-pen	Working principle	Indentation/applanation
	Relation with cornea	Contact
	Corneal biomechanics	Same as GAT
	Clinical application	Underestimates IOP value Highly variable and poor repeatability
	Availability/cost	Moderately available Expensive
DCT	Working principle	Contour matching
	Relation with cornea	Contact
	Corneal biomechanics	Independent of corneal properties
	Clinical application	Precise but difficult to use Needs high patient cooperation
	Availability/cost	Not available easily Expensive
ORA	Working principle	Applanation
	Relation with cornea	Non-contact
	Corneal biomechanics	Provides information on corneal biomechanics and IOP corrected for corneal biomechanical property
	Clinical application	Useful in post-refractive surgery; self-calibration possible Provides a quality index, but there is limited evidence for application
Corvis ST	Availability/cost	Expensive
	Working principle	Indentation/applanation
	Relation with cornea	Non-contact
	Corneal biomechanics	Provides information on corneal biomechanics and IOP corrected for corneal biomechanical property
	Clinical application	Useful in post-refractive surgery cases and glaucoma cases Tends to underestimate the GAT values
	Availability/cost	Expensive
iCare Rebound tonometer	Working principle	Rebound principle using a ballistic probe
	Relation with cornea	Contact
	Corneal biomechanics	Influenced by corneal properties
	Clinical application	Can be used for screening purposes and in GA cases
	Availability/cost	Expensive but feasible to use
Bioresonator ART	Working principle	Applanation, based on the acoustic impedance
	Relation with cornea	Contact
	Corneal biomechanics	Affected by corneal properties
	Clinical application	No need for fluorescein, self-calibrated, provides a quality index Has a learning curve to measuring IOP
	Availability/cost	Expensive
Sensimed Triggerfish	Working principle	Scleral stretch monitoring
	Relation with cornea	Contact
	Corneal biomechanics	Affected by corneal biomechanics
	Clinical application	Used for continuous 24-h IOP monitoring Does not provide direct IOP (only an estimate)
	Availability/cost	Expensive

17.4 Ocular Response Analyzer (ORA)

Technology—ORA measures the biomechanical properties of the cornea. It rapidly delivers a puff of air to the cornea that deforms/indents the corneal surface [15–18]. The ORA measures two key parameters of the cornea's response to this puff: (a) corneal hysteresis (CH) and (b) corneal resistance factor (CRF).

The CH measures the cornea's ability to absorb and dissipate energy during deformation. It reflects the cornea's elasticity or "bounce-back," and a low CH may indicate a stiffer cornea associated with a higher risk of developing glaucoma [16]. The CRF is a measure of the overall resistance of the cornea to deformation. A higher CRF value suggests the cornea's ability to resist deformation, which may be protective against glaucoma.

Clinical Application—ORA measurements help identify individuals at increased risk of developing glaucoma, even if their IOP is within the normal range; this can aid in early and more individualized interventions.

Over the years, the design and technology of ORAs have evolved. The most recent version, the ORA G3 (2016), features a waveform analysis that provides more detailed information on the corneal response to the puff of air. The ORA G3 also includes a more user-friendly interface and a redesigned, easy-to-use probe that is less prone to operator error. Other improvements in the ORA G3 include individualized measurement protocols and the ability to integrate with optical coherence tomography (OCT). The proposed developments in ORA technology that may improve its accuracy and reliability and expand its diagnostic capabilities include corneal biomechanical imaging [16, 18], artificial intelligence integration [19–22], and improved waveform analysis.

The ORA and Goldmann applanation tonometer differ in their approaches to measuring IOP and the information they provide. In certain conditions, ORA may be more accurate and reliable, but GAT remains the gold standard for measuring IOP in most patients.

17.5 Telemetric 24-h IOP Monitoring

Technology—Telemetric 24-h screening of IOP is a non-invasive method for measuring IOP over an extended period, typically 24 h [23–27]. This method uses a tiny wireless sensor implanted inside the eye to transmit data to an external receiver/recorder. The data is then analyzed to obtain a comprehensive profile of the fluctuations in the patient's IOP over 24 h.

Currently, there are several modes/types of telemetric 24-h screening of IOP for monitoring glaucoma. These include (a) continuous recording mode: the sensor records the IOP continuously over 24 h, (b) pulsatile mode: the sensor records the IOP at intervals during the cardiac cycle, allowing for the detection of IOP fluctuations related to changes in blood pressure, (c) triggered mode: the sensor is triggered by a specific event or activity, such as physical activity or changes in posture, to record the IOP during that specific period, (d) hybrid mode: a combination of two or more of the above modes to provide a more comprehensive profile of the patient's IOP fluctuations over the 24 h. The choice of a specific telemetric mode depends on the specific research question or clinical need.

Telemetric 24-h screening of IOP in glaucoma is a growing area of research and clinical practice, with potential applications in the early detection and management of glaucoma and other eye diseases. Several investigators are currently working on the development and commercialization of such devices. Here are some examples:

1. Eyemate-SC (Implantable Ophthalmic Products, Germany): The system consists of a tiny pressure sensor implanted inside the eye and a wireless handheld device reading the sensor's data. The pressure sensor is implanted in a minimally invasive surgical procedure under local anesthesia. The device is powered by a small battery that can last up to 5 years, after which the device can be easily replaced. It is used with the EyeMate Reader, a handheld device that wirelessly

reads the data from the pressure sensor. The data from the Eyemate-SC system is transmitted to a secure cloud-based platform where physicians and other healthcare professionals can analyze it. The Eyemate-SC system has received regulatory approval in Europe and is currently undergoing clinical trials in the USA [28].

2. Triggerfish (Sensimed AG, Switzerland) [26]: This device uses "continuous monitoring of ocular dimensional changes" (CMOD) technology, which measures changes in the diameter of the eye over 24 h. Changes in the diameter of the eye are directly related to changes in IOP. During the monitoring period, the patient wears a contact lens with the sensor, and the data is recorded by a portable recorder that can be worn on a belt or carried in a pocket. The data is then transferred to a computer for analysis. The Triggerfish device has been approved by the US Food and Drug Administration (FDA) and is available in the USA and several other countries.
3. EyeSeal (Bausch + Lomb, USA): The EyeSEAL is a small, disposable patch worn on the skin around the eye. The patch contains a tiny wireless sensor capable of measuring changes in the shape of the eye due to changes in IOP. The sensor wirelessly transmits the data to a small portable device worn by the patient and can store up to 24 h of data. The device is currently undergoing clinical trials and is not yet commercially available.
4. IOP Watcher (NovaSight, Israel): The system consists of a small wireless sensor placed on the skin near the eye and a mobile app that wirelessly reads the data from the sensor. It provides a comprehensive view of a patient's IOP over 24 h. It can also help identify the peak and trough times in IOP values, which can be used to determine the most effective time for administering glaucoma medications. The IOP Watcher system has been approved for use in Europe and is currently undergoing clinical trials in the USA.

17.5.1 Clinical Application of Telemetric IOP Monitoring

While 24-h monitoring of IOP can provide valuable information for diagnosing and managing glaucoma, this technology has safety concerns and pitfalls. These include an increased risk of infection, damage to the cornea, false positive or negative results [22], high cost, and the possibility of poor patient compliance. Currently, there is also limited evidence of the utility of this form of monitoring. The clinical application of 24-h monitoring in glaucoma practice may take time to evolve and will need radical ways of dealing with the enormous amount of data from such measurements. Novel AI-based algorithms may help incorporate the data into clinical treatment decisions in glaucoma practice in the future.

17.6 Rebound Tonometer

Technology—A rebound tonometer is a portable handheld tonometer that uses a disposable probe propelled from the tonometer toward the cornea by an electrical-pulse generator to create a magnetic field via a solenoid. The speed with which the probe returns to the device changes the magnetic field, and the tonometer uses this value to calculate the IOP [29, 30]. In patients with higher IOPs, the probe touches the cornea for a shorter time and therefore rebounds into the tonometer faster.

Clinical Application—This tonometer does not require topical anesthesia, making it useful for IOP measurements in less cooperative patients and children [31]. It is also used for IOP monitoring at home for patients who cannot follow-up regularly but require frequent IOP assessment [2]. The other advantages of this tonometer are lightweight and portable, easy to use, there is no need for staining with fluorescein, and there is a lower risk of eye infections since it uses a disposable probe [31]. In addition, this tonometer can also measure IOP in people with corneal abnormalities [32]. However, the disadvantages of this device are its high cost and that the IOP measurements made with the device may vary with variations in eyelid position.

17.7 Corvis ST

Technology—The Corvis ST combines tonometry with corneal imaging to provide a more comprehensive assessment of the eye. It uses a high-speed Scheimpflug camera to capture images of the cornea as it responds to a puff of air. The camera captures over 4300 images per second, allowing for a detailed analysis of the corneal responses. In this device, an all-blue UV-free light (of wavelength 455 nm) covers an 8.5 mm horizontal slit that evaluates the dynamic corneal deformation resulting in 140 images captured during the 30 ms after a puff of air is directed at the cornea. The bidirectional corneal deformation by the air puff is recorded during the entire process [33]. When a puff of air is directed at the cornea, it causes the cornea to applanate (A1 or first applanation) and then deform (to the point of highest concavity or HC) and then recover with second applanation (A2 or second applanation) before it returns to the primary position. With the help of algorithms, this device identifies the anterior and posterior limits of the deformation, and the IOP is measured at A1.

Clinical Application—The Corvis ST provides parameters related to the shape of the cornea, IOP, and depth, like deformation amplitude (DA), timing, and velocity [34, 35]. The advantages of this device are its ease of use (specially trained personnel not required), it is non-contact (reduces the risk of eye infection and contamination), has diverse applicability (can be used for ectatic corneas like those in patients with keratoconus or glaucoma), and is accurate (not affected by the central corneal thickness (CCT)). The disadvantages of the device include its high cost and currently limited evidence of precise IOP measurement.

17.8 Tono-Pen

Technology—The Tono-pen is a handheld device that works on the principles of applanation and indentation. The Tono-pen XL and the more recent Tono-pen Avia (Reichert Ophthalmic Instruments, Depew, NY, USA) are portable battery-operated devices. The measured IOP is displayed on the digital screen with a standard deviation of an average of 10 consecutive readings.

Clinical application—The Tono-pen is commonly used in clinical practice because it is a portable and easy-to-use device that can quickly and accurately measure IOP. However, the variability in intra-session measurements is quite high (±4.3 mmHg) [36]. It is particularly useful when traditional GAT is difficult or impossible to use, such as in patients with corneal abnormalities or those who cannot sit upright. However, CCT is known to impact the IOP measurements by the Tono-pen [37]. The advantages of the Tono-pen include its portability, ease of use, quick and accurate measurements, and reduced risk of corneal infection since the device uses a disposable latex cap. The disadvantages of the device include its high cost, the need for calibration before every use, and regular maintenance requirements. Studies have also shown that the Tono-pen consistently underestimates IOP in high ranges (at IOP values >30 mmHg) [38]. Recent advances in Tono-pen technology have focused on improving its accuracy, reliability, and ease of use. For example, newer models may include automatic calibration, data storage, and improved algorithms for calculating IOP. Additionally, some devices may incorporate additional diagnostic tools, such as pachymetry and/or imaging.

17.9 Schiotz Tonometry in Today's Practice

Introduced by the Norwegian ophthalmologist Professor Magne Schiotz in 1905 [39], Schoitz tonometry has since been widely used in ophthalmic practice. **Technology**—The footplate of the tonometer is placed on the anaesthetized cornea with known standard weights via a plunger that indents the cornea. The indentation distorts the globe with aqueous displacement inside the anterior chamber. The movement of the plunger from its "0" position is correlated to the deformation of

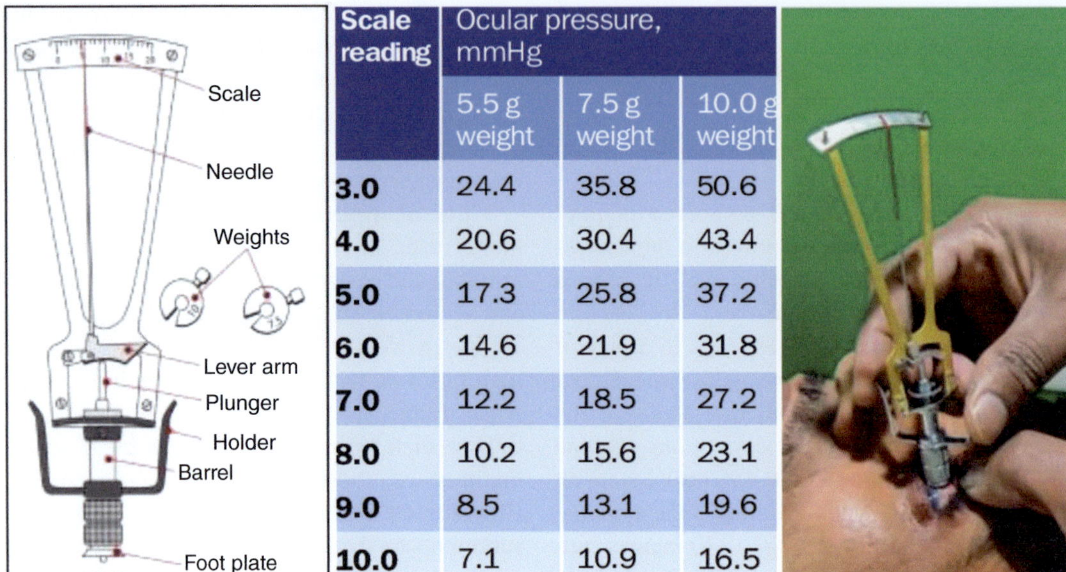

Scale reading	Ocular pressure, mmHg		
	5.5 g weight	7.5 g weight	10.0 g weight
3.0	24.4	35.8	50.6
4.0	20.6	30.4	43.4
5.0	17.3	25.8	37.2
6.0	14.6	21.9	31.8
7.0	12.2	18.5	27.2
8.0	10.2	15.6	23.1
9.0	8.5	13.1	19.6
10.0	7.1	10.9	16.5

Fig. 17.2 Schiotz tonometer. Left panel: the device; middle panel: the nomogram to translate the scale reading to intraocular pressure in mmHg; right panel: the tonometer in use. (Source for left and middle panels: Understanding and caring for a Schiotz tonometer. Comm Eye Health, 2014; 27(87): 57. Ismael Cordero. Copyright 2014, used under the Creative Common Attribution 2.0 license)

the cornea and can be translated via a calibrated scale read with the help of the lever that indicates it. Friedewald's formula relates to it and needs a constant "K," which is the ocular rigidity coefficient [39]. The IOP can be obtained from the table, which calculates this value using the weight and the scale reading (Fig. 17.2).

Technique—After the cornea is adequately anesthetized, the mid-temporal sclera (3 mm from the temporal corneoscleral limbus) is tested by asking the patient to look at the medial side for good exposure; in other cases, the extreme temporal gaze is used with a point midway between the medial canthus and medial corneoscleral limbus. The readings are taken with 5.5 g weights. If the reading is less than 4, the weight is increased to 7.5 g, and the IOP is measured again. The measured reading is converted to IOP using the nomogram. Figure 17.2 (right panel) shows Schiotz tonometry performed on the Kpro eye at an extreme temporal gaze while the nasal sclera is widely exposed for tonometry.

Clinical applications—Senthil et al. (2019) showed that the IOP values recorded using scleral Schiotz tonometry had better agreement with GAT [40]. The main advantages of this method are that it is simple to use, affordable, can be used in people in supine position, and does not require other equipment like a slit lamp. The disadvantages of this method are that it is operator dependent, needs frequent calibration, and may cause corneal abrasion and infection. Due to these limitations, Schiotz tonometry has been replaced by the current gold standard, GAT, and the other newer tonometers due to their greater accuracy and reproducibility. However, there are certain situations where GAT/newer tonometers are unreliable or cannot be used, such as post-keratoprosthesis, post-keratoplasty, or in scarred irregular corneas where the central cornea cannot be used for the measurement of the IOP.

Modifications and advances in Schiotz tonometry include (a) a digital scale to measure the force required to indent the cornea, thus eliminating the need for the operator to read the scale manually, and (b) the use of a disposable plunger, which reduces the risk of transmitting infections between patients.

17.10 Bioresonator Applanation Resonance Tonometer (ART)

Technology—Eklund et al. (2003) proposed a new tonometer based on the resonance principle. It estimates IOP by a simultaneous continuous sampling of the force needed to applanate the cornea and the corresponding area of contact [41]. It is commercially available as the Bioresonator ART (Medical sensors and Instruments, BioResonator AB, Sweden) in manual and automatic versions. In the manual (BioResonator ART manual) version, the sensor is pushed manually toward the cornea, and in the automatic version (BioResonator ART servo), this motion is servo-controlled(with a small motor that controls the sensor movement). The instrument gives the median of multiple IOP measurements and a quality score that denotes the standard deviation of the recordings.

A sensor and a transducer continuously measure the contact force along with the area of contact. A cylindrical piezoelectric element in the resonance sensor has a known resonance frequency. When it comes in contact with the cornea, the acoustic impedance changes the resonance frequency with a shift in the frequency proportional to the area of contact between the sensor and the cornea. The IOP is calculated using a complex formula that considers the slope of the relationship between the force and frequency in a specific frequency shift with respect to the applanation area interval between 4.3 and 11.0 mm^2 [41]. The entire apparatus is slit-lamp mounted like in GAT, or can be handheld. It warrants all usage precautions that apply to GAT; i.e., local anesthesia must be applied before IOP measurements can be taken, and the probe must be thoroughly sterilized before use.

The advantages of this technique are as follows: (a) there is no need for the fluorescein dye, (b) contact time with the cornea is less than that for GAT (hence, the chances of corneal abrasion damage are reduced) [42], (c) it is portable, and (d) it is self-calibrated.

The disadvantages of this technique are: (a) the patient needs to remain still during measurement, (b) IOP may be overestimated at higher ranges and if the alignment is off-center [42, 43], (c) it needs adequate surface moisture on the cornea to get good acoustic impedance (therefore, it is difficult to use in people with dry eye and ocular surface disorders) [42]. In addition, ART is also affected by CCT and other corneal biomechanical factors [43].

17.11 Conclusion

There are numerous commercially available tonometers, each with advantages and disadvantages. However, the IOP measurements of these are not interchangeable. Despite several recent developments and promising early reports, none of the alternative tonometers have gained widespread use in routine clinical practice. The Goldmann applanation tonometer remains the gold standard despite some limitations in its use in certain clinical settings. Although an ideal tonometer does not exist, it is preferable to get consistent and reliable readings every time with the same type of equipment for each patient to diagnose and treat people with glaucoma.

Funding Hyderabad Eye Research Foundation, Hyderabad, India

Disclosure Ramyashri S: None; Aparna Rao: None; Sardar M Khan: None.

References

1. Da Silva F, Lira M. Intraocular pressure measurement: a review. Surv Ophthalmol. 2022;67:1319–31.
2. Okafor KC, Brandt JD. Measuring intraocular pressure. Curr Opin Ophthalmol. 2015;26:103–9.
3. Garcia-Feijoo J, Martinez-de-la-Casa JM, Morales-Fernandez L, et al. New technologies for measuring intraocular pressure. Prog Brain Res. 2015;221:67–79.
4. ElMallah MK, Asrani SG. New ways to measure intraocular pressure. Curr Opin Ophthalmol. 2008;19:122–6.
5. Goldmann H, Schmidt T. Über Applanationstonometrie. Acta Ophthalmol. 1957;134:221–42.

6. Stamper RL. A history of intraocular pressure and its measurement. Optom Vis Sci. 2011;88:e16–28.
7. Kotecha A, White E, Schlottmann PG, Garway-Heath DF. Intraocular pressure measurement precision with the Goldmann applanation, dynamic contour, and ocular response analyzer tonometers. Ophthalmology. 2010;117:730–7.
8. Brandt JD, Beiser JA, Kass MA, Gordon MO. Central corneal thickness in the Ocular Hypertension Treatment Study (OHTS). Ophthalmology. 2001;108:1779–88.
9. Whitacre MM, Stein R. Sources of error with use of Goldmann-type tonometers. Surv Ophthalmol. 1993;38:1–30.
10. Punjabi OS, Kniestedt C, Stamper RL, Lin SC. Dynamic contour tonometry: principle and use. Clin Experiment Ophthalmol. 2006;34:837–40.
11. Kamppeter BA, Jonas JB. Dynamic contour tonometry for intraocular pressure measurement. Am J Ophthalmol. 2005;140:318–20.
12. Kanngiesser HE, Kniestedt C, Robert YC. Dynamic contour tonometry: presentation of a new tonometer. J Glaucoma. 2005;14:344–50.
13. Willekens K, Rocha R, Van Keer K, et al. Review on dynamic contour tonometry and ocular pulse amplitude. Ophthalmic Res. 2015;55:91–8.
14. Moghimi S, Torabi H, Fakhraie G, et al. Dynamic contour tonometry in primary open angle glaucoma and pseudoexfoliation glaucoma: factors associated with intraocular pressure and ocular pulse amplitude. Middle East Afr J Ophthalmol. 2013;20:158–62.
15. Sullivan-Mee M, Billingsley SC, Patel AD, et al. Ocular response analyzer in subjects with and without glaucoma. Optom Vis Sci. 2008;85:463–70.
16. Terai N, Raiskup F, Haustein M, et al. Identification of biomechanical properties of the cornea: the ocular response analyzer. Curr Eye Res. 2012;37:553–62.
17. Asano S, Asaoka R, Yamashita T, et al. Visualizing the dynamic change of ocular response analyzer waveform using variational autoencoder in association with the peripapillary retinal arteries angle. Sci Rep. 2020;10:6592. https://doi.org/10.1038/s41598-020-63601-8.
18. Aoki S, Murata H, Matsuura M, et al. The relationship between the waveform parameters from the ocular response analyzer and the progression of glaucoma. Ophthalmol Glaucoma. 2018;1:123–31.
19. Ting DSW, Pasquale LR, Peng L, et al. Artificial intelligence and deep learning in ophthalmology. Br J Ophthalmol. 2019;103:167–75.
20. Nair M, Tagare S, Venkatesh R, Odayappan A. Artificial intelligence in glaucoma. Indian J Ophthalmol. 2022;70:1868–9.
21. Yousefi S, Pasquale LR, Boland MV. Artificial intelligence and glaucoma: illuminating the black box. Ophthalmol Glaucoma. 2020;3:311–3.
22. Chaurasia AK, Greatbatch CJ, Hewitt AW. Diagnostic accuracy of artificial intelligence in glaucoma screening and clinical practice. J Glaucoma. 2022;31:285–99.
23. Yuan X, Zhang J. Real-time monitoring of intraocular pressure in glaucoma patients using wearable Mobile medicine devices. J Healthc Eng. 2022;2022:2271937. https://doi.org/10.1155/2022/2271937.
24. Yang C, Huang X, Li X, et al. Wearable and implantable intraocular pressure biosensors: recent Progress and future prospects. Adv Sci (Weinh). 2021;8:2002971. https://doi.org/10.1002/advs.202002971.
25. Shah JV, Albors GO, Williams J, et al. Clinical study of the IOPTx™ system—an electroceutical wearable to lower intraocular pressure. Curr Eye Res. 2021;46:1531–8.
26. Beltran-Agulló L, Buys YM, Jahan F, et al. Twenty-four-hour intraocular pressure monitoring with the SENSIMED triggerfish contact lens: effect of body posture during sleep. Br J Ophthalmol. 2017;101:1323–8.
27. Ittoop SM, SooHoo JR, Seibold LK, et al. Systematic review of current devices for 24-h intraocular pressure monitoring. Adv Ther. 2016;33:1679–90.
28. Szurman P, Gillmann K, Seuthe AM, et al. EYEMATE-SC Study Group. EYEMATE-SC trial: twelve-month safety, performance, and accuracy of a Suprachoroidal sensor for telemetric measurement of intraocular pressure. Ophthalmology. 2023;130:304–12.
29. Nakakura S. Icare® rebound tonometers: review of their characteristics and ease of use. Clin Ophthalmol. 2018;12:1245–53.
30. Liu J, De Francesco T, Schlenker M, Ahmed II. Icare home tonometer: a review of characteristics and clinical utility. Clin Ophthalmol. 2020;23(14):4031–45.
31. Fayed MA, Chen TC. Pediatric intraocular pressure measurements: tonometers, central corneal thickness, and anesthesia. Surv Ophthalmol. 2019;64:810–25.
32. Chui WS, Lam A, Chen D, Chiu R. The influence of corneal properties on rebound tonometry. Ophthalmology. 2008;115:80–4.
33. Vinciguerra R, Ambrósio R Jr, Elsheikh A, et al. Detection of keratoconus with a new biomechanical index. J Refract Surg. 2016;32:803–10.
34. Vinciguerra R, Elsheikh A, Roberts CJ, et al. Influence of pachymetry and intraocular pressure on dynamic corneal response parameters in healthy patients. J Refract Surg. 2016;32:550–61.
35. Ruberti JW, Sinha Roy A, Roberts CJ. Corneal biomechanics and biomaterials. Annu Rev Biomed Eng. 2011;13:269–95.
36. Tonnu PA, Ho T, Sharma K, et al. A comparison of four methods of tonometry: method agreement and interobserver variability. Br J Ophthalmol. 2005;89:847–50.
37. Tonnu PA, Ho T, Newson T, et al. The influence of central corneal thickness and age on intraocular pressure measured by pneumotonometry, non-contact tonometry, the Tono-Pen XL, and Goldmann applanation tonometry. Br J Ophthalmol. 2005;89:851–4.
38. Gopesh T, Camp A, Unanian M, et al. Rapid and accurate pressure sensing device for direct measure-

ment of intraocular pressure. Transl Vis Sci Technol. 2020;9:28. https://doi.org/10.1167/tvst.9.3.28.
39. Albert DM, Keeler R. The pressure: before and after Schiøtz. Ophthalmol Glaucoma. 2020;3:409–13.
40. Senthil S, Chary R, Ali MH, et al. Schiotz scleral intraocular pressure readings predict Goldmann applanation readings better than rebound tonometry. Cornea. 2019;38:1117–23.
41. Eklund A, Hallberg P, Lindén C, Lindahl OA. An applanation resonator sensor for measuring intraocular pressure using combined continuous force and area measurement. Invest Ophthalmol Vis Sci. 2003;44:3017–24.
42. Mulak M, Czak WA, Mimier M, Kaczmarek R. A comparison of intraocular pressure values obtained using a Goldmann applanation tonometer and a handheld version of applanation resonance tonometer: a preliminary report. Adv Clin Exp Med. 2018;27:481–5.
43. Salvetat ML, Zeppieri M, Tosoni C, Brusini P. Repeatability and accuracy of applanation resonance tonometry in healthy subjects and patients with glaucoma. Acta Ophthalmol. 2014;92:e66–73.

Gonioscopy

18

Arnav Panigrahi, Shikha Gupta, and Viney Gupta

18.1 Introduction

Gonioscopy is necessary when testing for glaucoma. It enables the visualization and magnification of the iridocorneal angle and helps identify its configuration, thereby aiding a proper diagnosis. The primary purpose of this test is to distinguish between angle closure and open-angle glaucoma and help diagnose the various open and closed angle varieties of secondary glaucoma by identifying the characteristics specific to these conditions. Currently, intraoperative gonioscopy is increasingly being used in angle-based surgeries. Although a simple technique, it takes years of practice to master the art of gonioscopy. Hence, practicing this technique as frequently as possible is advisable.

18.2 The Optics of Gonioscopy and Lenses Used

Gonioscopy entails the visualization of angle structures. The main problem with the direct visualization of angle structures is that it is difficult to ascertain the position of the angle with respect to the eye due to the sudden rarefication of the refractive index when the light rays pass from the cornea ($\mu = 1.33$) into the air ($\mu = 1.0$). Since the critical angle at the cornea–air interface is about 46°, only the rays that are incident on the cornea at an angle of <46° can emerge from the anterior chamber into the air, allowing the direct visualization of the angle. This is usually not possible in eyes with normal anatomy (Fig. 18.1a) but might be possible in pathological conditions like distorted corneal contour, keratoconus, and keratoglobus, where the angle structures may be directly visible without any aid. In normal scenarios, this problem can be circumvented in two ways. One entails the use of a thick concavo-convex lens placed on the cornea, with a power higher than the corneal dioptric power, to prevent the phenomenon of total internal reflection; this allows most of the rays to pass out of the cornea following refraction (Fig. 18.1b) (the principle behind direct gonioscopy). The second entails using a plano-concave lens with a coupling agent to nullify the difference in refractive index between the two media, hence avoiding total internal reflection such that the emergent light can then be brought onto the central frame using plane mirrors placed at a specific angle (Fig. 18.1c) (the principle behind indirect gonioscopy).

The commonly used gonioscopes for slit-lamp angle visualization utilize indirect optics. The prototype for such a lens is the Goldmann single mirror gonioscope. It consists of a plano-concave lens at the base, the corneal interface, and a single

A. Panigrahi · S. Gupta · V. Gupta (✉)
Dr. Rajendra Prasad Centre for Ophthalmic Sciences, AIIMS, New Delhi, India

T. Das, P. Satgunam (eds.), *Ophthalmic Diagnostics*, https://doi.org/10.1007/978-981-97-0138-4_18

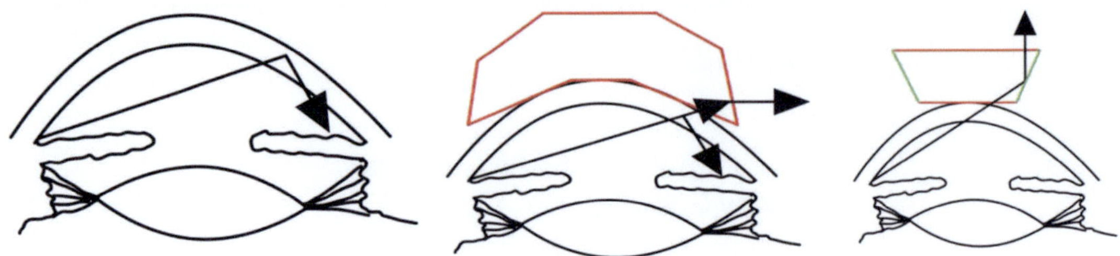

Fig. 18.1 The schematic diagram shows the transmission of light rays originating from the anterior chamber angle, with and without the aid of a goniolens. In the natural state, all the light rays undergo total internal reflection, and none emerges from the eye (left). A direct (middle) or indirect (right) goniolens allows the light rays to exit the eye, allowing the observer to visualize the angle structures. The green lines indicate the placement of the mirrors

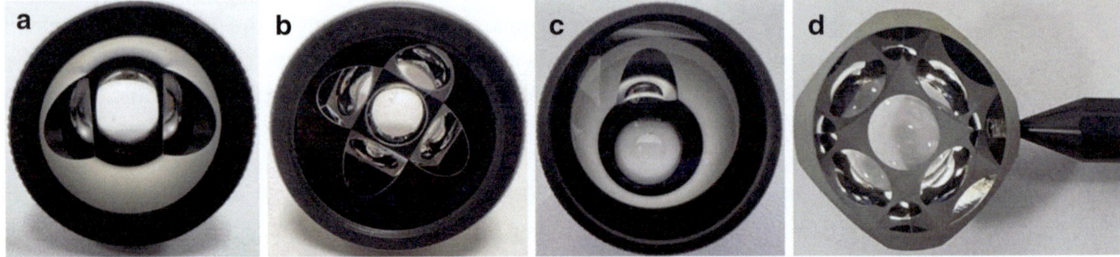

Fig. 18.2 Indirect gonioprisms commonly used for angle evaluation: (**a**) the Goldmann 2-mirror lens; (**b**) Goldmann 4-mirror lens; (**c**) Latina selective laser trabeculoplasty lens; and (**d**) Posner gonioprism with a handle

plane mirror placed within the body of the gonioscope at 62°, which reflects the emergent light rays out of the cornea almost perpendicular to the lens. The base is larger than the corneal diameter (12 mm for the Goldmann-type lens). These lenses require a coupling agent to ensure homogenous contact between the lens and the cornea, thus accounting for the sudden change in curvature at the corneoscleral junction. These lenses are considered indirect as the visualization of the structures occurs after reflection by a plane mirror. The placement of the mirror is such that the image obtained is reversed but not crossed. For example, the inferior angle can be visualized by ensuring superior placement of the mirror, but the image on the right side of the mirror is still the right side of the concerned angle. Other lenses with similar builds are the Goldmann 2-mirror (Fig. 18.2a), 3-mirror, 4-mirror lenses (Fig. 18.2b) and the Allen Thorpe goniolens. The Goldmann 3-mirror lens has a mirror placed at 59° for the gonioscopic visualization of the opposite angle. The other two mirrors, placed at 67° and 73°, are for visualizing the equatorial and peripheral retina, respectively. The Allen Thorpe lens uses 4 prisms instead of plane mirrors. The central lens in each of these variants can be used to evaluate the posterior pole. This allows for complete glaucoma evaluation, simultaneously assessing the disc and the angle. It can also be used to stabilize the globe, hence ensuring a more accurate examination, especially in eyes with nystagmus. The Latina selective laser trabeculoplasty (SLT) gonio laser lens (Fig. 18.2c) is a modification of a single mirror Goldmann-type goniolens specially designed to deliver laser light during laser trabeculoplasty. It consists of a single plane mirror placed at an angulation of 63° and utilizes indirect optics to visualize angle structures. It has a 1× magnification; hence the size of the beam emitted by the laser machine and that visualized by the observer is the same. It may also incorporate a special lid flange that prevents the lens from slipping due to the resistance caused by squeezing the patient's eyelids. A special modification includes the five high-contrast bars imaged over the trabecular meshwork (TM). The bars are spaced at 400 μm, providing a guide for delivering 10 laser spots, five corresponding to and five between the aforementioned bars. The bar can be rotated 10 times to complete a full circle around the angle, allowing for the accurately spaced delivery of 100 laser spots to the TM.

A modification to conventional indirect gonioscopy involves the use of goniolens with a base smaller than the cornea. This allows these lenses to use the precorneal tear film as a coupling agent by excluding the steep curvature change at the corneoscleral junction from its contact surface. This obviates the need for external coupling agents like methylcellulose. The smaller diameter of these lenses also allows for diagnostic and therapeutic maneuvers during gonioscopy. Pressing the lens on the central cornea displaces the aqueous humor from the central anterior chamber (AC) toward the periphery, pushing the iris root posteriorly and opening up the angle structures. This maneuver, called "dynamic gonioscopy" or "indentation gonioscopy," helps differentiate between appositional and synechial closure. This maneuver can also be therapeutic as it helps decongest the AC by partially opening up the angle during an acute angle closure (AAC) attack. The prototype for such a lens is the Zeiss 4 mirror goniolens. It uses a plano-concave lens of 9 mm diameter as its base and 4 mirrors inclined at 64° as the primary reflecting surface. All 4 quadrants are visible simultaneously, with a rotation of merely 11° allowing for the areas between the adjacent mirrors to be viewed. The Posner (Fig. 18.2d) and Sussman lens are other prototypes used for indentation gonioscopy. A comparison between the various types of indirect gonioprisms is given in Table 18.1.

Direct gonioscopy utilizes a thick convex lens placed on the cornea to nullify the rarefication of the refractive index when the light emerges from the cornea into the air. This prevents total internal reflection and allows the direct visualization of the angle. These may come with or without handles. Since a single lens is used, and there is no provision of plane mirrors to make the emergent light perpendicular to the cornea, the patient's head must be tilted away from the observer to allow the emergent rays to reach the observer's cornea. These lenses can be used for diagnostic purposes but are more commonly used as surgical goniolens for the intraoperative visualization of angle structures during procedures like goniotomy and gonioscopic-assisted transluminal trabeculotomy (GATT). Koeppe lens (Fig. 18.3a) and Swan Jacob lens (Fig. 18.3b) are prototypes for direct goniolenses. Other examples are the Barkan lens, Thorpe lens, and Mori lens. The Mori upright surgical goniolens incorporates a two-mirror design that redirects the oblique emergent rays to the coaxial position perpendicular to the cornea, hence obviating the need for tilting the patient's head during surgery. This allows for 360° visualization of angle structures while the head is supine, without requiring intraoperative maneuvers like head tilting.

Table 18.1 Comparison of indirect gonio prisms

Lens type	Goldmann Single mirror	Goldmann Three mirrors	Zeiss Four mirrors
Diameter of corneal contact	12 mm	12 mm	9 mm
Overall diameter	15 mm	18 m	9 mm
Rim size	1.5 mm	3 mm	None
Mirror angulation	62°	59°	64°
Mirror height	17 mm	12 mm	12 mm
Distance from central cornea	3 mm	7 mm	5 mm
Radius of curvature	7.4 mm	7.4 mm	7.85 mm
Coupling fluid	Required	Required	Not required
Dynamic gonioscopy	Manipulation	Manipulation	Indentation

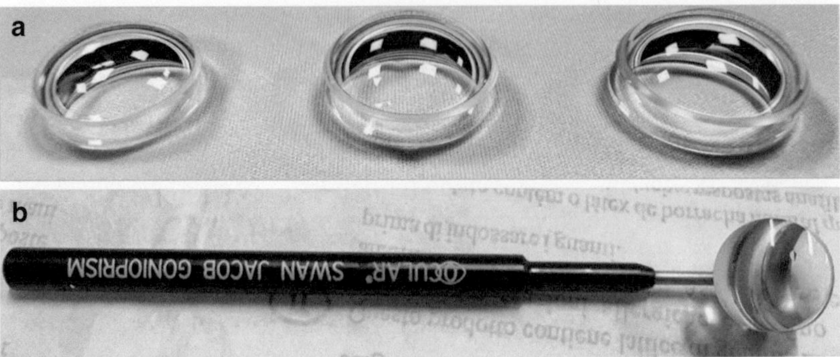

Fig. 18.3 The direct goniolenses commonly used in routine glaucoma practice: (**a**) Koeppe lenses of varying sizes and (**b**) a Swan Jacob lens with a handle

18.3 Techniques Used in Gonioscopy

18.3.1 Indirect Lenses

There is no defined standardized technique for performing indirect gonioscopy. Here is a simple method for performing gonioscopy using an indirect handheld gonioprism without a handle. The readers are advised to experiment with different gazes and gonioprisms to find the technique most suitable for them.

Explain the procedure thoroughly to the patient and take verbal consent. Anesthetize the eye with 0.5% proparacaine eye drops. Ask the patient to sit upright at the slit lamp, with the forehead pressed firmly against the headrest. If a Goldmann-type lens is used, put 2–3 drops of coupling agent (generally methylcellulose) on the corneal surface of the lens. Indentation goniolenses do not require coupling agents for performing gonioscopy. Ask the patient to look down and gently elevate the upper eyelid. Dock the corneal surface of the gonioscope onto the inferior fornix and firmly appose it against the cornea to prevent the formation of air bubbles in the interface, which impedes clear visualization of angle structures. Rotation of the lens and intermittent pressure on the goniolens against the cornea also helps remove air bubbles if present. Ask the patient to look straight ahead and direct an oblique beam of 3–4 mm in length at an angle of 30°–45° onto the mirror of interest. Move the slit lamp back and forth until the angle structures are visible, and rotate the lens to visualize the whole angle in the primary position.

If indentation gonioscopy is performed, gently pressing the goniolens against the cornea opens up the angle structures, allowing one to differentiate between appositional and synechial closure. Contrary to traditional belief, similar maneuvers are also possible with the Goldmann-type goniolenses, although the process is far more complicated. To open up the angle visible in the superior mirror, which is the inferior angle, the patient is asked to look superiorly, and gentle pressure is applied on the superior rim of the contact surface of the goniolens. This maneuver displaces the fluid in the superior angle inferiorly, thereby opening the inferior angle if appositional closure is present. This “opening up” is visualized in the superior mirror. Hence, to open the angle seen in one of the mirrors of the Goldmann goniolens, the patient is asked to look toward the direction of the mirror, and the pressure is applied on the sclera adjacent to the mirror.

18.3.2 Direct Lenses

Direct goniolenses are primarily used for intraoperative gonioscopy. The patient’s head is tilted away from the observer, and the globe is pushed toward the nasal bridge (to visualize the nasal angle), with the observer seated in a temporal position. A surgical visco-dispersive ophthalmic viscoelastic device (OVD), like HPMC 2%, is placed on the contact surface of the surgical goniolens. The lens is held with a handle and gently placed on the nasal limbus without any undue pressure not to induce any corneal folds. This allows clear visualization of the nasal angle, the site of most angle surgeries, without apparent image distortion.

Direct goniolenses, like the Koeppe lens, may also come without a handle. They are held at the equator between the thumb and index finger of the right hand for right eye examination, the left hand for the left eye, and the head tilted toward the angle being visualized. The space between the lens and the eye is filled with a coupling agent. The light source is provided either by the operating microscope or a handheld slit lamp.

18.4 Structures Seen on Gonioscopy

Figure 18.4 shows an open angle in a normal eye, where all the angle structures are visible. From anterior to posterior, the angle structures seen are Schwalbe's line (SL), anterior trabecular meshwork (ATM), posterior trabecular meshwork (PTM), scleral spur (SS), and ciliary body band (CBB). The condensation of collagen fibers forms the SL and marks the termination of Descemet's membrane (DM). Identification of the SL is important because the labeling of the angle structures begins from the SL and continues posteriorly toward the CBB. Hence, identifying the SL is crucial, especially in cases with featureless angles, where none of the angle structures are seen. In these cases, the SL usually provides a landmark from which the point labeling of the angle structures can begin. The identification of the SL, although difficult in these cases, can be aided by the "corneal wedge" technique as follows: direct a narrow beam of light from the slit lamp obliquely on the cornea; the beam is split into an outer part (corresponding to the corneal epithelium) and an inner part (corresponding to the corneal endothelium); a fusion of both these parts marks the termination of the DM, which is the landmark for the SL.

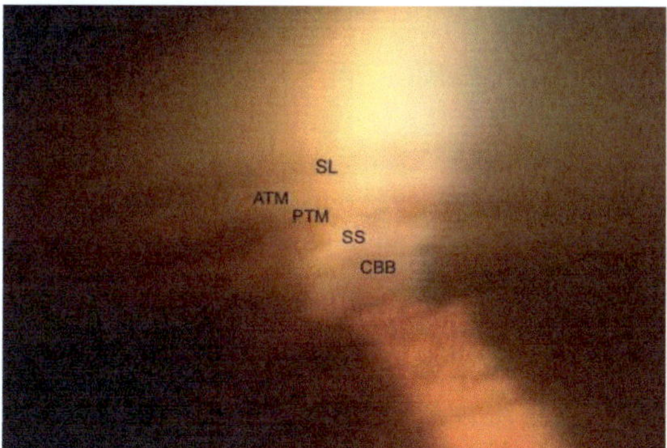

Fig. 18.4 Goniophotograph of a normal wide open angle. Structures seen, from anterior to posterior, are Schwalbe's line (SL), anterior trabecular meshwork (ATM), posterior trabecular meshwork (PTM), scleral spur (SS), and ciliary body band (CBB)

The trabecular meshwork (TM) can be divided into two parts: the anteriorly placed nonfunctional anterior TM (ATM) and the posteriorly placed functional TM (PTM). ATM forms the structural scaffold and has almost no outflow function owing to the lack of Schlemm's canal (SC) behind it. It is lightly pigmented or nonpigmented in appearance. Its posterior extent marks the site of an incision during *ab interno* angle surgeries like goniotomy and GATT. The PTM, on the other hand, forms the site of maximum resistance to aqueous outflow. Due to the SC behind it, it marks the site of conventional outflow, also known as pressure-dependent outflow or trabecular outflow. It also indicates the incision site for inserting minimally invasive glaucoma drainage devices, like iStent and Hydrus implants. It is relatively easier to identify due to its pigmented nature. This might not be the case in pediatric eyes, where pigmentation is sparse, and a featureless angle may also be a possibility. The PTM in the superior angle usually exhibits less pigmentation than in the inferior angle. Any change in the intensity of pigmentation, or its distribution, may provide a clue to underlying pathologies. Figure 18.5a shows a densely pigmented TM in a patient with pigmentary glaucoma.

Another important landmark to identify in the angle is the SS. It is a ridge formed by the condensation of the collagen tissue of the sclera, and it is the site of attachment of longitudinal fibers of the ciliary muscle. Identifying the SS is relatively easy; the white band is immediately posterior to the PTM. Identifying the SS is very important, as it allows us to differentiate between open and closed angles. Due to the attachment of

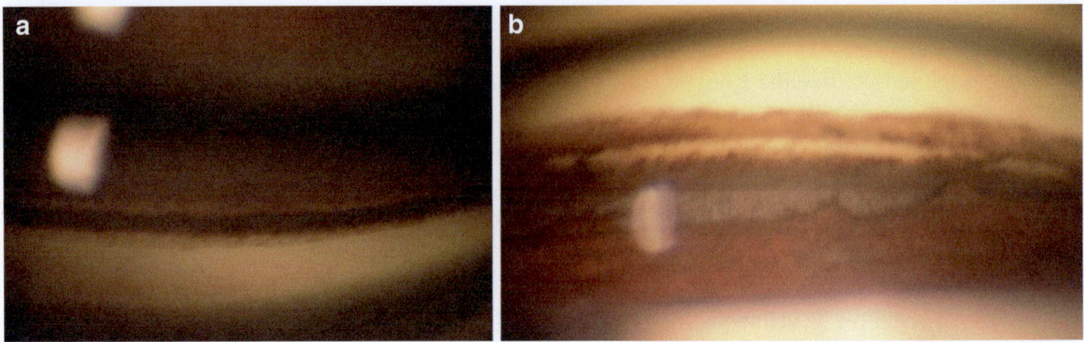

Fig. 18.5 Goniophotograph of a patient with (**a**) pigment dispersion syndrome, showing a densely pigmented trabecular meshwork of the superior angle; (**b**) angle recession, showing an irregularly widened ciliary body band

the ciliary muscle, contraction due to light-induced miosis pulls the SS posteriorly, which may artefactually open the angle. Hence, a preliminary examination of the angle structures is advised under low illumination to avoid the abovementioned phenomenon and falsely label the angle as open. Occasionally, the scleral spur might be covered by fine projections of uveal tissue known as the iris processes. These do not cross the SS, are found in about one-third of healthy individuals, and are not associated with an increased risk of glaucoma.

The CBB forms the posterior-most part of the angle and lies adjacent to the iris root. It is wide in eyes with high myopia, trauma, posteriorly subluxated lens, pseudophakia, or aphakia. It is narrow in hyperopic eyes and those with an anterior insertion of the iris. A unilateral abnormally widened CBB, especially with the history and other signs and symptoms of ocular trauma, with or without an associated cyclodialysis cleft (Fig. 18.5b), is usually pathognomonic of post-traumatic angle recession.

18.5 Identifying Occludability

Numerous systems have been devised to grade the occludability of the angle based on the number of structures seen on the gonioscopy. The nomenclature systems currently in clinical use have been developed by Scheie, Spaeth, Becker, and Shaffer-Kanski; the latter is the most practical and commonly used. Scheie [1] used a system based on the visibility of angle structures, allotted with a higher number of narrower angles (range: I–IV). Emphasizing the complexity of angle structures, Spaeth [2, 3] proposed a system incorporating multiple parameters limited to the angle. These include iris insertion (range A–E), iris configuration, iris angulation (range 10°–40°) (Fig. 18.6), and pigmentation of PTM (range 0–4). Various combinations of these parameters give a more accurate representation of the angle [4]. Becker limited his classification to 2 important angle parameters: the width of the trabecular zone (the space between the SL and SS, represented by numbers) and the distance between the SS and iris root (represented by letters). Shaffer-Kanski has devised the most clinically relevant and practically useful system. It is a modification of the system originally developed by Shaffer [5] (Table 18.2). It incorporates two parameters: iris angulation and visibility of structures. Combining both parameters can help the clinician estimate the risk of angle closure. The readers are directed to consult additional sources for a detailed discussion of these nomenclature systems.

It is important to document the findings clearly and concisely, which, even if elaborate, must impart as much information as possible and be easily understandable by fellow ophthalmologists. This helps avoid repeat examinations and hence saves time in clinics. A simple example of a diagrammatic representation of gonioscopy findings is given in Fig. 18.7. Divide the eye into

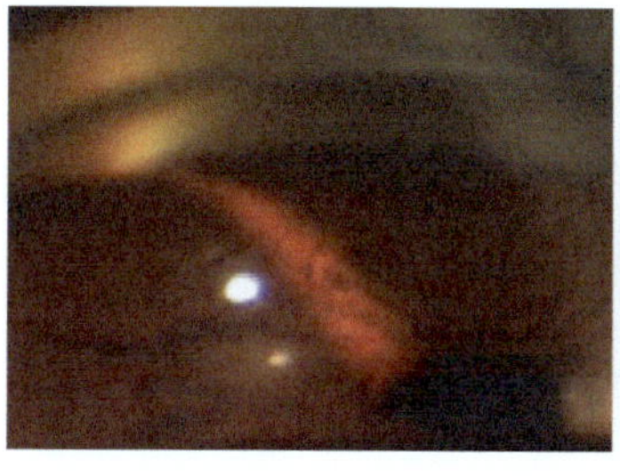
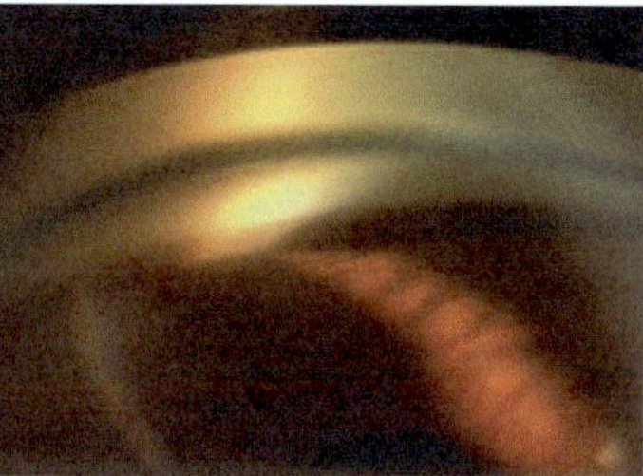
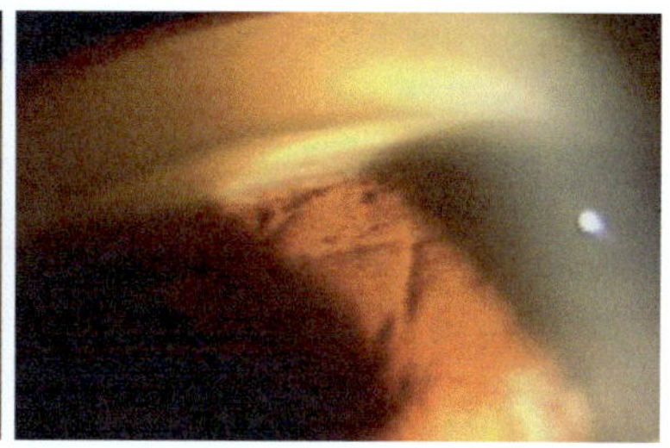

Fig. 18.6 Varying degrees of angle recess and occludability as classified according to the Spaeth system: the left and middle panels show occludable angle recesses of 10° and 20°, respectively. The right panel shows a wide open angle with a 30° angle recess

Table 18.2 Classification and clinical application of anterior chamber angle

Grade	Angle width	Description	Risk of closure
4	45°–35°	Wide-open	Impossible
3	35°–20°	Wide-open	Impossible
2	20°	Narrow	Possible
1	<10°	Extremely narrow	Probable
Slit	Slit	Narrow to slit	Probable
0	0°	Closed	Closed

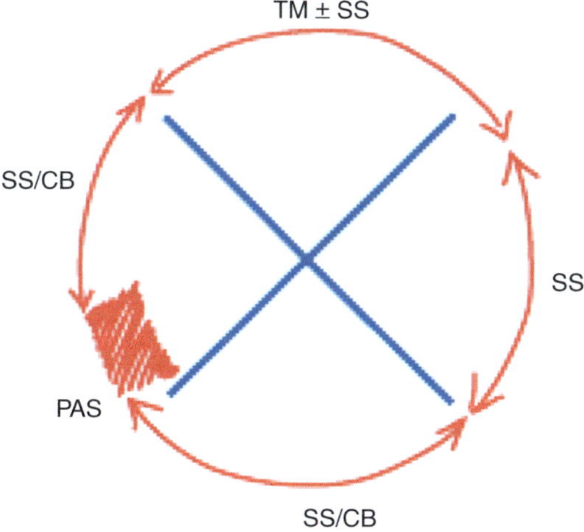

Fig. 18.7 Schematic representation of angle findings in the right eye of a patient. The double-headed arrows represent a dynamic gonioscopy being performed. The furthest structure seen on the baseline condition and maximal illumination and manipulation are marked for each corresponding quadrant. Any special findings, like inferotemporal peripheral anterior synechiae (PAS) at 8 clock hours in this figure, are also drawn

four quadrants using two oblique lines intersecting at an angle of 90°. The four quadrants correspond to the part of the eye being examined, as seen by the examiner. The deepest part of the angle seen under the baseline conditions in each quadrant is marked. If an indentation or "manipulation" gonioscopy is performed, the quadrants are designated with doubled-ended arrows, and the part seen after the maneuver mentioned above is also marked. Additional information regarding the iris insertion, configuration, and angle pigmentation can be added per the Spaeth nomenclature. Special details, like PAS, cyclodialysis, and new vessels, can be drawn at their location to give a complete diagrammatic representation of the angle.

18.6 Look Beyond What You See

Although gonioscopy seems simple, mastering it requires optimal vigilance and years of practice. Gonioscopic findings, on their own, may be of limited importance; but in conjecture with the relevant history and associated anterior segment findings, may provide a lot of information. Let's consider this example:

Case report: A 42-year-old male with proliferative diabetic retinopathy in both eyes was referred to the glaucoma clinic because of high IOP in both eyes. Anterior segment evaluation showed the presence of neovascularization of the iris in the left eye; the right eye appeared normal, except for a temporally pulled pupillary ruff (Fig. 18.8a). Hence, right eye primary open-angle glaucoma and left eye neovascular glaucoma (NVG) were diagnosed. A detailed gonioscopic evaluation revealed the presence of a single strand of neovascularization at the angle in the temporal angle corresponding to the site of the pulled pupillary ruff, visible only at higher magnifications (Fig. 18.8b). The diagnosis was eventually changed to NVG for both eyes. Thus, a detailed gonioscopic evaluation helped make an appropriate diagnosis.

Other important uses of gonioscopy are identifying angle occludability, staging angle closure, and proper management. Labeling an occludable angle open after a brief screening under high illumination by a novice is a common mistake. Misdiagnosing angle closure glaucoma (ACG) as open-angle glaucoma (OAG) can be catastrophic, considering the aggressive course and potentially blinding nature of ACG. Most iridotrabecular contact in ACG occurs during pupil dilation when the risk of a pupillary block is the highest and the amount of iridotrabecular contact is maximum. This results in progressive damage to the PTM, resulting in outflow dysfunction and elevated IOP. Hence, it is valuable to simulate this aggravating condition as closely and safely as possible to assess the actual risk of development and progression of glaucoma. To assess angle closure, it is important to determine the angle structures under the thinnest slit and dimmest illumination possible (Fig. 18.9a and b), which permits a proper estimation of the occludability.

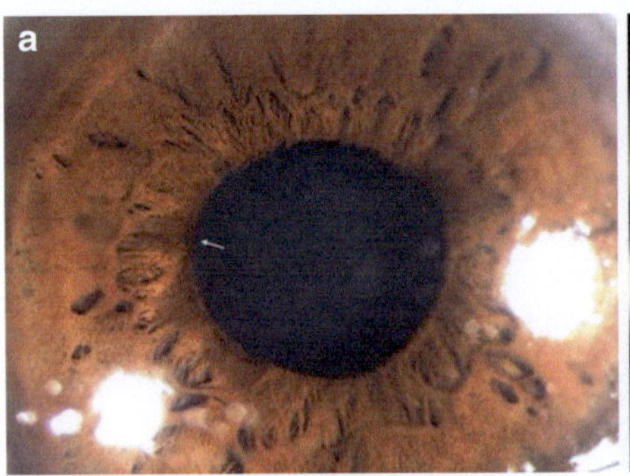
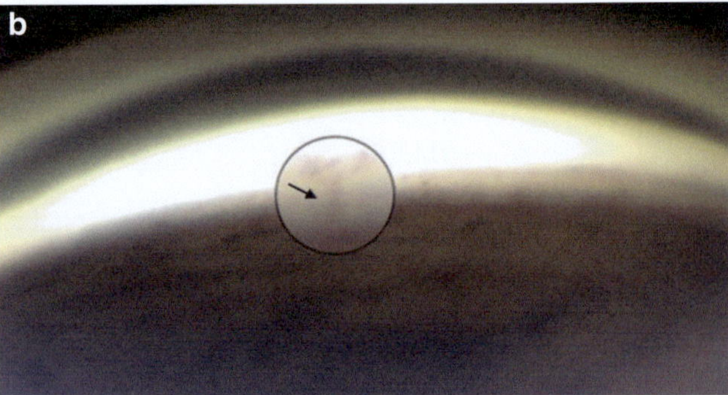

Fig. 18.8 An anterior segment photograph of the patient's right eye (**a**) shows ruff atrophy with early ectropion uvea in the temporal pupillary margin (white arrow). Right (**b**): gonioscopic examination revealed an open angle with the presence of a single new vessel (black arrow), crossing the scleral spur to reach Schwalbe's line

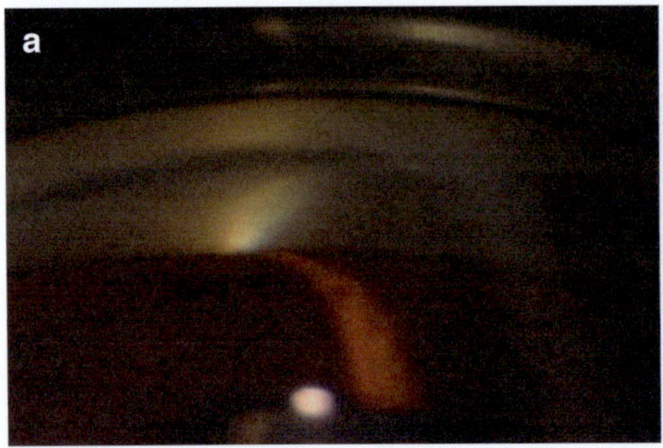
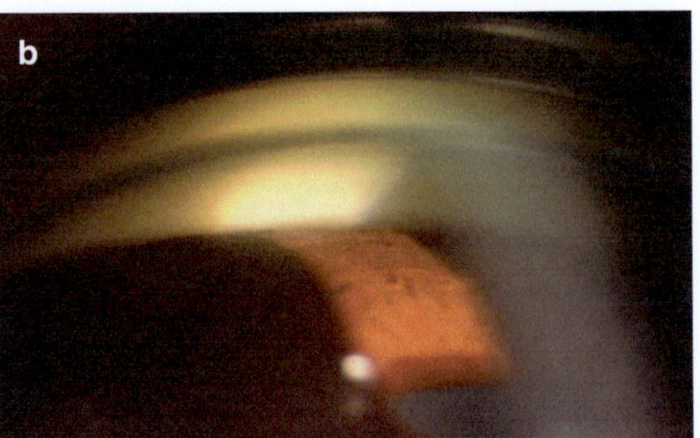

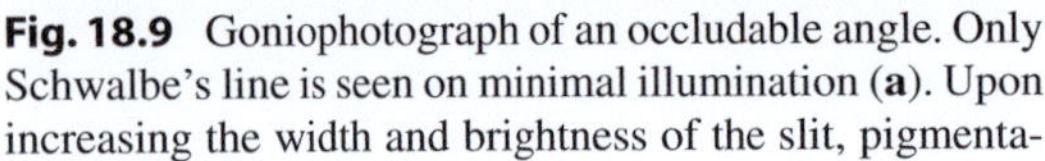

Fig. 18.9 Goniophotograph of an occludable angle. Only Schwalbe's line is seen on minimal illumination (**a**). Upon increasing the width and brightness of the slit, pigmentation of the posterior trabecular meshwork can be seen (**b**), signifying occludability with appositional closure

18.7 Systems for Automated Goniophotography

Recently, systems for goniophotography have been developed to image the anterior chamber angle without using a conventional gonioscope, thus reducing human variations and errors. These systems utilize a contact lens system and coupling agent, similar to a conventional gonioscope system. Examples of such specialized systems include the following.

1. RetCam, NGS-1 automated gonioscope, the GonioPEN, and axicon lens-assisted gonioscopy [6]. The RetCam (Natus Medical Incorporated, Pleasanton, CA) is a handheld retinal and angiographic camera primarily developed to screen retinopathy of prematurity. It can also visualize the anterior chamber angle using its B1200 lens with a 120° field of view. It has shown good sensitivity, specificity, and excellent diagnostic performance for detecting gonioscopic angle closure, especially when using the definition of two-quadrant angle closure for diagnosis [7].
2. The NGS-1 automated gonioscope (Nidek, Gamagori, Japan) is a recently commercialized contact-based automated goniophotography device that can capture 16 sections over a 360° angle in less than 1 min [8, 9]. The main advantage of this system is the shorter image capture time and learning curve compared to manual gonioscopy. However, poor resolution of the trabecular meshwork due to defocus remains a problem. Hence, the jury is still not out regarding using this system in routine clinical practice.
3. The GonioPEN combines a miniaturized charge-coupled diode camera with a light-emitting diode, both integrated into a probe that can be used as a slit-lamp attachment. It is placed near the limbus to visualize structures of the opposite iridocorneal angle [10].
4. The axicon lens-assisted gonioscopy is a potential alternate mechanism for gonioscopic visualization and imaging, which is currently under development. It integrates the concept of Bessel beam microscopy, which enables accurate imaging of the anterior chamber angle to a spatial resolution of 3 μm. It has been used to visualize the anterior chamber angle in bovine [11] and rabbit [12] eyes; further studies are needed to validate this technology for use in human eyes.

18.8 Technological Adjuncts to Gonioscopy

Ultrasound biomicroscopy (UBM) was one of the first devices to aid in gonioscopic diagnosis. It employs high-frequency ultrasonic waves, which help in the detailed imaging of the anterior chamber and angle structures. It is instrumental in visualizing the morphology of the ciliary body. It is useful in detecting angle closure glaucoma, especially differentiating between the major subgroups of primary angle closure glaucoma (PACG). Iridotrabecular contact with a convex iris configuration suggests a pupillary block mechanism (Fig. 18.10a). A deep central and a shallow peripheral anterior chamber due to an anteriorly rotated ciliary body (Fig. 18.10b), with partial or complete obliteration of the iridociliary sulcus, suggests a plateau iris configuration. A ciliary body cyst may be present, causing an anterior shift in the ciliary body (Fig. 18.10c). This leads to an appearance similar to the plateau iris configuration and is termed as pseudo plateau iris configuration. The latter two can be gonioscopically identified based on the presence of "sine wave iris configuration" and "lumpy, bumpy appearance," respectively. Differentiation between the three groups is necessary, as the pupillary block mechanism is amenable to laser iridotomy, whereas the other two are refractory. Occasionally, a ciliary body melanoma may be noted, leading to secondary angle closure. UBM is also used in children with hazy corneas to evaluate the angle of closure. This allows differentiation between primary congenital glaucoma and secondary glaucoma, aiding in prognostication and decision-making.

Recently, swept-source anterior segment optical coherence tomography (AS-OCT) has been used in the stratification of the risk of develop-

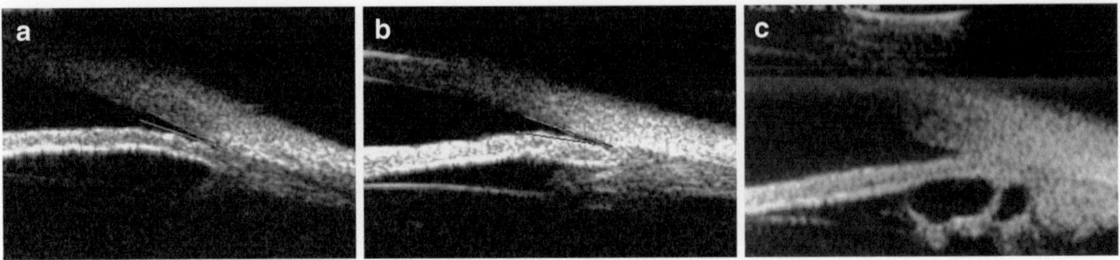

Fig. 18.10 Ultrasound biomicroscopy (UBM) findings of the three mechanisms of primary angle closure mechanism: pupillary block (**a**), plateau iris configuration (**b**), and pseudo plateau iris configuration due to multiple ciliary body cysts (**c**)

ment of PACG. It employs a beam of longer wavelength (1310 nm) and lower penetration than retinal OCT, hence facilitating the detailed imaging of the AC. Recent studies have shown that the detection of the anatomic angle closure by AS-OCT parameters like angle opening distance and trabecular iris space area is more strongly correlated to the risk of progression to glaucoma, as compared to gonioscopic angle closure [13–15]. This result is not an anomaly; where human evaluation is tainted with variations due to illumination, pressure, eye movement, and the individuality of the examiner, machines are highly automated with the ability to simulate the optimal conditions for imaging. A 360° evaluation of the angle using AS-OCT to rule out any form of iridotrabecular contact before delaying the institution of laser iridotomy may help prevent progression and thereby reduce the burden of angle closure disease.

18.9 Gonioscopy and Using Artificial Intelligence

With the latest technological advancement, artificial intelligence is increasingly used for classifying medical images, often performing better than manual grading [16, 17]. It is used in aiding gonioscopic diagnosis of open-angle and angle closure glaucoma. Both these diagnoses are enabled by sequential and segmental SS-OCT scans, which are further analyzed by various deep learning (DL) models. The efficacy of these DL models is assessed by the area under curve (AUC) enclosed by the receiver operator characteristic curves, with a higher AUC indicating a more accurate model.

Many DL models have been used in assessing and further classifying angle closure disease. Earlier models used scans obtained on UBM [18], or a single AS-OCT [19] or SS-OCT [20] scan obtained over either meridian, where the vertical scans were more accurate than the horizontal scans for detecting angle closure. The latest advancements include the circumferential assessment of angle using SS-OCT scans obtained over 360° of the anterior chamber angle (Casia 2, Tomey Corporation, Japan). A recent study using a novel DL algorithm using circumferential SS-OCT scans has noted that the cut-off of ≥35° of circumferential iridotrabecular contact was the most accurate for diagnosing gonioscopic angle closure, with high sensitivity and specificity [21]. A lower cut-off value, although more sensitive, has extremely low specificity for diagnosing angle closure. Similarly, a higher cut-off has very low sensitivity for diagnosing angle closure, despite being extremely specific. Interestingly, the AUC noted in this study with a 35% cut-off was similar to the performance of a semiautomated built-in software called the "ITC index" [22]. Calculation of this ITC index depends on the manual marking of the scleral spur by the operator; hence, it is prone to inter-observer variability and aberrant results. On the other hand, DL models are entirely automated and do not require manual marking of the scleral spur, resulting in a faster and more accurate assessment of gonioscopic angle closure.

DL models also can classify different morphological patterns of juvenile open-angle glaucoma (JOAG) into various clusters. These clusters can be divided by the iris and gonioscopic features, age of onset, and baseline IOP. A recent study revealed that abnormal iris morphology and a high iris insertion correlate more closely with a higher IOP and worse visual prognosis [23]. Such a phenotypic classification of JOAG can help in the stratification of severity when screening such patients.

18.10 Conclusion

This chapter explored the optics and techniques of gonioscopy and highlighted its significance in evaluating and managing glaucoma. The technological advances discussed can assist manual gonioscopy for better diagnoses and management of glaucoma but cannot replace it. Hence, mastery of this technique is essential. Gonioscopy is an acquired art, and optimal utilization of the procedure requires considerable personal experience. However, awareness of the sources of error and the proper interpretation of the findings would result in a shorter learning phase.

Funding None.

Disclosure None.

References

1. Scheie HG. Width and pigmentation of the angle of the anterior chamber; a system of grading by gonioscopy. AMA Arch Ophthalmol. 1957;58(4):510–2.
2. Spaeth GL. The normal development of the human anterior chamber angle: a new system of descriptive grading. Trans Ophthalmol Soc U K. 1971;91:709–39.
3. Spaeth GL. Gonioscopy: uses old and new. The inheritance of occludable angles. Ophthalmology. 1978;85(3):222–32.
4. Spaeth GL, Azuara-Blanco A, Araujo SV, Augsburger JJ. Intraobserver and interobserver agreement in evaluating the anterior chamber angle configuration by ultrasound biomicroscopy. J Glaucoma. 1997;6(1):13–7.
5. Shaffer RN. Primary glaucomas Gonioscopy, ophthalmoscopy and perimetry. Trans Am Acad Ophthalmol Otolaryngol Am Acad Ophthalmol Otolaryngol. 1960;64:112–27.
6. Porporato N, Bell KC, Perera SA, Aung T. Non-optical coherence tomography modalities for assessment of angle closure. Taiwan J Ophthalmol. 2022;12(4):409–14.
7. Perera SA, Baskaran M, Friedman DS, Tun TA, Htoon HM, Kumar RS, et al. Use of EyeCam for imaging the anterior chamber angle. Invest Ophthalmol Vis Sci. 2010;51(6):2993–7.
8. Matsuo M, Mizoue S, Nitta K, Takai Y, et al. Intraobserver and interobserver agreement among anterior chamber angle evaluations using automated 360-degree gonio-photos. Huang J, editor. PLoS One. 2021;16(5):e0251249.
9. Teixeira F, Sousa DC, Leal I, Barata A, et al. Automated gonioscopy photography for iridocorneal angle grading. Eur J Ophthalmol. 2020;30(1):112–8.
10. Shinoj VK, Murukeshan VM, Baskaran M, Aung T. Integrated flexible handheld probe for imaging and evaluation of iridocorneal angle. J Biomed Opt. 2015;20(1):016014.
11. Perinchery SM, Shinde A, Fu CY, et al. High resolution iridocorneal angle imaging system by axicon lens assisted gonioscopy. Sci Rep. 2016;6:30844.
12. Hong XJJ, Suchand Sandeep CS, et al. Noninvasive and noncontact sequential imaging of the Iridocorneal angle and the cornea of the eye. Transl Vis Sci Technol. 2020;9(5):1.
13. Gupta B, Angmo D, Yadav S, et al. Quantification of Iridotrabecular contact in primary angle-closure disease. J Glaucoma. 2020;29(8):681–8.
14. Zhang X, Guo PY, Lin C, et al. Assessment of iris trabecular contact in eyes with Gonioscopic angle-closure. Ophthalmology. 2023;130(1):111–9.
15. Xu BY, Friedman DS, Foster PJ, et al. Ocular biometric risk factors for progression of primary angle closure disease: the Zhongshan angle closure prevention trial. Ophthalmology. 2022;129(3):267–75.
16. Carin L, Pencina MJ. On deep learning for medical image analysis. JAMA. 2018;320(11):1192–3.
17. Grzybowski A, Brona P, Lim G, et al. Artificial intelligence for diabetic retinopathy screening: a review. Eye Lond Engl. 2020;34(3):451–60.
18. Shi G, Jiang Z, Deng G, et al. Automatic classification of anterior chamber angle using ultrasound biomicroscopy and deep learning. Transl Vis Sci Technol. 2019;8(4):25.
19. Fu H, Baskaran M, Xu Y, et al. A deep learning system for automated angle-closure detection in anterior segment optical coherence tomography images. Am J Ophthalmol. 2019;203:37–45.
20. Xu BY, Chiang M, Chaudhary S, et al. Deep learning classifiers for automated detection of Gonioscopic angle closure based on anterior segment OCT images. Am J Ophthalmol. 2019;208:273–80.

21. Porporato N, Tun TA, Baskaran M, et al. Towards "automated gonioscopy": a deep learning algorithm for 360° angle assessment by swept-source optical coherence tomography. Br J Ophthalmol. 2022;106(10):1387–92.
22. Baskaran M, Ho SW, Tun TA, et al. Assessment of circumferential angle-closure by the iris–trabecular contact index with swept-source optical coherence tomography. Ophthalmology. 2013;120(11):2226–31.
23. Birla S, Gupta D, Somarajan BI, et al. Classifying juvenile onset primary open angle glaucoma using cluster analysis. Br J Ophthalmol. 2020;104(6):827–35.

Optic Disc Photography

19

K. Gowri Pratinya, Aparna Rao, Pallavi Ray, and Bhoomi Thakkar

19.1 Introduction

Ophthalmic disc photography is a valuable tool in glaucoma care. It allows precise documentation and analysis of the optic disc, which is crucial for glaucoma evaluation. The history parallels the evolution of imaging technology and contributed significantly to diagnosing and managing glaucoma and several other ocular conditions. Using specialized software installed in the cameras, it provides accurate optic disc images for objective quantification and characterization of the disc for enhanced patient care. This chapter explores the historical developments, equipment, techniques, image interpretation, clinical applications, and future directions of optic disc photography.

19.2 History of Ophthalmic Photography

The history of ophthalmic photography dates back to the mid-nineteenth century when Jackman and Webster published the first retinal image of a living human subject [1]. The optic disc was faintly visible due to strong reflexes from the cornea. It was not until the twentieth century that fundus photography became an established technique for optic disc imaging [2]. In 1911, a large reflex-free ophthalmoscope invented by Alvar Gullstrand viewed the fundus through the upper pupil reducing unwanted reflexes from the cornea [3]. the Zeiss-Nordenson camera was designed and introduced in 1925 using this principle [4]. These cameras allowed for more accurate and standardized optic disc measurements. The advent of digital imaging in the 1990s enabled good-quality optic disc photography.

19.3 Optic Nerve Photography

Optic disc photography has become an important part of glaucoma screening for objective and quantitative measurements enabling early detection and management. It also plays a vital role in telemedicine.

19.3.1 Monoscopic Color Fundus Photography

Monoscopic color fundus photography is a widely used technique for capturing detailed retina and optic disc images. Monoscopic photography pro-

K. G. Pratinya · A. Rao (✉)
Kallam Anji Reddy Campus, L V Prasad Eye Institute, Hyderabad, India
e-mail: kolipaka.pratinya@lvpei.org; aparna@lvpei.org

P. Ray · B. Thakkar
Mithu Tulsi Chanrai Campus, L V Prasad Eye Institute, Bhubaneswar, India
e-mail: pallavi.ray@lvpei.org; bhoomi.Thakkar@lvpei.org

T. Das, P. Satgunam (eds.), *Ophthalmic Diagnostics*, https://doi.org/10.1007/978-981-97-0138-4_19

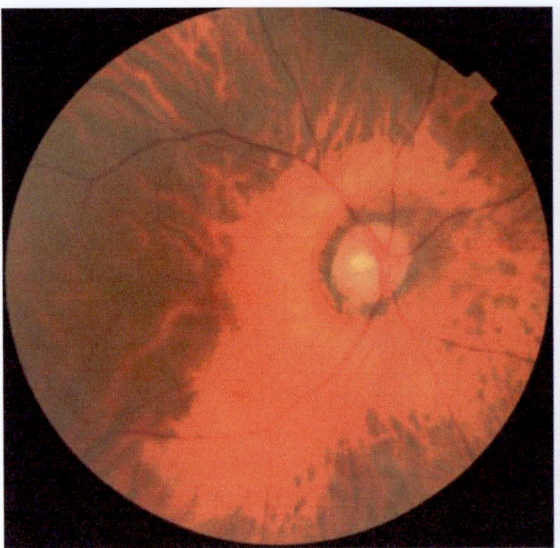

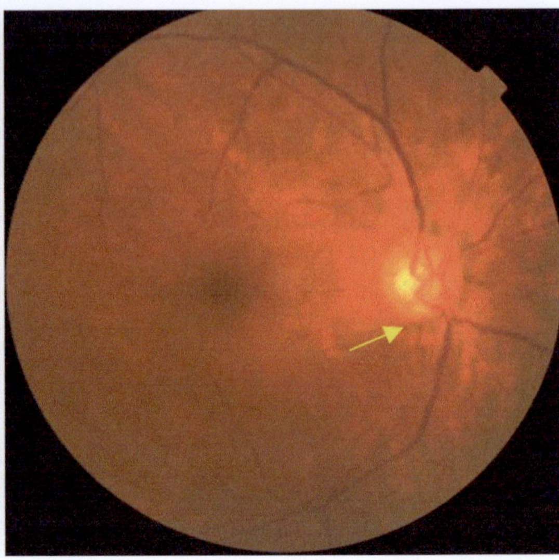

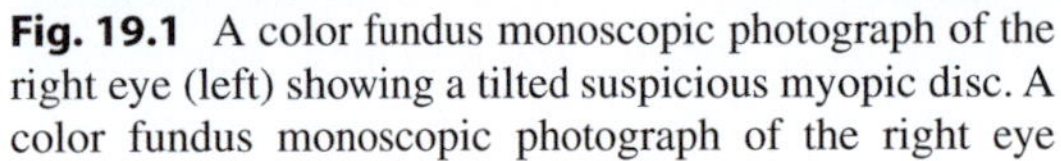

Fig. 19.1 A color fundus monoscopic photograph of the right eye (left) showing a tilted suspicious myopic disc. A color fundus monoscopic photograph of the right eye (right) showing a glaucomatous disc with inferior excavation and inferior nerve fiber layer thinning (yellow arrow)

duces a two-dimensional optic disc image by employing a single-lens camera system. This technique provides quick images for reference, but due to the inability of the technique to capture the three-dimensional structure of the optic disc, at times, assessing the depth and contour of the optic nerve head is often challenging. This is more acutely observed in myopic disc assessment, where the cupping can be very shallow (Fig. 19.1).

19.3.2 Red-Free Photography

Red-free photography, also known as green or blue filter photography, is an imaging technique to visualize the retinal nerve fiber layer (RNFL). It captures images of the optic disc and retina with a specific filter that blocks red light, allowing only green or blue light to pass. In red-free photography, the RNFL appears as a darker shade against the background of the retinal layers. Since the RNFL contains melanin, a pigment that absorbs green and blue light more than red light, eliminating red light (which is predominantly absorbed by the other retinal layers) can selectively accentuate the RNFL, making it easier to detect defects; this is red-free photography.

Clinical application: Red-free photography reduces the visibility of the blood vessels by minimizing their background contrast, allowing the identification of the RNFL (Fig. 19.2).

19.3.3 Stereoscopic Images

Stereoscopic images of the optic disc are obtained by taking two images of the optic disc from slightly different angles, mimicking the binocular vision that our eyes naturally provide. In the stereoscopic camera system, either two camera lenses or two separate cameras are positioned slightly apart horizontally. This simultaneous capture of the optic disc from slightly different angles creates the necessary parallax and enables the brain to perceive the depth. Once the two images are captured, they can be viewed together using a stereoscope or a specialized device that allows the observer to merge the two images into a single, three-dimensional perception (Fig. 19.3). The stereoscope typically contains lenses that direct each image to the corresponding eye, allowing the brain to fuse the images and perceive the three-dimensional structure of the optic disc.

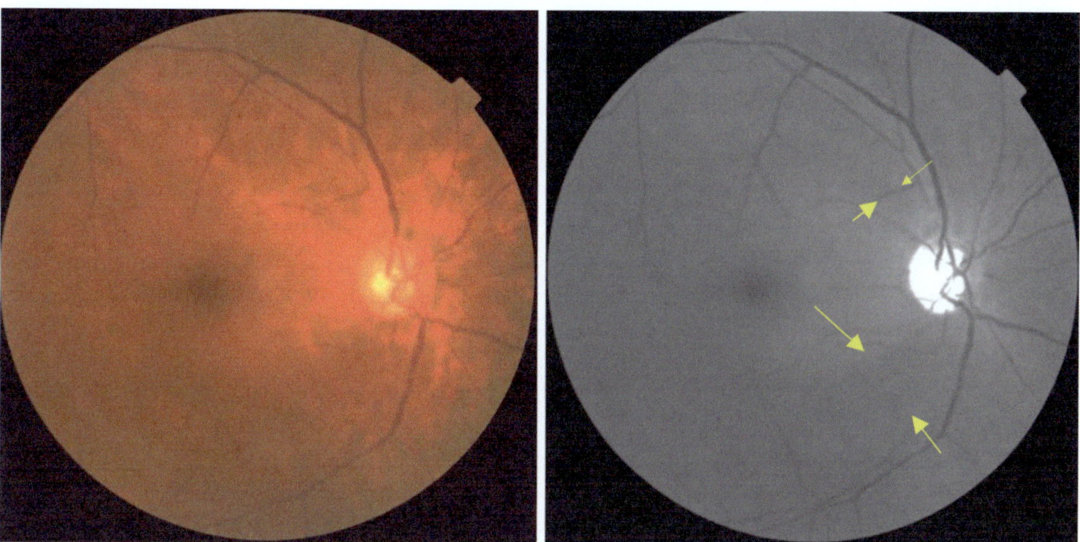

Fig. 19.2 Color fundus (left) and red-free (right) monoscopic photographs of the right eye with inferior and superior retinal nerve fiber layer defects; the defects are more clearly visible in the red-free photographs (yellow arrows)

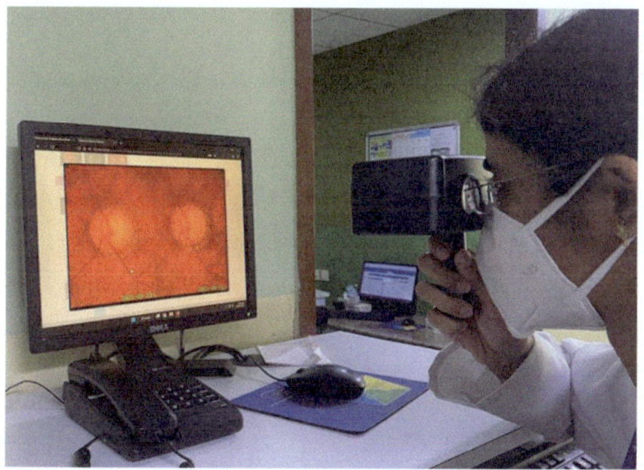

Fig. 19.3 Examining the stereoscopic optic disc photographs with a stereoscope

Clinical application: With these stereoscopic images, clinicians gain a better understanding of features of cup-to-disc ratio, neuroretinal rim abnormalities, and other structural changes for better diagnosis and management of glaucoma. However, stereoscopic optic disc imaging may provide higher estimates of the cup-disc ratio and lower estimates of the neuroretinal rim area [5].

Morgan et al. [6] compared monoscopic and stereoscopic images of the optic disc using software for the digital stereoscopic analysis of optic disc stereo pairs and found that digital stereoscopic optic disc assessment provides higher levels of interobserver agreement than monoscopic assessments. Parkin et al. [7] and Varma et al. [5] have evaluated the intraobserver and interobserver agreement for evaluating the optic disc for glaucoma under monoscopic and stereoscopic conditions; the agreement was similar under both conditions, Yang et al. [8] have reported better performance with stereoscopic images among general ophthalmologists.

19.4 Retinal Camera for Optic Disc Photography

19.4.1 Non-mydriatic Fundus Cameras

Non-mydriatic fundus cameras are designed to capture high-resolution images of the fundus, including the optic disc, without pupil dilation. They combine optical elements to capture clear and detailed images of the fundus. These optical components typically include lenses, mirrors, and filters. The lenses focus the light onto the retina, and the mirrors are used to direct the light to form the image. Filters enhance contrast and selectively capture specific wavelengths of light. Non-mydriatic fundus cameras employ pupil detection and alignment systems to ensure accurate and centered imaging. Infrared light is commonly used as it causes less discomfort for the patient and allows better visualization of fundus structures. The camera's software then adjusts the focus and alignment to capture the desired region, typically the optic disc, with high precision and clarity. By eliminating the need for pupil dilatation, these cameras provide a more convenient and patient-friendly approach to fundus imaging without compromising the quality of the image [9].

19.4.2 Handheld Fundus Cameras

Handheld fundus cameras are portable and compact imaging devices used to capture an image of the optic disc and retina. These are lightweight, compact, and portable, allowing effortless maneuverability and use in various clinical settings. They typically consist of a camera unit, an imaging module, a light source, a display screen, and controls for image capture and adjustment. Handheld fundus cameras offer various methods for image capture. They may have a built-in camera module or use attachments that can be connected to smartphones or other mobile devices. Some cameras feature a live-view display that shows real-time images as the operator aligns the camera with the patient's eye. Images can be captured with a hand-operated button or by activating a foot pedal. The image quality may be variable due to operator variability. Additionally, the field of view may be narrower than larger cameras, requiring multiple images to obtain an image of the entire fundus. However, they address the growing demand for retinal imaging in different clinical scenarios like those for screening children, school screenings, and screening of bed-ridden patients [10]. Integrating smartphone technology and miniature tabletop versions make these cameras increasingly portable, convenient, and accessible (Fig. 19.4).

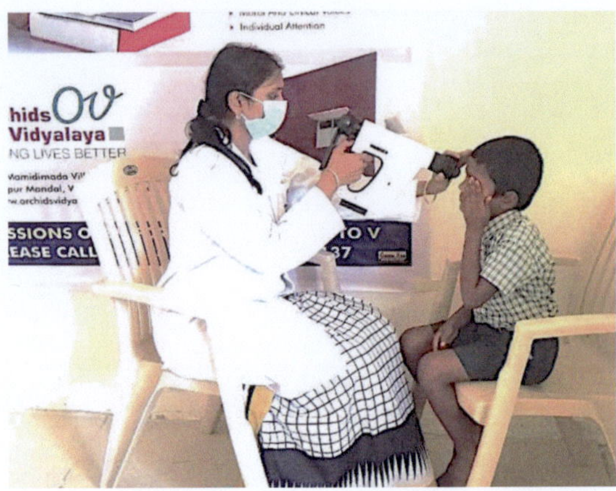

Fig. 19.4 Fundus photography in a school screening using a handheld non-mydriatic smartphone-integrated fundus camera (Remidio, Bangalore, India)

19.5 Technology Assessment

Bak et al. [11] compared the RNFL defect measurements obtained from red-free fundus photography and optical coherence tomography (OCT) en face imaging vis-à-vis the functional outcomes in terms of mean and pattern standard deviation. They reported that the en face RNFL defect showed a higher correlation with the severity of visual field loss than the red-free RNFL defect. Watanabe et al. [12] evaluated the accuracy of glaucoma screening using fundus photography combined with OCT. They found that the diagnostic accuracy of glaucoma screening significantly increased when the OCT was added to the fundus imaging.

19.6 Deep Learning-Based Enhanced Optic Disc Photography

This refers to the applications of artificial intelligence (AI) techniques, specifically deep learning algorithms, to improve the quality and interpretation of optic disc photographs. These

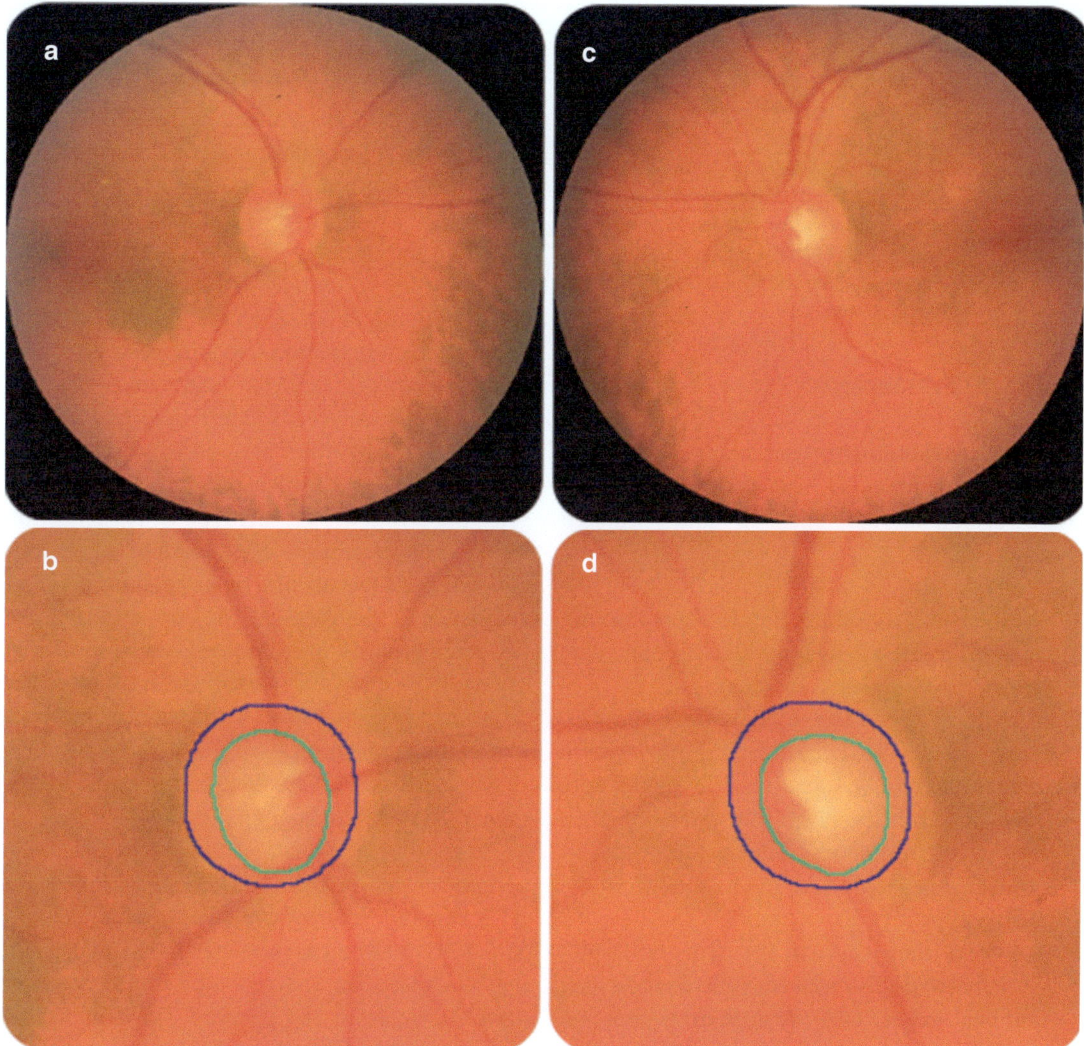

Fig. 19.5 Color fundus photograph and artificial intelligence showing the segmentation of the optic disc boundary of the right eye (**a** and **b**) and the left eye (**c** and **d**) (original photograph)

algorithms are trained on large datasets of annotated images to learn patterns and features that aid in image enhancement, segmentation, and analysis. These algorithms can extract features from images and perform complex tasks, such as enhancing image quality, sharpness, contrast, and clarity without relying on explicit instructions, and identify and correct common image artifacts, such as noise, blurriness, and uneven illumination. These can be trained to automatically segment the optic disc region and accurately delineate the borders, enabling precise measurements (Fig. 19.5).

Over the years, optic disc image analysis has witnessed significant advancements (Table 19.1), beginning with early studies in the early 2000s involving regression analysis and machine learning techniques. Subsequent developments focused on applying AI frameworks for optic disc segmentation, enabling accurate estimation of parameters such as vertical cup-to-disc ratio (VCDR) and RNFL analysis. More recently, deep learning algorithms have been employed for automated abnormality detection, enabling the identification of glaucoma-related features and providing valuable insights for clinical decision-making.

Table 19.1 Showing the evolution of the deep learning-based optic disc image analysis

Study	Method
Sihota et al. [20]	Moorfields regression analysis
Almazrao et al. [21]	Deep learning-based segmentation algorithms
Park et al. [22]	Deep learning-based vCDR estimation
Lee et al. [23]	Deep learning-based RNFL analysis

19.6.1 AI Framework

There are two commonly used approaches in the AI framework for optic disc analysis and glaucoma detection: the one-step and two-step frameworks.

1. One-step framework: A single deep learning model is trained to directly classify optic disc images as normal or glaucomatous in the one-step framework. The model takes the raw input images and performs both feature extraction and classification in a single step. This approach leverages the ability of deep learning algorithms to automatically learn relevant features and make predictions from the raw data.
2. Two-step framework: In the two-step framework, the optic disc analysis process is divided into two distinct steps: feature extraction and classification.

   Step 1: Feature extraction:

   - Deep learning models extract features from the optic disc images, such as optic disc cupping, rim thickness, vessel characteristics, or other relevant parameters associated with glaucoma.
   - The feature extraction step aims to capture informative representations of the optic disc that can be used for subsequent classification.

   Step 2: Classification:

   - The extracted features are fed into a separate classification algorithm or model, such as a support vector machine (SVM) or random forest classifier, to perform the final classification task.
   - The classifier uses the extracted features as input and determines whether the optic disc is normal or shows signs of glaucoma.

While the one-step framework simplifies the workflow by combining feature extraction and classification into a single model, reducing complexity and computational requirements, the two-step framework allows extracting specific features relevant to glaucoma detection. These features can be further analyzed and interpreted by clinicians, and it also provides flexibility in selecting different classifiers for the classification step; it thus enables the use of various algorithms depending on the specific requirements and characteristics of the dataset. The superiority of the two-step process over the one-step process in optic disc analysis for glaucoma detection depends on various factors and the specific context of the application [13].

Various studies were done to assess the agreement of AI with manual grading [14–19].

For example, Shroff et al. [14] studied the agreement of vCDR measured by an offline AI-integrated smartphone fundus camera with SD-OCT vCDR measurements and manual grading by experts on a stereoscopic fundus camera on 473 eyes from 244 patients. They found that the offline AI had an excellent agreement and correlation with the SD-OCT and manual grading. MacCormik et al. [18] studied a glaucoma detection algorithm that segments and analyzes color photographs to quantify optic nerve rim consistency around the entire disc at 15-degree intervals. They found that it accurately distinguished glaucomatous and healthy discs on internal and external validation with an area under the ROC of 99.6% and 91.0%, respectively.

Deep learning algorithms can assist in glaucoma screening and diagnosis by analyzing optic disc photographs. By analyzing the enhanced images and comparing them with a vast database of reference images, the system can highlight potential abnormalities, suggest follow-up tests, or provide risk stratification for glaucoma [13].

Future directions: Ongoing research and development in AI and deep learning continue to advance the field of enhanced optic disc photography. Efforts are being made to incorporate multimodal imaging data, such as combining optic disc photographs with OCT or visual field data, to improve diagnostic accuracy further. Additionally, integrating AI algorithms into portable and handheld imaging devices opens up the possibilities for point-of-care screening and remote monitoring [14].

19.7 Conclusion

Optic disc photography has played a pivotal role in the screening and diagnosing glaucoma, contributing to the early detection and management of this sight-threatening disease. Technological advancements have revolutionized optic disc image analysis from its historical roots in the early twentieth century to the modern era. AI-powered frameworks have emerged as transformative tools for automated segmentation and abnormality detection. These developments have enabled large-scale, low-cost screening, and extended eye care services to remote areas lacking access to qualified ophthalmologists. As research in this field continues, we anticipate further innovations that will enhance the accuracy and accessibility of glaucoma screening and management, offering a brighter outlook for patients worldwide.

Funding Hyderabad Eye Research Foundation.

Disclosure Nil.

References

1. Panwar N, Huang P, Lee J, et al. Fundus photography in the 21st century—a review of recent technological advances and their implications for worldwide healthcare. Telemed J E Health. 2016;22(3):198–208.
2. Yannuzzi LA. The retinal atlas. Elsevier Health Sciences; 2010. p. 929.
3. Keeler R, Singh AD, Dua HS. Reflecting on reflections: Gullstrand's large reflex-free ophthalmoscope. Br J Ophthalmol. 2010;94(7):826–6.
4. Myers J, Fudemberg S, Lee D. Evolution of optic nerve photography for glaucoma screening: a review: evolution of disc photos for screening. Clin Experiment Ophthalmol. 2018;46(2):169–76.
5. Varma R, Steinmann WC, Scott IU. Expert agreement in evaluating the optic disc for glaucoma. Ophthalmology. 1992;99(2):215–21.
6. Morgan JE, Sheen NJL, North RV, et al. Digital imaging of the optic nerve head: monoscopic and stereoscopic analysis. Br J Ophthalmol. 2005;89(7):879–84.
7. Parkin B, Shuttleworth G, Costen M, Davison C. A comparison of stereoscopic and monoscopic evaluation of optic disc topography using a digital optic disc stereo camera. Br J Ophthalmol. 2001;85(11):1347–51.
8. Yang J, Qu Y, Zhao J, et al. Stereoscopic vs. monoscopic photographs on optic disc evaluation and glaucoma diagnosis among general ophthalmologists: a cloud-based real-world multicenter study. Front Med (Lausanne). 2022;9:990611.
9. Varshney T, Parthasarathy DR, Gupta V. Artificial intelligence integrated smartphone fundus camera for screening the glaucomatous optic disc. Indian J Ophthalmol. 2021;69(12):3787–9.
10. Das S, Kuht HJ, De Silva I, et al. Feasibility and clinical utility of handheld fundus cameras for retinal imaging. Eye (Lond). 2023;37(2):274–9.
11. Bak E, Choi HJ. Structure-function relationship in glaucoma: optical coherence tomography en face imaging vs. red-free fundus photography. Eye (Lond). 2023;37(14):2969–76.
12. Watanabe T, Hiratsuka Y, Kita Y, et al. Combining optical coherence tomography and fundus photography to improve glaucoma screening. Diagnostics (Basel). 2022;12(5):1100.
13. Coan L, Williams B, Venkatesh KA, et al. Automatic detection of glaucoma via fundus imaging and artificial intelligence: a review. Surv Ophthalmol. 2023;68(1):17–41.
14. Shroff S, Rao DP, Savoy FM, et al. Agreement of a novel artificial intelligence software with optical coherence tomography and manual grading of the optic disc in glaucoma. J Glaucoma. 2023;32(4):280–6.
15. Yousefi S. Clinical applications of artificial intelligence in glaucoma. J Ophthalmic Vis Res. 2023;18(1):97–112.
16. Mvoulana A, Kachouri R, Akil M. Fully automated method for glaucoma screening using robust optic nerve head detection and unsupervised segmentation based cup-to-disc ratio computation in retinal fundus images. Comput Med Imaging Graph. 2019;77:101643.
17. Bajwa MN, Malik MI, Siddiqui SA, et al. Two-stage framework for optic disc localization and glaucoma classification in retinal fundus images using deep learning. BMC Med Inform Decis Mak. 2019;19(1):136.
18. MacCormick IJC, Williams BM, Zheng Y, et al. Accurate, fast, data efficient and interpretable glaucoma diagnosis with automated spatial analy-

sis of the whole cup to disc profile. PLoS One. 2019;14(1):e0209409.

19. Zhao R, Chen X, Liu X, et al. Direct cup-to-disc ratio estimation for glaucoma screening via semi-supervised learning. IEEE J Biomed Health Inform. 2020;24(4):1104–13.
20. Sihota R, Gulati V, Agarwal HC, et al. Variables affecting test-retest variability of Heidelberg retina Tomograph II stereometric parameters. J Glaucoma. 2002;11(4):321–8.
21. Almazroa A, Burman R, Raahemifar K, Lakshminarayanan V. Optic disc and optic cup segmentation methodologies for glaucoma image detection: a survey. J Ophthalmol. 2015;2015:180972.
22. Park K, Kim J, Lee J. Automatic optic nerve head localization and cup-to-disc ratio detection using state-of-the-art deep-learning architectures. Sci Rep. 2020;10(1):5025.
23. Lee T, Jammal AA, Mariottoni EB, Medeiros FA. Predicting glaucoma development with longitudinal deep learning predictions from fundus photographs. Am J Ophthalmol. 2021;225:86–94.

20 OCT in Glaucoma

K. Gowri Pratinya, Aparna Rao, Pallavi Ray, and Bhoomi Thakkar

20.1 Introduction

Glaucoma is a chronic progressive optic neuropathy characterized by optic nerve head changes due to the progressive loss of retinal ganglion cells. Diagnosing this structural damage early is crucial in managing glaucoma. Though it can be clinically assessed by optic nerve head (ONH) and peripapillary retinal nerve fiber layer (RNFL) examinations, the introduction of optical coherence tomography (OCT) has allowed for supplemental objective and quantitative evaluation of ONH and RNFL changes. OCT is a noninvasive, noncontact technique that uses the differences in the optical properties of tissue structures to create an "optical biopsy" thereby providing high-resolution and cross-sectional imaging of the ONH, RNFL, and macula [1].

20.2 Technology

Optical coherence tomography is based on the principle of the Michelson low-coherence interferometry. This imaging technique directs waves to the tissue under examination, where the waves echo off the tissue structure. The reflected waves are analyzed, and their delay is measured to document the depth at which the reflection occurred. OCT uses light in the near infrared. The delay of the reflected waves cannot be measured directly, so a reference measurement is used. In an interferometer, part of the light is directed to the sample, and another portion is sent to a reference arm with a well-known length. These techniques were adapted into time domain (TD) OCT and evolved into Fourier domain-OCTs.

20.2.1 Time-Domain OCT

The first commercial TD-OCT was OCT 1 by Carl Zeiss Meditec (Dublin, CA, USA) [2]. The light of a low-coherence source is guided to the interferometer. The input beam is split into the sample and reference beams by a beam splitter. The reference beam travels to a mirror on a translational stage and is reflected back. The light reflected from the eye is compared with that reflected from the reference mirror using a low-coherence interferometry system. The reference mirror is moved mechanically from the beam splitter to estimate the depth of the reflection within the tissue. Multiple axial scans are created to construct B-scans. Final 2D or 3D images are created by computer systems in the OCT devices either in grayscale or false colors.

K. G. Pratinya · A. Rao (✉)
Kallam Anji Reddy Campus, L V Prasad Eye Institute, Hyderabad, India
e-mail: kolipaka.pratinya@lvpei.org; aparna@lvpei.org

P. Ray · B. Thakkar
Mithu Tulsi Chanrai Campus, L V Prasad Eye Institute, Bhubaneswar, India
e-mail: pallavi.ray@lvpei.org; bhoomi.Thakkar@lvpei.org

T. Das, P. Satgunam (eds.), *Ophthalmic Diagnostics*, https://doi.org/10.1007/978-981-97-0138-4_20

20.2.2 Spectral-Domain OCT

Spectral-domain (SD) OCT techniques use Fourier domain transformation [3]. Fourier transformation helps transform the signals between two different domains, from the time- or spatial domain to the frequency domain [4]. Using the Fourier transformation, the technology from the original method of TD-OCT, the SD-OCT, was developed. While the TD-OCT encoded the location of each reflection in the time information relating the position of a moving reference mirror to the location of the reflection, SD-OCT, instead, acquires all data in a single axial scan through the tissue simultaneously by evaluating the frequency spectrum of the interference between the reflected light and a stationary reference mirror. Zeiss Cirrus HD-OCT (Carl Zeiss Meditec, Dublin, CA, USA), Heidelberg Engineering Spectralis OCT (Heidelberg Engineering, Heidelberg, Germany) Optovue RTVue (Optovue Inc., Fremont, CA, USA), and Topcon 3D OCT 2000 (Topcon Medical Systems, Oakland, NJ) use the SD-OCT system.

Advantages of SD-OCT over TD-OCT:

- It uses a fixed reference mirror, which acquires 18,000–70,000 A-scans/s compared to the 400 A-scans/s TD-OCT acquires. Hence, SD-OCT systems are 200–400 times faster than TD-OCT systems.
- Increased scanning speed results in a higher axial resolution (around 5 μm).
- Due to increased scanning speed, the artifacts caused by eye movements are reduced.

20.2.3 Swept-Source OCT

Swept-source OCT is based on the Fourier domain principles. It combines the advantages of TD-OCT and SD-OCT. The light source used in SS-OCT is of a narrow bandwidth, which changes and sweeps the wavelength across a narrow band in time. The variation in frequency with time encodes different echo delay times in the light beams [5]. The light source in the SS-OCT is divided into a spectrum using a swept-source laser; therefore, unlike SD-OCT, a spectrometer is not required. In SS-OCT, high-speed detectors detect interference signals in time and measure echo delays using Fourier transformation [6].

20.3 Clinical Utility of OCT in Glaucoma

The use of SD-OCT for glaucoma diagnosis is an increasingly common practice. While progressive neuro-retinal rim changes such as thinning and excavation are more specific for glaucoma, the RNFL changes are more sensitive for detecting glaucoma. OCT plays a key role in detecting early glaucoma not detected by the perimetric examination.

20.3.1 Glaucoma Diagnosis

Standard automated perimetry is widely used for the diagnosis, staging, and monitoring of glaucoma, but it is only likely to detect functional deficits after at least 20–40% of retinal ganglion cells (RGCs) are lost [7, 8]. Additionally, visual field testing requires patient cooperation and understanding and is often variable [9]. Picking up the early glaucomatous structural damage, such as thinning of the RNFL and inner retinal layers, is fundamental for early diagnosis and prevention of vision loss.

The diagnostic capabilities of SD-OCT depend on the severity/stage of glaucoma; it performs better when discriminating healthy from advanced disease rather than early stages of glaucoma [10].

Taking multiple parameters into account, such as peripapillary RNFL, ONH, and macular parameters, OCT is useful for diagnosing early glaucoma (Fig. 20.1a–c), staging the severity of glaucoma, and evaluating risk in glaucoma suspects [11]. Although using multiple parameters could increase false-positive results, structural damage may be present in one parameter and not the other, and thus it is helpful to have information from the macula, ONH, and RNFL in glaucoma diagnosis [10].

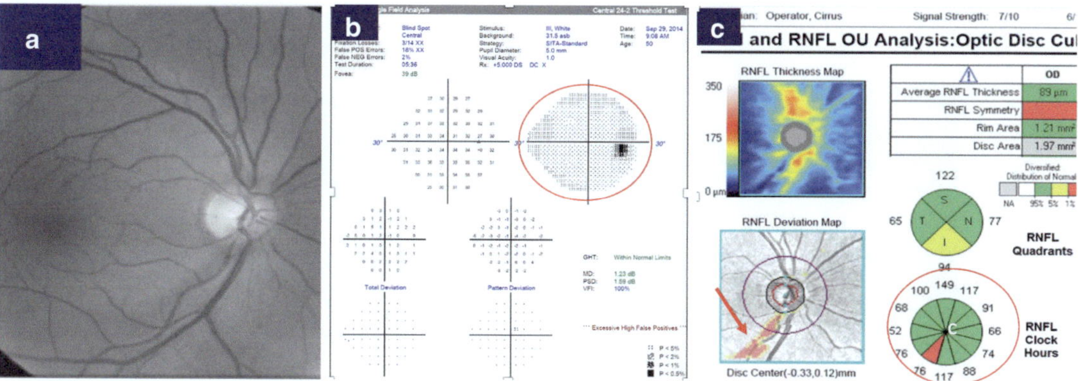

Fig. 20.1 (**a**) Red-free fundus photograph of the RE showing a disc indicative of glaucoma with inferior nerve fiber layer defect. (**b**) Humphrey visual field print out of the same eye showing a normal field. (**c**) OCT (ONH and RNFL analysis) showing inferior RNFL thinning on deviation and clock hour map (red arrow and red circle)

20.3.2 Glaucoma Progression

To assess the progression of glaucoma with the RNFL thickness obtained by OCT, we need to be aware of a few factors: (a) thinning due to normal aging; (b) the floor effect of this parameter; (c) thinning suggestive of glaucoma progression, both globally and within a sector; and (d) correlation of RNFL loss with visual field loss.

The RNFL undergoes attrition with age in healthy eyes at a mean rate of −0.48 μm/year in Cirrus and −0.60 μm/year in Spectralis images. Glaucoma progression, on the other hand, has a faster rate of RNFL thinning, ranging from −0.98 μm/year for the Cirrus to −2.12 μm/year for the Spectralis images. RNFL measurement continues to decrease as glaucoma advances, but does not go to zero, a phenomenon known as the "floor effect." This is because the architectural support of the Müller cells, astroglia, microglia, and blood vessels do not allow the structure of the RNFL to degenerate completely with the retinal ganglion cell axons. Average RNFL floor values range from 49.2 μm for the Spectralis to 57 μm for the Cirrus to 64.7 μm for the RTVue images. Once the RNFL thickness reaches the floor, progression can still occur but cannot be detected by OCT. Therefore, the clinician should consider using macular OCT and the Humphry Visual Field (HVF, Carl Zeiss, Dublin, CA, USA) to monitor the progression of advanced glaucoma.

Each OCT device provides progression analysis, which can be event- or trend-based. The event-based analysis measures the difference between baseline and follow-up measurements. A decrease of >5 μm in average RNFL thickness indicates glaucoma progression, while a decrease of 7–8 μm or more in a sector also suggests progression. The trend-based analysis identifies progression by monitoring the slope of RNFL thickness over time. Cirrus provides a glaucoma progression algorithm based on events and trend, comparing the RNFL thickness of individual pixels between baseline and follow-up images. Pixels are coded yellow if there is test–retest variability between a follow-up and baseline image, while red indicates the same change on three consecutive scans. In Spectralis, the system looks for specific patterns in retinal structures to position the retest scan in the same location automatically; RNFL thickness change and trend reports are plotted over time to compare the rate of change. The RTVue system offers a trend-based analysis, which includes side-by-side comparisons of global RNFL thicknesses, six sectorial thickness analyses, and a regression line to determine the slope and standard error. Although progression analysis software can be a great tool, especially in a busy clinic, one should always review the original scans and the sectors, as subtle changes in a small area can be easily missed.

Although SD-OCT has significantly increased signal-to-noise ratio and decreased motion artifacts than TD-OCT, both are prone to image artifacts. These artifacts include speckle noise, segmentation errors (Fig. 20.2a, b), alignment errors, low signal quality, software problems, and

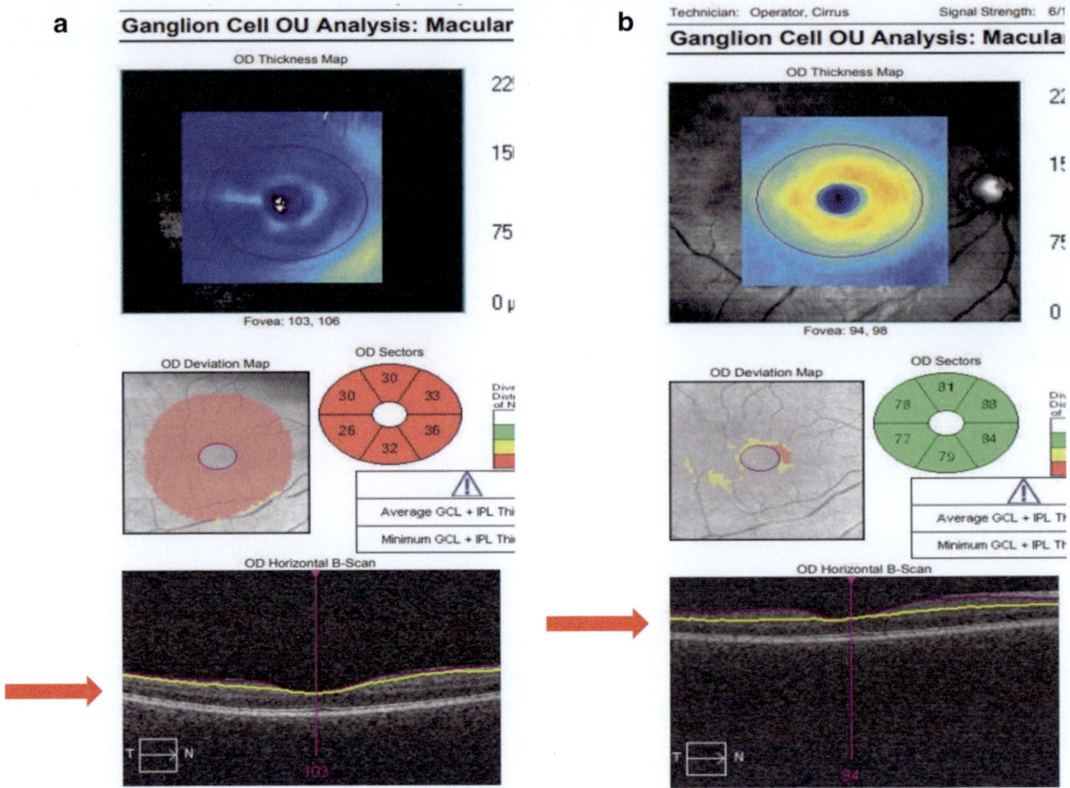

Fig. 20.2 (**a**) Ganglion cell analysis showing false thinning over the macular region due to improper segmentation (red arrow). (**b**) Repeat OCT of the same patient with proper segmentation (red arrow) and normal macular thickness

media opacities, such as reduced corneal clarity or cataracts. Fixational eye movements, such as ocular tremors, drift, and microsaccades, can further reduce image quality.

While SD-OCT devices still require a trained imaging technician to minimize artifacts, it is comparatively less operator dependent than TD-OCT devices. Clinicians should be cautious in interpreting these OCT findings and avoid overtreating people with false-positive results.

20.4 New Advances in Glaucoma OCT

20.4.1 Adaptive Optics in OCT

As mentioned earlier, the diagnostic capacity of OCT is dependent on the severity of glaucoma. The OCT is more effective in discriminating healthy from moderate and advanced diseases than early glaucoma. In addition, wide anatomic variations of the optic nerve head, several sources of error, and the database having a limited number of subjects of any single ethnicity limit the diagnostic performance of OCT in detecting glaucoma [12]. Adaptive optics (AO) could fill this gap in retinal imaging for the early diagnosis of glaucoma by compensating for ocular aberrations. It has been combined with a fundus camera, scanning laser ophthalmoscope, and OCT to help with a better understanding of the disease process (Fig. 20.3). The OCT system has an excellent axial resolution, and with the addition of AO, its lateral resolution improves dramatically [13]. The AO-OCT system has the best spot size (in terms of axial and lateral resolution) among all the other AO systems.

AO-OCT can be used in the following ways:

1. To quantify morphological changes in the photoreceptor cells in the abnormal areas of the cone-mosaic.

2. To detect optic nerve head changes and abnormalities for monitoring glaucoma progression.
3. Imaging subtle changes in the RNFL at the preclinical stage and visualization of the individual RNFL bundles in vivo could help detect and monitor glaucoma progression early.

Adaptive optics is an evolving technology; it is not without limitations. Its greatest limitation is the narrow field of imaging; only 0.225 mm is covered in a single image [14]. The technology is adversely affected by media opacity, dry eye, poor pupillary dilatation, and high refractive error. The focal plane of reference needs adjustment each time to obtain images at a particular depth. In addition, ocular motion artifacts can affect the quality of images. The technology demands expertise, and acquiring images can be time-consuming.

20.4.2 Enhanced Depth Imaging and Artificial Intelligence Application in OCT Glaucoma

Enhanced depth imaging (EDI) is used in OCT imaging to enhance the visualization of the deeper structures within the eye, particularly the optic nerve head and the lamina cribrosa [15–18]. EDI-OCT imaging allows for a more detailed and accurate assessment of the optic nerve head and the lamina cribrosa, both critical structures in the development and progression of glaucoma (Fig. 20.4). EDI-OCT imaging has proven to be a valuable tool in the early detection and monitoring of glaucoma and is increasingly used in clinical practice.

20.4.2.1 Principle

The principle behind EDI-OCT imaging is similar to that of traditional OCT imaging. However, EDI-OCT uses a specialized technique to enhance

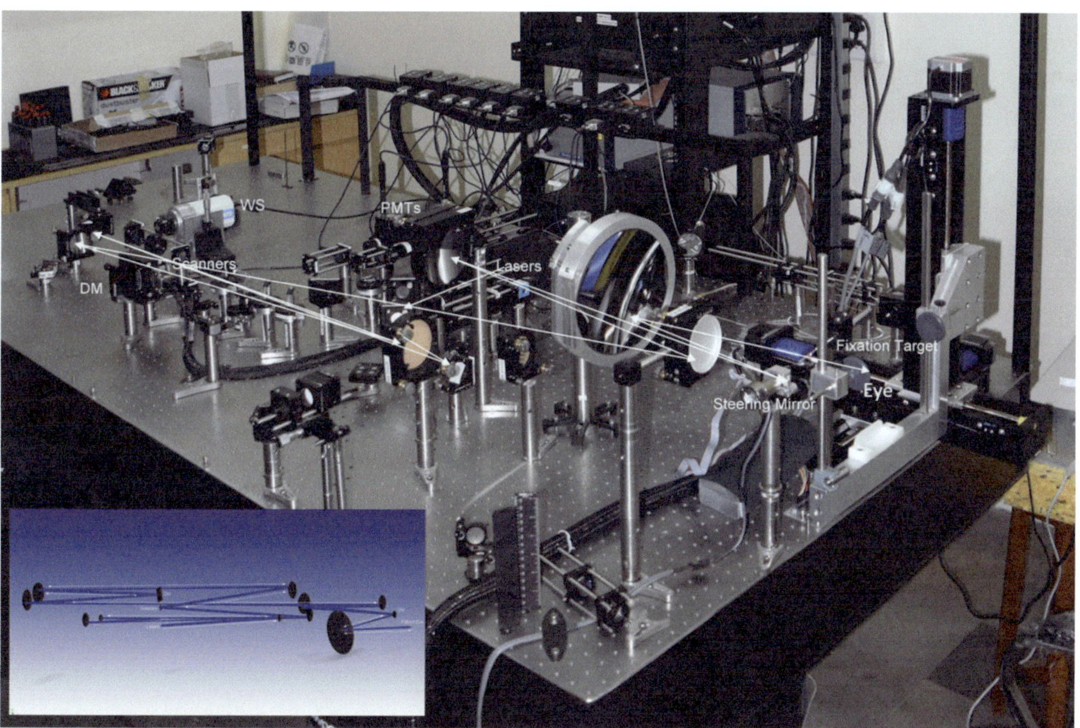

Fig. 20.3 Adaptive optics (prototype) setup at L V Prasad eye institute, Hyderabad, India

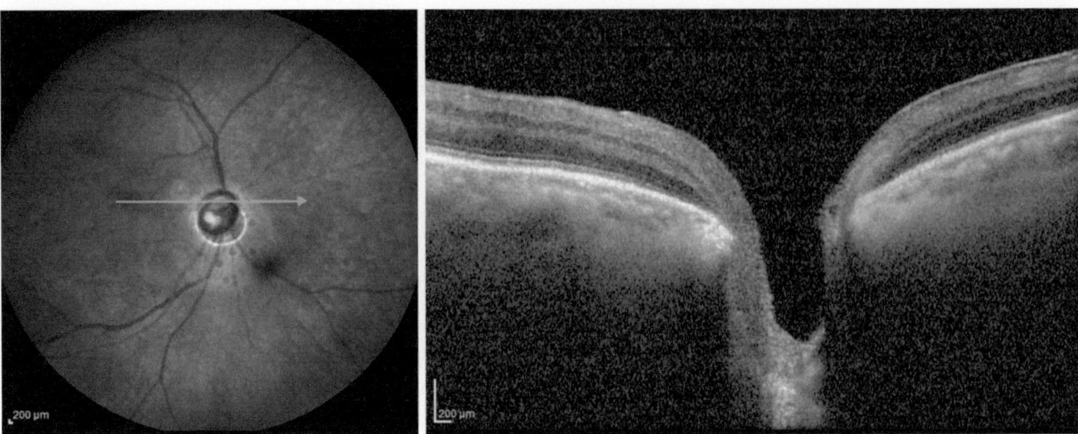

Fig. 20.4 An EDI Spectralis image through the optic disc showing segmentation of various retinal layers (original photograph)

the depth resolution of the image, allowing for better visualization of deeper structures. In EDI-OCT, the light source used to produce the image is positioned closer to the eye, bringing the deeper portion so the eye is closer to the zero-delay line of the highest sensitivity. This enables greater penetration of the light into the tissues. This results in a sharper and more detailed image of the deeper structures, such as the optic nerve head and the lamina cribrosa.

In contrast, high-penetration OCT is an OCT imaging technique that uses longer wavelength light to increase the depth of penetration of the OCT signal. This technique allows for better visualization of deeper structures in the eye, such as the choroid and sclera.

Some of the commercially available OCT systems that offer EDI imaging are Spectralis OCT (Heidelberg Engineering), Cirrus HD-OCT (Carl Zeiss Meditec), Topcon 3D OCT-1 Maestro (Topcon Medical Systems), RTVue XR Avanti (Optovue), Triton Swept Source OCT (Topcon Medical Systems), AngioVue OCT (Optovue), DRI OCT Triton Plus (Topcon Medical Systems), and Envisu R2210 OCT (Bioptigen, Inc.).

EDI-OCT imaging is a powerful tool for studying the complex anatomical and physiological changes associated with glaucoma and is increasingly used in clinical practice and research.

20.4.2.2 Clinical Applicability of EDI Imaging on OCT

A. EDI-OCT imaging is very useful for studying laminar bowing. In this phenomenon, the lamina cribrosa (a thin, sieve-like structure within the optic nerve head) bows inward or outward in response to changes in intraocular pressure. Laminar bowing is an important factor in the development and progression of glaucoma, and understanding this phenomenon is critical for diagnosing and managing the disease. EDI-OCT imaging allows better visualization of the lamina cribrosa, located deep within the eye and difficult to see using other imaging techniques [15–17]. This can help to understand the mechanisms underlying laminar bowing better and may lead to improved diagnostic and treatment approaches for glaucoma.
B. EDI-OCT imaging is used to evaluate other structural changes within the optic nerve head and the surrounding tissues, such as changes in the size and shape of the optic cup and the presence of fluid-filled spaces within the retina.
C. EDI-OCT imaging can also be used to evaluate the efficacy of glaucoma treatments by monitoring changes in the optic nerve head, lamina cribrosa, RNFL, and ganglion cell layer (GCL) over time. The early detection of

changes in these structures can enable clinicians to adjust treatment plans to manage the disease better and improve patient outcomes.

The following laminar parameters can be studied using EDI imaging on OCT in glaucoma:

1. *Lamina cribrosa depth* is the distance between the anterior surface of the lamina cribrosa and the reference plane, usually the Bruch's membrane or the retinal pigment epithelium. A deeper lamina cribrosa is associated with an increased risk of glaucoma progression.
2. *Lamina cribrosa thickness* is the thickness of the lamina cribrosa at its thinnest point. A thinner lamina cribrosa is associated with an increased risk of glaucoma progression.
3. *Lamina cribrosa position* is its position relative to the optic nerve head rim. A more posteriorly positioned lamina cribrosa is associated with an increased risk of glaucoma progression.
4. *Lamina cribrosa curvature* is the curvature of the lamina cribrosa surface. A more curved lamina cribrosa is associated with an increased risk of glaucoma progression.
5. *Pre-laminar tissue thickness* is the thickness of the tissue anterior to the lamina cribrosa, including the retinal nerve fiber layer and the pre-laminar tissue. Thinning of the pre-laminar tissue is associated with an increased risk of glaucoma progression.

20.5 Artificial Intelligence (AI) Applications in Glaucoma OCT

1. AI has several potential applications in OCT imaging for glaucoma [16, 18–20]. AI algorithms can be trained to detect subtle changes in the optic nerve head and surrounding tissues that may indicate glaucoma. This can help clinicians identify patients at risk of developing the disease and initiate appropriate monitoring and treatment.

   AI in OCT imaging for glaucoma is useful in monitoring disease progression. AI algorithms can analyze longitudinal datasets of OCT images to identify changes in the optic nerve head and surrounding tissues over time. This can help clinicians detect subtle changes that may indicate disease progression.

   AI can also be used to assist in the management of glaucoma by predicting the efficacy of different treatment options. By analyzing datasets of OCT images from patients who have undergone different treatment modalities, AI algorithms can predict the likelihood of success for different treatments in individual patients.
2. New developments in AI-based applications on OCT in glaucoma are listed below.
   (a) Multimodal imaging: Combining different types of imaging modalities, such as OCT, fundus photography, and visual fields, can provide a more comprehensive view of the eye and improve the accuracy of glaucoma diagnosis and monitoring.
   (b) Personalized medicine: AI algorithms can analyze large datasets of patient information and OCT images to identify individualized risk factors for glaucoma and tailor treatment plans accordingly.
   (c) Real-time monitoring: Real-time monitoring of RNFL parameters using AI-based algorithms can help to identify changes in disease progression earlier and adjust treatment plans accordingly.
   (d) Big data analysis: AI-based algorithms can analyze large datasets of OCT images and patient data to identify trends and patterns indicative of glaucoma. This can help improve our understanding of the disease and guide future research.
   (e) Automated reporting: AI algorithms can generate automated reports based on the analysis of OCT images, reducing the need for manual interpretation by clinicians.
3. Several AI platforms exist for OCT analysis of RNFL, optic disc, and macula for glaucoma. Some of the novelties in different AI platforms are listed below.

(a) *DeepGlaucoma:* This AI uses quantitative measurements of RNFL thickness, optic disc morphology, and macular thickness to predict the likelihood of developing glaucoma.
(b) *iWellnessScan:* This AI provides a report summarizing the results and compares the patient's measurements to a normative database.
(c) *Optovue:* This AI platform includes the "Ganglion Cell Complex Map," which displays the location of the ganglion cell complex in a color-coded map.
(d) *Topcon:* This AI platform includes the "Glaucoma Asymmetry Analysis," which compares the measurements of both eyes to identify asymmetry.

20.6 Conclusion

OCT is an important imaging tool for generating high-resolution cross-sectional images. Medicine and technology keep evolving hand-in-hand. New OCT variants, moving from time-domain acquisition to frequency domain measurement of spectral interference, have facilitated greater acquisition speed and tissue contrast in the images. A patient can be followed over time using their baseline values. Clinicians should understand the limitations of this imaging technology and correlate clinically with IOP, ONH, and RNFL appearance, visual field data, and quantitative data to detect glaucoma and its progression. AI has the potential to revolutionize OCT imaging for glaucoma by improving the accuracy of diagnosis, monitoring disease progression, and optimizing treatment options. Further research is needed to develop and validate AI algorithms for clinical use in glaucoma.

Funding Hyderabad Eye Research Foundation.

Disclosure Nil.

References

1. Fercher AF, Drexler W, Hitzenberger CK, Lasser T. Optical coherence tomography—principles and applications. Rep Prog Phys. 2003;66:239.
2. Schuman JS, Hee MR, Arya AV, et al. Optical coherence tomography: a new tool for glaucoma diagnosis. Curr Opin Ophthalmol. 1995;6(2):89–95.
3. Chen TC, Cense B, Pierce MC, et al. Spectral domain optical coherence tomography: ultra-high speed, ultra-high resolution ophthalmic imaging. Arch Ophthalmol. 2005;123(12):1715–20.
4. Bouma BE, Yun SH, Vakoc BJ, et al. Fourier-domain optical coherence tomography: recent advances toward clinical utility. Curr Opin Biotechnol. 2009;20(1):111–8.
5. Choma MA, Hsu K, Izatt JA. Swept source optical coherence tomography using an all-fiber 1300-nm ring laser source. J Biomed Opt. 2005;10(4):044009.
6. Choma M, Sarunic M, Yang C, Izatt J. Sensitivity advantage of swept source and Fourier domain optical coherence tomography. Opt Express. 2003;11(18):2183–9.
7. Quigley HA, Dunkelberger GR, Green WR. Retinal ganglion cell atrophy correlated with automated perimetry in human eyes with glaucoma. Am J Ophthalmol. 1989;107(5):453–64.
8. Wollstein G, Schuman JS, Price LL, et al. Optical coherence tomography longitudinal evaluation of retinal nerve fiber layer thickness in glaucoma. Arch Ophthalmol. 2005;123(4):464–70.
9. Kuang TM, Zhang C, Zangwill LM, et al. Estimating lead time gained by optical coherence tomography in detecting glaucoma before development of visual field defects. Ophthalmology. 2015;122(10):2002–9.
10. Dong ZM, Wollstein G, Schuman JS. Clinical utility of optical coherence tomography in glaucoma. Invest Ophthalmol Vis Sci. 2016;57(9):OCT556–67.
11. Gracitelli CPB, Abe RY, Medeiros FA. Spectral-domain optical coherence tomography for glaucoma diagnosis. Open Ophthalmol J. 2015;9:68–77.
12. Rao HL, Kumbar T, Addepalli UK, et al. Effect of spectrum bias on the diagnostic accuracy of spectral-domain optical coherence tomography in glaucoma. Invest Ophthalmol Vis Sci. 2012;53(2):1058–65.
13. Williams DR. Imaging single cells in the living retina. Vis Res. 2011;51(13):1379–96.
14. Kotcharlakota D, Choudhari NS. Role of adaptive optics in early diagnosis of glaucoma from a Clinician's perspective. Semin Ophthalmol. 2023;38(1):44–51.
15. Park HY, Jeon SH, Park CK. Enhanced depth imaging detects lamina cribrosa thickness differences in normal tension glaucoma and primary open-angle glaucoma. Ophthalmology. 2012;119:10–20.

16. Park SC, De Moraes CG, Teng CC, et al. Enhanced depth imaging optical coherence tomography of deep optic nerve complex structures in glaucoma. Ophthalmology. 2012;119:3–9.
17. Lee EJ, Kim TW, Weinreb RN, et al. Visualization of the lamina cribrosa using enhanced depth imaging spectral-domain optical coherence tomography. Am J Ophthalmol. 2011;152:87–95.
18. Dell'Omo R, Costagliola C, Di Salvatore F, et al. Enhanced depth imaging spectral-domain optical coherence tomography. Retina. 2010;30(2):378–9.
19. Yazdanpanah A, Hamarneh G, Smith B, Sarunic M. Intra-retinal layer segmentation in optical coherence tomography using an active contour approach. Med Image Comput Comput Assist Interv. 2009;12(Pt 2):649–56.
20. Xiong J, Li F, Song D, et al. Multimodal machine learning using visual fields and peripapillary circular OCT scans in detection of glaucomatous optic neuropathy. Ophthalmology. 2022;129(2):171–80.

21 Visual Field

Avik K. Roy, Ramyashri Shastry, and Aparna Rao

21.1 Introduction

Visual field testing is indispensable in diagnosing and managing glaucoma. Over the past 50 years, computerized visual field testing with standard automated perimetry (SAP) has become the standard method for assessing visual function in glaucoma. SAP measures threshold sensitivity at specific test locations of the subject's retina using white stimuli on a white background and provides a method for estimating visual field abnormalities by comparing these to a normative database. This chapter will briefly describe the historical development of the "field test" and cover important new advances in the technology, technique, and clinical applications.

A. K. Roy
Mithu Tulsi Chanrai Campus, L V Prasad Eye Institute, Bhubaneswar, India
e-mail: dravik@lvpei.org

R. Shastry
Drishti Eye Centre, Hyderabad, India

A. Rao (✉)
Kallam Anji Reddy Campus, L V Prasad Eye Institute, Hyderabad, India
e-mail: aparna@lvpei.org

21.2 History

The visual field test began with Aubert and Forster developing the arc perimeter in the 1860s [1]. It helped map peripheral neurologic and advanced glaucomatous visual field abnormalities. The first modern kinetic perimetry was described in 1920 [2]. The tangent screen kinetic perimetry was introduced by Traquair a few years later [3]. The "bowl perimeter" design by Goldmann was widely accepted by ophthalmologists by 1945 [4]. The standardization of the background illumination and varying degrees of test stimuli remained the clinical benchmark. Since then, automated perimetry has progressed rapidly over the past few decades, courtesy the works of Fankhauser [5], Heijl and Krakau [6], and Flammer et al. [7].

21.3 Current Test

The Humphrey Visual Field Analyzer (HVFA) is the current gold standard of visual field testing [8]. It includes varying test strategies like the suprathreshold, full-threshold, efficient threshold, and the latest SITA (the Swedish Interactive Thresholding Algorithm) [9].

The various test programs are 30-2, 24-2, 10-2, macular, and the most recent, 24-2C program. There are two numbers for the test; "30"

T. Das, P. Satgunam (eds.), *Ophthalmic Diagnostics*, https://doi.org/10.1007/978-981-97-0138-4_21

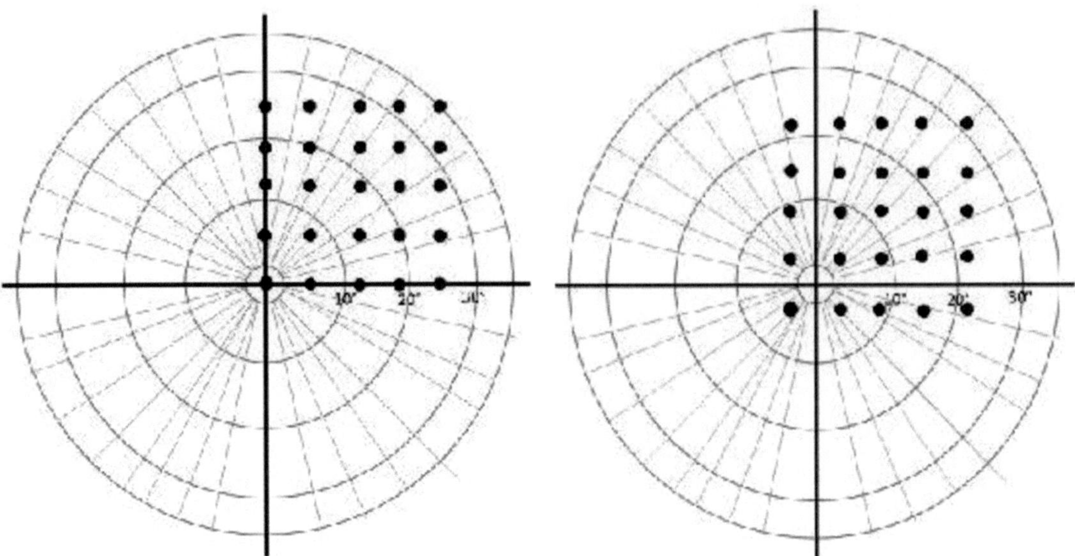

Fig. 21.1 The locations of the stimuli in the visual field analysis. Left: in the threshold test "1", the stimuli are placed 6° apart in the x- and y-axes. Right: in the threshold test "2", the stimuli are placed 3° apart in the x- and y-axes. (Source: http://www.healio.com)

(or 24 and 10) refers to the visual field 30° extending from the fixation; it is 30° in all four directions. Thus, it is 60° of the subject's visual field (similarly 48° for "24" and 20° for "10").

The second number of the test is "2", which denotes the second pattern of the developed threshold test. It varies from the first pattern, "1", by the configuration of the stimuli in the x- and y-axes. In "2", the stimuli are 3° apart in contrast to the 6° apart in "1" (Fig. 21.1).

Thus a "30-2" field means testing the field 30° from the fixation point in all directions where the stimuli are presented 3° apart. Appropriate changes apply for the 24-2 and 10-2 tests. The normal visual field is widest horizontally, extending over 90° temporally, 60° nasally and superiorly, and 70° inferiorly.

21.4 Technique of Humphry Visual Field (HVF) Tests

A particular number (based on the "program") of (usually) white-colored stimuli of a standard size (III or V) but with varying intensity (based on the "strategy") are presented on a white background of a fixed brightness. Each eye is tested one at a time. The subject must click on a mouse to register a response as and when the subject sees the stimulus. The 30-2, 24-2, 10-2, and macular programs test the central 30° (with 76 points locations), 24° (with 54 points locations), 10° (with 68 points locations), and 5° (with 16 points locations), respectively. The details of the procedures and interpretation of findings are elaborated in manuals and textbooks (Fig. 21.2) [8].

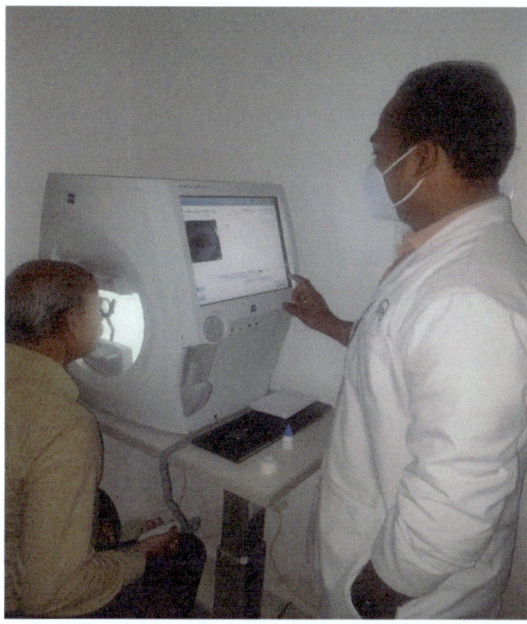

Fig. 21.2 The subject sits comfortably facing the dome of the device and places the chin on the chin rest. The room is dimly illuminated (mesopic condition), with the background illumination fixed at 31.5 apostilbs. The average time taken for the SITA standard (most commonly used) 24-2 test for one eye is approximately 8–10 min

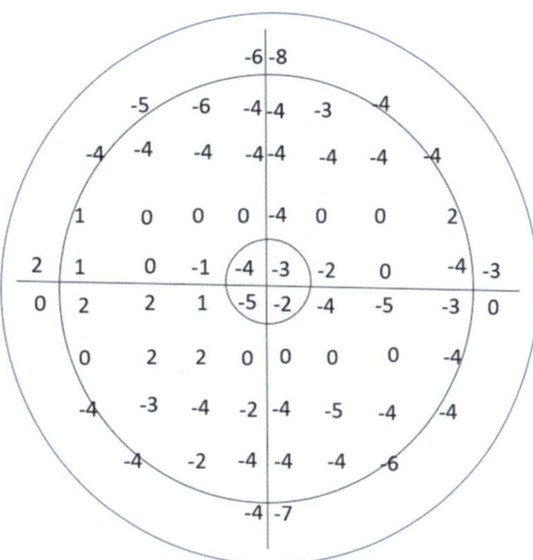

Fig. 21.3 Central Visual Field. The central most ring (2° of eccentricity) was allotted a weight of 8.0, the second ring was assigned a weight of 2.5, and the outermost ring was assigned a weight of 2.0

21.5 Technology

21.5.1 Visual Field Index (VFI)

The HVFA provides the mean deviation (MD) for the 24-2 and 10-2 programs as a global index of the subject's visual function. This is calculated by averaging the age-corrected threshold sensitivities at all test locations after adjusting for the variability of each test location and eccentricity from the fovea. The MD is subject to alterations secondary to any media opacity—most commonly, the senile cataract that might co-exist with glaucoma. There is a significant change in MD after cataract surgery in the presence or absence of glaucomatous damage. To address this and other issues, Bengtsson and Heijl [10] described a new global index for 24-2 and 30-2 programs, the Visual Field Index (VFI). It summarizes the visual field information into a number (percentage) that measures the visual field status and changes over time. The VFI ranges from 100 (normal) to 0 (perimetrically blind).

21.5.1.1 Clinical Application

VFI is an extremely useful tool in diagnosing glaucoma and monitoring disease progression. This is also less sensitive to cataract and its removal.

21.5.2 Central Field Index (CFI)

The VFI is a global measure of the subject's visual function in the 24 or 30° visual fields. There was no similar analytic tool for the central 10° visual field. The macula corresponds to only 10° of the visual field, but it is represented a much larger (approx. 60%) area of the visual cortex [11]. Central field disturbances are significantly related to deterioration in vision-related quality of life [12]. de Moraes et al. [13] introduced a novel global index for the central 10° of the visual field, the Central Field Index (CFI). It follows almost the same methodology as that of Bengtsson and Heijl [10] but divides the 10-2 printout into three smaller concentric rings, instead of five for the VFI calculation, with increasing weight from the center toward the periphery (Fig. 21.3).

These values were obtained from a study by Qiu et al. [14] on estimating linear cortical magnification in the human primary visual cortex. Finally, the weighted averages of the CFI value of all 68 test locations of the 10-2 visual field printout are calculated for each visual field examination of each patient's sequence of 5 or more examinations. The result is a global index that ranges from 0% (central blindness) to 100% (normal central vision). The calculation is primarily based on the 10-2 pattern deviation probability plots, already adjusted for diffuse sensitivity loss resulting from media opacities. Hence the discrimination between glaucomatous field defects and those that result from media opacity, mainly cataract, is relatively easy.

21.5.2.1 Clinical Application

CFI varies less than VFI in stable eyes. Hence, incorporating CFI calculation for monitoring advanced disease in eyes with central defects could be valuable [15]. However, as of now, there is no commercially available software designed specifically to detect and measure rates of progression in the central field.

21.5.3 Swedish Interactive Thresholding Algorithm (SITA) Faster

In the late 1990s, two modes of Swedish Interactive Thresholding Algorithm (SITA) were introduced: the SITA Standard and SITA Fast (Fig. 21.4) [9]. The SITA Faster (Fig. 21.5) was introduced in 2019 by Heijl et al. [16] to expedite testing time without compromising the quality.

Seven adjustments were made to the SITA Fast algorithm. These were: (1) the use of age-corrected normal threshold values for starting stimulus intensity (without conventional staircase method for cardinal points), (2) requiring only one staircase test reversal at primary test points, (3) using the distribution of SITA Fast normal values to determine when testing can stop at each test point location, (4) performing no false-negative catch trials, (5) rechecking the physiologic blind spot, (6) accounting for the delay in stimulus timing, and (7) performing a second check of points in which the test individual did not respond to a stimulus of maximum intensity.

21.5.3.1 Clinical Application

Heijl et al. [16] reported that the SITA Faster test time was 30.4% shorter the SITA Fast and 53.5% shorter than the SITA Standard. Furthermore, there were no differences in MD or VFI between these strategies. However, on comparing the 24-2 SITA Standard and SITA Faster, Phu et al. [17] reported that the latter was significantly less reliable, mainly due to high false-positive rates and a type of artifact the authors named as "seeding point errors." These are errors in determining threshold sensitivity in the initial phase of the visual field when the four cardinal locations were tested. Despite these shortcomings, SITA Faster can be considered when frequent visual field testing and more data are desired.

21.5.4 The 24-2C SITA Faster Algorithm

An accumulating body of evidence demonstrates that the retinal ganglion cells residing in the macula are lost, even in the early stages of glaucoma, and this has important clinical implications [18]. Detection of central visual field loss is therefore important in the management of glaucoma although it is unclear whether patients should be evaluated with dedicated 10-2 visual field tests instead of or in addition to 24-2 visual field tests. The 24-2 visual field test points are spaced 6° apart, with 13 points in the central 10° when foveal sensitivity is included. On the contrary, 10-2 visual field test points are spaced 2° apart, with 68 points in the central 10°. Therefore, the 24-2 test may not detect central damage that would have otherwise been detected with 10-2 visual fields [19]. Moraes et al. [20] found that 61.5% of glaucomatous eyes and 39.5% of glaucoma-suspect eyes had depressed points on 10-2 tests, which were earlier considered normal on cluster criteria on the 24-2 tests.

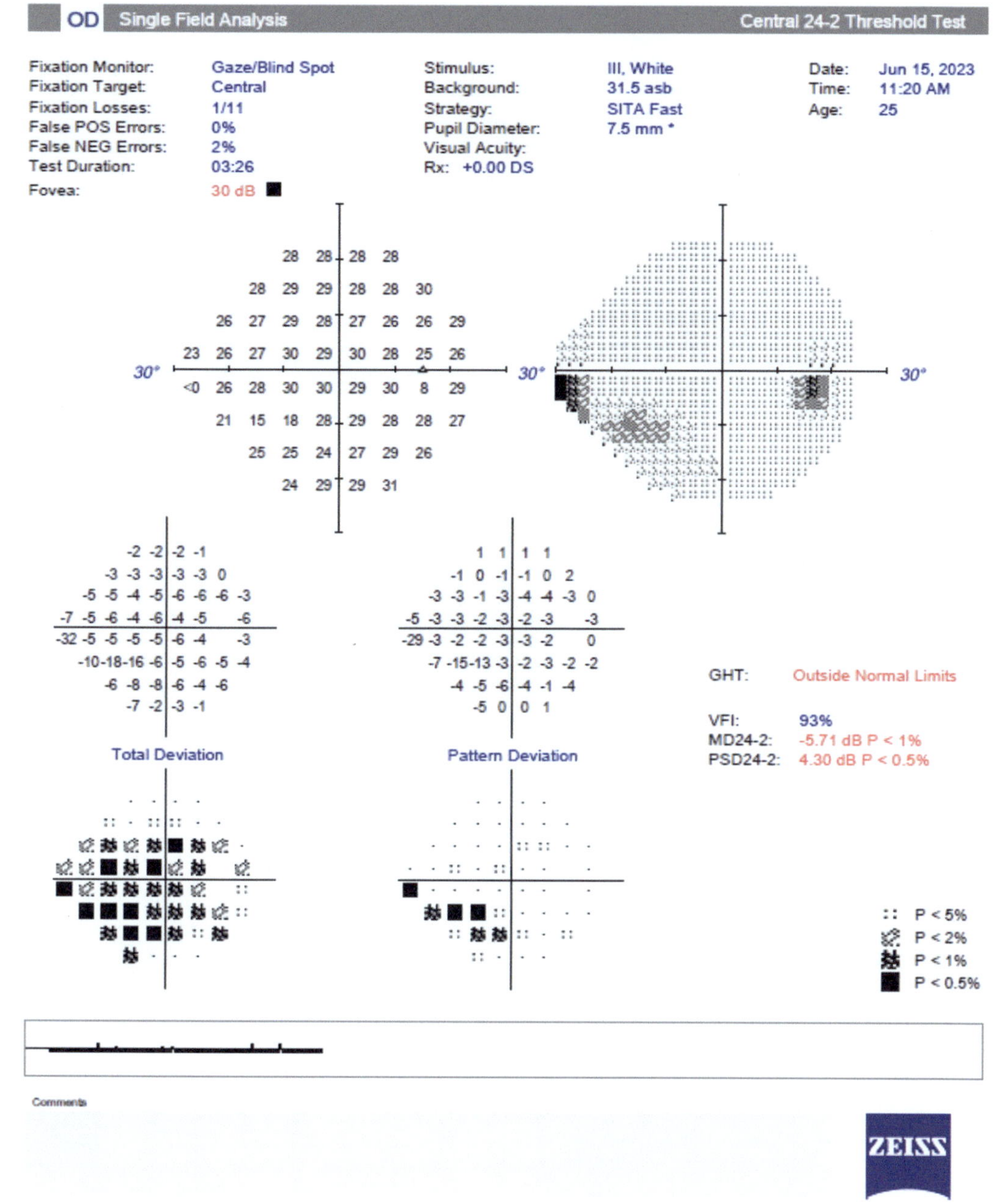

Fig. 21.4 SITA Fast. An HVF single field printout of a 25-year-old subject's right eye, with reliable indices, with the 24-2 program and the SITA Fast strategy showing significantly depressed points in both, the total deviation and pattern deviation maps (the total duration of the test was 3 min and 26 s)

21.5.5 Technology

Leveraging the time saved using the SITA Faster algorithm, ten additional testing locations are added in the central 10° in the 24-2C SITA Faster algorithm (Fig. 21.6). Preliminary studies have shown that the 24-2C SITA Faster is 18.3% faster than the 24-2 SITA Fast, but 17.5% slower than the 24-2 SITA Faster in glaucoma [21].

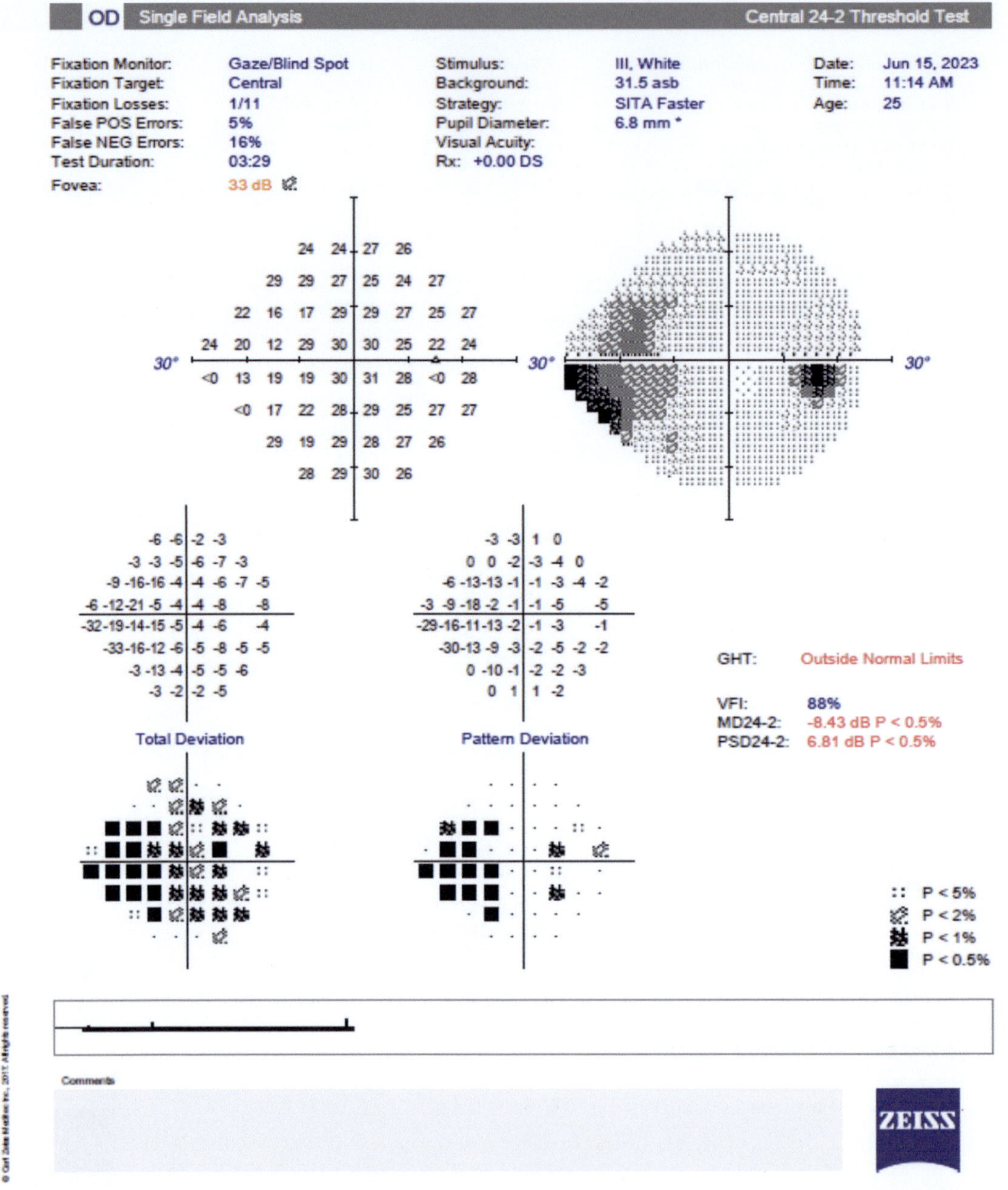

Fig. 21.5 SITA FASTER. An HVF single field printout of a 25-year-old subject's right eye, with reliable indices, with the 24-2 program and the SITA Faster strategy showing significantly depressed points in both, total deviation and pattern deviation maps (more than the previously demonstrated SITA Fast). The total duration of the test was 3 min and 29 s

21.5.5.1 Clinical Application

In a larger, prospective cross-sectional study, Phu et al. [22] compared global visual field indices, test duration, and pattern standard deviation results of glaucoma patients and glaucoma suspects who underwent both, the 24-2 and 24-2C SITA Faster tests. In their study, the 24-2C SITA Faster and 24-2 SITA obtained similar global

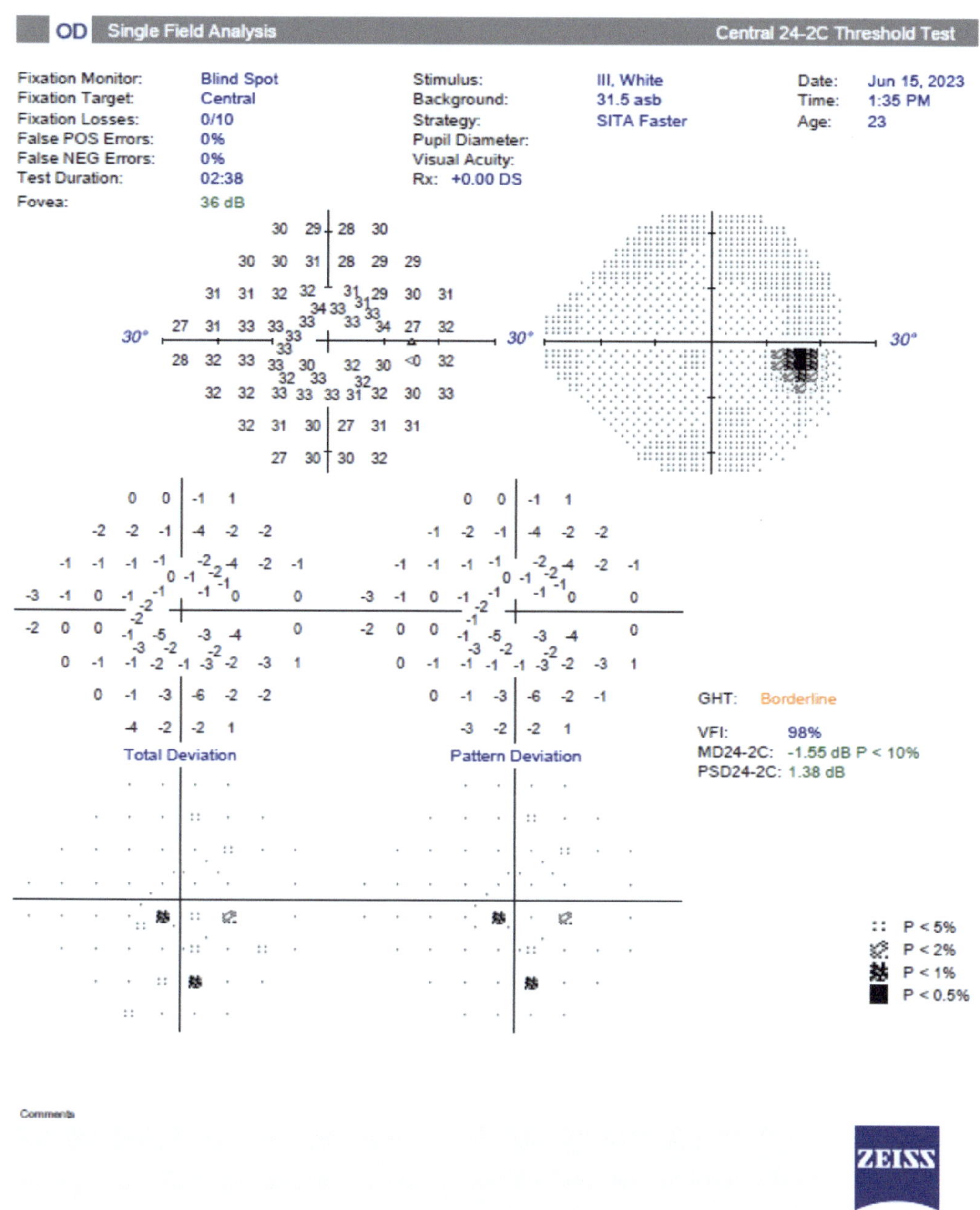

Fig. 21.6 The SITA Faster 24-2C HVF single field printout of a 23-year-old subject's right eye, with reliable indices, with the 24-2C program and SITA Faster strategy, showing few scattered non-significantly depressed points in both, total and pattern deviation maps. The total duration of the test was 2 min and 38 s

indexes, but the former test identified more clusters of central defects (though this was not statistically significant). Thus, the 24-2C SITA Faster may be a reasonable alternative when central defects are suspected. It can be done to avoid performing 10-2 tests routinely.

21.6 Recent Advances in Octopus Perimetry

The first automated static perimeter, the Octopus 201, was developed by Franz Fankauser and colleagues in 1974 [23]. Since then, various improvements have been made to the original test, such as the G program, M program, direct projection system, and different testing strategies with software to analyze early progression on visual fields, as elaborated in the user manual (Octopus Digest, 8th Edition [23]). Recent studies report that the HFA and Octopus have similar efficacies and performance [24]. The newer Octopus 900 offers several technical advancements over the earlier Octopus 600 model; it has static and kinetic perimetry algorithms and seamless integration with the patented EyeSuite Software for more effective data analysis.

21.7 Home-Based Portable Perimeter

Portable perimeters are visual field-testing devices that are lightweight, compact, and easily transportable. These are ideal for use in remote or underserved areas with limited access to specialized eye care equipment. Portable perimeters are typically battery-powered and may use different stimuli, such as white or colored lights, to test the patient's visual field. They may also use different testing strategies, such as static or kinetic perimetry. Portable perimeters offer several advantages over traditional tabletop perimeters, including greater flexibility and portability, reduced cost, and the ability to perform visual field testing in various settings. These are also ideal for screening programs, where many patients must be tested quickly and efficiently. The limitations of these include limited testing range and the need for frequent calibration and maintenance. Currently, three platforms are available for portable perimeters, namely, tablet-based, laptop-based, and head-mounted virtual reality.

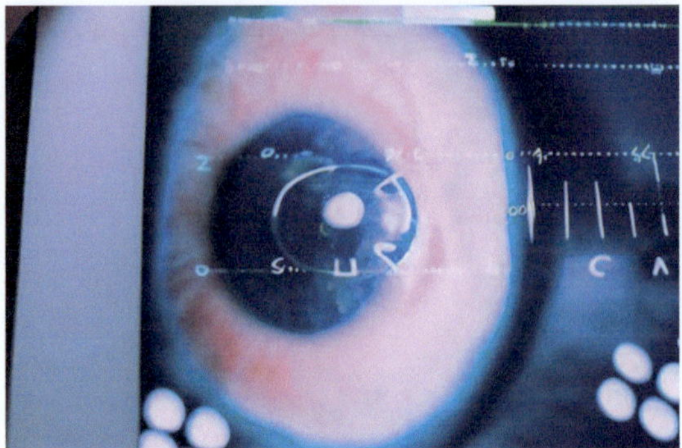

Fig. 21.7 This is a representative picture of a portable perimeter that enables visual field testing on portable tablet devices

21.7.1 Tablet-Based or iPad-Based Perimetry

Tablet/iPad-based perimetry involves using a tablet or smartphone with a specialized application to perform visual field testing (Fig. 21.7). While these are portable, flexible, and less expensive, their limitations include reduced testing accuracy and the need for frequent calibration and maintenance.

Some examples of tablet-based/smartphone-based perimeters used in glaucoma are:

(a) **Visual Fields Easy (VFE)** [25]: Designed by Konan Medical, it uses a standardized testing protocol and provides a range of testing options, including threshold and supra-threshold perimetry. The VFE runs on a small smartphone screen (iPhone) which must be held steady in the hands throughout the test. The VFE is a reliable and effective tool for glaucoma telescreening. The average testing time is under 3 min.
(b) **Peristat** [26] is an online visual field test. It is based on Adobe/Flash technology and runs on a web browser.
(c) **Melbourne Rapid Fields (MRF)** [27]: This iPad-based perimetry app is reportedly similar to the SITA Fast in speed, with an intra-class coefficient value of 0.7–0.88 over 6 months of follow-up visits. The MRF tests 66 locations over 28° × 18° by having the

patient vary fixation. The MRF tests include 10-2, 24-2, and 30-2, and interact with the patient during the screening process. The results of the MRF are saved to either cloud-based storage or can be integrated into the hospital's electronic record system for easy storage and retrieval.

(d) **Eyecatcher** [28]: This VR-based platform found good acceptance by 20 patients for home visual field testing with good concordance between visual fields measured at home and in the clinic. The median test duration was 4.5 min, with the ambient illumination in the patient's surroundings not affecting visual field measurements.

21.7.2 Laptop-Based Perimetry

Portable laptop perimeters are small and lightweight versions of traditional tabletop perimeters [29, 30]. These are ideal for screening programs and remote locations with limited access to specialized equipment. Laptop-based perimeters typically use static stimuli, such as lights of different intensities and colors, to test the patient's visual field. They may also use different testing strategies, such as threshold and suprathreshold perimetry, to evaluate the patient's visual field. Some examples of laptop-based perimeters used in glaucoma testing include the Medmont M700 Automated Perimeter, [29] the Oculus Easyfield Perimeter, [30] and the Octopus 900 Perimeter.

21.7.2.1 Clinical Applications

The advantages of laptop-based perimeters over traditional tabletop perimeters include greater flexibility and portability, reduced cost, and the ability to test in various settings. The limitations are reduced testing accuracy, limited testing range, and the need for frequent calibration and maintenance. One study [31] found a reasonable ROC curve for a home-based visual field examination method using a PC monitor or virtual reality (VR) glasses using the suprathreshold algorithm for the central 24° and the HVFA.

21.7.2.2 Head-Mounted or VR Technology

Head-Mounted or VR Technology is an emerging method for visual field testing in glaucoma. In VR visual field testing, patients wear a VR headset that displays stimuli in a 360° virtual environment.

The virtual environment can be customized to simulate real-world scenarios such as driving, walking, or navigating through a crowded area. The stimuli are presented aerodynamically and interactively, which can help reduce patient fatigue and improve the accuracy of results [32–37]. It is reportedly more sensitive, [32, 33] and equally reliable [36, 37]. VR technology can also potentially improve patient engagement and satisfaction with visual field testing. Because the testing environment is more interactive and engaging, patients may be more likely to comply with testing instructions and complete the test accurately. The challenges, however, are its cost (which could be a barrier to widespread use) and technology (setting it up and calibrating it are difficult). Further research is needed to determine the optimal design and implementation of VR visual field testing in clinical practice. One such device is described in Chap. 35.

21.8 Artificial Intelligence (AI) in Visual Field Measurement

In recent years, there has been growing interest in using artificial intelligence (AI) to automate and improve the analysis of visual field data. Several AI platforms have been developed [38–44]. The Advanced Glaucoma Intervention Study (AGIS) group developed the Progression Analysis Tool (PAT) that used a statistical algorithm to analyze visual field data and detect changes over time that may indicate disease progression. More recently, deep learning algorithms have been applied to analyze visual fields in glaucoma. These algorithms use artificial neural networks to analyze large datasets of visual field data and identify patterns and trends that traditional methods may miss. One example is the Glaucoma Deep

Learning Detection (GDD) system developed by researchers at Google. The GDD uses a deep learning algorithm to analyze visual field data and provide an objective measure of glaucomatous damage.

21.8.1 Pros and Cons of AI for Visual Field in Glaucoma

Pros

1. AI may improve the accuracy and consistency of visual field testing, as it analyzes data objectively and without inter-observer variability.
2. AI algorithms may be able to detect early signs of glaucomatous damage that may be missed by traditional methods, thus enabling earlier diagnosis and treatment.
3. AI algorithms can analyze large visual field datasets and provide detailed and nuanced information on the patient's visual field status.
4. The recent introduction of amalgamating structural parameters to predict functional visual field indices and parameters is a new development that may change how glaucoma is monitored over time.

Cons

1. AI algorithms may be less transparent and interpretable than traditional methods, making it difficult for clinicians to understand the analysis process, which may affect their ability to interpret the test results.
2. AI algorithms may be less accurate than traditional methods in certain patient populations, such as those with advanced glaucoma or those with poor fixation stability.
3. Using AI algorithms may raise ethical concerns about patient privacy and data security.

21.9 Pediatric Perimetry

The pediatric perimeter is a device that shows promise as a clinical device to map visual fields in infants and patients with special needs [45]. Although a lot of research is currently being done to develop pediatric perimetry, this subject is out of the scope of this chapter.

21.9.1 The Future of Visual Field Testing

Visual field testing is an integral part of glaucoma management. Recent advances have improved the efficiency, accessibility, and reliability of visual field testing. The future developments include multifocal steady-state visual-evoked potentials (mfSSVEP) [46] and adaptive optics scanning laser ophthalmoscopy (AOSLO) [47, 48]. The mfSSVEP is a portable brain-computer interface (BCI) designed to assess visual field damage objectively. The AOSLO technology uses a wavefront sensor that records ocular wavefront aberrations and calculates the distortion degree as light passes from the cornea and retina and back into the cornea. The amount of distortion is calculated and corrected to give a high-resolution image captured through a CCD camera system. Additionally, novel testing modalities such as portable devices, tablets, and VR headsets may improve the ease of testing for both, remote and in clinical settings, for patients with glaucoma and other related disorders.

Funding Hyderabad Eye Research Foundation, Hyderabad, India.

Disclosure NA.

References

1. Forster C. Vorzeigung des Perimeter. Klin Monatsbl Augenheilk. 1869;7:411–22.
2. Lang BT. Perimetry: the methods, means, and manner of determining the size of a field or scotoma. Br J Ophthalmol. 1920;4:489–503.
3. Traquair H. An introduction to clinical Perimetry, vol. 21. London: Kimpton; 1927. p. 250.
4. Goldmann H. Demonstration unseres neuen Projektionskugelperimeters samt theoretischen und klinischen Bemerkung über Perimetrie [Demonstration of our new projection ball perimeter

with theoretical and clinical remark about perimetry]. Ophthalmologica. 1946;111:187–92. (Germany).
5. Fankhauser F. Background illumination and automated perimetry. Arch Ophthalmol. 1986;104:1126.
6. Heijl A, Krakau CE. An automatic perimeter for glaucoma visual field screening and control. Construction and clinical cases. Albrecht Von Graefes Arch Klin Exp Ophthalmol. 1975;197:13–23.
7. Flammer J, Drance SM, Augustiny L, Funkhouser A. Quantification of glaucomatous visual field defects with automated perimetry. Invest Ophthalmol Vis Sci. 1985;26:176–81.
8. Anderson DR, Patella VM. Automated static perimetry. 2nd ed. St Louis: Mosby; 1999.
9. Bengtsson B, Heijl A, Olsson J. Evaluation of a new threshold visual field strategy, SITA, in normal subjects. Swedish interactive thresholding algorithm. Acta Ophthalmol Scand. 1998;76:165–9.
10. Bengtsson B, Heijl A. A visual field index for calculation of glaucoma rate of progression. Am J Ophthalmol. 2008;145:343–53.
11. Prasad S, Galetta SL. Anatomy and physiology of the afferent visual system. Handb Clin Neurol. 2011;102:3–19.
12. Murata H, Hirasawa H, Aoyama Y, et al. Identifying areas of the visual field important for quality of life in patients with glaucoma. PLoS One. 2013;8:e58695. https://doi.org/10.1371/journal.pone.0058695.
13. de Moraes CG, Furlanetto RL, Ritch R, Liebmann JM. A new index to monitor central visual field progression in glaucoma. Ophthalmology. 2014;121:1531–8.
14. Qiu A, Rosenau BJ, Greenberg AS, et al. Estimating linear cortical magnification in human primary visual cortex via dynamic programming. NeuroImage. 2006;31:125–38.
15. Rao A, Padhy D, Mudunuri H, et al. Central field index versus visual field index for central visual function in stable glaucoma. J Glaucoma. 2017;26:1–7.
16. Heijl A, Patella VM, Chong LX, et al. A new SITA perimetric threshold testing algorithm: construction and a multicenter clinical study. Am J Ophthalmol. 2019;198:154–65.
17. Phu J, Khuu SK, Agar A, Kalloniatis M. Clinical evaluation of Swedish interactive thresholding algorithm-faster compared with Swedish interactive thresholding algorithm-standard in normal subjects, glaucoma suspects, and patients with glaucoma. Am J Ophthalmol. 2019;208:251–64.
18. Hood DC, Raza AS, de Moraes CG, et al. Glaucomatous damage of the macula. Prog Retin Eye Res. 2013;32:1–21.
19. Traynis I, De Moraes CG, Raza AS, et al. Prevalence and nature of early glaucomatous defects in the central 10 degrees of the visual field. JAMA Ophthalmol. 2014;132:291–7.
20. de Moraes CG, Hood DC, Thenappan A, et al. 24-2 visual fields miss central defects shown on 10-2 tests in glaucoma suspects, ocular hypertensives, and early glaucoma. Ophthalmology. 2017;124:1449–56.
21. Yu S, Lee GC, Callan T, et al. Comparison of SITA faster 24-2C test times to legacy SITA tests (abstract). Invest Ophthalmol Vis Sci. 2019;60:2454.
22. Phu J, Kalloniatis M. Ability of 24-2C and 24-2 grids in identifying central visual field defects and structure-function concordance in glaucoma and suspects. Am J Ophthalmol. 2020;219:317–31.
23. https://www.haag-streit.com/fileadmin/Haag-Streit_USA/Diagnostics/Visual_Field_Digest_8th_eng_.pdf. Accessed 15 June 2023.
24. Bevers C, Blanckaert G, Van Keer K, et al. Semi-automated kinetic perimetry: comparison of the octopus 900 and Humphrey visual field analyzer 3 versus Goldmann perimetry. Acta Ophthalmol. 2019;97:e499–505.
25. "VisualFields Easy": an iPad application as a simple tool for detecting visual field defects. Philippine J Ophthalmol. paojournal.com. Accessed 15 June 2023.
26. Peristat: test - keep your sight. kysvision.com. Accessed 15 June 2023.
27. Kumar H, Thulasidas M. Comparison of perimetric outcomes from Melbourne rapid fields tablet perimeter software and Humphrey field analyzer in glaucoma patients. J Ophthalmol. 2020;2020:8384509. https://doi.org/10.1155/2020/8384509.
28. Jones PR, Campbell P, Callaghan T, et al. Glaucoma home monitoring using a tablet-based visual field test (Eyecatcher): an assessment of accuracy and adherence over 6 months. Am J Ophthalmol. 2021;223:42–52.
29. M700 Automated Perimeter | Medmont International Pty Ltd. Accessed 15 June 2023.
30. Easyfield® - Perimetry - Highlights - OCULUS, Inc. Accessed 15 June 2023.
31. Tsapakis S, Papaconstantinou D, Diagourtas A, et al. Home-based visual field test for glaucoma screening comparison with Humphrey perimeter. Clin Ophthalmol. 2018;12:2597–606. https://doi.org/10.2147/OPTH.S187832.
32. Razeghinejad R, Gonzalez-Garcia A, Myers JS, Katz LJ. Preliminary report on a novel virtual reality perimeter compared with standard automated perimetry. J Glaucoma. 2021;30:17–23.
33. Stapelfeldt J, Kucur SS, Huber N, et al. Virtual reality-based and conventional visual field examination comparison in healthy and glaucoma patients. Transl Vis Sci Technol. 2021;10(12):10. https://doi.org/10.1167/tvst.10.12.10.
34. Montelongo M, Gonzalez A, Morgenstern F, et al. Virtual reality-based automated perimeter, device, and pilot study. Transl Vis Sci Technol. 2021;10:20. https://doi.org/10.1167/tvst.10.3.20.
35. Groth SL, Linton EF, Brown EN, et al. Evaluation of virtual reality perimetry and standard automated perimetry in normal children. Transl Vis Sci Technol. 2023;12(1):6. https://doi.org/10.1167/tvst.12.1.6.
36. Narang P, Agarwal A, Srinivasan M, Agarwal A. Advanced vision analyzer-virtual reality perimeter: device validation, functional correlation and comparison with Humphrey field analyzer. Ophthalmol

Sci. 2021;1(2):100035. https://doi.org/10.1016/j.xops.2021.100035.

37. Odayappan A, Sivakumar P, Kotawala S, et al. Comparison of a new head mount virtual reality perimeter (C3 field analyzer) with automated field analyzer in neuro-ophthalmic disorders. J Neuroophthalmol. 2023;43:232–6.
38. Zheng C, Johnson TV, Garg A, Boland MV. Artificial intelligence in glaucoma. Curr Opin Ophthalmol. 2019;30:97–103.
39. Salazar H, Misra V, Swaminathan SS. Artificial intelligence and complex statistical modeling in glaucoma diagnosis and management. Curr Opin Ophthalmol. 2021;32:105–17.
40. Thompson AC, Jammal AA, Medeiros FA. A review of deep learning for screening, diagnosis, and detection of glaucoma progression. Transl Vis Sci Technol. 2020;9(2):4. https://doi.org/10.1167/tvst.9.2.42.
41. Kucur S, Holló G, Sznitman R. A deep learning approach to automatic detection of early glaucoma from visual fields. PLoS One. 2018;13(11):e0206081. https://doi.org/10.1371/journal.pone.0206081.
42. Ting DSW, Pasquale LR, Peng L, et al. Artificial intelligence and deep learning in ophthalmology. Br J Ophthalmol. 2019;103:167–75.
43. Li F, Wang Z, Qu G, et al. Automatic differentiation of glaucoma visual field from non-glaucoma visual filed using deep convolutional neural network. BMC Med Imaging. 2018;18(1):35. https://doi.org/10.1186/s12880-018-0273-5.
44. Asaoka R, Murata H, Iwase A, Araie M. Detecting preperimetric glaucoma with standard automated perimetry using a deep learning classifier. Ophthalmology. 2016;123:1974–80.
45. Satgunam P, Datta S, Chillakala K, et al. Pediatric perimeter-a novel device to measure visual fields in infants and patients with special needs. Transl Vis Sci Technol. 2017;6(4):3. https://doi.org/10.1167/tvst.6.4.3.
46. Kuba M, Kremláček J, Vít F, et al. VEP examination with new portable device. Doc Ophthalmol. 2023;146:79–91.
47. Vilupuru AS, Rangaswamy NV, Frishman LJ, et al. Adaptive optics scanning laser ophthalmoscopy for in vivo imaging of lamina cribrosa. J Opt Soc Am A Opt Image Sci Vis. 2007;24:1417–25.
48. Huang G, Gast T, Luo T, et al. Imaging retinal nerve fiber loss in glaucoma using adaptive optics scanning laser ophthalmoscopy (abstract). Invest Ophthalmol Vis Sci. 2013;54(15):1451.

22 Retinal Nerve Fiber Layer

Aparna Rao and Niladri B. Puhan

22.1 Introduction

The retinal nerve fiber layer (RNFL) is a thin layer of nerve fibers originating from the ganglion cells in the retina and converging to form the optic nerve, which serves as a conduit for visual signals from the retina to the brain [1–3]. One of the earliest and most pathognomonic features of glaucoma is RNFL [2, 4, 5]. Structural loss of the RNFL layer precedes visual field damage by many years; this is crucial for diagnosing pre-perimetric glaucoma and monitoring disease progression [5, 6]. Thus, RNFL is an important biomarker for glaucoma diagnosis and monitoring disease progression. The RNFL thickness can be measured using a variety of techniques, including optical coherence tomography (OCT), scanning laser polarimetry (SLP), and confocal scanning laser ophthalmoscopy (CSLO) [2, 5–7]. While technological developments have improved the resolution and accuracy of imaging modalities used for RNFL measurements, artificial intelligence (AI) has emerged as a promising tool for detecting and measuring RNFL defects in glaucoma. This chapter will elaborate on the anatomical characterization of the RNFL and its relevance in glaucoma while detailing methods to assess them. This chapter will also discuss using AI-based tools for RNFL assessment using fundus imaging.

A. Rao (✉)
Kallam Anji Reddy Campus, L V Prasad Eye Institute, Hyderabad, India
e-mail: aparna@lvpei.org

N. B. Puhan
Indian Institute of Technology Bhubaneswar, Bhubaneswar, India
e-mail: nbpuhan@iitbbs.ac.in

22.2 History

The retinal nerve fiber layer was first described in the scientific literature in the early nineteenth century. The Italian anatomist Giovanni Battista Betti is credited with identifying optic nerve fibers in animal and human retinas in 1823. In the early twentieth century, investigators could observe and study the RNFL in living human eyes using the ophthalmoscope and slit lamp. Over the following decades, researchers have used various imaging and diagnostic techniques, such as fundus photography and visual field testing, to study the RNFL [5–7]. The invention of OCT in the 1990s revolutionized our ability to visualize and measure the RNFL with unprecedented accuracy and detail. Further technological advancements, including the nerve fiber layer analyzer and retinal tomography, have marked a paradigm shift in glaucoma imaging [5, 6]. In the past few years, this has been augmented exponentially using AI in the interpretation and analysis of RNFL thickness and measurements in glaucoma monitoring and progression.

T. Das, P. Satgunam (eds.), *Ophthalmic Diagnostics*, https://doi.org/10.1007/978-981-97-0138-4_22

22.3 Revisiting RNFL Anatomy and New Insights from Technology

The anatomy of the RNFL is described by its location, composition, and organization [2, 3, 8–10]. The RNFL is located just below the inner limiting membrane (ILM) of the retina and above the ganglion cell layer (GCL) (Fig. 22.1). The RNFL consists of unmyelinated axons of the ganglion cells, which are bundled together to form the nerve fiber layer [1–3, 8, 9]. The axons are surrounded by glial cells called astrocytes, which provide support and insulation. The RNFL also contains blood vessels that supply the retina with nutrients and oxygen.

22.3.1 Organization

The RNFL is thickest in the peripapillary region, which is the area around the optic nerve head, and gradually thins towards the retinal periphery [1–3, 8]. The axons in the RNFL, are organized into bundles that converge towards the optic nerve head, and exit the eye to form the optic nerve. The organization of the RNFL is also influenced by the distribution of the ganglion cells in the retina. Different types of ganglion cells detect different types of visual information, such as color, contrast, and motion [1, 3, 8]. The ganglion cells are not evenly distributed across the retina but are clustered in specific regions known as retinal subfields. These subfields correspond to different regions of the visual field and have distinct connectivity patterns with other parts of the visual system.

In glaucoma, the loss of retinal ganglion cells and their axons occurs in a characteristic pattern. These axon bundles are aligned in a radial pattern around the optic nerve head, with the thickest bundles located in the superior and inferior regions of the retina (Fig. 22.2). Knowledge of the organization of the retinal nerve fiber layer (RNFL) is critical for understanding the topographic localization of nerve damage in glaucoma.

22.3.2 Topographic Localization and its Relevance in Glaucoma

Retinal ganglion cells are organized into distinct subtypes, which differ in their spatial distribution and functional properties [1–3]. Each ganglion cell subtype receives input from specific photoreceptors and processes visual information differently. The axonal fascicles are organized in a distinct and orderly manner as they enter the optic nerve, and this topographic localization changes as they exit the eye to the lateral geniculate body and visual cortex. The retinotopic localization determines the

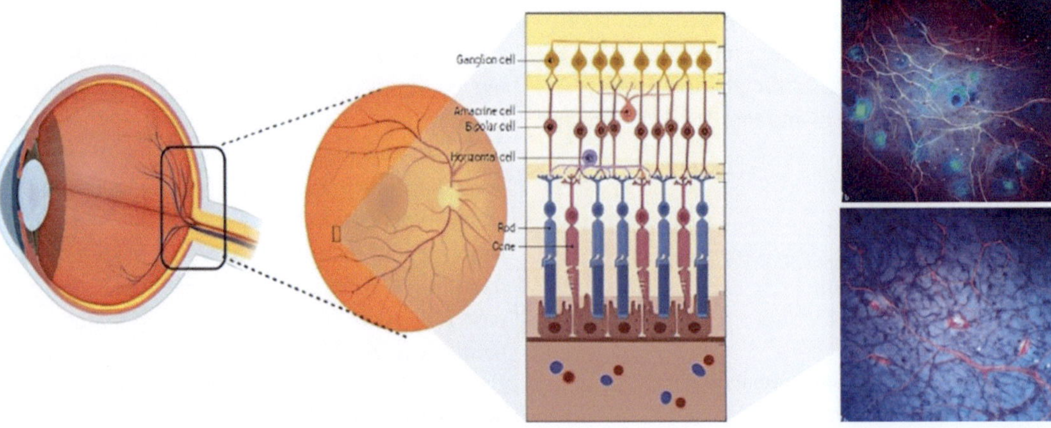

Fig. 22.1 Anatomy and composition of the retinal nerve fiber layer. (Original image created in BIORENDER https://www.biorender.com/ and Free AI generator)

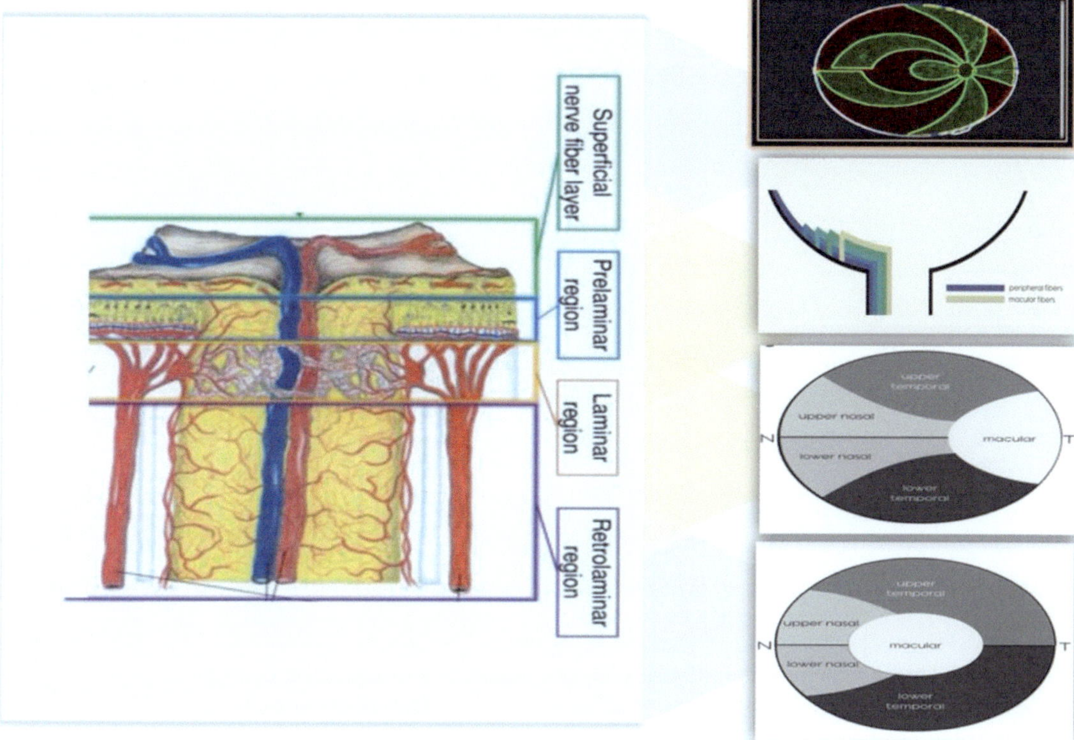

Fig. 22.2 Structural attributes of the retinal nerve fiber layer. The left panel shows the different regions of the optic nerve; the right panel shows the positions of the axons from different regions of the retina as they course from the optic nerve to the brain. (Original image created in BIORENDER https://www.biorender.com/)

spatial integrity and continuity of signals from the retina to the brain. While the bundles arch from the peripheral retina superiorly and inferiorly, the papillomacular bundle approaches the optic nerve directly (Fig. 22.2) [1, 2, 8, 11–14]. The peripheral fibers arising from the arcuate regions are located deeply in the prelaminar portion of the optic nerve, and the macular fibers closer to the optic nerve are placed more superficially. This notable shift in arrangement is seen in the papillomacular bundle fibers that course from the temporal part of the laminar region to the central part in the retrolaminar portion of the optic nerve. The papillomacular bundle is organized such that the most central fibers, which correspond to the fovea, are located in the center of the bundle, with progressively more peripheral fibers arranged around the periphery of the bundle. This arrangement of macular fibers and specific attributes of the ganglion cells in the macula makes the papillomacular bundle more susceptible to intraocular pressure (IOP)-dependent damage than ischemic/vascular damage in glaucoma [11, 14].

The other notable change is the rearrangement of the nasal and temporal fibers as these travel through the optic nerve. In the retina, the nasal fibers (from the nasal part of the retina) cross over to the opposite side of the brain at the optic chiasm, and the temporal fibers (from the temporal part of the retina) remain on the same side of the brain. After the fibers cross at the optic chiasm, the axons continue as the optic tracts, which extend from the chiasm to the brain. The axons in the optic tracts are arranged in a distinct and orderly manner, with those from the temporal retina located in the lateral portion of the tract and those from the nasal retina located in the medial portion of the tract. As the axons continue into the brain, they form synapses with neurons in the lateral geniculate nucleus of the thalamus.

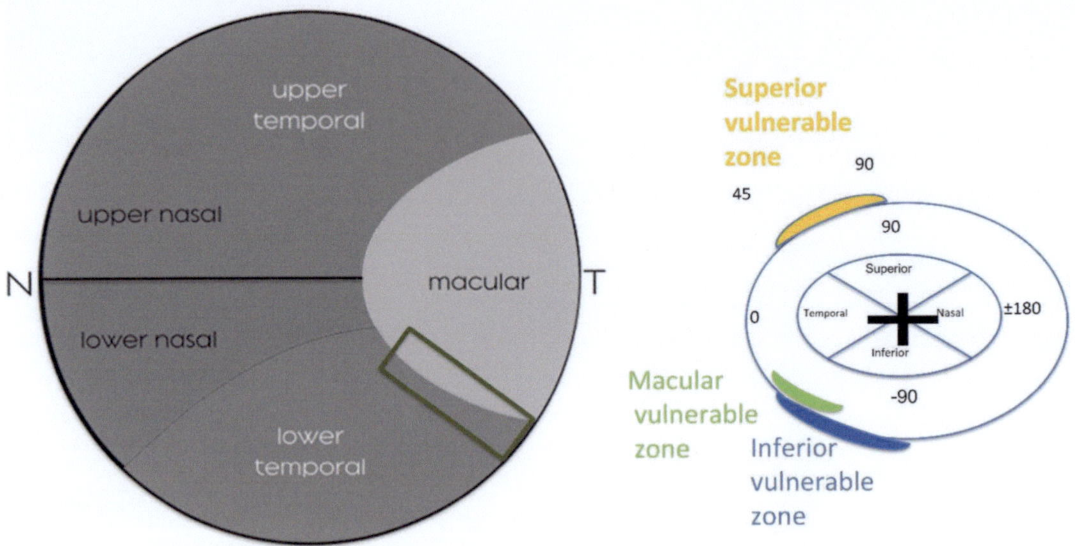

Fig. 22.3 Location of the macular vulnerable zone, which is particularly vulnerable to early glaucoma damage

The spatial arrangement of the fibers typically confers different susceptibility patterns of loss in early or established glaucoma [1, 3, 11, 13, 14]. Different zones have been identified on the optic nerve head and macular regions that may be affected early in glaucoma. Of particular interest is the macular vulnerable zone [15, 16]. It is a strip of fibers between 295 and 322° on the inferior optic disc, which results in a paracentral visual field defect (Fig. 22.3) [6, 16]. This area is most vulnerable to damage and contains axons from the temporal part of the inferior macula that projects towards the optic nerve above the inferior arcuate fibers. An RNFL defect in this region should alert the clinician to the possibility of central involvement, requiring 10-2 visual fields for documenting early glaucomatous defects.

22.4 Techniques of RNFL Detection and Quantification

There are several ways to detect and quantify the RNFL in glaucoma [6, 7, 11, 12, 17–24]. Some of the most common techniques are described below:

22.4.1 Fundus Slit Lamp Biomicroscopy

This is the most common method currently used in clinics. The RNFL defect is visible as a wedge-shaped dark area with loss of normal white striations, fanning out from the optic disc towards the arcuate area, and may sometimes reach close to the macula [1–3, 17–19].

Technique: While using a +78 or +90D lens on the slit lamp, ensure the patient is seated comfortably, and focus the view on the optic disc margins superiorly and inferiorly. Now move the gaze towards the vessels along the supertemporal and inferotemporal arcade and look for disruption of the normal "light-dark-light" pattern of RNFL striations. In the presence of an RNFL defect, this pattern is interrupted by a focal or diffuse dark area along the superior or inferior arcades. Once identified, follow the dark pattern and mark its location with respect to its proximity to the fovea and adjacent vessel trunks for visual quantification and clinical drawings (Fig. 22.4).

Clinical application: A meticulous hand-drawing of the extent and size of the RNFL defect can be very useful in low-resource settings where

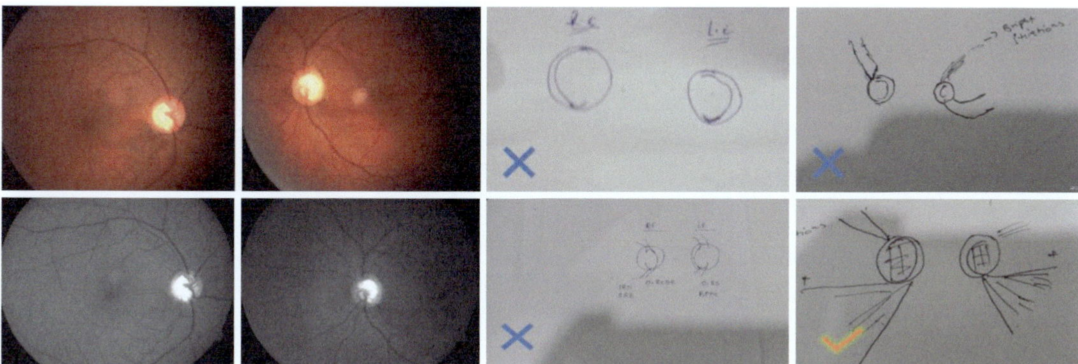

Fig. 22.4 Example of hand drawings from clinical slit lamp biomicroscopy to denote the exact location and extent of RNFL defects and their distance from landmarks like vessels or fovea. The right panel now shows the incorrect (blue cross) and the correct method (yellow tick) of hand-drawing for depicting rim findings and the location/ extent of nerve fiber layer defects

other imaging modalities or fundus photography are unavailable (Fig. 22.4).

22.4.2 Fundus Photography

Fundus photography uses a specialized camera to obtain high-resolution retinal images.

Clinical application: By analyzing the images, fundus photography can provide measurements of RNFL thickness and overall health [1, 3, 17–19]. This is an economical way for low-resource countries where all imaging modalities may not be available. These photographs can be two- or three dimensional; the latter is used for stereoscopic view. These can also be used for analysis using software like Image J for analyzing vessel diameter, rim/disc area, torsion, or any other quantitative fundus parameters. Figure 22.5 shows representative non-stereoscopic fundus pictures depicting focal or diffuse RNFL defects detectable using the above technique.

22.4.3 Optical Coherence Tomography (OCT)

OCT is widely used to measure RNFL thickness in glaucoma.

Technology: OCT is a non-invasive imaging technique that uses light waves to create high-resolution retina images. It is based on the principle of low-coherence light interferometry [6, 7].

Clinical application: OCT provides precise measurements of the thickness of the RNFL in different regions of the retina. Spectral-domain OCT (SD-OCT) is more popular than time-domain OCT (TD-OCT) owing to its superior axial resolution (3–6 μm versus 8–10 μm with TD-OCT) while enabling 3D volumetric analysis of the optic nerve.

22.4.4 Scanning Laser Polarimetry (SLP)

Technology: SLP (GDx, Carl Zeiss Meditec, Dublin, CA) uses a laser to measure the polarization of light as it passes through the RNFL and utilizes the birefringent nature of the RNFL [3, 6, 7, 21–24]. By analyzing the polarization patterns and extent of retardation as the light passes through the RNFL of varying thickness, SLP measures RNFL and the overall extent of optic nerve damage. Recent versions (GDx VCC [Variable Corneal Compensator], GDx ECC [Enhanced Corneal Compensator], and GDx PRO) now have adjusted for and provided compensations for birefringence of the cornea and macula for superior reproducible measurements of RNFL thickness. The RNFL thickness measured by this instrument is currently more reliable than other devices.

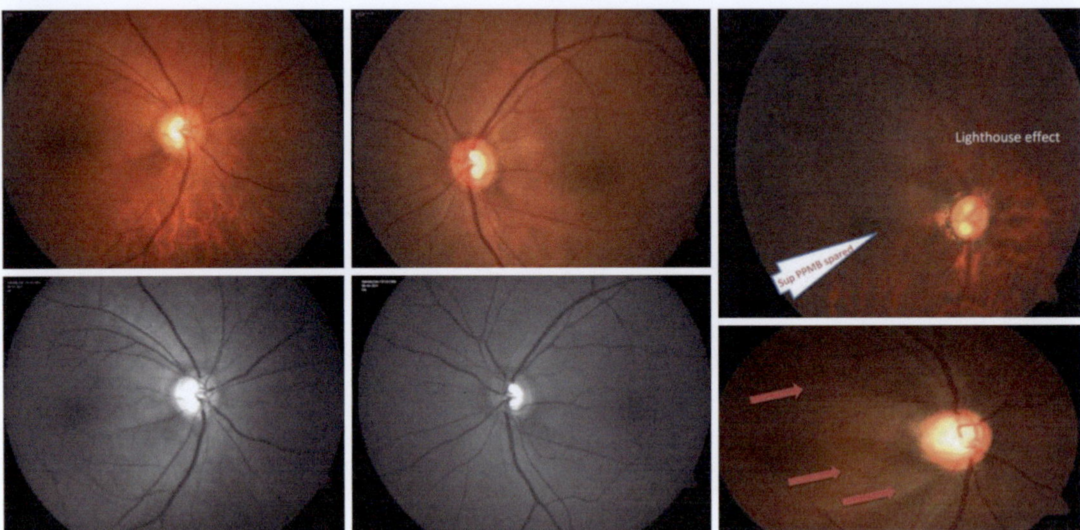

Fig. 22.5 Fundus images of patients with retinal nerve fiber layer defects. Note the focal or diffuse dark-colored and wedge-shaped defect with the prominence of the vessels that appear darker with contrasting background choroidal tessellation

22.4.5 Confocal Scanning Laser Ophthalmoscopy (CSLO)

The CSLO (Heidelberg Retina Tomograph, HRT, Heidelberg Engineering, Heidelberg, Germany) uses a laser to create high-resolution images of the optic nerve head and RNFL [3, 21, 22, 24–26]. It provides measurements of RNFL thickness across different regions of the optic nerve and a volumetric three-dimensional topography of the optic nerve.

Clinical application: CSLO could detect RNFL changes longer than 5 years before evident visual field damage in the ocular hypertension treatment study [22, 23]. The newer versions have expanded the normative database with improved accuracy and analytical tools that help discriminate between healthy and glaucomatous eyes with the glaucoma probability score (GPS).

Limitations: While most of the above imaging modalities help quantitate optic nerve parameters (and macula in OCT) and provide a means for objective monitoring of the disease progression, the progression algorithms using imaging modalities raise concerns about the utility of the structural information vis-a-vis the clinical treatment paradigms. These are also subject to errors by increased "RNFL thickness" reported by the instrument owing to surface gliosis and hence cannot be applied to patients with media opacities or high refractive errors [22–26]. These devices are not feasible for bedridden patients. Additionally, the information or analysis these machines applies only to people of age and race included in the normative database [6, 7, 19, 22, 23, 26]. Though these are widely reported to have utility in clinics, their sensitivity decreases as the specificity increases [26]. The discriminatory abilities using the best parameters of all these instruments have been reported to be similar and comparable to those of subjective evaluation by glaucoma experts. The structure–function correlation is better with the SD-OCT than with SLP or CSLO.

22.5 Artificial Intelligence-Based Early RNFL Defect Methodologies

The past decade has seen a huge increase in AI (Artificial Intelligence)-based tools for RNFL defect detection and quantification using fundus images and AI-based analysis of optic nerve head parameters [27–42].

Technology: Several early techniques were used to find RNFL defect patches in a fundus image without needing OCT imaging [30, 31]. However, these early methods failed to demarcate the RNFL defect boundary explicitly. Oh et al. suggested a new method for localizing the RNFL defect boundaries [32]. In their approach, the RNFL defect edges were first detected by incorporating Canny's operator, and then lines were fitted using the Hough transformation. The false positives were reduced using decision rules based on the average intensity, vertical length, and angular placement among the observed lines.

However, false positives are not entirely eliminated with this method. After removing the retinal blood vessels, Muramatsu et al. [33] utilized Gabor filtering for augmented detection of the RNFL defect. The mean and standard deviation of neighborhood intensities are used to locate the candidate RNFL defect boundary pixels. The ANN (Artificial Neural Network) classifier is then used to reduce the false positives. The primary drawback of this method is that it defines the relationship between the RNFL defect boundary and neighborhood intensities by utilizing several empirically established image processing-based factors.

Recent Machine and Deep Learning-Based RNFL Defect Detection. Several methods for detecting RNFL defects are proposed (Table 22.1). Some of these are mentioned below.

Table 22.1 Summary of all methods for retinal nerve fiber layer defect (RNFLD) analysis in fundus images

1	Recurrent neural network-based retinal nerve fiber layer defect detection in early glaucoma	Methodology	Recurrent neural network (RNN)
		Dataset	Dataset from LV Prasad Eye Institute, Bhubaneswar, India
		Model parameter	No. of hidden layers: 5 Input patch size: 11 × 11 pixels
		Performance measure	Euclidean distance
		Advantages	Accomplishes accurate RNFLD detection for the newly developed dataset.
2	Automated retinal nerve fiber layer defect detection using fundus imaging in glaucoma	Methodology	Random forest classifier
		Dataset	Dataset from LV Prasad Eye Institute, Bhubaneswar, India
		Model parameter	Input patch size: 11 × 11 pixels Cluster size: 0.4 times the maximum cluster size No. of trees: 30 Max. depth of tree: 20
		Performance measure	Sensitivity vs. false positives per image (FPI) and AUC
		Advantages	It measures the angular width of the RNFLD region, which can be used to track the progression of glaucoma
3	Deep convolutional neural network-based patch classification for retinal nerve fiber layer defect detection in early glaucoma	Methodology	CNN and random sample consensus (RANSAC)-based line fitting algorithm
		Dataset	Dataset from LV Prasad Eye Institute, Bhubaneswar, India
		Model parameter	Batch size: 64 No. of epochs: 100 Learning rate: 0.0001
		Performance measure	Sensitivity vs. false positives per image (FPI) and AUC
		Advantages	Learning of patch-based image features directly using a CNN, as opposed to the classifiers learning from manually created features

(continued)

Table 22.1 (continued)

4	A large-scale database and a CNN model for attention-based glaucoma detection	Methodology	AG-CNN
		Dataset	LAG and RIM -ONE
		Model parameter	Batch size: 8 Optimizer: Adam Learning rate: 0.00001
		Performance measure	Accuracy, sensitivity, specificity, AUC and F2-score
		Advantages	The deployed attention maps emphasize the most crucial regions for glaucoma detection
5	A novel adaptive weighted loss design in adversarial learning for retinal nerve fiber layer defect segmentation	Methodology	Conditional adversarial shuffle U-shaped network (CASU-Net)
		Dataset	Dataset from Beijing Tongren Hospital, China
		Model parameter	Learning rate: 0.0001 Optimizer: Adam Shuffle module, p: 0.8 Threshold: 0.5
		Performance measure	AUC, F-score, MAP, M-IoU, sensitivity, and specificity
		Advantages	It analyzes the overall geometric and pixel-level discrepancies between the RNFLD prediction result and ground truth
6	Retinal nerve fiber layer defect detection with position guidance	Methodology	Position-Guided Network (PGN)
		Dataset	Dataset from the Department of Ophthalmology, Peking Union Medical College Hospital, China
		Model parameter	Optimizer: Stochastic Gradient Descent Momentum: 0.9 Weight decay: 0.0001 Learning rate: 0.02 No. of epochs: 20
		Performance measure	Accuracy, specificity, sensitivity, and F1-score
		Advantages	The suggested method can be applied to other position-related diseases and is particularly useful for detecting RNFLD since it can sense position in both input data and the network
7	Retinal nerve fiber layer defect detection using machine learning on optic disc photograph	Methodology	Gaussian SVM, kNN, and ensemble RUSBoosted Trees
		Dataset	Dataset from King Chulalongkorn Memorial Hospital, Thailand
		Model parameter	–
		Performance measure	Sensitivity, specificity, accuracy, and AUC
		Advantages	This technique did not require complex image processing; therefore, it may be suited for image capture and classification using a mobile phone
8	Detecting retinal nerve fiber layer using gray level co-occurrence matrix and machine learning approach	Methodology	Random forest classifier
		Dataset	Private dataset
		Model parameter	
		Performance measure	Accuracy, precision, and recall
		Advantages	The method obtained excellent results on the used private dataset.

Table 22.1 (continued)

9	Active transfer learning network for retinal nerve fiber layer (RNFL) loss/ defect diagnosis from digital fundus images	Methodology	Active transfer learning-based framework with VGG16
		Dataset	Dataset from All-India Institute of Medical Sciences (AIIMS), New Delhi, India
		Model parameter	Dropout: 0.1 Activation function: ReLU Optimizer: Adam Learning rate: 0.000001 Batch size: 32 No. of epochs: 50
		Performance measure	Accuracy, AUC, sensitivity vs. false positive per image
		Advantages	Existing methods typically considers high-gradient regions with noisy information, which can distract an RNFL loss diagnosis system. This problem is resolved by the proposed method

22.5.1 Recurrent Neural Network (RNN)

It utilizes fundus images using a patch feature-driven recurrent neural network [34]. The essential steps in this method are (1) blood vessel inpainting and contrast enhancement; (2) finding the initial set of RNFL defect boundary pixels by examining concentric 1-D intensity profiles around the optic disc; and (3) determining the true boundary by using the recurrent neural networks (RNN) classifier. The mean Euclidean distance between the detected boundary pixels and the actual boundary is used to measure the accuracy of the method. The proposed method achieved high accuracy for the newly created fundus image datasets [34].

22.5.2 Contrast-Limited Adaptive Histogram Equalization (CLAHE) [35]

The one-dimensional intensity profiles derived from several concentric circles around the optic disc region are subjected to wavelet-based local minima analysis to identify the possible RNFL defect boundary pixels. In addition to Shannon and Tsallis entropy and intensity-based features, novel features like Cumulative Zero Count Local Binary Pattern (CZC-LBP) and Directional Differential Energy (DDE) have been developed. For precise RNFL defect localization, the feature vectors train the random forest classifier. The Random Sample Consensus (RANSAC) algorithm is used to line-fit the detected boundary pixels to calculate the RNFL defect's angular width. However, sometimes this method generates false-positive results in the presence of hemorrhages or dark pigmentation at the macula.

22.5.3 Deep Convolutional Neural Network (CNN)

In this approach, after blood vessel inpainting, contrast enhancement, and disc localization, a region of interest is first chosen around the optic disc [36]. The first step is to examine the one-dimensional intensity profiles on concentric circles surrounding the optic disc to obtain the initial set of RNFL defect boundary pixels. By creating a CNN that is trained on a large number of image patches, the true border pixels are retained. Unlike other methods, the proposed architecture directly learns the important features from many fundus image patches. Figure 22.6 shows the RNFL defect boundary detection outputs for multiple test fundus images.

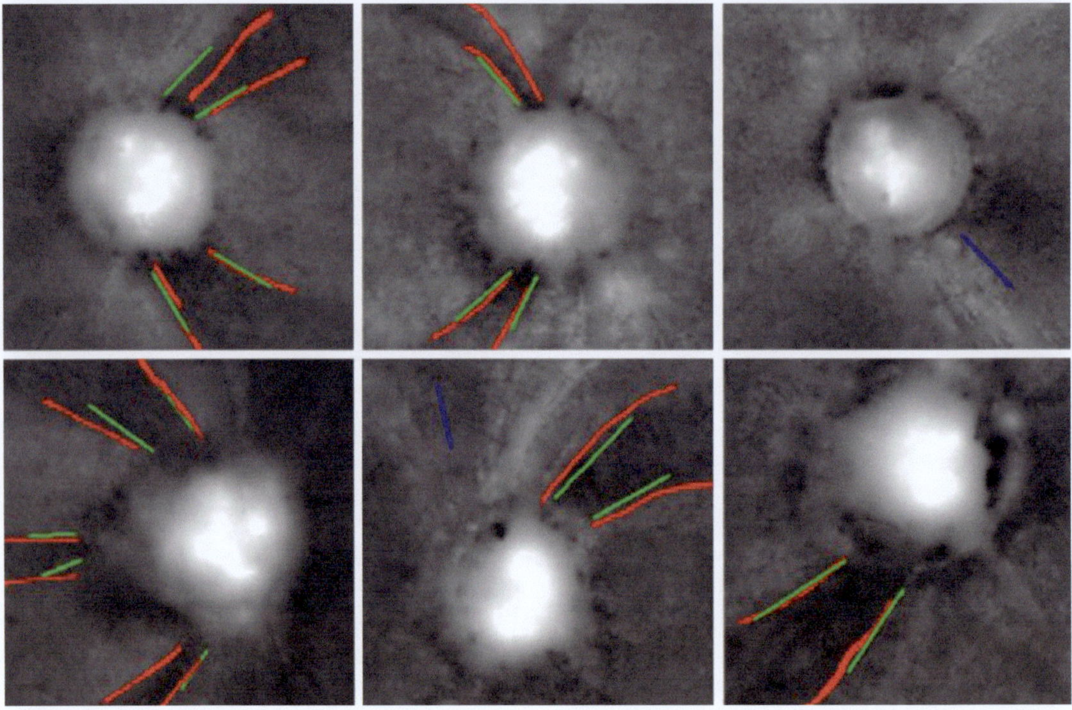

Fig. 22.6 RNFL defect boundary detection results (Red: ground truth, Green: truly detected RNFL defect (TP), Blue: falsely detected RNFLD (FP)) [36]

22.5.4 Attention-Based Convolutional Neural Network (AG-CNN) [37]

To build this dataset, the attention maps for 5824 of 11,760 fundus images were collected from ophthalmologists as part of a simulated eye-tracking experiment. Then, an attention prediction subnet, a pathological area localization subnet, and a glaucoma classification subnet were designed as part of a new AG-CNN structure. Under a weakly supervised training method, the attention prediction subnet predicted the attention maps to highlight the salient regions for glaucoma detection. Finally, tests were run on the existing RIM-ONE and the new LAG datasets. This technique effectively reduced high levels of redundancy in fundus images for glaucoma identification, improving the accuracy and reliability of glaucoma detection. The attention maps employed in building the AG-CNN were enhanced to highlight the most important area for glaucoma detection.

22.5.5 Conditional Adversarial Shuffle U-Shaped Network (CASU-Net) [38]

It comprises a generator and a discriminator to segment the RNFL defect region in the fundus images. This technique combines an adversarial loss and an adaptive weighted segmentation loss to provide a mixed loss for the generator. The CASU-Net increases the segmentation accuracy at the pixel level and brings the geometry of the target area closer to the ground truth. An adaptive weighted (AW) segmentation loss is created for the generator. The proposed network is focused on the pixel-level and overall geometry differences between the RNFL defect prediction output and the ground truth.

22.5.6 Alternative Methods

Some alternative methods are described below.

22.5.6.1 Position-Consistent Data Pre-processing and a Position-Guided Network [39]

It pre-processes input images using a constant coordinate system to give the absolution positions of pixels in fundus images. A location-guided network, which considers the physiological location and global dependencies of RNFL in fundus images, is created for sector classification. The suggested method senses positions in both the input data and the network; as a result, it is particularly useful for detecting RNFL defects and can be applied to other position-related disorders. Additionally, it deals with the noise labels that the RNFL defect experiences and which cause low generalization errors.

A machine learning classifier on the color information of the RNFL distinguishes between RNFL defects (d-RNFL) and intact RNFLs (i-RNFL) on the images of optic discs [40]. With this technique, a semi-circle drawn on the disc photos distinguishes the i-RNFL and d-RNFL. The RGB intensities and various color spaces of both profiles are gathered. Finally, five classifiers' classification efficacies are compared using fivefold cross-validation. The accuracy of a new feature was examined using a semi-automated technique that required an ophthalmologist to select a region and let the algorithm determine the presence/absence of the RNFL. This technique used simple image processing, making it potentially appropriate for screening when utilizing a mobile phone to take the image and identify it. However, the applicability of this technology may be constrained by variations among different fundus cameras.

22.6 Random Forest and Gray Level Co-occurrence Matrix (GLCM) [41]

The main steps for this method are: (1) defining the region of interest by segmentation with K-means clustering and segmenting the fundus image into 12 sub-sectors; (2) forming the area of feature extraction; (3) pre-processing by making the image grayscale; (4) feature extraction using gray level co-occurrence matrix; and (5) classification using random forest classifier. The authors reported high-performance measures using this technique on various fundus image datasets.

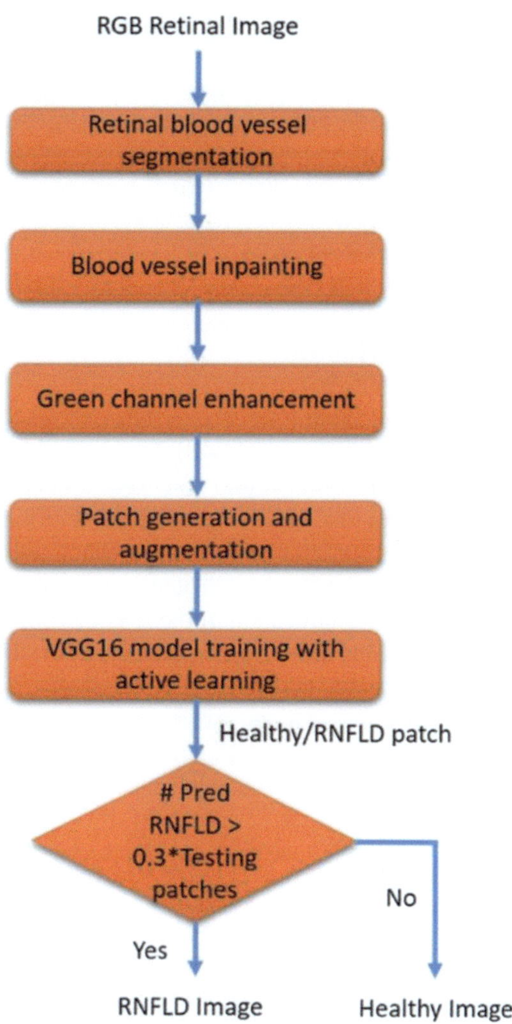

Fig. 22.7 Block diagram of the active transfer learning-based RNFL defect detection method [42]

Sharma et al. have proposed an automated method for the early diagnosis of RNFL loss using fundus images (Fig. 22.7) [42]. It aims to find RNFL defect patches using an active transfer learning-based framework (with the VGG16 pre-trained network as the backbone). In a limited labelled training scenario, RNFL loss diagnosis is accounted for by combining active and transfer learning. The patch-based sampling method performs RNFL loss detection for the entire image while using patches for the deep neural network. The current methods frequently consider targeted regions (high-gradient regions) but ultimately consider noisy information, which confuses an RNFL loss detection system. The suggested technique could resolve this issue.

22.7 Conclusion

Examining the retinal nerve fiber layer in glaucoma is of utmost importance in diagnosing and monitoring glaucoma progression. Recent developments in the imaging and quantification of the retinal nerve fiber layer using newer technologies and artificial intelligence enable automated detection and quantification of the RNFL, which will be a valuable asset if incorporated into existing fundus imaging systems. Such evolving paradigms will allow remote screening, diagnosis, and monitoring of glaucoma, which may be part of glaucoma telemedicine diagnostics.

Funding Hyderabad Eye Research Foundation, Hyderabad, India (2023).

Disclosure None.

References

1. Hood DC, Kardon RH. A framework for comparing structural and functional measures of glaucomatous damage. Prog Retin Eye Res. 2007;26:688–710.
2. Sommer A. Retinal nerve fiber layer. Am J Ophthalmol. 1995;120:665–7.
3. Sommer A, Katz J, Quigely HA, et al. Clinically detectable nerve fibre atrophy precedes the onset of glaucomatous field loss. Arch Ophthalmol. 1991;109:77–83.
4. Kotowski J, Wollstein G, Ishikawa H, Schuman JS. Imaging of the optic nerve and retinal nerve fiber layer: an essential part of glaucoma diagnosis and monitoring. Surv Ophthalmol. 2014;59:458–67.
5. Greenfield DS. Optic nerve and retinal nerve fiber layer analyzers in glaucoma. Curr Opin Ophthalmol. 2002;13:68–76.
6. Zangwill LM, Bowd C. Retinal nerve fiber layer analysis in the diagnosis of glaucoma. Curr Opin Ophthalmol. 2006;17:120–31.
7. Zangwill LM, Bowd C, Weinreb RN. Evaluating the optic disc and retinal nerve fiber layer in glaucoma. II: Optical image analysis. Semin Ophthalmol. 2000;15:206–20.
8. Radius RL, Anderson DR. The course of axons through the retina and optic nerve head. Arch Ophthalmol. 1979;97:1154–8.
9. Rao A, Mukherjee S. Anatomical attributes of the optic nerve head in eyes with Parafoveal scotoma in Normal tension glaucoma. PLoS One. 2014;9:e90554. https://doi.org/10.1371/journal.pone.0090554.
10. Curcio CA, Allen KA. Topography of ganglion cells in human retina. J Comp Neurol. 1990;300:5–25.
11. Rao A, Mukherjee S, Padhy D. Optic nerve head characteristics in eyes with papillomacular bundle defects in glaucoma. Int Ophthalmol. 2015;35:819–26.
12. Silver J, Sidman RL. A mechanism for the guidance and topographic patterning of retinal ganglion cell axons. J Comp Neurol. 1980;189:101–11.
13. Gierer A. Model for the retinotectal projection. Proc R Soc Lond B. 1983;218(1212):77–93.
14. Radius RL, de Bruin J. Anatomy of the retinal nerve fiber layer. Invest Ophthalmol Vis Sci. 1981;21:745–9.
15. Hood DC, Raza AS, de Moraes CGV, et al. The nature of macular damage in glaucoma as revealed by averaging optical coherence tomography data. Trans Vis Sci Tech. 2012;1:1–15. https://doi.org/10.1167/tvst.1.1.3.
16. Hood DC, Raza AS, de Moraes CG, et al. Glaucomatous damage of the macula. Prog Retin Eye Res. 2013;32:1–21.
17. Hoyt WF, Schlicke B, Eckelhoff RJ. Funduscopic appearance of a nerve fibre bundle defect. Br J Ophthalmol. 1972;56:577–83. https://doi.org/10.1136/bjo.56.8.577.
18. Airaksinen PJ, Nieminen H, Mustonen E. Retinal nerve fiber layer photography with a wide angle fundus camera. Acta Ophthalmol. 1982;60:362–8.
19. Quigley HA, Katz J, Derick RJ, et al. An evaluation of optic disc and nerve fiber layer examinations in monitoring progression of early glaucoma damage. Ophthalmology. 1992;99:19–28.
20. Hood DC, La Bruna S, Tsamis E, et al. Detecting glaucoma with only OCT: implications for the clinic, research, screening, and AI development. Prog Retin Eye Res. 2022;90:101052. https://doi.org/10.1016/j.preteyeres.2022.101052.
21. Weinreb RN. Evaluating the retinal nerve fiber layer in glaucoma with scanning laser polarimetry. Arch Ophthalmol. 1999;117:1403–6.
22. Harwerth RS, Anderson DR, Varma R, et al. Linking structure and function in glaucoma. Prog Retin Eye Res. 2010;29:249–71.
23. Caprioli J. Correlation of visual function with optic nerve and nerve fiber layer structure in glaucoma. Surv Ophthalmol. 1989;33(Suppl):319–30.
24. Weinreb RN, Zangwill L. Retinal nerve fiber layer evaluation in glaucoma. J Glaucoma. 2001;10(5 Suppl 1):S56–8.

25. Johnson CA, Cioffi GA, Liebmann JR, et al. The relationship between structural and functional alterations in glaucoma: a review. Semin Ophthalmol. 2000;15:221–33.
26. Fanihagh F, Kremmer S, Anastassiou C, et al. Optical coherence tomography, scanning laser polarimetry and confocal scanning laser ophthalmoscopy in retinal nerve fiber layer measurements of glaucoma patients. Open Ophthalmol J. 2015;9:41–8. https://doi.org/10.2174/1874364101509010041.
27. Saini C, Shen LQ, Pasquale LR, et al. Assessing surface shapes of the optic nerve head and Peripapillary retinal nerve fiber layer in glaucoma with artificial intelligence. Ophthalmol Sci. 2022;2:100161. https://doi.org/10.1016/j.xops.2022.100161.
28. Ramesh PV, Subramaniam T, Ray P, et al. Utilizing human intelligence in artificial intelligence for detecting glaucomatous fundus images using human-in-the-loop machine learning. Indian J Ophthalmol. 2022;70:1131–8.
29. Wang P, Shen J, Chang R, et al. Machine learning models for diagnosing glaucoma from retinal nerve fiber layer thickness maps. Ophthalmol Glaucoma. 2019;2:422–8.
30. Joshi GD, Sivaswamy J, Prashanth R, Krishnadas SR. Detection of peri-papillary atrophy and RNFL defect from retinal images. In: Lecture notes in computer science. Springer; 2012. p. 400–7.
31. Lamani D, Manjunath TC, Mahesh M, Nijagunarya YS. Early detection of glaucoma through retinal nerve fiber layer analysis using fractal dimension and texture feature. Int J Res Eng Technol. 2014;3:158–63.
32. Oh JE, Yang HK, Kim KG, Hwang JM. Automatic computer-aided diagnosis of retinal nerve fiber layer defects using fundus photographs in optic neuropathy CAD of RNFL defects in optic neuropathy. Invest Ophthalmol Vis Sci. 2015;56:2872–9.
33. Muramatsu C, Hayashi Y, Sawada A, et al. Detection of retinal nerve fiber layer defects on retinal fundus images for early diagnosis of glaucoma. J Biomed Optics. 2010;15:160–216.
34. Panda R, Puhan NB, Rao A, et al. Recurrent neural network based retinal nerve fiber layer defect detection in early glaucoma. In: IEEE international symposium biomedical imaging. 2017. p. 692–95.
35. Panda R, Puhan NB, Rao A, et al. Automated retinal nerve fiber layer defect detection using fundus imaging in glaucoma. Comp Med Imag Graph. 2018;66:56–65.
36. Panda R, Puhan NB, Rao A, et al. Deep convolutional neural network based patch classification for retinal nerve fiber layer defect detection in early glaucoma. J Med Imag. 2018;5:044003–8. https://doi.org/10.1117/1.JMI.5.4.044003.
37. Li L, Liu H, Li Y, et al. A large-scale database and a CNN model for attention-based glaucoma detection. IEEE Trans on Med Imag. 2020;39:413–24.
38. Lu S, Hu M, Li R, Xu Y. A novel adaptive weighted loss design in adversarial learning for retinal nerve fiber layer defect segmentation. IEEE Access. 2020;8:132348–59. https://doi.org/10.1109/ACCESS.2020.30094.
39. Ding F, Yang G, Ding D, Cheng G. Retinal nerve fiber layer defect detection with position guidance. In: MICCAI 2020: medical image computing and computer assisted intervention—MICCAI 2020. 2020. p. 745–54.
40. Manassakorn K, Khamwan D, Owasirikul R, et al. Retinal nerve fiber layer defect detection using machine learning on optic disc photograph. In: 2021 IEEE EMBS international conference on biomedical and health informatics (BHI). 2021. p. 1–4.
41. Septiarini H, Hamdani E, Setyaningsih S, et al. Detecting retinal nerve fiber layer using gray level co-occurrence matrix and machine learning approach. In: 2022 International Conference on Information Technology Research and Innovation (ICITRI). 2022. p. 173–78.
42. Sharma M, Agrawal S, Roy D, Gupta V. Active transfer learning network for retinal nerve fiber layer (RNFL) loss/defect diagnosis from digital fundus images. Image Vis Comput. 2022:1–10.

23 Ultrasound Biomicroscopy

Mona Khurana and Vedvati Hemant Albal

23.1 Introduction

The term "ultrasound biomicroscopy" (UBM) was coined due to its similarity to optical biomicroscopy, that is, observing living tissues at a microscopic resolution. It utilizes ultrasound frequencies in the 40–100 MHz range to allow non-invasive in vivo examinations of anterior segment structures in the eye [1–5]. Images produced by UBM have a resolution similar to those of a low-power light microscope [3]. UBM can help in imaging structures posterior to the iris pigment epithelium, which does not allow light to pass through but allows sound to pass through. This makes UBM an investigation of choice to assess the posterior chamber structures, including the lens zonules, ciliary body, and anterior choroid, compared to anterior segment optical coherence tomography (AS-OCT) (Table 23.1). UBM has multiple clinical applications, particularly in evaluating corneal diseases, glaucoma, anterior segment tumors, and trauma [4].

Table 23.1 Comparison of Ultrasound Biomicroscopy and Anterior Segment-Optical Coherence Tomography

Features	Ultrasound biomicroscopy (UBM)	Anterior segment optical coherence tomography (AS-OCT)
Operating system	Ultrasound waves	Near-infrared light
Resolution	Axial: 20–25 μm Lateral: 40–50 μm	Axial: 5–10 μm Lateral: 15–25 μm
Tissue penetration	4–5 mm	3–6 mm
Procedure	Contact	Non-contact
Acquisition time	Long (approximately 15 minutes) [6]	Fast (up to 50,000 A-scans/s) [7]
Ocular tissue	Cornea: It gives an approximate measurement of corneal thickness	Cornea: Excellent visualization of all layers of cornea and reliable measure of corneal thickness
	Visualization of the ciliary body, posterior chamber, lens, and zonules	Poor visualization of the ciliary body and posterior chamber Partial visualization of the lens
Specific advantage	Imaging non-pigmented iris tumors, ciliary body neoplasm	Imaging ocular surface squamous neoplasia, cornea

M. Khurana (✉) · V. H. Albal
Shri Nathmal Singhvi Jadhavbhai Glaucoma Services, Sankara Nethralaya, Medical Research Foundation, Chennai, India

T. Das, P. Satgunam (eds.), *Ophthalmic Diagnostics*, https://doi.org/10.1007/978-981-97-0138-4_23

23.2 History

The concept of acoustic imaging was introduced by Marmor, who imaged sections of the retina and iris in 1977 [8]. Pavlin et al. conducted in vitro studies to assess the use of high-frequency ultrasound (50–100 MHz) for ophthalmic imaging and developed the first commercial instrument for clinical use in 1989. UBM uses a 50 MHz transducer to provide a good balance between resolution and depth of tissue penetration [1]. The 50 MHz probe has a resolution of 37 μm and a 4–5 mm depth of tissue penetration [1].

23.3 Technology

Ultrasound consists of acoustic waves generated by oscillating particles within a medium. Ophthalmic ultrasound imaging utilizes higher frequencies, 8–80 MHz, compared to other diagnostic medical ultrasounds (2–6 MHz). This provides increased resolution to evaluate ocular structures which are more superficial [4]. As the frequency of ultrasound increases, the acoustic waves are more strongly attenuated, limiting the depth of penetration. Higher frequencies (7–10 MHz) can be used to image smaller parts of the body, such as the eye, where a penetration of 4–5 cm is sufficient [1]. The higher the frequency, the higher the resolution.

The three tissue properties important in ultrasound imaging are attenuation, reflectivity, and the speed of sound. *Attenuation* is any interaction that removes energy from the ultrasound beam. It can be divided into absorption and reflectivity [1]. The absorbed energy is converted to thermal energy. *Reflectivity* is subdivided into specular and scatter components.

Th*e speed of ultrasound* depends on the tissue composition. Given their high water content, the speed of sound in soft tissues is similar to that in water. The highest speed of ultrasound is in the sclera (1622 m/s), and comparatively lower speeds are seen in the ciliary muscle (1554 m/s) and iris (1542 m/s) [1, 9]. An ideal material with uniform elastic properties will allow an ultrasound wave to propagate undisturbed, and any material with differing elastic properties will partly transmit and partly reflect the wave. Tissues have structures that reflect ultrasound, for example, organ boundaries, blood vessels, and cellular and intracellular structures. When the difference in the tissue interface is larger than the ultrasound wavelength, the reflection is specular, like a partially reflecting mirror. When the interface is similar to or smaller than the ultrasound wavelength, the reflected wave is called "scatter" [1].

23.3.1 Scanner Design

Commercially available machines use frequencies of 35 and 50 MHz, whereas higher frequency probes (80 MHz) are used to image the cornea, ocular surface, and anterior chamber [3], with a 2 mm penetration depth. The transducer is excited by a monocycle high voltage pulse of 40–100 MHz. It is linearly moved over the imaging field. Using a time-gain circuit, the transducer receives a reflected radiofrequency signal from the tissues, further amplified in proportion to the depth at which it originated. This compensates for the attenuation of the ultrasound beam occurring in deeper tissues.

After processing the received signal to enhance low-level signals, a section of the detected signal corresponding to the focal zone is digitized by a high-speed scan converter, and the real-time image is displayed on a video monitor [1, 2].

23.3.2 Transducers

High-resolution images can be obtained using ultrasound with a higher frequency and shorter focal length. However, the penetration is poor, and deeper structures are not imaged clearly. Imaging smaller tissues requires high-frequency ultrasound, which in turn requires high-frequency transducers. Thus, the transducer is an important component in an ultrasound imaging system responsible for image resolution, contrast, and sensitivity. The transducer transforms electrical energy to acoustic energy and back. It contains active piezoelectric material that vibrates at the scanner materials' resonant frequency [1]. The transducer is mounted on the backing. There is an acoustic matching layer and an electric matching circuit.

The range of depth over which the ultrasound beam remains reasonably well focused is called the depth of field. The focusing characteristics of the transducer are selected such that the tissue of interest lies within the depth of field [1]. The quality of the image depends upon the transducer, the frequency of ultrasound, f-number (ratio of the focal length to the transducer diameter), and length of the pulse. The axial resolution depends upon the speed of sound in the tissue and the sound speed constant used in the transducer. The lateral resolution is determined by the distribution of ultrasound in the field of the transducer.

23.3.3 Scan Acquisition

The transducer has an oscillating probe without a cover. A water bath is required to acquire scans. A monocycle high voltage pulse excites the transducer. A 40–100 MHz ultrasound pulse is transmitted to the scanned tissue. The transducer is moved along the image field (4–5 mm). It collects radiofrequency data at 512 equally spaced lines (8 μm apart). This signal is amplified nonlinearly in proportion to its depth of origin based on the time-gain compensation. Signals from deeper structures with more attenuation are enhanced more than those from superficial structures. A scan is produced from the detected signal, converted to a digital format, and transferred to a high-speed scan converter. The image is displayed on a video monitor at 5–10 frames per second and stored. The transducer direction can be assessed by looking at the image on the screen, and the probe can be maneuvered to scan different tissue sections. Images are stored electronically on an attached computer with compatible software.

23.4 Technique

UBM is performed under topical anesthesia with the patient in a reclining or supine position. A fluid-immersion technique is used. Specially designed scleral shells are available in various sizes to hold the eyelids apart and serve as a reservoir for the coupling agent. Water (distilled water) is effective as a coupling agent. The fluid level should be maintained throughout the scanning procedure. Air bubbles should be avoided as air is a poor medium for sound transmission. Methylcellulose (1%), an alternative coupling agent, has low sound attenuation and greater viscosity, thus minimizing fluid loss during the procedure [1, 4]. The UBM probe does not have a membrane over the probe tip, as it would cause significant sound attenuation at the higher frequencies used. Thus, care must be taken to avoid touching the cornea with the probe (Fig. 23.1).

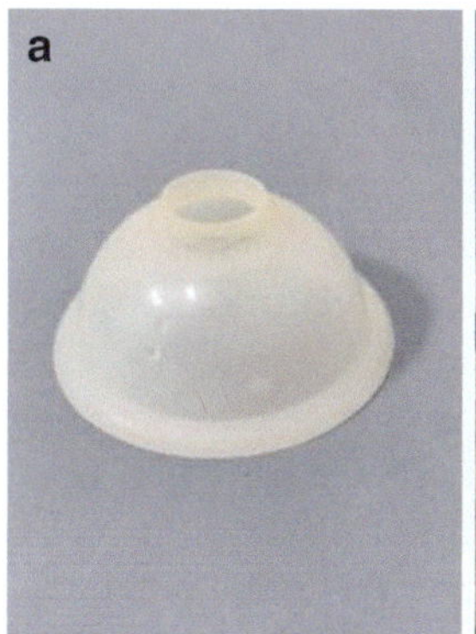

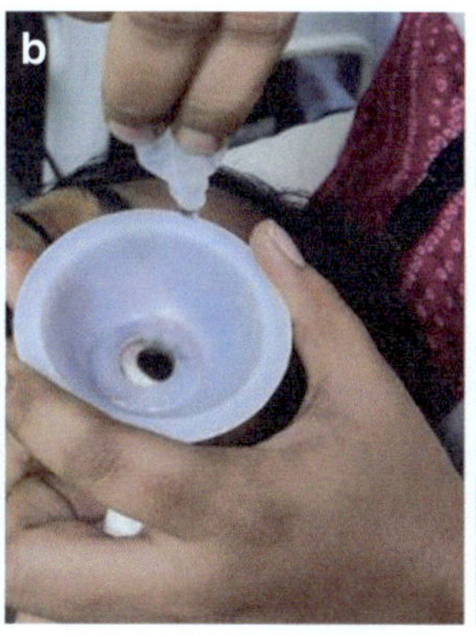

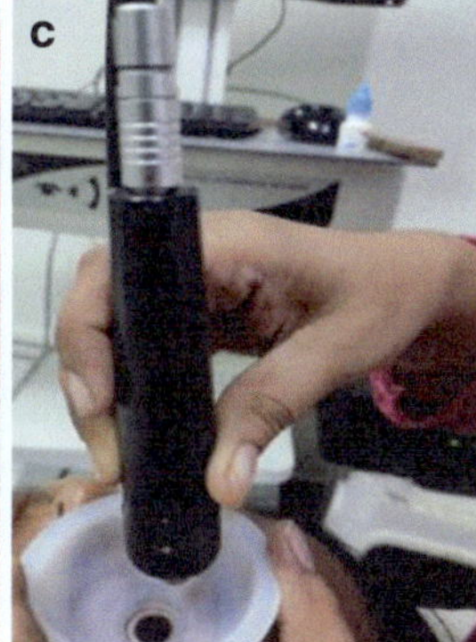

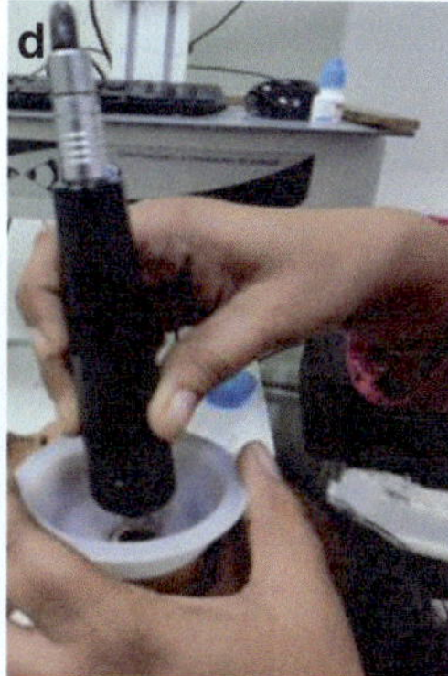

Fig. 23.1 (**a**) Scleral shell used during ultrasound biomicroscopy (UBM); (**b**) The scleral shell is positioned with the patient in a reclining position. The scleral shell is placed over the eye under topical anesthesia and is filled with coupling fluid; (**c**) UBM probe with the marker; (**d**) UBM scan is acquired by dipping the oscillating tip of the probe in the scleral shell filled with coupling fluid. The acquired scans are displayed and stored in the accompanying computer

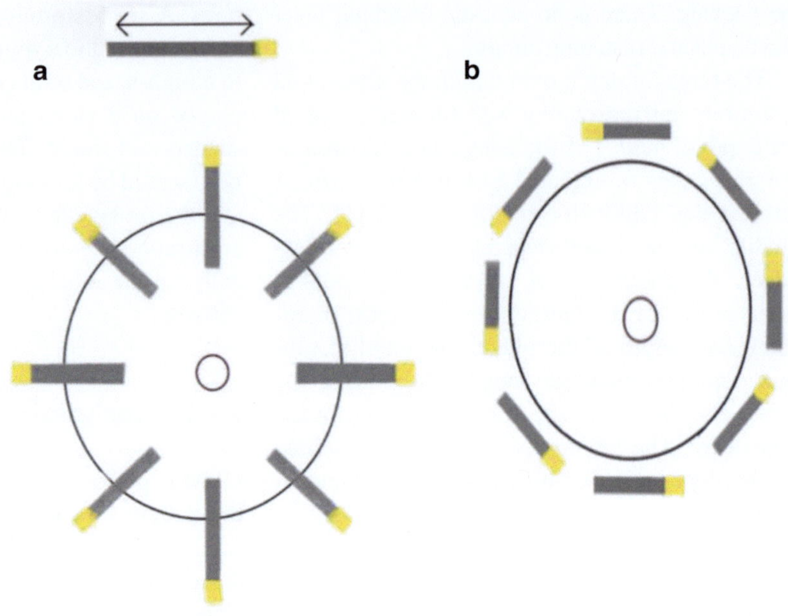

Fig. 23.2 A diagrammatic representation of probe position during UBM scanning. The highlighted yellow part shows the mark on the probe (**a**) radial scan (**b**) transverse scan

Table 23.2 Scan types in UBM

Type	Technique	Remark
Axial	Probe is placed perpendicular to the corneal surface over the pupil – Horizontal scan: marker is oriented nasally – Vertical scan: marker is oriented superiorly	Good for assessing – anterior chamber depth – orientation of displaced or tilted intraocular lenses
Radial (longitudinal)	Probe is placed perpendicular to the limbus at each clock hour	It is the most common scan used in UBM examinations. Good for imaging the following: – anterior chamber angle, identification of the scleral spur, ciliary body – anterior to posterior extent of mass lesions of the iris and ciliary body
Transverse	Probe placed parallel to the limbus – Central scan: over the cornea and iris – Peripheral scan: over the limbus	Ideal for the evaluation of: – lateral extent of iris and ciliary body masses – ciliary processes

ClearScan® is a single-use UBM probe tip cover consisting of a fine acoustically invisible film that can be filled with water. It eliminates the chances of ocular injury with the moving transducer and the need for a scleral shell [10]. This allows the scan to be performed in a sitting or reclining position.

To perform the examination, the probe is placed directly over the ocular structures to be imaged. The penetration of the ultrasound through the skin is not as good as through the conjunctiva, as the keratinized epithelium attenuates the ultrasound beam.

The cornea, iris, and crystalline lens can be imaged in any plane. Radially orientated images through the limbus provide a cross-sectional view of the anterior chamber angle (Fig. 23.2, Table 23.2). To image the conjunctiva, anterior sclera, ciliary body, and ora, the patient is asked to look 180° away from the clock hour of interest. Images are brightest when the probe is perpendicular to the surface examined, and the reflected sound is returned directly to the transducer [1].

The top of the UBM display screen corresponds to the front of the transducer. A marker along the probe's side helps in the orientation of

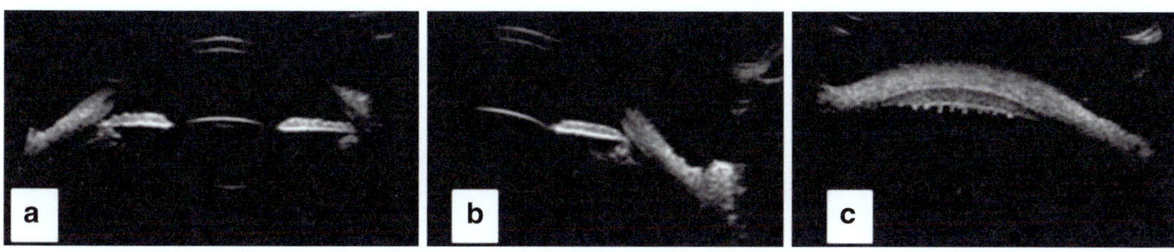

Fig. 23.3 Types of scans in UBM. Left (**a**): an axial scan. Middle (**b**): longitudinal (radial) scan showing the angle of the anterior chamber. Right (**c**): transverse scan showing the ciliary processes

transducer movement and the image formed. The far left of the display screen corresponds to the area toward the marker, and the far right of the display screen corresponds to the area away from the marker [4]. In the image, structures at the top of the display screen are closest to the probe tip, and those at the bottom are the farthest (Fig. 23.2). Measurements within the scanned area can be carried out with the software provided with the machine (Fig. 23.3) [1].

23.5 Clinical Applications of Ultrasound Biomicroscopy

UBM is useful in assessing the anterior segment, with details of the anatomical structure, pathology, and pathophysiology of various ocular diseases. UBM is contraindicated in penetrating ocular trauma. Here, we describe the clinical application of UBM in diagnosing and managing different ocular conditions.

23.5.1 Ocular Surface

UBM helps identify the extent of ocular surface tumors [11], invasion of adjacent structures, and the posterior limit. It is useful in imaging in the presence of corneal opacities and pigmented lesions (Figs. 23.4 and 23.5).

23.5.2 Cornea

In UBM, the corneal epithelium has a smooth reflection; Bowman's membrane and Descemet's membrane-endothelial layer are highly reflective lines with a hypoechoic stroma in between. UBM helps in imaging corneal edema (microcystic and stromal) and Descemet's membrane detachment in the presence of corneal haze or opacity. The anterior segment status in eyes with corneal opacity can be assessed for any iridocorneal touch, anterior synechiae, and iridolenticular contact (Fig. 23.6).

23.5.3 Sclera

UBM can be useful in imaging the sclera anterior to the equator. In episcleritis, a localized hyperreflective thickened area is seen in the episcleral tissue with normal reflectivity of the scleral stroma. In scleritis, both episcleral and scleral stroma appear hyperechoic.

23.5.4 Lens and Zonules

1. Normal zonules appear as medium reflective lines extending from the ciliary processes to the lens margin [9, 10]. UBM helps in identifying areas of zonular abnormalities. Increased lenticular sphericity is seen in areas of zonular abnormality. Direct signs of zonular abnormality include the absence of zonular fibers, increased zonular fiber length, and the presence of zonular remnants on the lens capsule. Ciliary body flattening and increased lens–ciliary body distance can also be seen (Fig. 23.7) [11].
2. **Position of the intraocular lens**: UBM can detect the position of the posterior chamber intraocular lens (IOL) in eyes with pseudophakic pigment dispersion and uveitis glau-

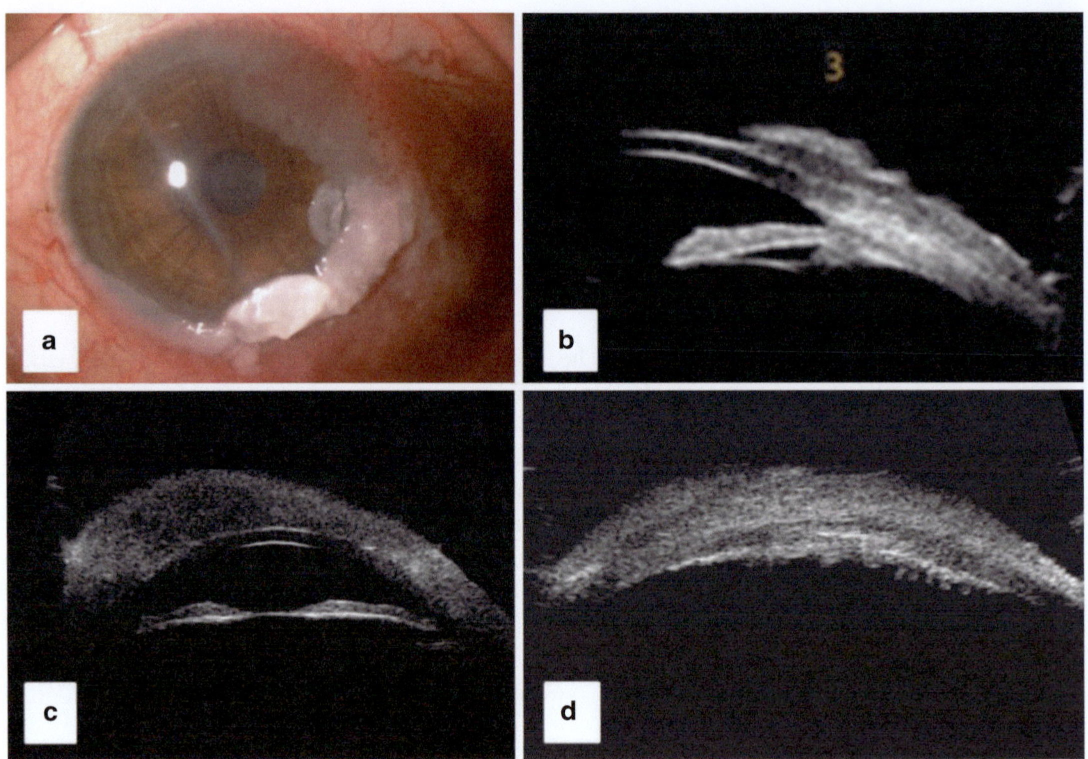

Fig. 23.4 (**a**) A diffuse slit lamp photograph of ocular surface squamous neoplasia. It is seen as a mass lesion extending from the cornea to the conjunctiva across the limbus without any episcleral or scleral involvement. (**b**–**d**) are UBM images of ocular surface neoplasia without underlying corneal involvement

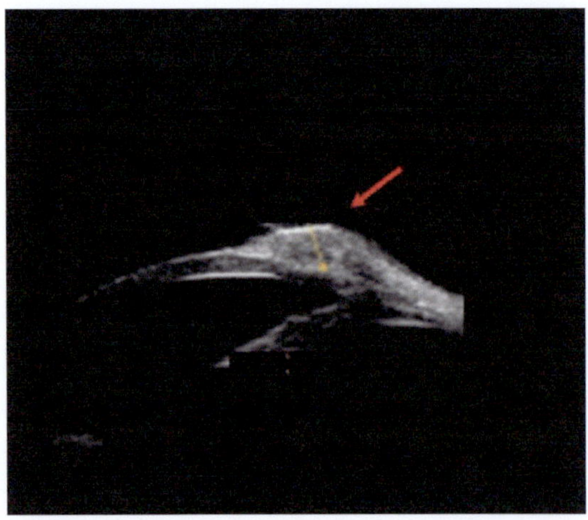

Fig. 23.5 A UBM image of a limbal dermoid. The lesion is well-defined without any corneal involvement

coma hyphema (UGH) syndrome. A single-piece square edge or plate-haptic IOL placed in the ciliary sulcus can cause pigment dispersion. UBM helps detect the position of the posterior chamber IOL (Fig. 23.8) [4]. UBM can localize the haptic position in eyes with UGH syndrome, where the haptics erode the iris and ciliary process and cause uveitis, glaucoma, and hyphema [4].

3. **Microphakia and spherophakia**: The equatorial and anterior-posterior diameter of the crystalline lens can be determined with UBM in eyes with microspherophakia and spherophakia (Fig. 23.8).
4. **Trauma to lens**: Anterior and posterior capsule status can be determined in traumatic cataract. Position of the crystalline lens and zonular status can be imaged [12, 13] (Fig. 23.8).

23.5.5 Glaucoma

UBM provides qualitative and quantitative information regarding primary and secondary glaucoma pathophysiology. It is useful in imag-

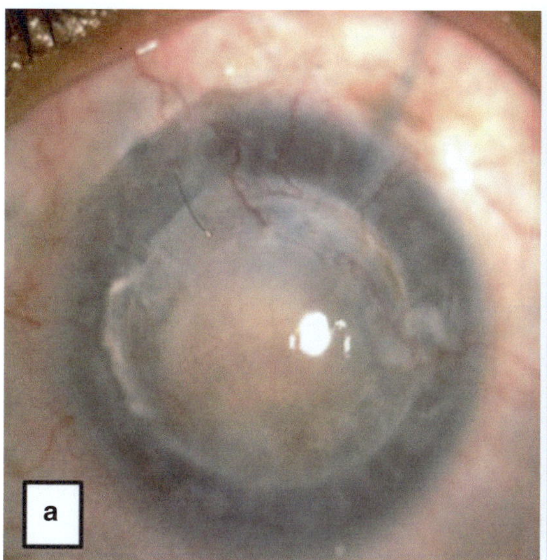

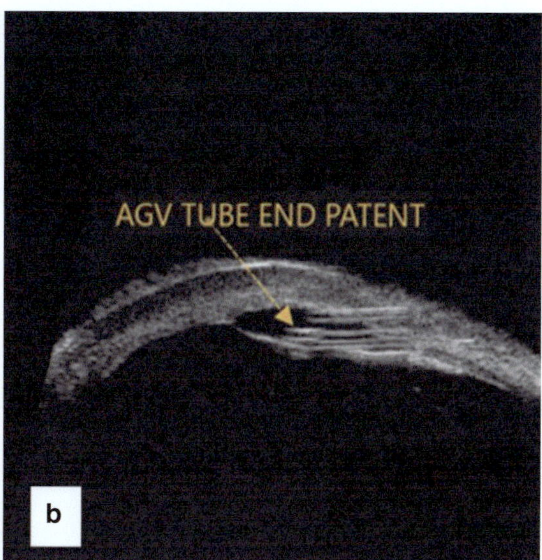

Fig. 23.6 (**a**) A diffuse slit lamp photograph of an eye with a failed graft following penetrating keratoplasty, secondary angle closure glaucoma, and Ahmed glaucoma valve (AGV) implantation. (**b**) UBM image of the same eye shows a patent AGV tube, which is not visible clinically. Iridocorneal adhesions [anterior synechiae] can also be appreciated

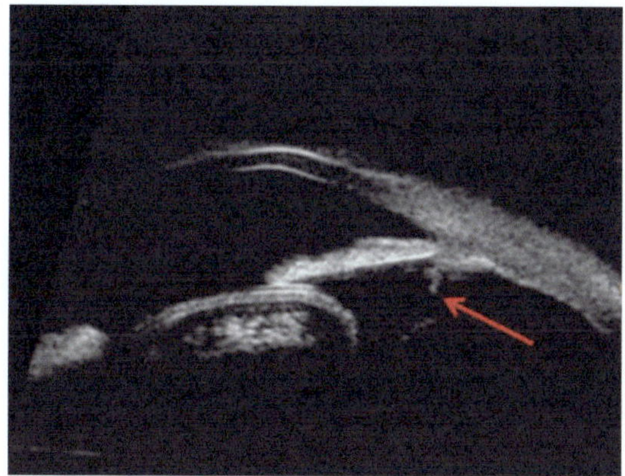

Fig. 23.7 A UBM image illustrating zonular dehiscence (arrow) in an eye with blunt trauma and subluxation of a cataractous crystalline lens. The rounding of the lens edge is seen due to a lack of zonular support

ing the angle of the anterior chamber, iris and lens configuration, and ciliary body, helping diagnose and plan the management [1, 4, 6, 14–22].

23.5.5.1 Angle Closure Disease

UBM helps identify and understand the various mechanisms of angle closure disease because it can image the ciliary body and lens. Identification of the scleral spur as a landmark is important in assessing the angle morphology. The various mechanisms of angle closure are (Fig. 23.9) as follows:

(a) **Lens iris diaphragm configuration**: A convex iris configuration, shallow anterior chamber, and iridotrabecular contact are seen in angle closure disease due to a relative pupillary block (Fig. 23.9).

(b) **Plateau iris configuration**: An anteriorly directed ciliary processes pushing the peripheral iris and causing iridotrabecular contact is present (Fig. 23.9) [1–4, 15]. The ciliary sulcus is absent, the iris root is short or thick, and a steep iris root from its point of insertion followed by a downward angulation is present along with a flat iris plane. The central anterior chamber depth is normal.

(c) **Pseudoplateau iris with cysts of iris and ciliary body epithelium**: On UBM, these multiple neuroepithelial cysts of the ciliary body have a well-delineated wall without a solid component. They push the peripheral iris leading to iridotrabecular contact (Fig. 23.9) [1–4, 16].

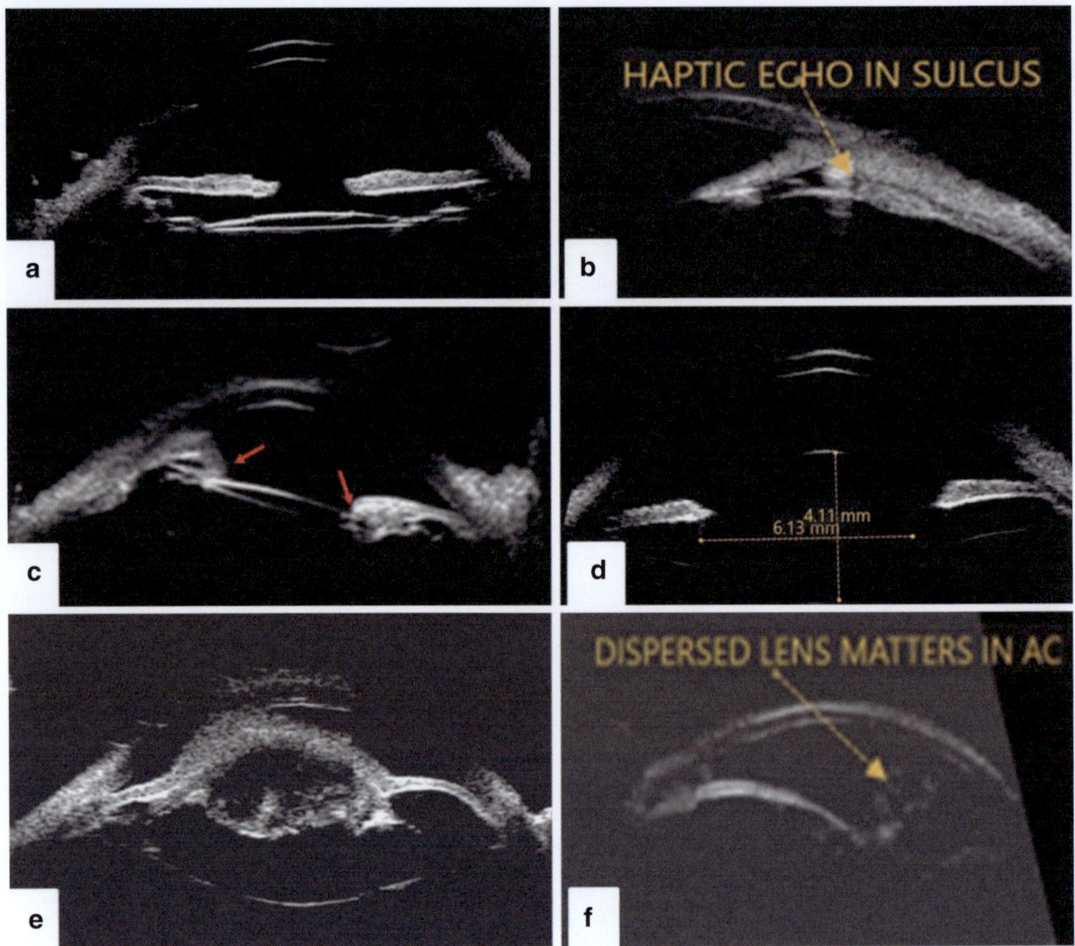

Fig. 23.8 Top left (**a**): an axial UBM image of a normal pseudophakic eye showing a posterior chamber intraocular lens in the capsular bag. The haptic's echo in the bag is visible. Top right (**b**): a UBM image showing a posterior chamber intraocular lens (IOL) with one haptic placed in the ciliary sulcus (arrow). Middle left (**c**): a UBM image of a pseudophakic eye showing an anteriorly tilted posterior chamber IOL touching the iris (arrow) with the formation of posterior synechiae. Middle right (**d**): an axial UBM scan of an eye with microspherophakia and angle closure disease. Bottom left (**e**): an axial UBM image of an eye of a child with a traumatic cataract with a ruptured anterior capsule. Bottom right (**f**): longitudinal UBM images of the eye of a child with blunt trauma, corneal scar, and secondary glaucoma taken during examination under anesthesia. Posterior synechiae with iris bombe were present. A ruptured anterior lens capsule with lens matter in the anterior chamber was demonstrated (arrow)

(d) **Phacomorphic glaucoma**: An intumescent cataract and an increased anteroposterior lens thickness result in a pupillary block with subsequent angle closure (Fig. 23.9). It can also occur in eyes with an anteriorly subluxated lens or zonular laxity or loss, which can be imaged with UBM.

(e) **Aqueous misdirection syndrome**: The UBM shows an anterior rotation of ciliary processes, iridotrabecular contact and shallow central and peripheral anterior chamber depth (Fig. 23.9) [1–4].

(f) **Supraciliary effusions**: In eyes with secondary angle closure due to a push mechanism, UBM helps in identifying supraciliary effusions which may not be clinically detectable.

23.5.5.2 Secondary Open-Angle Glaucoma

UBM is useful in the following situations in secondary open-angle glaucoma

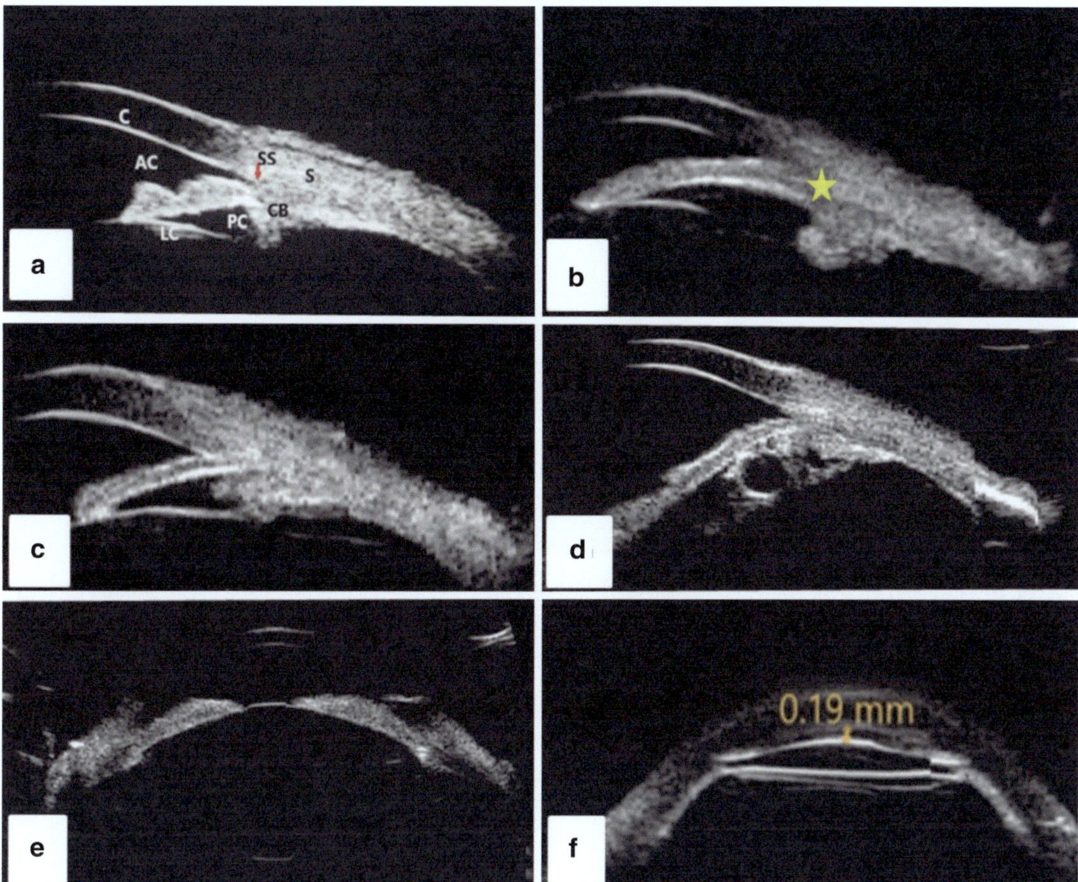

Fig. 23.9 Top: left (**a**): structures of the anterior chamber angle and anterior segment as seen on UBM. C = cornea, S = sclera, SS = scleral spur (scleral spur is where the trabecular meshwork meets the ciliary body and scleral interface; a change in curvature is seen), LC=lens capsule, CB = ciliary body, AC = anterior chamber, PC = posterior chamber. Top right (**b**): a UBM image of a longitudinal scan of an eye with primary angle closure glaucoma showing iridotrabecular contact (asterix) due to pupillary block indicated by the bowing of the iris. Middle left (**c**): a UBM image of a longitudinal scan of an eye with plateau iris configuration showing iridotrabecular contact, absence of a ciliary sulcus, and an anteriorly placed ciliary process. Middle right (**d**): a UBM image of a longitudinal scan of an eye with ciliary body cysts showing iridotrabecular contact, absence of a ciliary sulcus, and a ciliary body cyst. Bottom left (**e**): a UBM image of a case of phacomorphic glaucoma. The intumescent cataractous lens is pushing the iris anteriorly, causing angle closure. An increase in the lens thickness (anterior-posterior diameter) with iridolenticular contact and a shallow anterior chamber is present. Bottom right (**f**): a UBM image of an axial scan in an eye with aqueous misdirection (malignant glaucoma) showing uniform shallowing of the anterior chamber and anteriorly rotated ciliary processes due to a push mechanism in a pseudophakic eye. The anterior chamber depth is 0.19 mm

(a) **Pigment dispersion syndrome (PDS) and pigmentary glaucoma (PG)**: In eyes with PDS and PG, a deep anterior chamber with posterior bowing of the mid-peripheral iris, causing a reverse pupillary block is seen (Fig. 23.10). The posterior insertion of the iris root and iris-zonular apposition are responsible for the pigment dispersion from the posterior pigmented epithelium of the iris can be imaged [19].

(b) **Angle recession**: Deepening of the angle recess and a tear of the ciliary processes from the scleral spur can be detected (Fig. 23.10).

(c) **Pseudoexfoliation (PXF)**: Zonular abnormality and lens position can be imaged in patients with PXF [14]. The PXF material can be seen on the zonules and peripheral lens capsule.

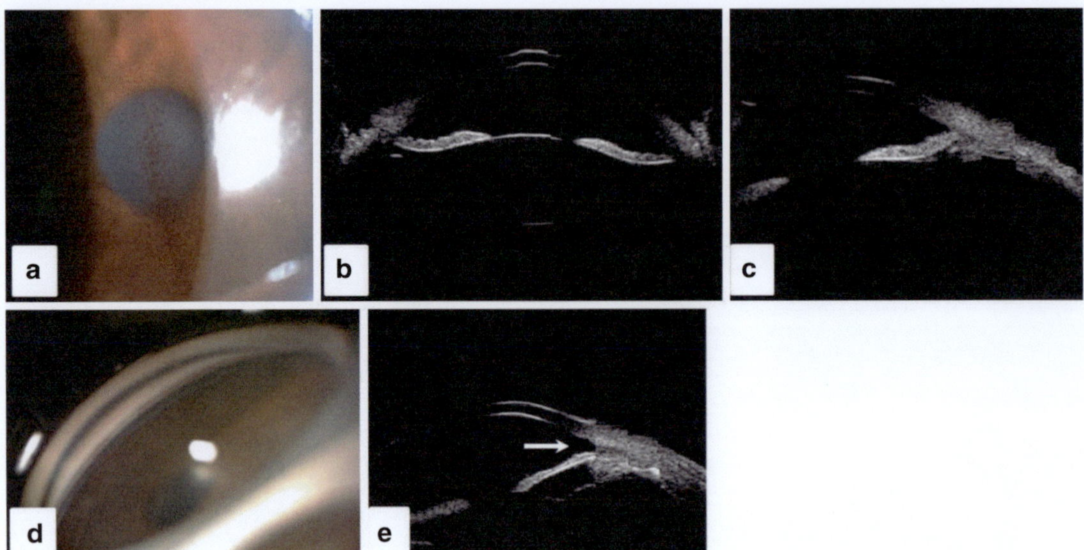

Fig. 23.10 Top left (**a**): a slit lamp photograph of an eye with pigment dispersion syndrome (PDS) showing a Krukenberg's spindle. Top right (**b**): a UBM axial image of the eye with PDS showing posterior bowing of mid-peripheral iris. Bottom left (**c**): a UBM image of an eye with PDS showing iridozonular contact. Bottom right (**d**): a gonioscopic photograph showing angle recession in a closed globe injury and angle recession glaucoma. Bottom left (**e**): a UBM longitudinal angle scan in an eye with blunt trauma demonstrating angle recession (arrow)

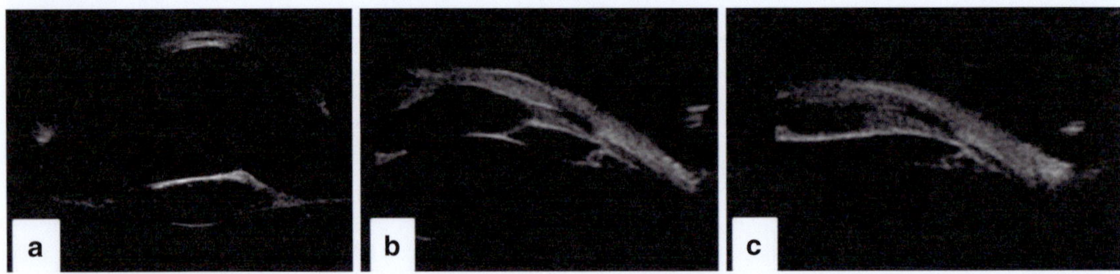

Fig. 23.11 Left (**a**): a UBM image of an eye of a child with uveitic glaucoma with buphthalmos. The UBM image shows anterior synechiae with the iris plastered to the cornea. Middle (**b**) and right (**c**) UBM images of an eye with anterior segment dysgenesis in a child with corneal opacity and congenital glaucoma; the iris is seen to be adherent to the cornea

(d) **Childhood glaucoma**: In childhood glaucoma with corneal haze or opacity, UBM can image the anterior segment (Fig. 23.11). UBM is helpful in imaging eyes and understanding the pathophysiology of primary and secondary childhood glaucoma [20]. The lens status can also be assessed in eyes with spherophakia (Fig. 23.11).

23.5.5.2.1 Quantitative Measurements

Quantitative measurements of the angle of the anterior chamber, anterior chamber, lens, and ciliary body can be performed (Fig. 23.12, Table 23.3). Pavlin described certain parameters, taking the scleral spur as the reference point [21].

23.5.5.2.2 Glaucoma Surgery

(a) **Glaucoma drainage devices (GDDs)**: UBM can localize the position of tube of GDDs in the anterior chamber (Fig. 23.13), ciliary sulcus, or vitreous cavity (Fig. 23.13). It can also help assess tube patency and identify the cause of the blockage, such as by the iris or

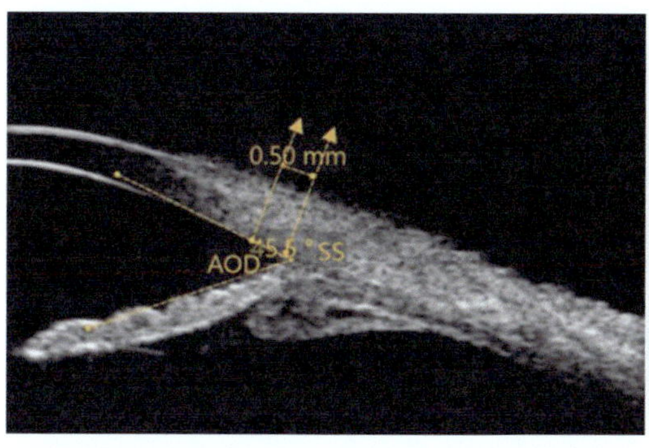

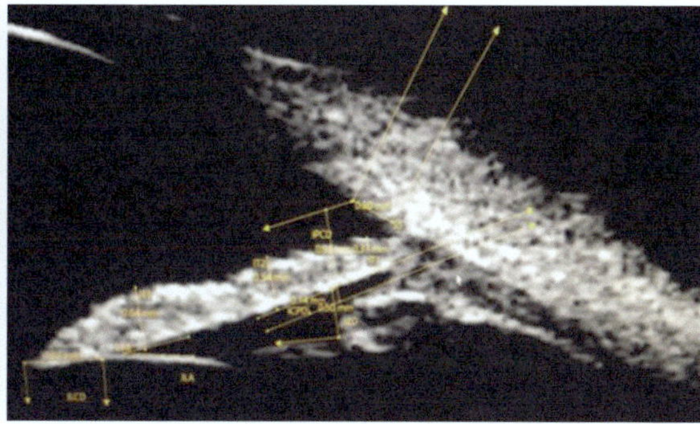

Fig. 23.12 Left: UBM scans illustrating the quantitative measurements of the anterior chamber angle described in Table 23.3. Right: UBM scans illustrating the quantitative measurements of the anterior chamber (lens thickness and anterior chamber depth) and the lens vault

Table 23.3 Quantitative measurements of the anterior chamber using UBM

Quantitative parameters	Description
Angle opening distance (AOD) – 500 – 750	Measured perpendicular distance between the iris and the trabecular meshwork at a point either 500 μm or 750 μm anterior to the scleral spur
Trabecular iris angle (TIA)	The apex of the angle is in the angle recess: the arms of the angle pass through a point on the trabecular meshwork at 500 μm from the scleral spur and the point on the iris perpendicularly opposite
Trabecular ciliary process distance (TCPD)	Measured distance between the ciliary process and the trabecular meshwork at a point 500 μm anterior to the scleral spur on a line perpendicular through the iris
Iris thickness – ID1 – ID2 – ID3	Measured thickness of the iris: – 500 μm anterior to scleral spur – 2 mm from iris root – at pupillary edge
Iris ciliary process distance (ICPD)	Measured distance between iris and ciliary body (carried forward along the line of TCPD)
Iris zonular distance (IZD)	Measured distance between iris and lens zonules (carried forward along the line of TCPD)
Iris-lens contact distance (ICLD)	Measured distance of iridolenticular contact
Iris-lens angle	Angle formed by the anterior lens surface with the iris at the pupillary margin

emulsified silicon oil (Fig. 23.10). UBM can help detect a tube-corneal touch in eyes with corneal decompensation (Figs. 23.6 and 23.13).

(b) **Trabeculectomy**: UBM can be used to assess the patency of trabeculectomy stoma and bleb morphology (Fig. 23.13) [22]. Cyclodialysis cleft can be detected in cases of postoperative hypotony (Fig. 23.13).

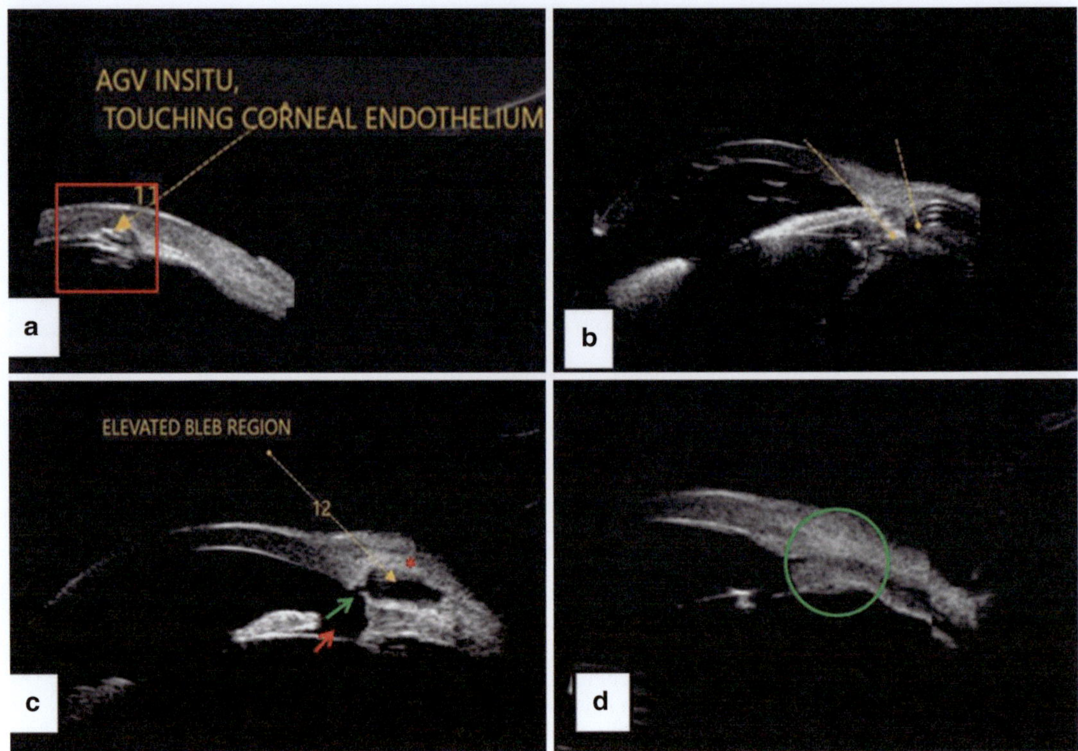

Fig. 23.13 Top left (**a**): a UBM image of an eye following Ahmed glaucoma valve implantation with the tube in the anterior chamber and showing the tube touching the corneal endothelium. Top right (**b**): a UBM image of an eye with silicone oil-induced glaucoma with Ahmed glaucoma valve implantation (pars plana tube insertion) with emulsified silicon oil bubbles blocking the tube lumen (arrow). Bottom left (**c**): a UBM image of an eye with an encapsulated bleb following trabeculectomy. A patent trabeculectomy stoma (green arrow) and peripheral iridectomy can be seen (red arrow). A large bleb with a thick wall (asterisk) is present. Bottom right (**d**): a UBM image showing a cyclodialysis cleft with supraciliary effusion

23.6 Uveitis

UBM helps detect the pathophysiology of glaucoma in eyes with uveitic glaucoma, for example, pupillary block glaucoma (Fig. 23.14) and secondary angle closure due to non-pupillary block mechanisms like uveal effusions. It can image the status of the ciliary processes (Fig. 23.14), supraciliary effusions, and cyclitic membranes in eyes with hypotony (Fig. 23.14).

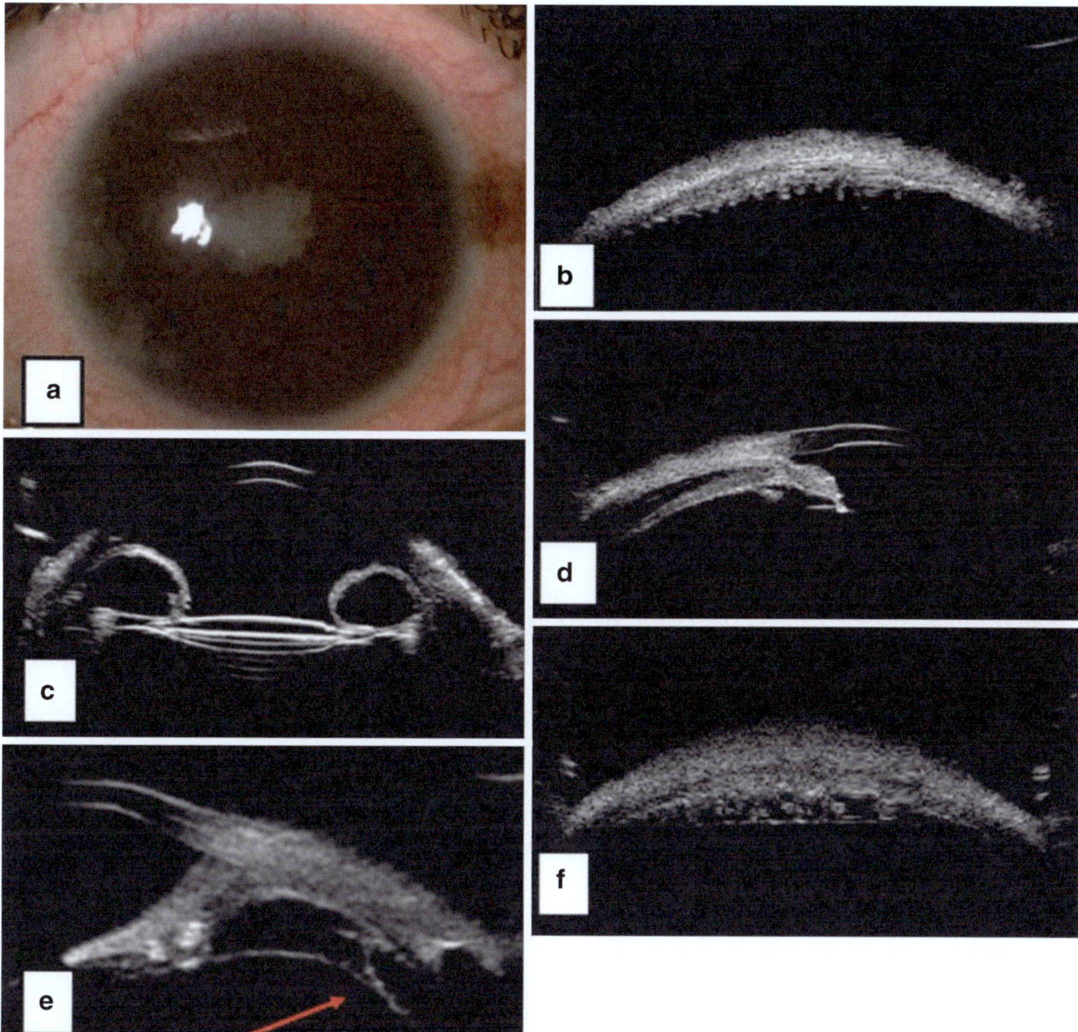

Fig. 23.14 Top left (**a**): a diffuse slit lamp photograph of an eye with panuveitis and secondary angle closure with hypotony. Top right (**b**): a UBM transverse section image of the same eye showing thin, sparse, and short ciliary processes with supraciliary effusion. Middle left (**c**): a UBM image (axial scan) in a pseudophakic eye with anterior uveitis and posterior synechiae showing iris bombe and secondary angle closure. Middle right (**d**): a UBM image showing a supraciliary effusion. Bottom left (**e**): an axial UBM image of a patient with chronic uveitis showing cyclitic membranes (arrow) and peripheral anterior synechiae. Bottom right (**f**): a transverse UBM image of a case of chronic uveitis with cyclitic membranes

23.7 Vitreo Retinal Surgery

UBM is useful in identifying fibrovascular proliferation (Fig. 23.15) and complications at the sclerotomy sites following pars plana vitrectomy [23].

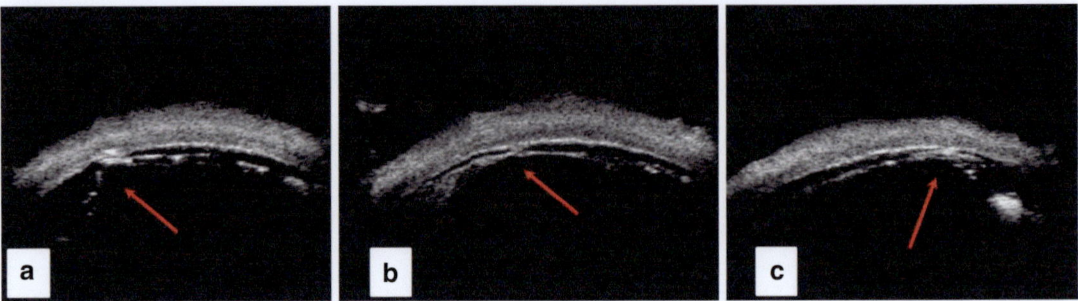

Fig. 23.15 (**a**, **b**, **c**) UBM images of the eyes of a patient post vitrectomy for non-resolving vitreous hemorrhage, showing fibrovascular proliferation at the sclerotomy sites (arrows)

23.8 Intraocular Tumors

23.8.1 Iris and Ciliary Body Cysts

Multiple ciliary body cysts can be seen in radial and transverse scans on UBM. They have a hyperechoic wall and an anechoic center (Fig. 23.16). Inflammatory lesions of the uveal tract may present as a mass (Fig. 23.16).

23.8.2 Uveal Mass Lesions

Uveal melanoma: A high correlation has been reported between UBM [24] and histopathological features of anterior uveal melanomas. The extent of the tumor can be defined, which helps in planning the management (Fig. 23.17). UBM helps differentiate suspected iris melanomas from neuroepithelial cysts, traumatic cysts, and vascular malformations. A peripheral neuroepithelial cyst shows a hyperechoic thin wall with an anechoic center. An iris melanoma appears as a solid irregular iris mass with variable internal reflectivity due to differences in vascularity. Distortion of surrounding structures is usually present. The posterior iris plane may show a convexity. Invasion of the iris root is a risk factor for metastasis. The mass shows progressive enlargement on serial biometry [16].

23.8.3 Ciliary Body Melanoma

It appears as an oval-shaped mass centered on the ciliary body (Fig. 23.17). It is primarily solid with low to medium internal reflectivity although some cavitation may be seen. The area of invasion of adjacent tissues appears to have reduced reflectivity compared to the surrounding ciliary body or iris [16].

23.8.4 Retinoblastoma

UBM helps in evaluating the anterior extents of retinoblastomas [25]. High-resolution imaging of the anterior retina, ciliary body, and the angle of the anterior chamber of the eye can be done to assess the extent of involvement and tumor extension beyond the retina (Fig. 23.18). Retinoblastomas have reflectivity similar to those of the ciliary body. A fine line of high reflectivity may help in identification. The anterior vitreous face, which is usually challenging to image, may be imaged if outlined with tumor or inflammatory cells (Fig. 23.18).

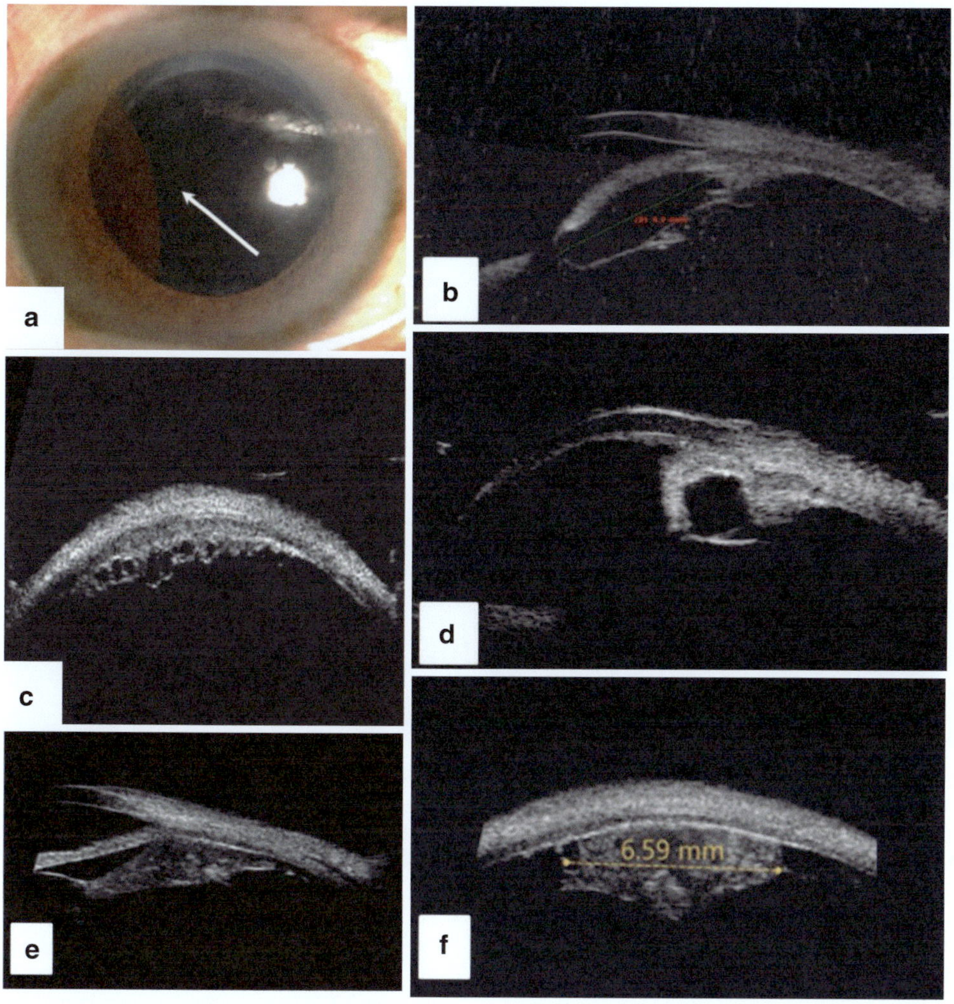

Fig. 23.16 Top left (**a**): a slit lamp photograph showing an iris cyst. Top right (**b**): a UBM of the iris cyst, measuring about 4.2 mm in diameter, with a hypoechoic lumen. Middle left (**c**): a UBM transverse scan image showing multiple ciliary body cysts. Middle right (**d**): a longitudinal UBM image showing a large iridociliary cyst causing secondary angle closure. Bottom left (**e**): radial; and bottom right (**f**): transverse scan UBM images of an eye of a patient with intermediate uveitis with an inflammatory ciliary body mass

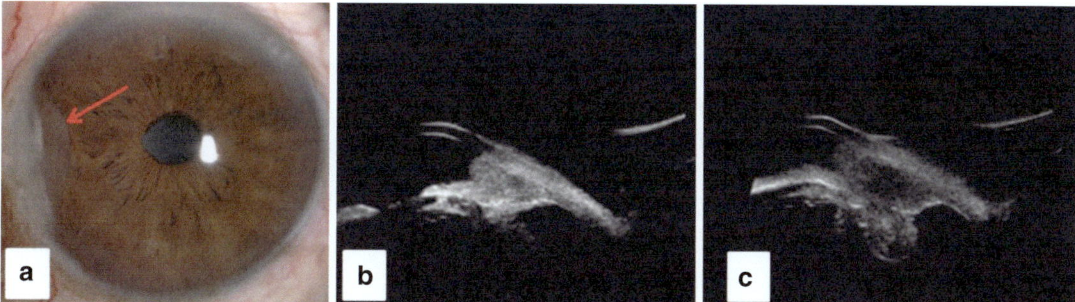

Fig. 23.17 Left (**a**): A slit lamp photograph of an eye with an iris mass (arrow). Middle (**b**) and right (**c**): UBM images showing the mass as a hyperechoic iridociliary lesion suspected as a melanoma

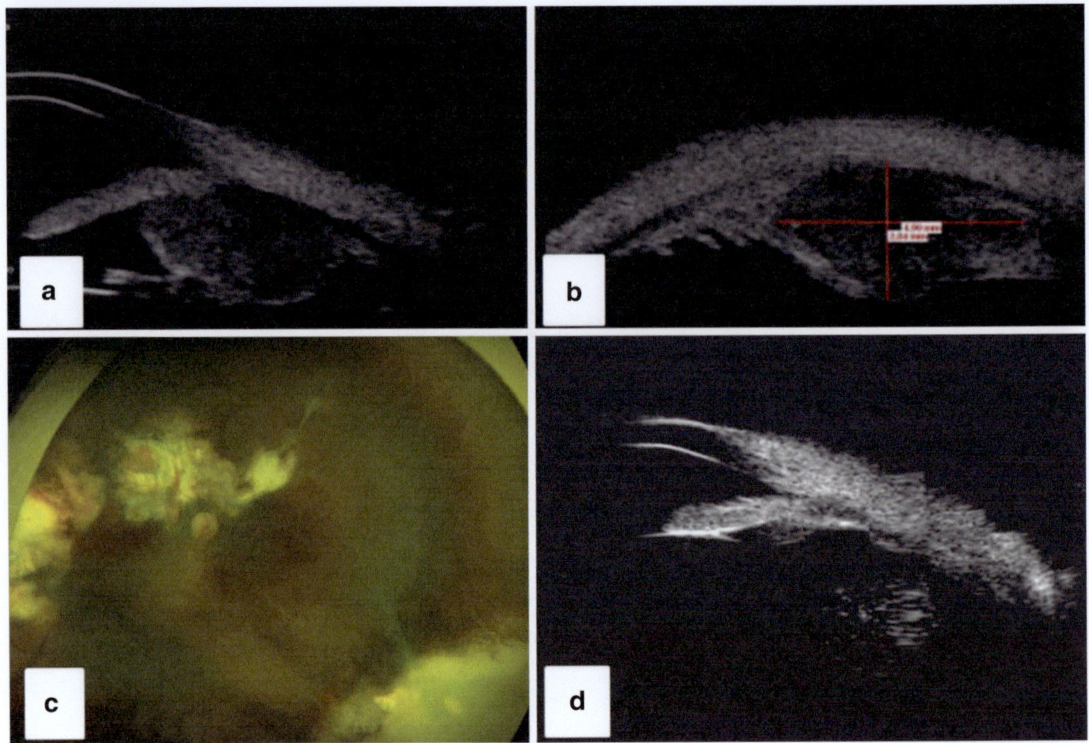

Fig. 23.18 Top: UBM images of an eye of a child with retinoblastoma showing a ciliary body mass. The other eye had undergone enucleation. Left (**a**): a radial scan, and right (**b**): transverse scans. Bottom left (**c**): a wide-field fundus photograph of an eye with retinoblastoma (under treatment) showing the tumor mass and inferior vitreous seeds. Bottom right (**d**): a UBM image of the eye with retinoblastoma showing vitreous seeds at the 6 o'clock position (arrow)

23.9 Conclusion

UBM is a vital non-invasive modality for imaging the anterior segment, with its main strength being the ability to visualize structures behind the iris. It provides high-resolution images of the anterior segment even in the presence of corneal opacity. It is an important tool in understanding the ocular anatomy, its pathophysiologies and in planning the management of many conditions like glaucoma, uveitis, cyclodialysis clefts, specific types of trauma, pediatric ocular diseases, and anterior segment tumors. UBM is an important tool in our armamentarium for patient management.

References

1. Pavlin CJ, Harasiewicz K, Foster FS. Ultrasound biomicroscopy of anterior segment structures in normal and glaucomatous eyes. Am J Ophthalmol. 1992;113:381–9.
2. Ishikawa H, Schuman JS. Anterior segment imaging: ultrasound biomicroscopy. Ophthalmol Clin N Am. 2004;17:7–20.
3. Nolan W. Anterior segment imaging: ultrasound biomicroscopy and anterior segment optical coherence tomography. Curr Opin Ophthalmol. 2008;19:115–21.
4. Allingham RR, Damji KF, Freedman S, et al. Shields textbook of glaucoma. 6th ed. Lippincott: William and Wilkins, Wolters Kluwer; 2011.
5. Byrne SF, Green RL. Ultrasound of the eye and orbit. 2nd ed. Jaypee Brothers Medical Publishers (P) Ltd; 2010.

6. Pavlin CJ, Foster FS. Ultrasound biomicroscopy in glaucoma. Acta Ophthalmol Suppl. 1992;70(S204):7–9.
7. CASIA2 Cornea/Anterior segment Optical Coherence Tomography Brochure, Tomey.
8. Marmor MF, Wickramasinghe HK, Lemons RA. Acoustic microscopy of the human retina and pigment epithelium. Invest Ophthalmol Vis Sci. 1977;16:660–6.
9. Ye SG, Harasiewicz KA, Pavlin CJ, Foster FS. Ultrasound characterization of normal ocular tissue in the frequency range from 50 MHz to 100 MHz. IEEE Trans Ultrason Ferroelectr Freq Control. 1995;42(1):8–14.
10. Sadaka A, Prager T, Beaver H, Malik A. A novel use of ultrasound biomicroscopy. Eye (Lond). 2018;32(2):474–5.
11. Pavlin CJ, McWhae JA, McGowan HD, Foster FS. Ultrasound biomicroscopy of anterior segment tumors. Ophthalmology. 1992;99:1220–8.
12. McWhae JA, Crichton ACS, Rinke M. Ultrasound biomicroscopy for the assessment of zonules after ocular trauma. Ophthalmology. 2003;110:1340–3.
13. Ozdal MP, Mansour M, Deschênes J. Ultrasound biomicroscopic evaluation of the traumatized eyes. Eye (Lond). 2003;17:467–72.
14. Marchini G, Pagliarusco A, Toscano A, et al. Ultrasound biomicroscopic and conventional ultrasonographic study of ocular dimensions in primary angle-closure glaucoma. Ophthalmology. 1998;105(11):2091–8.
15. Barkana Y, Dorairaj SK, Gerber Y, et al. Agreement between gonioscopy and ultrasound biomicroscopy in detecting iridotrabecular apposition. Arch Ophthalmol. 2007;125:1331–5.
16. Narayanaswamy A, Vijaya L, Shantha B, et al. Anterior chamber angle assessment using gonioscopy and ultrasound biomicroscopy. Jpn J Ophthalmol. 2004;48:44–9.
17. Kumar RS, Baskaran M, Chew PT, et al. Prevalence of plateau iris in primary angle closure suspects an ultrasound biomicroscopy study. Ophthalmology. 2008;115(3):430–4.
18. Marigo FA, Esaki K, Finger PT, et al. Differential diagnosis of anterior segment cysts by ultrasound biomicroscopy. Ophthalmology. 1999;106:2131–5.
19. Potash SD, Tello C, Liebmann J, Ritch R. Ultrasound biomicroscopy in pigment dispersion syndrome. Ophthalmology. 1994;101:332–9.
20. Alexander JL, Wei L, Palmer J, et al. A systematic review of ultrasound biomicroscopy use in pediatric ophthalmology. Eye. 2021;35:265–76.
21. Pavlin CJ, Ritch R, Foster FS. Ultrasound biomicroscopy in plateau iris syndrome. Am J Ophthalmol. 1992;113(4):390–5.
22. Yamamoto T, Sakuma T, Kitakawa Y. An ultrasound biomicroscopic study of filtering blebs after mitomycin C trabeculectomy. Ophthalmology. 1995;102:1770–6.
23. Bhende M, Agraharam SG, Gopal L, et al. Ultrasound biomicroscopy of sclerotomy sites after pars plana vitrectomy for diabetic vitreous hemorrhage. Ophthalmology. 2000;107:1729–36.
24. Conway RM, Chew T, Golchet P, et al. Ultrasound biomicroscopy: role in diagnosis and management in 130 consecutive patients evaluated for anterior segment tumours. Br J Ophthalmol. 2005;89:950–5.
25. Vasquez LM, Giuliari GP, Halliday W, et al. Ultrasound biomicroscopy in the management of retinoblastoma. Eye (Lond). 2011;25:141–7.

24 Ophthalmic Ultrasound

Suganeswari Ganesan, Sashwanthi Mohan, Debarati Dasgupta, and Muna Bhende

Ocular ultrasonography was first introduced in the 1950s by Mundt and Hughes. They described the A-scan. Baum and Greenwood described the B-scan in 1958, and Purnell and Coleman further improved it [1–4]. Standardization was done in the 1960s by Ossoinig, and other modifications such as immersion, contact B-scan, and anterior segment imaging were introduced two to three decades later [5, 6].

24.1 Physics

B-scan ultrasound uses high-frequency sound waves to generate a two-dimensional topographic image of the eye [7]. It uses a pulse-echo system that generates an oscillatory signal transmitted to the piezoelectric crystal in the ultrasound probe. The piezoelectric crystal then generates an ultrasonic sound wave of high-frequency (8–10 MHz) projected onto the ocular tissue. The reflected echo is then collected by the transducer and transmitted to the receiver, which amplifies the echoes and displays a 2D image of the eye called an echogram. Several technical terms are used to describe B-scans (Table 24.1).

Table 24.1 Important B-scan terms

Term	Definition
Echoes	Produced at the junction of two media with different acoustic impedance
Acoustic impedance	Difference in the strength of the returning echoes between two tissues with different acoustic interfaces
Angle of incidence	Angle at which the sound strikes an interface: the more perpendicular the beam, the stronger the returning echo will be
Resolution	Ability to distinguish between two different echoes
Amplification	This occurs before the reflected sound beam is displayed, which can be linear, logarithmic, or S curve
Absorption	Sound wave is absorbed through mediums which it passes through; the denser the medium, the more the absorption
Gain	Procedure of increasing or decreasing the amplitude of echoes; higher gain can detect weaker echoes
Time gain compensation	Technique used to enhance returning echoes from deeper structures by decreasing the ones from structures closer to the surface

S. Ganesan (✉) · M. Bhende
Medical Research Foundation, Sankara Nethralaya, Chennai, India
e-mail: drgsi@snmail.org; drmuna@snmail.org

D. Dasgupta
Greater Lions Eye Hospital, Siliguri, India

S. Mohan
Medcare Eye Centre, Dubai and Rajan Eye Care Hospital, Chennai, India

T. Das, P. Satgunam (eds.), *Ophthalmic Diagnostics*, https://doi.org/10.1007/978-981-97-0138-4_24

24.2 Technique

Ultrasound is usually performed in the supine or reclining position. The sitting position is utilized for gas or oil-filled eyes and to look for shifting fluid in exudative retinal detachments. The ultrasound probe is either placed over closed eyelids or directly placed over the conjunctiva or cornea with a coupling solution, which reduces sound attenuation by air. Documentation should be done with both stationary and dynamic images.

24.2.1 Probe Positions

The ultrasound probe has a marking. The marking denotes the upper part of the scan.

Depending on how the probe is oriented, there are three different positions [7]:

1. Axial: This passes through the center of the lens and optic nerve.
2. Transverse: This gives the lateral extent of the lesion and covers the 6-clock hour.
3. Longitudinal: This covers the anteroposterior extent of the lesion and covers the 1-clock hour.

24.2.2 Performing the Scans

24.2.2.1 Axial Scan

An axial scan is performed with the eye in the primary position and the probe centered on the cornea. Axial scans can be vertical, horizontal, or oblique. For vertical axial scans, the probe marker is directed superiorly; for horizontal axial scans, the probe marker is directly nasally; for oblique axial scans, the probe marker is directed towards the upper of the two meridians scanned. In the vertical axial scan, the retina is seen above, the optic disc is seen below, and the macula is not visualized. Axial length is measured in the horizontal axial scan, where the macula will be below the optic disc when the probe marker is directed nasally.

24.2.2.2 Transverse Scan

In transverse scans, the eye is directed towards the area of interest. The probe is parallel to the limbus on the opposite side. The probe marker is conventionally directed nasally for examining superior and inferior quadrants and superiorly for examining temporal and nasal quadrants. Transverse scans measure the lateral extent of a lesion and cover the 6-clock hour in one scan.

24.2.2.3 Longitudinal Scans

In longitudinal scans, the eye is directed towards the area of interest, with the probe perpendicular to the limbus on the opposite side. The probe marker is perpendicular to the limbus towards the meridian of interest. Longitudinal scans measure the anteroposterior extent of a lesion and cover the 1-clock hour.

24.2.3 Limbus to Fornix Approach

To examine the entire retina from the posterior part to the anterior part, the limbus to fornix approach is used, where the former position shows the posterior pole and the latter shows the anterior portion of the retina.

24.2.4 Special Examination Techniques

The topographic technique helps determine the location, shape, and extent of a lesion. The quantitative technique shows the reflectivity, internal structure, and sound attenuation of a lesion. Kinetic echography shows the motility, i.e., after-movement; vascularity, i.e., fast spontaneous motion; and convection motion, i.e., slow spontaneous motion.

24.3 Indications

Ultrasound B-scan is indicated in both clear and opaque ocular media. Table 24.2 gives the list of clinical indications for ophthalmic ultrasound.

Table 24.2 Indications of ultrasound B-scan

Clear ocular media	Opaque ocular media	Others
Iris and ciliary body tumors	Corneal opacity	Ocular trauma
Retinal detachment	Pupillary membrane	
Choroidal detachment (serous vs. hemorrhagic)	Hyphema/hypopyon	
Intraocular tumors	Dense cataracts	
Optic disc anomalies	Non-dilating pupils	
Intraocular foreign body	Vitreous hemorrhage	
Posterior scleritis	Vitritis	
	Retinal detachment	
	Intraocular foreign body	

24.4 Clinical Applications

24.4.1 Anatomy of a Normal Ultrasound (Fig. 24.1)

- Lens: An oval, highly reflective structure with intralesional echoes based on the degree of lens opacity. It is best seen with the standoff or immersion technique.
- Vitreous: Usually echo-lucent but can have low reflective echoes with age, secondary to syneresis.
- Retina, choroid, sclera: Seen as a single highly reflective structure which can only be differentiated when there is a pathology such as retinal detachment, choroidal detachment, and posterior scleritis.
- Optic nerve head: Wedge-shaped echo-lucent area in the retrobulbar area in the axial scan. It is best visualized in the vertical transverse scan.
- Extraocular muscles: Low reflective fusiform structures within the orbit.

24.4.2 Asteroid Hyalosis (Fig. 24.1)

Asteroid hyalosis (AH) is a degenerative condition where calcium-lipid complexes are suspended throughout the collagen fibrils of the vitreous. On ultrasound, they appear as multiple bright homogenous, densely packed dot echoes with medium to high reflectivity with a clear zone between the echoes and the retina [8].

24.4.3 Vitreous Hemorrhage (Fig. 24.1)

Vitreous hemorrhage (VH) is the extravasation of blood into the vitreous cavity secondary to conditions like proliferative diabetic retinopathy, retinal vein occlusion, trauma, retinal breaks, etc. On ultrasound, fresh VH appears as multiple mobile dot echoes and short lines of low reflectivity in the vitreous on the A-scan. When the hemorrhage gets organized, it appears as membranous echoes with higher reflectivity on the A-scan. In dense VH, there is an increase in the echoes with high reflectivity. Ultrasound is a useful tool for diagnosis, prognosis, and monitoring in cases of VH [9, 10].

24.4.4 Posterior Vitreous Detachment (Fig. 24.1)

Posterior vitreous detachment (PVD) is the detachment of the posterior hyaloid from the neurosensory retina, which can be complete or incomplete. On ultrasound, it appears as a membranous echo with low to moderate reflectivity on the A-scan. An incomplete PVD is attached to the optic nerve head, whereas a complete PVD is freely mobile and not attached to the optic nerve head; a PVD usually has good after-movements on kinetic scans. Hemorrhagic PVD has a thicker membranous echo with a higher reflectivity on the A-scan. To differentiate PVD from retinal detachment (RD), different portions of the PVD should be examined to look for decreased reflectivity, which is suggestive of the vitreous membrane [7].

24.4.5 Retinal Detachment (Fig. 24.2)

Rhegmatogenous RD is a separation of the neurosensory retina from the retinal pigment epithelium secondary to a full-thickness retinal

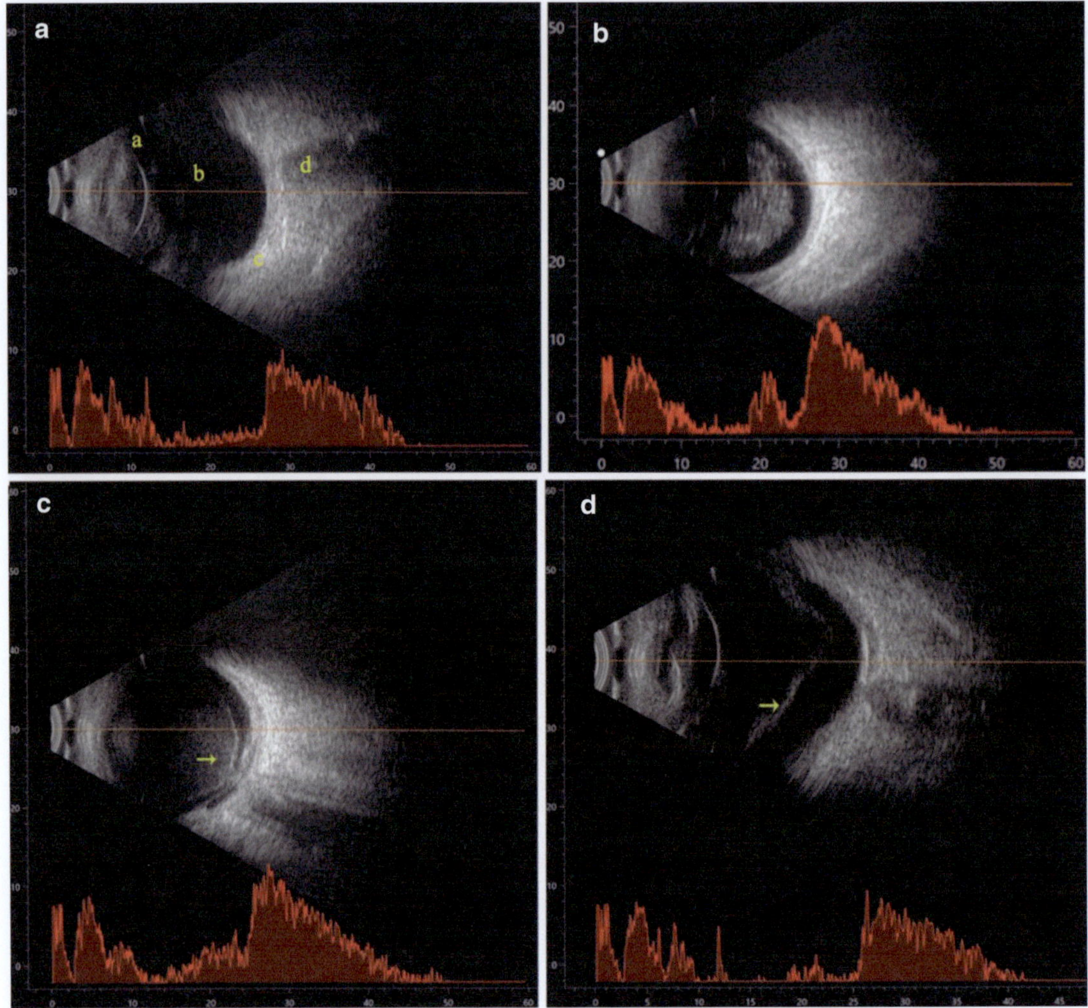

Fig. 24.1 **Top left**: Normal USG. Lens echo (a) seen with the anechoic vitreous cavity (b). Retina attached with normal retinal-choroidal-scleral (RCS) complex (c); the optic nerve head shadow appears normal (d). **Top right**: In asteroid hyalosis, the vitreous shows plenty of moderate to high reflective dot echoes with clear spaces between these echoes and the RCS complex. **Bottom left**: In vitreous hemorrhage, the vitreous cavity shows a moderate number of low reflective dot echoes and moderate reflective membranous echoes attached to the optic nerve head (arrow). A low reflective membrane echo attached to the optic nerve head suggests incomplete posterior vitreous detachment. **Bottom right**: A low reflective membrane echo not attached to the optic nerve head (arrow) suggests complete posterior vitreous detachment

break. It is the most common type of RD. On ultrasound, it appears as a bright, continuous membrane with close to 100% reflectivity, higher than ocular coats on the A-scan. On the B-scan, it is attached to the optic nerve head. It has poor after-movements on kinetic scans and is always less mobile than the vitreous membranes [11].

24.4.6 Tractional RD (Fig. 24.2)

Tractional RD is detachment of the neurosensory retina secondary to traction in retinal vascular diseases such as proliferative diabetic retinopathy, retinal vein occlusions, retinopathy of prematurity, and trauma. On ultrasound, it appears as a concave membrane with high reflectivity on

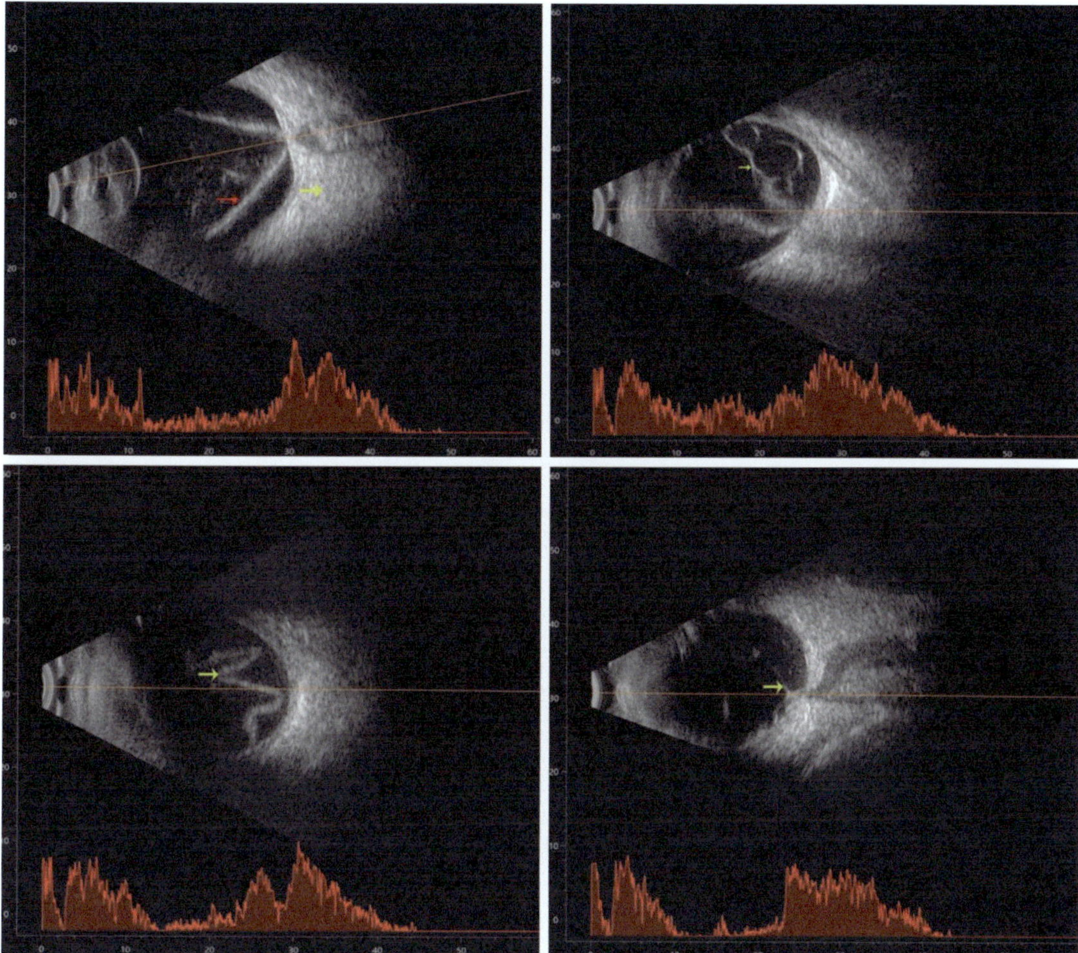

Fig. 24.2 **Top left**: Total retinal detachment. Red Arrow: A highly reflective membrane is attached to the optic nerve head to the periphery with subretinal echoes; Yellow Arrow: Subtle retinochoroidal sloping is noted behind the RD. **Top right**: Chronic RD. A highly reflective membrane echo is attached from the optic nerve head to the periphery, with underlying cystic changes (arrow) and subretinal echoes are present. **Bottom left**: Giant retinal tear with RD. Highly reflective convoluted membranous double linear echo (arrow). **Bottom right**: Tractional RD. A partially detached posterior hyaloid is noted with multiple attachments causing focal tractions at numerous points (arrow)

the A-scan with varying extents of vitreous adhesions. It can have a tented or table-top configuration which does not extend to the ora serrata with a vitreous band connected to the anterior surface. They have lesser mobility than rhegmatogenous RDs because of traction on the retina [12].

24.4.7 Exudative RD (Fig. 24.3)

Exudative RD is an accumulation of fluid in the subretinal space without retinal breaks and occurs secondary to inflammations, infections, neoplasms, etc. On ultrasound, it appears as a bullous membranous echo with high reflectivity on the A-scan and a smooth surface without rugae in the B-scan. It has a characteristic "shifting fluid" appearance that can be noted by changing the patient's head position, which changes the configuration of the exudative detachment. Depending on the underlying condition, associated findings can include retinochoroidal thickening, choroidal masses, etc.

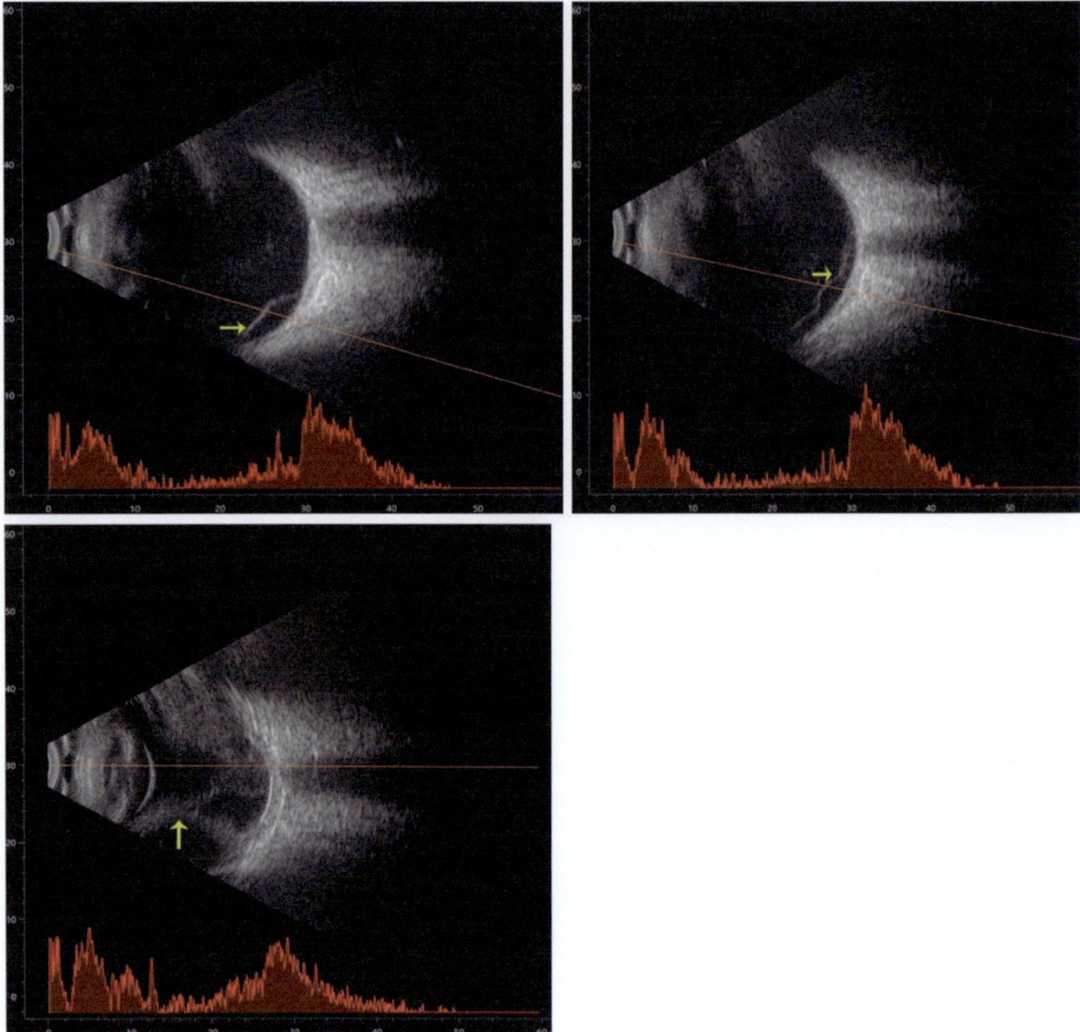

Fig. 24.3 **Top row**: Exudative retinal detachment. A moderately high reflective membrane echo (arrow) is noted located only inferiorly initially (left) but involving the posterior pole in the supine position, suggestive of shifting fluid (right). **Bottom row**: Choroidal detachment. Total retinal detachment with dome-shaped elevation and hypo-echoic space beneath it suggests serous choroidal detachment (arrow)

24.4.8 Choroidal Detachment (CD) (Fig. 24.3)

A CD is defined as the detachment of the choroid from the sclera due to the accumulation of fluid or hemorrhage in the suprachoroidal space. It is bound by uveoscleral solid attachments. On ultrasound, it appears as a smooth, dome-shaped membrane with a double highly reflective spike on the A-scan, called the "M spike." The "M spike" refers to the echoes from the choroid and retina.

The CD is not attached to the optic nerve head and has no after-movements on kinetic scans. When CDs touch each other, it is called "kissing choroidals." Serous CDs have an echo-lucent space behind the membrane, and hemorrhagic CDs have multiple mild to moderate reflective dot echoes behind the membrane. Shallow peripheral CDs appear flat or concave and not dome-shaped [13]. Ultrasound helps monitor clot lysis in cases of hemorrhagic CDs and helps in deciding the time and location of drainage.

Table 24.3 Ultrasound findings in PVD, RD, and CD

Characteristic	PVD	RD	CD
Echogenicity and reflectivity	Low reflective membranous echo with a corresponding low reflective A-scan spike	High reflective membranous echo with a corresponding high A-scan spike	High reflective membranous echo with a corresponding high reflective double or M spike on A-scan
Amplitude of echo	Less than 100%	100% compared to choroid and sclera	100%
Attachment to the optic nerve head	Complete: Not attached to the optic nerve head Incomplete: Attached to the optic nerve head	Attached to the optic nerve head	Not attached to the optic nerve head
Mobility	Good after-movements	Poor after-movements	No after-movements
Low gain	Disappears	Persists	Persists

Table 24.3 details the differences between PVD, RD, and CD.

24.4.9 Retinoschisis

Retinoschisis splits the retinal layers into inner and outer ones with cystic spaces in between. It appears as a thin immobile membrane with a convex and smooth configuration on ultrasound. It is usually located in the inferotemporal quadrant in patients with hypermetropia. Retinoschisis must be differentiated from RD. Retinoschisis is usually of lower amplitude and thinner than RD [14]. The height of retinoschisis does not decrease on indentation, while the height of RD decreases on indentation.

24.4.10 Retinal Tear

Retinal tears are breaks in the retina secondary to PVD and vitreous traction. Ultrasound has over 90% sensitivity and specificity in detecting small retinal tears [15]. On ultrasound, a retinal tear appears as focal retinal elevations with high reflectivity and an adherent vitreous strand with lower reflectivity. They do not have good movements on kinetic scans. In a low gain setting, only the retinal component will remain visible. A giant retinal tear is a retinal tear that is more than 3-clock hours of the retina. On ultrasound, it appears as two membranes attached to the optic disc; the first echo is the inverted posterior flap of the tear, and the second echo is the detached retina [16, 17].

24.4.11 Endophthalmitis/Panophthalmitis (Fig. 24.4)

Endophthalmitis is inflammation of the intraocular fluids (vitreous/aqueous) secondary to infection after surgery, trauma, etc. Panophthalmitis is purulent inflammation of all coats of the eyeball and intraocular structures. On ultrasound, vitreous inflammation appears as point echoes in the vitreous cavity and mild to moderate reflectivity on A-scan. Ultrasound findings can also include vitreous debris and loculations. There is associated retinochoroidal thickening and associated RD and CD in some cases. Thickening of the scleral coats and collection of fluid in the sub-Tenon's space called the "T sign" is typically seen in panophthalmitis [18].

24.4.12 Vogt-Koyanagi Harada Syndrome (Fig. 24.4)

Vogt-Koyanagi Harada (VKH) syndrome is a bilateral granulomatous panuveitis with associated central nervous system, auditory, and skin involvement. On ultrasound, there are mild to moderately low reflective vitreous echoes (Fig. 24.4; lower left panel) and no PVD. There is choroidal thickening with low to medium reflectivity of the choroid (Fig. 24.4; lower right panel)

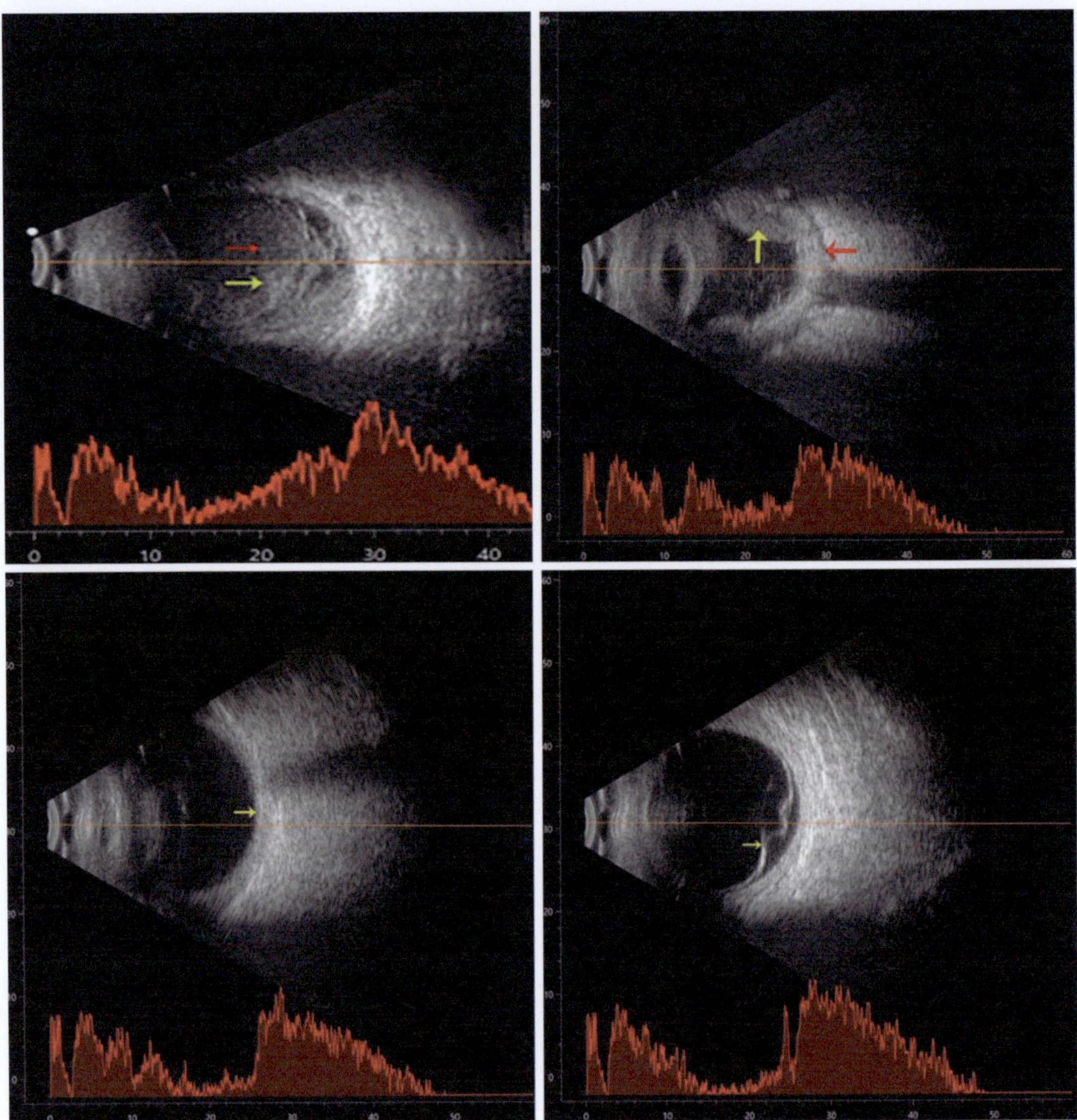

Fig. 24.4 **Top left**: Endophthalmitis. The vitreous cavity shows plenty of low reflective dot echoes (red arrow) and membranous echoes (yellow arrow) with thickening of the RCS complex. **Top right**: Panophthalmitis. Multiple vitreous cavity echoes with subretinal low reflective dot echoes suggest a subretinal abscess (yellow arrow) with a prominent hypo-echoic space behind the ocular coat called the T-sign (red arrow). **Bottom**: VKH. The vitreous shows a moderate number of low reflective dot echoes with a moderate reflective membrane extending from the optic nerve head to the inferior periphery, suggesting retinal detachment (right) and diffuse choroidal thickening (left)

[7, 19]. Serous RDs can be seen inferiorly or at the posterior pole. Ultrasound is useful in monitoring response to corticosteroid treatment by evaluating serous RDs and choroidal thickening in eyes with opaque media.

24.4.13 Posterior Scleritis

Posterior scleritis is a painful inflammation of the sclera posterior to the equator. On ultrasound, there is a thickening of ocular coats, episcleral

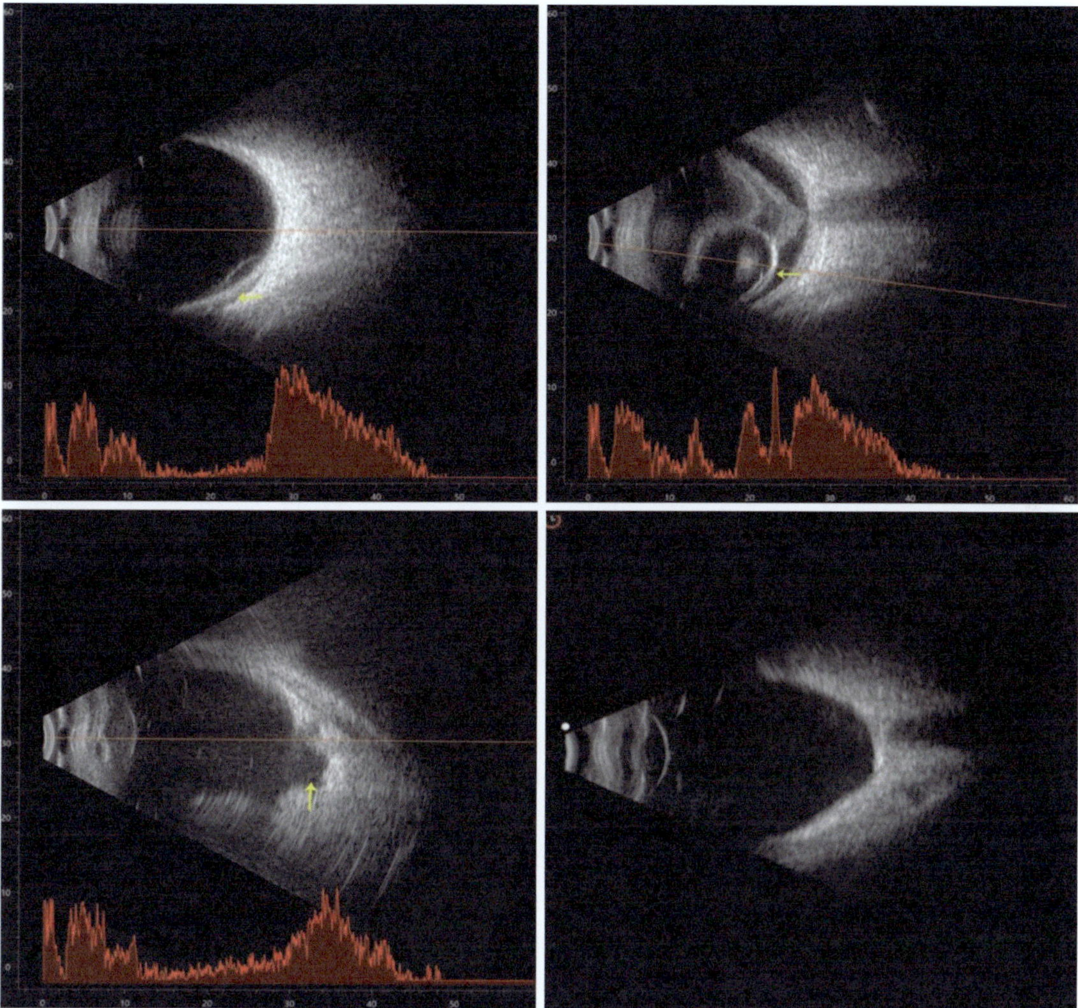

Fig. 24.5 **Top row; left**: Posterior scleritis. A localized, highly reflective membrane echo is noted in posterior pole. Peripapillary choroid and choroid adjacent to retinal detachment are thickened with hypo-echoic space beneath them. **Top row; right**: RD with cysticercosis. A moderately high reflective membrane echo with large cystic lesions and intracystic hyper-reflective clump echoes is noted. **Bottom row; left**: Retinochoroidal coloboma. A retinochoroidal excavation is noted with sharp edges is suggestive of RC coloboma involving the disc and macula. **Bottom row; right**: Posterior staphyloma. A retinochoroidal excavation with smooth edges in the posterior pole in an eye with increased axial length suggests posterior staphyloma

space fluid, enlargement of the optic nerve shadow, and exudative RD. A pathognomic sign is the "T-sign," i.e., fluid accumulation in the sub-Tenon's space, i.e., between the optic nerve and the sclera, seen as hypo-echo-lucency continuous with the optic nerve head. A recent study has suggested a new criterion of scleral thickness of >1.7 mm and a difference of 20% or more in scleral thickness between two eyes of a patient for the diagnosis of posterior scleritis [20].

24.4.14 Cysticercosis (Fig. 24.5)

Cysticercosis is a parasitic infection caused by *Cysticercus cellulosae*, the larval form of *Taenia solium,* which affects various parts of the eye. When present in the posterior segment, it can be seen on ultrasound as a well-defined round to oval echo-lucent cyst with a dense echogenic nodule attached to the inner wall of the cyst is suggestive of scolex and exhibits movements on kinetic scanning [21]. Dead cysts cause inflammation, leading to vitreous dots, membranous echoes, and possible RD.

24.4.15 Choroidal Coloboma (Fig. 24.5)

Colobomas occur due to the failure of closure of the embryonic fissure and are typically located in the inferonasal part of the fundus. On ultrasound, there is excavation of varying depths involving the retina, choroid, and/or optic disc [21]. It has a smooth contour or outpouching. The edge is overhanging, sharp, or shelved. The intercalary membrane can be visualized in some cases across the coloboma.

24.4.16 Posterior Staphyloma (Fig. 24.5)

Posterior staphyloma is an outpouching of the wall of the eye that has a radius of curvature lesser than the surrounding curvature of the wall of the eye seen in pathological myopia. On ultrasound, an excavation with smooth edges is noted at the posterior pole in an eye with increased axial length [21].

24.4.17 Phthisis Bulbi

Phthisis bulbi is an end-stage ocular disease related to scarring, inflammation, atrophy, and disorganization of the globe and intraocular contents. On ultrasound, the eye has a grossly reduced axial length, distorted globe structure, and ocular coat calcification [22].

24.4.18 Trauma

Ocular trauma secondary to blunt or penetrating injuries can damage the eye, with the severity ranging from minor injuries to globe ruptures leading to temporary or permanent impairment of visual function. Ultrasound of the posterior segment helps assess the internal ocular damage in eyes with opaque media and detect various conditions such as dislocated crystalline lens/cataract or intraocular lens, PVD and vitreous hemorrhage, retinal tears and RDs, CDs, optic nerve avulsion, scleral rupture, incarcerated wounds, and intraocular foreign bodies (IOFBs) [21].

24.4.18.1 Dislocated Crystalline Lens/Intraocular Lens (Fig. 24.6)

Crystalline, cataractous, or intraocular lenses can dislocate posteriorly into the vitreous after trauma. On ultrasound, the dislocated lens is seen as a hyper-reflective globular shadow in the inferior vitreous, and the dislocated intraocular lens has a hyper-reflective surface with posterior reverberation echoes [21].

24.4.18.2 Intraocular Foreign Body (IOFB) (Fig. 24.6)

Ultrasound is used to localize the position and determine the number, size, and type of IOFB and associated complications such as vitreous hemorrhage and retinal detachment, especially in opaque media. In cases of clear ocular media, documentation of IOFB by ultrasound is important for medicolegal reasons. On ultrasound, IOFBs appear hyperechoic, bright, and acoustically opaque lesions with acoustic shadowing of ocular or orbital structures with a corresponding 100% reflective echo on the A-scan (Fig. 24.6 top right). IOFBs persist in low gain settings of 20 to 30 dB [21]. Spherical IOFBs characteristically have reverberations. Metal and stone foreign bodies have higher amplitude echoes than wood and vegetable matter. Glass IOFBs are challenging to locate on ultrasound unless the sound beam strikes perpendicular to the IOFB. Transverse scans can help locate the foreign body, while longitudinal scans are used for better exposure of the IOFB and accurately measure its dimensions. Mobility of the IOFBs can be assessed on kinetic scans, which can help assess if it is freely mobile in the vitreous or adherent to the underlying retina.

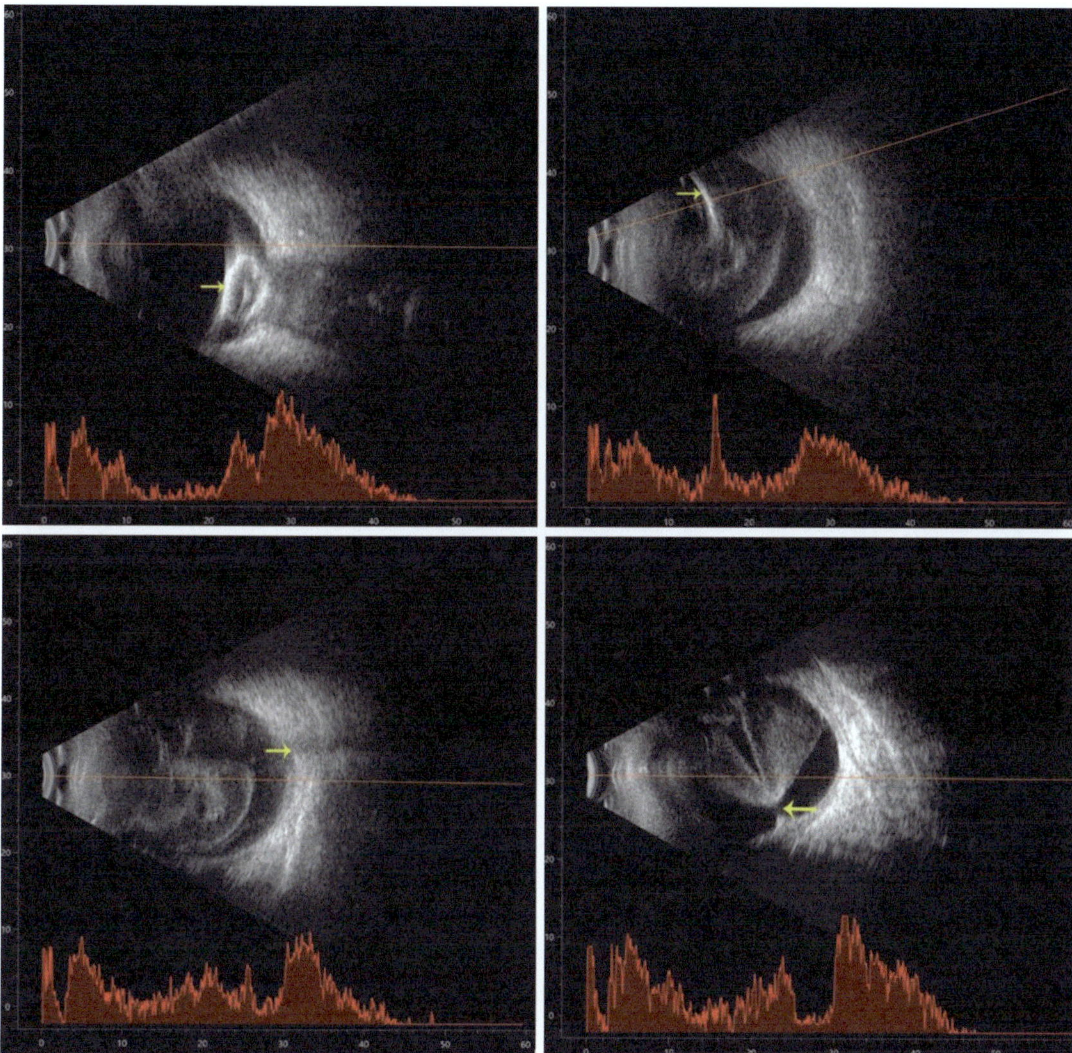

Fig. 24.6 **Top left**: Posterior dislocated lens. A highly reflective biconvex echo is noted inferiorly with back shadowing (arrow). **Top right**: Intra ocular foreign body. A high reflective linear echo is noted in the mid-vitreous cavity (arrow). **Bottom left**: Globe discontinuity. Vitreous incarceration is seen temporally with suspected discontinuity of the ocular coat (arrow). **Bottom right**: Vitreous incarceration. A variable reflective membrane echo is noted with good after-movement converging towards the ocular coats (arrow), causing possible incarceration

24.4.18.3 Optic Nerve Head Avulsion

Optic nerve head avulsion is a rare but serious effect of trauma and is described as the separation of optic nerve fibers from the globe at the level of the lamina cribrosa. It appears as hypolucency posterior to the optic nerve head on ultrasound. A corresponding A-scan may show marked widening of the nerve, suggesting hemorrhage and edema within the nerve sheath in addition to optic nerve avulsion [23].

24.4.18.4 Scleral Rupture (Fig. 24.6)

Scleral rupture can be difficult to detect clinically. On ultrasound, the rupture site appears as an area with decreased reflectivity, i.e., hypoechogenic with an irregular contour. Indirect signs include vitreous incarceration with VH and PVD, episcleral hemorrhage close to the rupture site, retinal tractional bands that converge at the site of rupture, RD, and CD [21].

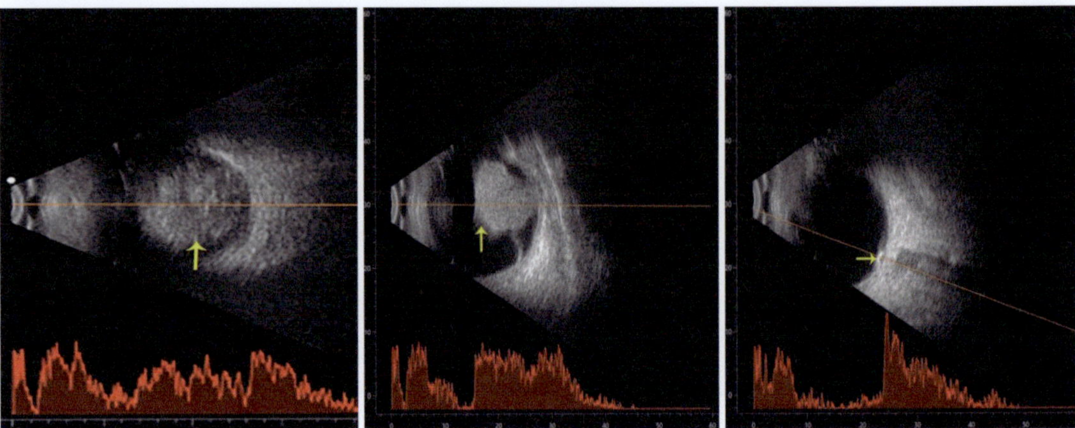

Fig. 24.7 **Left**: Retinoblastoma. The vitreous cavity shows an irregular hyperechoic mass with areas of high internal reflectivity, suggesting intralesional calcification. **Middle**: Choroidal melanoma. A homogenous mass lesion with moderate surface and internal reflectivity with associated localized retinal detachment. **Right**: Small choroidal hemangioma. A small mass lesion with a highly reflective surface echo and moderate reflective internal echo

24.4.19 Tumors

24.4.19.1 Retinoblastoma (Fig. 24.7)

Retinoblastoma is a rare childhood cancer of the retina arising due to biallelic mutations of the cone photoreceptor precursor. Worldwide, 8000 new cases are reported yearly, with most children presenting with the condition before 5 years of age. The hallmark of retinoblastoma is the presence of calcium. When calcium is present in large quantities, the mass has high internal reflectivity and causes intense back shadowing masking the structures behind it, like the choroid, sclera, and optic nerve, especially if the tumor is close to the optic nerve. Non-calcified tumors express low to medium reflectivity. If calcium is present in very less quantities, like specks, they are represented as tiny point areas of high internal reflectivity within areas of medium internal reflectivity [21]. The surface can vary from dome to irregular configuration. There can be associated exudative RD. Diffuse infiltrating retinoblastoma can present as a small elevation from the retina or irregular retinal thickening with no calcification.

24.4.19.2 Choroidal Melanoma (Fig. 24.7)

Choroidal melanoma arises from uveal melanocytes predominantly originating from the choroid located posterior to the equator. On ultrasound, it is commonly dome-shaped and, less commonly, can be collar button- or mushroom-shaped. Lobulated types and those with irregular surface contours have also been described. The tumor consistency is often solid, uniformly homogenous, with low to medium internal reflectivity except in areas of hemorrhage due to intervening necrosis. Choroidal excavation may also occur. Acoustic hollowing is secondary to the densely packed cellular nature of the tumor, causing decreased echogenicity at the tumor base compared with the adjacent choroid [24, 25]. Attenuation of the sound waves on the A-scan towards the base of the tumor is called angle kappa. Associated exudative RD can extend from the margins and not from the summit of the tumor. The adjoining sclera should be examined for the presence of extra-scleral invasion.

Table 24.4 lists the clinical and ultrasound findings of other choroidal tumors, such as choroidal hemangioma, osteoma, and metastasis.

24.4.20 Pediatric Retinal Disease

24.4.20.1 Retinopathy of Prematurity (ROP) (Fig. 24.8)

ROP is an abnormality of retinal blood vessels that occur in premature infants; when not treated in time, it can progress to RD. Indirect ophthal-

Table 24.4 Choroidal hemangioma vs. choroidal osteoma vs. choroidal metastasis [26]

Characteristic	Choroidal hemangioma	Choroidal osteoma	Choroidal metastasis
Clinical	Two types 1. Circumscribed: Red dome-shaped posterior pole choroidal elevation. 2. Diffuse: Tomato ketchup fundus associated with Sturge-Weber syndrome	Peripapillary yellow-white to orange-red colored benign ossifying flat and elevated choroidal lesion	Metastatic carcinoma of the choroid. Cream-colored single or multifocal lesions located in the posterior pole with an irregular surface. Choroidal elevations may be mild or moderate
Ultrasound	Circumscribed: Elevated dome-shaped acoustically solid mass, no choroidal excavation. High surface reflectivity and high internal reflectivity between 50 and 100% due to vascular channels. Diffuse: Diffuse thickening of choroid extending from the optic nerve head to the equator. Associated exudative RD	Mature bone causes high reflectivity with back shadowing of orbital tissues persisting at low gain, usually located over the posterior pole	Varying internal reflectivity from moderate to high with heterogenous internal structure. Associated exudative RD

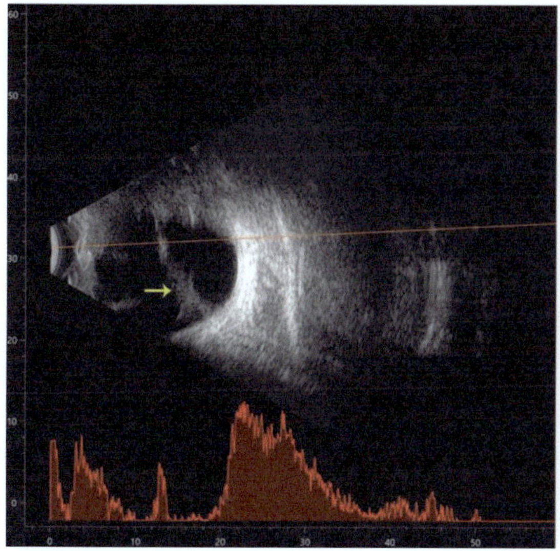

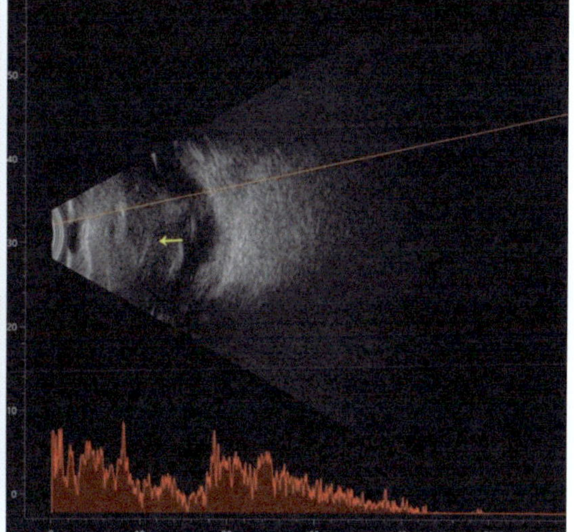

Fig. 24.8 **Left**: Stage 4 ROP. A highly reflective membranous echo (arrow) with moderate after-movements extending from the optic nerve head to the periphery in the temporal quadrant, suggestive of temporal falciform fold. **Right**: Stage 5 ROP. A moderate reflective membrane extending from the optic nerve head to the periphery suggests total retinal detachment with an open funnel configuration (arrow)

moscopic evaluation or fundus camera-based imaging are the conventional methods of evaluation. Ultrasonography is widely used in advanced stages of ROP. In circumstances like non-dilating pupils or the setting of cataracts on a preterm infant, ultrasound can be useful in assessing all the stages of ROP [27]. The demarcation line in Stage 1 is seen as a shallow ridge. Retinal thickening with a ridge is noted in stage 2. Stage 3 is seen as a giant ridge. Stage 4a is seen as an anteriorly drawn retina towards the lens margin with vitreous condensation. Stage 4b is seen as high reflective echoes of fibrovascular tissue pulling up the retina in a concave configuration with macular involvement. Further progression of this stage by cicatricial processes results in complete tractional retinal detachment, which appears as a funnel-shaped, highly reflective membrane attached to the optic disc in four different configurations, namely, open-open, close-open, open-close, and close-close. A peripheral trough signifies areas of the avascular retinal fold. The presence of subretinal echoes, suggestive of layering of subretinal hemorrhage or cholesterol, is considered to be prognostically poor. Axial length measurement is mandatory as reduced axial length can signify poor anatomical outcomes.

24.4.20.2 Coats Disease

Coats disease, the commonest cause of leukocoria characterized by an exudative retinal detachment, retinal telangiectasia, aneurysms, and exudation known to occur in males is an idiopathic ocular condition. The classical finding is the subretinal cholesterol appearing as subretinal echoes in ultrasound. Total RD is seen behind the crystalline lens but does not present with shifting fluid; less massive detachments are present with shifting fluid.

24.4.20.3 Persistence of Fetal Vasculature (PFV)

PFV occurs due to the failure of regression of the hyaloid vasculature in utero. The location of persistent vasculature remnants determines the spectrum of presentation. PFV is of three types: posterior, anterior, and hybrid. In posterior PFV, the hyaloidal stalk connects between the back surface of the lens and the optic nerve head, and on ultrasound, it presents as a variably reflecting thin vitreous band extending between the back surface of the lens and the optic nerve head with or without peripapillary tractional RD [28]. Anterior PFV presents with reduced axial length, cataract, prominent, elongated ciliary process, shallow anterior chamber, engorged iris vessels, and retrolental membrane. This presents as irregular thickening behind the posterior capsule, very often unilateral.

24.4.21 Silicon Oil-Filled Eye (Fig. 24.9)

The sound velocity in an eye filled with silicon oil (~987 m/s) is much slower than in a normal eye (~1532 m/s). Hence, an echogram of a silicon oil-filled eye shows an apparently enlarged eye in

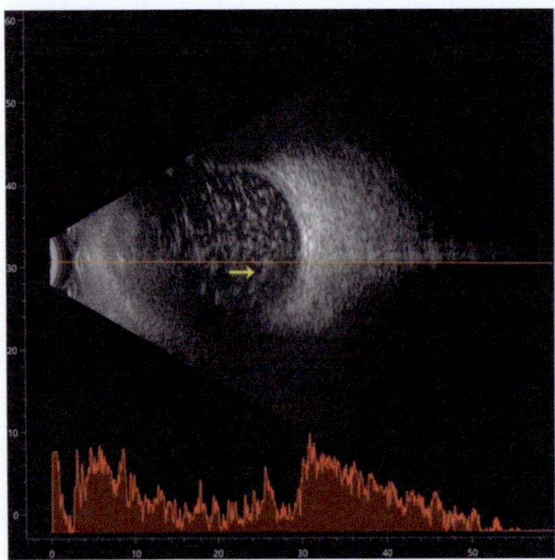

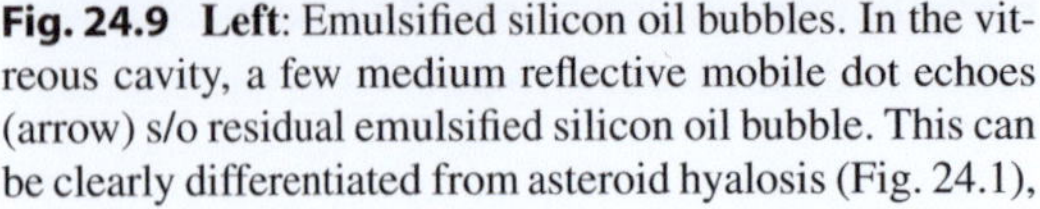

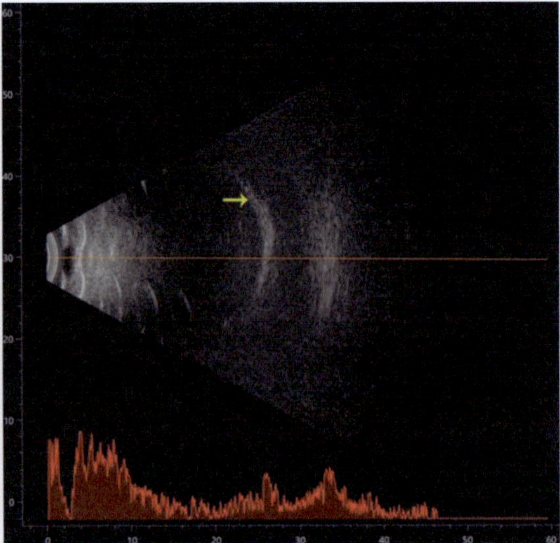

Fig. 24.9 **Left**: Emulsified silicon oil bubbles. In the vitreous cavity, a few medium reflective mobile dot echoes (arrow) s/o residual emulsified silicon oil bubble. This can be clearly differentiated from asteroid hyalosis (Fig. 24.1), where there is clear space behind it. **Right**: Silicon oil-filled eye with RD. Apparently, an enlarged globe with a highly reflective membrane-like echo was noted inferiorly, suggesting possible retinal detachment

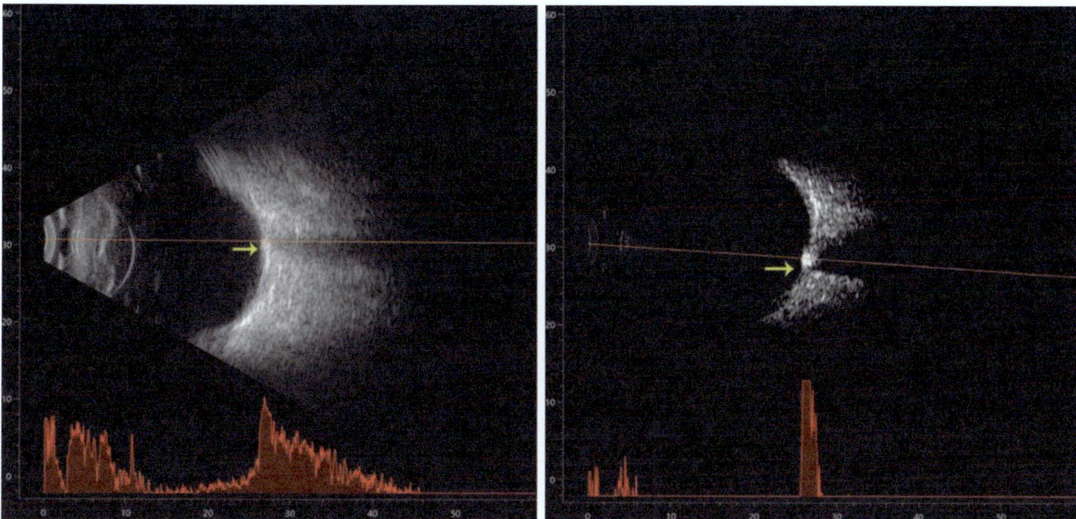

Fig. 24.10 Optic nerve head drusen. Localized very highly reflective clump echo (arrow) over the optic nerve head (left), persisting even in the low gain (right)

a supine position [29]. Retinal and choroidal status cannot be clearly defined, and detecting RD in these eyes is challenging due to high sound attenuation. A prone or sitting position is preferable to scan the normal ocular wall. Since the silicon oil moves towards the retina, in a prone position, the retina is identified with the help of a single spike when the retina is attached; in a detached retina, two spikes will be seen.

24.4.22 Common Optic Nerve Lesions

24.4.22.1 Papilledema

Papilledema is swelling of the optic disc secondary to increased intracranial pressure (ICP). On ultrasound, the optic nerve sheath diameter (ONSD) is used to assess ICP indirectly. Normal ONSD ranges from 2.2 to 5 mm. ONSD >5 mm is suggestive of ICP [30]. ONSD is measured 3 mm behind the posterior scleral surface of the eyeball [31]. The 30° test involves measuring the optic nerve head in primary gaze and when the patient's gaze is directed 30° laterally. A decrease of the optic nerve head by 10% in the lateral gaze is considered positive and indicates increased subarachnoid fluid [31].

24.4.22.2 Optic Disc Cupping

Optic disc cupping occurs in cases of advanced glaucoma or could be physiological. On ultrasound, it is seen as an excavation of the optic nerve head. It is best visualized on vertical transverse and longitudinal scans [32, 33]. A cup-disc ratio of a minimum of 0.5 is required for ultrasound detection of cupping.

24.4.22.3 Optic Disc Drusen (Fig. 24.10)

Optic disc drusen are calcified nodules within the optic nerve head. On ultrasound, drusen are seen as very high reflective echoes over the optic nerve head, which persists in low gain [21].

24.5 Conclusion

Ultrasound B-scan is a useful non-invasive tool in multiple posterior segment conditions. Clinical correlation is important while interpreting a B-scan.

Funding Nil.

Disclosure Nil.

References

1. Mundt G, Hughes W. Ultrasonics in ocular diagnosis. Am J Ophthalmol. 1956;41:488–98.
2. Baum G, Greenwood I. The application of ultrasonics locating techniques to ophthalmology*: heoretic considerations and acoustic properties of ocular media: part I. Reflective properties. Am J Ophthalmol. 1958;46(5):319–29.
3. Purnell EW. Ultrasound in ophthalmological diagnosis. In: Grossman C, Homes JH, Joyner C, Purnell EW, editors. Diagnostic ultrasound. New York: Plenum Press; 1966. p. 95–109.
4. Coleman DJ, Konig WF, Katz L. A hand-operated, ultrasound scan system for ophthalmic evaluation. Am J Ophthalmol. 1969;68:256–63.
5. Ossoinig K. Clinical echo-ophthalmology. In: Blodi FC, editor. Current concepts in ophthalmology, vol. III. St Louis: CV Mosby Co; 1972. p. 101–30.
6. Lizzi FL, Coleman DJ. History of ophthalmic ultrasound. J Ultrasound Med. 2004;23(10):1255–66. https://doi.org/10.7863/jum.2004.23.10.1255.
7. Green RL, Byrne SF. Chapter 14: Diagnostic ophthalmic ultrasound. In: Ryan SJ, editor. Retina. Philadelphia: Elsevier/Mosby; 2006. p. 265–350.
8. Allison KL, Price J, Odin LJ. Asteroid hyalosis and axial length measurement using automated biometry. Cataract Refract Surg. 1991;17(2):181–6.
9. Capeans C, Santos L, Tourino R, et al. Ocular echography in the prognosis of vitreous haemorrhage in type II diabetes mellitus. Int Ophthalmol. 1997;21(5):269–75.
10. Dawood Z, Mirza SA, Qadeer A. Role of B-scan ultrasonography for posterior segment lesions. JLUMHS; 2008.
11. Freyler H, Egerer I. Echography and histological studies in various eye conditions. Arch Ophthalmol. 1977;95(8):1387–94.
12. Jalkh AE, Avila MP, El-Markabi H, et al. Immersion A- and B-scan ultrasonography. Its use in preoperative evaluation of diabetic vitreous hemorrhage. Arch Ophthalmol. 1984;102(5):686–90.
13. Fledelius HC. Ultrasound in ophthalmology. Ultrasound Med Biol. 1997;23(3):365–75.
14. Hillman JS, Ridgway AE. Retinoschisis and retinal detachment, an ultrasonic comparison. Bibl Ophthalmol. 1975;83:63–7.
15. Nischal KK, James JN, McAllister J. The use of dynamic ultrasound B-scan to detect retinal tears in spontaneous vitreous haemorrhage. Eye. 1995;9(4):502–6.
16. DiBernardo C, Blodi B, Byrne SF. Echographic evaluation of retinal tears in patients with spontaneous vitreous hemorrhage. Arch Ophthalmol. 1992;110(4):511.
17. Jalkh AE, Jabbour N, Avila MP, et al. Ultrasonographic findings in eyes with giant retinal tears and opaque media. Retina. 1983;3(3):154–8.
18. Marchini G, Pagliarusco A, Tosi R, Castagna G. Ultrasonographic findings in endophthalmitis. Acta Ophthalmol Scand. 1995;73(5):446–9. https://doi.org/10.1111/j.1600-0420.1995.tb00306.x.
19. Byrne S, Green R. Ultrasound of the eye and orbit. 2nd ed. St Louis, MO: Mosby; 2002.
20. Maleki A, Ruggeri M, Colombo A, et al. B-scan ultrasonography findings in unilateral posterior scleritis. J CurrOphthalmol. 2022;34(1):93–9.
21. Bhende M, Kamat H, Krishna T, et al. Atlas of ophthalmic ultrasound and ultrasound biomicroscopy. JP Medical Ltd; 2013.
22. Coleman JD. Ultrasonography of eye and orbit. 2nd ed. Lippincott: Williams and Wilkins; 1977. p. 47–122.
23. Sawhney R, Kochhar S, Gupta R, et al. Traumatic optic nerve avulsion: role of ultrasonography. Eye. 2003;17(5):667–70.
24. Singh P, Singh A. Choroidal melanoma. Oman J Ophthalmol. 2012;5(1):3–9. https://doi.org/10.4103/0974-620X.94718.
25. Yeh PT. B-scan for the diagnosis of choroidal diseases. J Med Ultrasound. 2013;21(3):123–5.
26. Wang TJ, Yang CH, Liao SL, et al. Characteristic ultrasonographic findings of choroidal tumors. J Med Ultrasound. 2003;11(2):55–9.
27. Lee KF, Abdul Rahim A, Raja Azmi MN, et al. Ultrasonographic findings in eyes with retinopathy of prematurity in Malaysia. Med J Malaysia. 2013;68(1):39–43.
28. Prakhunhungsit S, Berrocal AM. Diagnostic and management strategies in patients with persistent fetal vasculature: current insights. Clin Ophthalmol. 2020;14:4325–35.
29. Abbas R. Ophthalmic ultrasonography and ultrasound biomicroscopy. Springer International Publishing; 2021.
30. Agrawal A, Cheng R, Tang J, Madhok DY. Comparison of two techniques to measure optic nerve sheath diameter in patients at risk for increased intracranial pressure. Crit Care Med. 2019;47(6):e495.
31. Kimberly HH, Shah S, Marill K, Noble V. Correlation of optic nerve sheath diameter with direct measurement of intracranial pressure. Acad Emerg Med. 2008;15(2):201–4.
32. Darnley-Fisch DA, Byrne SF, Huhges JR, et al. Contact B-scan echography in the assessment of optic nerve cupping. Am J Ophthalmol. 1990;109(1):55–61.
33. Özen Ö, Özer MA, Tosun A, Özen S. Evaluation of the optic nerve and scleral-choroidal-retinal layer with ultrasound elastography in glaucoma and physiological optic nerve head cupping. Med Ultrason. 2018;20(1):76–9.

Fundus Photography

25

Ashwini Kulkarni, Timothy Y. Y. Lai, Simon K. H. Szeto, and Niroj Kumar Sahoo

25.1 Introduction

Fundus photography is used to screen, diagnose, and monitor numerous treatable and preventable causes of blindness, particularly diabetic retinopathy, age-related macular degeneration, retinopathy of prematurity, etc. The quality of fundus photographs and the simplicity of imaging have substantially increased over time. Modern technologies can capture a 200° view of the posterior pole in a single acquisition, unlike older devices that can only capture 30–60° of the ocular fundus. The evolution of retinal imaging technology has led to the development of clearer images, pupil tracking, non-mydriatic cameras, ultra-wide field fundus imaging, smartphone fundus imaging, and artificial intelligence-integrated imaging. This chapter highlights the various fundus cameras available, fundus photography techniques, and the use of smartphones for fundus photography.

A. Kulkarni
Kode Venkatadri Chowdary Campus, LV Prasad Eye Institute, Vijayawada, India

T. Y. Y. Lai · S. K. H. Szeto
Department of Ophthalmology and Visual Science, The Chinese University of Hong Kong, Faculty of Medicine, Pok Fu Lam, Hong Kong
e-mail: tyylai@cuhk.edu.hk

N. K. Sahoo (✉)
Anant Bajaj Retina Institute, Kode Venkatadri Chowdary Campus, L V Prasad Eye Institute, Vijayawada, India

25.2 History

In 1886, Jackman and Webster [1] captured and published the first retinal images. Carl Zeiss made the first fundus camera in 1926, which had a 20° field of view (FOV) [2]; the company later produced cameras with a 30–50° FOV. Donaldson [3] reported that Metzger released stereoscopic fundus images in 1927 that were taken using the side-to-side shifting technique. Hansell and Beeson [4] successfully linked the electrical flash tube to the camera in 1953, allowing light to be focused through the pupil. The revolutionary Pomerantzeff Equator-Plus fundus camera debuted in 1960, and Behrendt and Wilson published the first study on nerve fiber layer photography using the conventional Carl Zeiss camera in 1965. According to Dobbins, in 1975, Steven Sasson of Eastman Kodak created the first digital camera, and the subsequent transition from analog to digital revolutionized medical record keeping. Confocal scanning laser ophthalmoscopy (cSLO) has become popular in recent years; it overcomes aberrations due to inadequate dilatation and helps obtain detailed, high-contrast images. Sharper images, non-mydriatic wide-field options, pupil monitoring, and portability have all been added to camera systems over time [5].

T. Das, P. Satgunam (eds.), *Ophthalmic Diagnostics*, https://doi.org/10.1007/978-981-97-0138-4_25

25.3 Technology

25.3.1 Optics of Fundus Photography

Technically, all fundus cameras are indirect ophthalmoscopes that operate on the same principles as Gullstrand's ophthalmoscope. Illumination and observation pathways traverse through different regions of the patient's pupil to avoid reflection off the patient's cornea and crystalline lens surfaces. Meanwhile, an inverted aerial image is created inside the fundus camera and projected onto the film plane.

Optical system: The illumination system, observation, and photography system together form the optical system of the fundus camera. Each part operates independently in the device, and only the front or ophthalmoscopic lens is shared with the other parts.

(a) **Illumination system**: A low-intensity incandescent bulb is used for the photographer to visualize the fundus and focus the device, and a high-intensity electronic flash tube is used to obtain images in flash-based fundus cameras (Fig. 25.1). These two light sources are optically merged by a semi-reflecting surface in the Zeiss fundus camera. In most commercial fundus cameras, the incandescent lamp and the electronic flashtube are mounted on the same base, and a transillumination technique is employed to combine the light paths of these two sources.

(b) **Observation and photographic system**: The size of the illuminated patch on the patient's retina is controlled by adjusting the diaphragm, which receives light from both the viewing lamp and the electrical flash through a common path. This light is projected onto a circular mirror after passing through a set of filters. After being reflected by this mirror, the light is focused by a set of lenses. The topmost lens has a mask that imparts a doughnut shape to the light. The doughnut-shaped light is reflected on a round mirror with a central hole, after which it passes through the objective lens before exiting the camera and then passes via the cornea into the subject's eye. If the illumination system and the image are properly positioned and focused, the resultant retinal image exits the subject's cornea through the center of the doughnut, which is not illu-

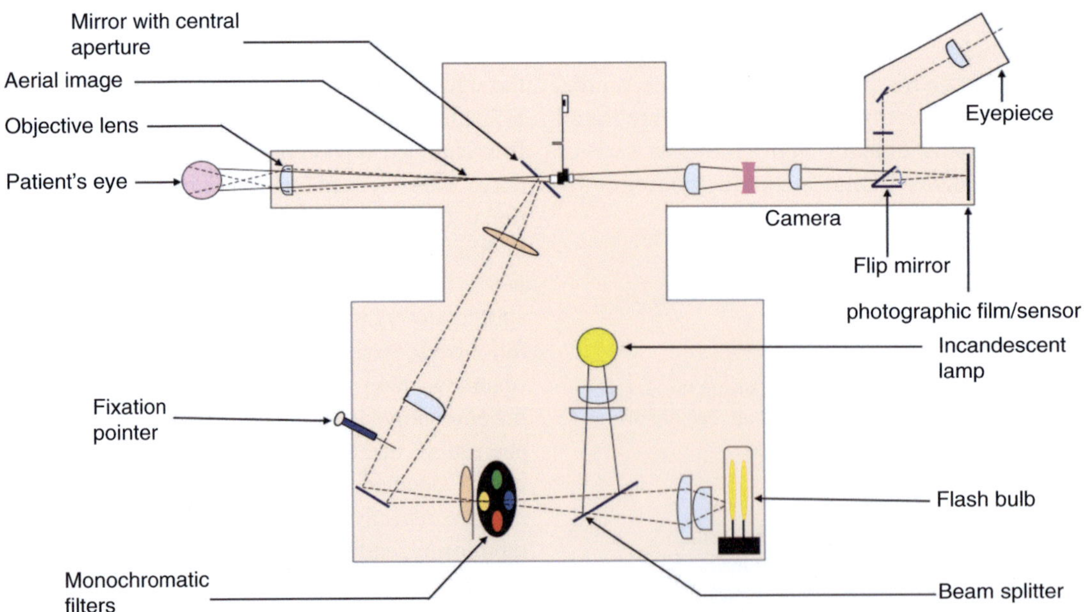

Fig. 25.1 Optics of a fundus camera. (https://www.aao.org/education/image/zeiss-fundus-camera © 2023 American Academy of Ophthalmology)

minated. As a result, the viewing and lighting paths split in the plane of the patient's pupil, freeing the device from unwanted reflexes that will result in glare and image degradation. The light travels through the holed mirror's central aperture, the astigmatic device, and the diopter compensating lenses before returning to the single-lens reflex camera system [6]. The ophthalmoscopic lens creates a fundus image between the holed mirror and the lens, which can be seen through the central aperture of the holed mirror using a compound microscope. An image of the fundus is projected by the microscope's objective using a flip mirror on a ground glass screen positioned at the focal point of the eyepiece. When the picture is taken, the flip mirror that normally directs the image into the eyepiece for observation swings out of the optical path, allowing the image to be projected onto the film for photography. Advances in image capture have significantly improved the quality of captured images.

25.3.2 Advances in Image Capture

25.3.2.1 Digital Imaging

Digital imaging is commonly used in color fundus photography (CFP), fluorescein angiography (FA), and indocyanine green angiography (ICGA). Digital imaging offers advantages over traditional film-based imaging, such as higher image resolution, ease of analysis, better storage, and instant access to images (Table 25.1). It aids in image reproducibility and exporting images for telemedicine. It aids in educating patients and their caretakers about their disease condition by allowing ophthalmologists to display and review the images on a computer monitor. Digital imaging can shorten the learning curve for beginner angiographers as immediate feedback on image quality and camera alignment are available, which improves the image-capturing technique. A digital camera obtains a single image of the retina using flashlight illumination. A digital camera captures true color images of the retina. However, flash intensity should be appropriately controlled to get the best details.

Table 25.1 Digital fundus camera versus confocal scanning laser ophthalmoscope (cSLO)

Digital fundus camera	Confocal scanning laser ophthalmoscope (cSLO)
Single flash of light used at maximum intensity to capture fundus image	Continuous scanning in a raster manner through a pin-hole aperture
Entire cone of light is used	Confocal system
True color image	Pseudo-color image
Bandwidth filters for excitation and emission are used	One excitation wavelength is used, which acts as a laser source
Slower image acquisition	Fast image acquisition
Poor image quality in opaque media and poorly dilated eyes	Good image, even in non-mydriatic pupils, penetrates opaque media; after-image processing decreases motion artifacts
Uses shorter wavelengths for FAF (fundus autofluorescence) and ICGA	Longer wavelength used, which gives better image quality in FAF (fundus autofluorescence) and ICGA

25.3.2.2 Confocal Scanning Laser Ophthalmoscope

The confocal scanning laser ophthalmoscope (cSLO) can be used for several retinal imaging modalities, such as FA, ICGA, and fundus autofluorescence (FAF). It uses monochromatic laser illumination and a confocal optical system to capture high-contrast images. Blue light and near-infrared illumination beams are commonly used for more efficient excitation of fluorescence for FA, FAF, and ICGA. A laser beam scans the retina point-by-point at speeds up to 24 ms in a raster pattern. Images obtained with a cSLO are characteristically rectangular due to the raster scanning pattern. A confocal aperture is positioned in front of the image detector at a focal plane conjugate to the retina, which blocks scattered light and chromatic aberration, enhancing image quality. The light reflected from each retinal point is captured by a photomultiplier. The photomultiplier output is recorded and displayed in a digital video format. Continuous high-speed representation of the flow dynamics of the retinal and choroidal vessels during angiography is also available. This is useful to document the early filling stages required for identifying feeder vessels of macular neovascularization (MNV), retinal angiomatous proliferation (RAP) lesions, etc. It also allows the measurement of capillary flow velocity. The flow velocity is calculated by measuring the transit time of blood between two points separated by a known distance on the video monitor. Simultaneous FA and ICGA can be performed with a single injection of both dyes. The crystalline lens forms the principal barrier for capturing fundus images as the lens is very fluorescent in the short-wavelength range (excitation between 400 and 600 nm results in peak emission at 520 nm). The major disadvantage of the cSLO is its inability to capture full real-color retinal images due to monochromatic illumination.

Several frames can be captured to produce a mean image using eye-tracking software with high acquisition speed (e.g., automatic retinal tracking (ART) mode in the Heidelberg system), and this improves exposure, decreases noise, and can overcome the effect of eye movement during imaging; after-image processing corrects movement artifacts. Sequential cSLO scans taken at increasing depths can create three-dimensional topographic images of the retina or optic disc for retinal thickness or optic nerve head topography assessment [7]. Table 25.1 highlights the differences between the digital fundus camera and cSLO.

In 2019, a panel of experts formally defined various terms based on the fundus FOV. According to these experts, the posterior pole is the area of the retina up to the outer edge of the major temporal vascular arcades and has a 50° FOV. The mid-periphery is the area of the retina from the vascular arcades to the posterior edge of the vortex vein ampullae, with an FOV from 60 to 100°. Wide-field imaging (WFI) produces a retinal image centered on the fovea, including all four retinal quadrants, and posterior to the vortex vein ampullae, i.e., the mid-periphery. In ultra-wide field imaging (UWFI), the retinal surface anterior to the vortex vein ampullae in each quadrant is captured with an FOV of 110–220° [8].

25.3.2.3 Adaptive Optics SLO

Standard fundus cameras cannot focus on individual cells or structures due to aberrations in the visual system. However, individual photoreceptors can be observed using adaptive optics, which uses deformable mirrors to overcome the wavefront distortions of the light reflected from the retinal surface. Recent research has demonstrated the capability of an adaptive optics-based system to image photoreceptor mosaics, arteriolar structures, and pathological lesions with a resolution of 2–3 μm. Its value in detecting decreases in the number of cone photoreceptors in retinitis pigmentosa has been demonstrated [9] (readers are encouraged to refer to Chap. 30 for more details).

25.3.2.4 Wide-Field and Ultra-wide Field Imaging

Wide Field Imaging (WFI) has an FOV of up to 50°, while UWFI systems can image over 80% of the retinal surface area (up to 200° FOV). The peripheral retina can be captured even without adequate mydriasis. The UWFI can be obtained using contact or non-contact systems. The Pomerantzeff camera (with an FOV of 148°), RetCam (with an FOV of 130°), and Panoret-1000™ camera (with an FOV of 130°) are contact-type UWFI cameras. The Optos®, Clarus® 500, and Heidelberg Spectralis with UWFI lens are non-contact UWFI cameras. The Heidelberg Spectralis captures images with an FOV of 105°, and with concomitant use of the Staurenghi lens, it can capture an image with an FOV of 150°; however, this requires a contact procedure.

25.3.3 Examples of Available Fundus Cameras (Table 25.2; Fig. 25.2)

25.3.4 Artifacts in Fundus Photography and Actions to Prevent These

The fundus camera can produce a variety of artifacts:

Illuminated iris: When the pupil is not sufficiently dilated, an illuminated iris causes an orange or bright crescent at the photo's margin.

Table 25.2 Descriptions of the currently available fundus camera

Type	Description	Field of view	Advantages	Disadvantages
Traditional Fundus Camera [10]	Montage with 19 images	96°		Patient cooperation and a skilled photographer required Dynamic studies like FA are not possible
Pomerantzeff Camera [10]	Contact lens-based system uses fiberoptic transpupillary illumination with scleral transillumination	148°		Limited resolution
Panoret [10]	Transscleral illumination with a handheld digital camera; uses contact lens	100°	Can be used in non-mydriatic pupils and lenticular opacity	Difficult to set up
Spectralis [9, 10]	Fundus imaging with spectral domain OCT with cSLO	105° 150° with Staurenghi contact lens	Multi-color imaging Spectral domain OCT with enhanced depth imaging (EDI) OCT, FAF, infrared reflectance, FA, ICGA can be performed simultaneously Reduced eyelash artifact Better imaging of the superior and inferior periphery	Topical anesthesia for contact lens placement required. Lenticular opacities can degrade image quality Needs an experienced photographer Pseudo-color images
Optos [9, 10]	UWF imaging system	200°	Can image through small optical apertures and non-mydriatic pupils. Faster image acquisitions Green-light FAF, FA, ICGA, and OCT (spectral domain [SD-OCT] and swept source) possible. Ultra-wide field angiography	Pseudo-color images Map distortion (when a 3D structure is projected onto a 2D surface) Does not provide a retinal vision before obtaining the image
Clarus [10]	Light-emitting diode (LED) and three distinct wavelength channels (red, green, and blue)	133°	True-color imaging Fewer lash and lid artifacts	Longer image acquisition times
Mirante [11]	SLO-based UWF imaging system	163° with a wide-field lens attachment	OCT angiography (OCTA), FA and ICGA, green and blue FAF, retro-modes, and high-definition OCT and confocal SLO (cSLO) available	Pseudo-color fundus images

(continued)

Table 25.2 (continued)

Type	Description	Field of view	Advantages	Disadvantages
RetCam [12]	Contact-based digital imaging system with an external fiberoptic light source	Portrait-external imaging, 130°—pediatric retina +adult anterior chamber, 120°—pediatric and young adult, 80°—high-contrast pediatric and adult, 30°—high magnification	High-resolution digital photos. Useful screening tool Useful in telemedicine	Lenticular opacities: Poor image quality
3Nethra Neo [12]	Compact and portable system Camera with integrated liquid lens system and LED lighting system	120°	High-resolution digital photos Useful screening tool Useful in telemedicine Color and contrast adjustments possible	Anterior segment photography is not possible
Navilas [13]	Target-locked frequency-doubled solid-state laser with a wavelength of 532 nm		Laser photocoagulation with color fundus photography, FA, and IR imaging available Eye-tracking technology available Ability to import and store multimodal pictures captured by other devices viz. FAF, OCT, ICG angiography images	Difficulty with moderate cataracts High cost of the machine Lack of ICGA and FAF imaging capabilities
Smartphone-based [14]	Smartphone fundus photography with a 20D condensing lens	25°: with i-Examiner 200°: with D-Eye adapter	Convenient, easy to learn, portable Contrast and color editing possible Useful for screening and telemedicine	Requires pupillary dilatation Poor resolution

Action: Move the joystick in the opposite direction. This directs the cone of light through the pupil and avoids the iris.

Eyelashes: The eyelashes cast hazy veils over some portions of the image.

Action: The eyelids should be kept open to prevent the lashes from obscuring the light.

Camera position: Depending on how close or distant the camera is from the eye, there is a haze and loss of detail.

Action: The eyepiece reticle should be adjusted before focusing. To capture the deepest tone of color of the fundus, the camera position and focusing knob should be adjusted till the aerial image of the fundus and the crosshairs appear sharp. The green filter can be used to improve contrast while focusing.

A spot in the same location will appear in images shot at various periods if there is a smudge in the system. This typically results from the patient touching the objective lens with their face, nose, or eyelashes.

Action: Clean the system of all debris or smudges [10].

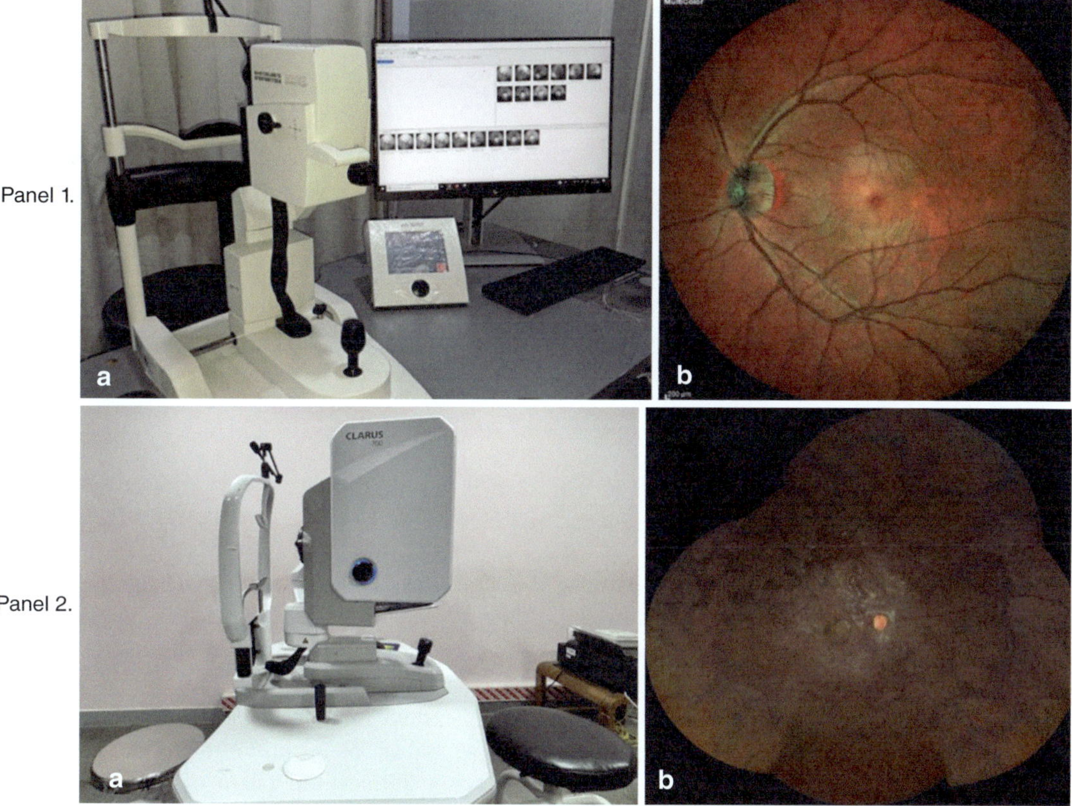

Fig. 25.2 Panel 1. (**a**) Heidelberg Spectralis fundus camera. (**b**) Multi-color imaging of a normal fundus obtained through the fundus camera. Panel 2. (**a**) Wide-field Clarus fundus camera. (**b**) A montage of fundus images of gyrate atrophy. Panel 3. (**a**) Ultra-wide field Optos fundus camera. (**b**) Fundus image of a patient with lasered proliferative diabetic retinopathy. Panel 4. Fundus images of a patient with retinopathy of prematurity (ROP) obtained using a RetCam. (**a**) Stage 1: demarcation line shown by a yellow arrow. (**b**) Stage 2: demarcation ridge. (**c**) Stage 3: extraretinal neovascular proliferation. (**d**) Stage 4A: partial retinal detachment with fovea sparing. (**e**) Aggressive retinopathy of prematurity F) Post-laser photocoagulation of avascular retina. (Picture provided by: Suman Sahu, MD)

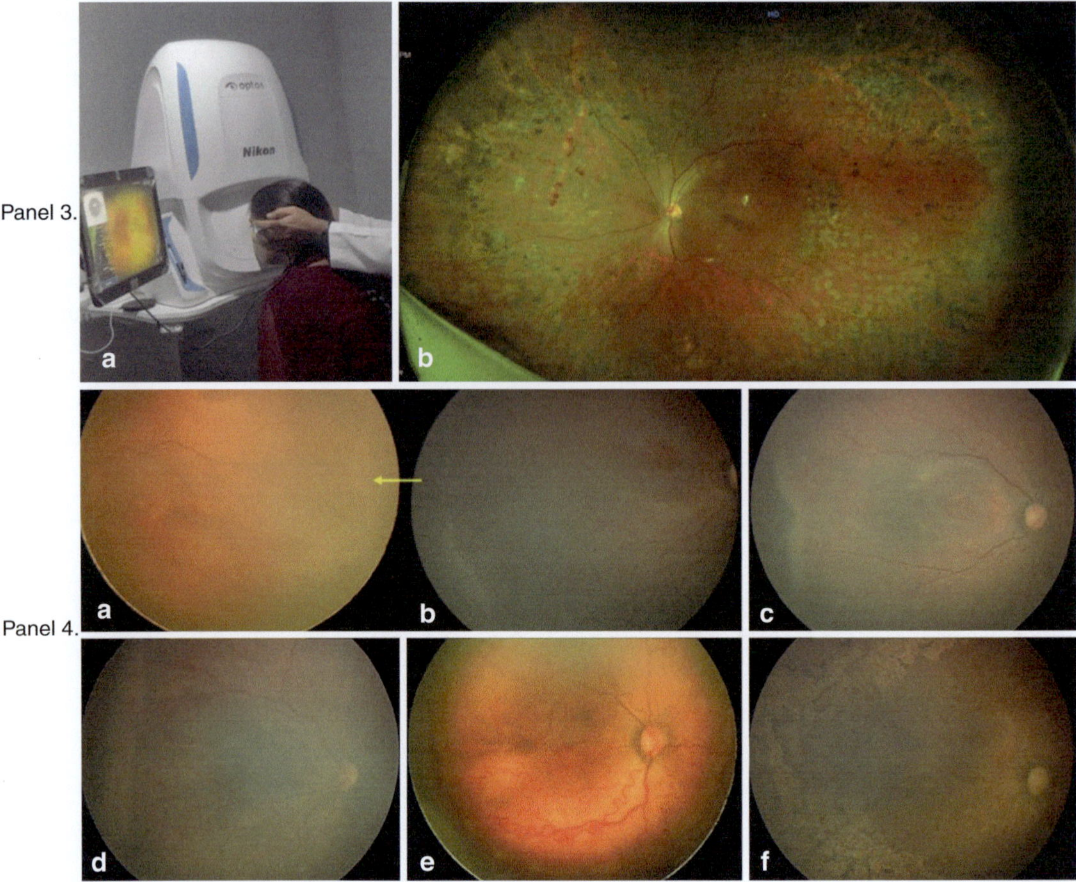

Fig. 25.2 (continued)

25.4 Types of Photography

Conventional flash-based fundus photography gives a true color image of the retina. However, several factors, like poor mydriasis, corneal scar, cataract, vitreous opacity, and background contrast, can all affect its ability to detect certain lesions. Several advances and modifications have been introduced to modern photography units to make them more robust in clinical practice.

25.4.1 Monochromatic Retinal Photography

Monochromatic photography includes capturing retina images under colored or monochromatic light. Vogt pioneered the usage of green light in 1925 to improve the visual contrast of anatomical features of the fundus. Fundus photography frequently employs this method. Using contrast filters to change the subject tones in monochrome images and limiting light scattering at shorter wavelengths are the foundations of monochromatic retinal imaging. It is possible to improve the visibility of specific fundus structures by reducing the spectral range of the illuminating source and limiting light scattering [15].

Blue light: The anterior retinal layers, typically almost transparent in white light, become more visible under blue light. Retinal pigmentation and blood vessels absorb blue light, creating a dark background that enhances specular reflections and scattering in the front layers of the fundus. The efficiency of these wavelengths can be restricted by scattering in the ocular media.

Short-wavelength illumination improves visualization of the semi-transparent scattering structures such as the retinal nerve fiber layer, internal limiting membrane, retinal folds, cysts, and epiretinal membranes. Blue-green (cyan) filters with a wavelength of 490 nm are frequently used because of the significant scattering at very short wavelengths. Scattering is also often seen due to cataract or corneal edema. Blue light imaging can be affected by simple procedures such as applanation tonometry or gonioscopy as it distorts the corneal surface and can produce slight corneal edema, enough to scatter blue light. After staining the cornea, residual fluorescein dye can also result in cumbersome fluorescence that can hamper the image quality [16].

Red-free: Although blood absorbs green light, retinal pigmentation reflects it more than blue light, creating the finest overall contrast and the ideal view of the retinal features. It improves the visibility of hemorrhages, drusen, exudates, and retinal vasculature. Green light has less scattering than the shorter wavelength blue light and can offer a better view of the fundus even in media opacities. Therefore, along with FA, green filter "red-free" pictures are frequently taken as baseline images [16].

Red light: In red light, retinal pigmentation gradually becomes lighter and more transparent, displaying a choroidal pattern with greater details. Red filters produce illumination in the 625–640 nm range, significantly reducing fundus contrast because many retinal structures are red-colored. The optic nerve appears to be exceedingly thin and practically featureless. Red light facilitates the imaging of pigmentary abnormalities, choroidal ruptures, choroidal nevi, and choroidal melanomas. Therefore, red light imaging is also known as the "poor man's ICGA." [16].

25.4.2 Autofluorescence: Blue, Green, and Near-Infrared

Fluorescein dye is used in FA to visualize retinal vasculature and diagnose and monitor retinal pathologies. During the advent of this technique, few ocular structures exhibited fluorescence without the presence of dye. Autofluorescence is the continuous emission of fluorescent light without fluorescein dye from ocular structures. Imaging of these autofluorescent structures aided the diagnosis of various retinal pathologies.

The continuous deposition of lipofuscin (LF) granules in the cytoplasm of retinal pigment epithelial (RPE) cells is a characteristic sign of aging. The continual phagocytosis of shed photoreceptor outer-segment discs is assumed to be the leading cause of this gradual LF accumulation. Once generated, the RPE cell cannot degrade or exocytose the LF material and granules into the extracellular space. These granules are then confined in the postmitotic RPE cells. A2-E (N-retinylidene-N-retinylethanol-amine) is the primary component of lipofuscin along with the precursors of A2-E, molecules created by the combination of oxygen-containing moieties within photo-oxidized A2-E, also known as bisretinoids [9]. The intrinsic autofluorescence of lipofuscin is utilized in FAF imaging. Lipofuscin accumulates excessively due to a disparity between lipofuscin synthesis and clearance caused by RPE dysfunction. The bisretinoids have different excitation wavelengths in the visible spectrum. The RPE cell will seem hyper-autofluorescent on FAF if its lipofuscin concentration is higher. Due to the absence of lipofuscin, atrophic or dead RPE cells exhibit extreme hypo-autofluorescence, whereas healthy cells exhibit varied levels of hyper-autofluorescence and lipofuscin [9].

When exposed to light, lipofuscin absorbs blue light of wavelength 470 nm and emits yellow-green light of 600–610 nm wavelength.

Blue auto-fluorescence (BAF) or shortwave autofluorescence (SWAF) are two terms used to describe autofluorescence based on lipofuscin. Melanin absorbs light at a wavelength of 787 nm and emits at a near-infrared wavelength. Near-infrared autofluorescence (NIRAF) is the autofluorescence based on melanin. The fovea in BAF is darker (hypo-autofluorescent) because of lesser lipofuscin content. On the other hand, the fovea in NIRAF is brighter (hyper-autofluorescent) as melanin is more concentrated at the fovea. Therefore, FAF is useful for the diagnosis and prognosis of many disorders, including central serous chorioretinopathy (CSC), age-related macular degeneration (AMD), retinal dystrophies, and uveitic entities such as choroiditis. A standard fundus camera with a 50–55° FOV can be used to capture FAF images of the retina. The Optos, Heidelberg Spectralis, Mirante, and Clarus all support UWF FAF [17].

Compared to confocal-based systems, which use continuous scanning with an excitation spectrum of 488 nm and acquire several images that are averaged to produce a final image with the highest resolution and contrast, modified fundus cameras use a single flash with an excitation range of 535–585 nm to acquire a single image. FAF imaging provides details on the metabolic changes occurring at the RPE level and aids in locating regions that could be particularly vulnerable to the onset of geographic atrophy or MNV. The green light of wavelengths 514 and 532 nm is used, which excites fluorophores with less absorption by macular pigments than BAF, thus making it more useful than BAF in detecting small atrophic patches near the fovea. Optic disc autofluorescence is higher in green reflectance (GR, 515 nm) than BAF, making GR more efficient for evaluating optic nerve head diseases. Green reflectance (515 nm) shows a higher autofluorescent signal at the disc than the fovea and blood vessels, unlike BAF, which shows a dark gray optic disc [18]. NIRAF uses infrared light for illumination. Red wavelengths are longer than the other wavelengths in the visible spectrum; they also scatter less and are less likely to be absorbed by blood and melanin. In contrast to shorter wavelengths in the visible spectrum, this results in a greater amount of reflected light to generate an image, making it a better technique for imaging deeper structures underneath the RPE.

25.4.3 Multi-color Imaging

Three reflectance pictures are simultaneously captured by multi-color imaging using cSLO: blue reflectance (BR; 488 nm), GR (515 nm), and near-infrared reflectance (IR; 820 nm). The inner retina is seen better with BR; the outer retina, including RPE abnormalities, is seen better with IR; and the retinal blood vessels and exudations in the retinal layers, if present, are seen better using GR. Given that IR is invisible and has higher penetration, it is more advantageous than flash-based retinal photography in imaging the eyes of children, people with photophobia, and people with media opacities such as dense cataracts. Additionally, IR imaging may offer a better view of the epiretinal membranes, cystoid macular edema, and deeper structures.

25.4.4 Retro-mode Imaging

Retro-mode imaging, based on the principles of retro illumination, is used by the F-10 confocal scanning laser ophthalmoscope (cSLO; Nidek, Gamagori, Japan) with an infrared laser to observe the retina. The F-10 is a recently created cSLO device with eight apertures (five confocal apertures and three apertures with a central stop) and four distinct wavelengths (blue, 490 nm; green, 532 nm; red, 660 nm; infrared, 790 nm). Direct backscattered light and additional dispersed light make up the reflected light from the fundus in the cSLO. Only the directly backscattered light from the confocal plane can pass through a confocal aperture. In the indirect (dark-field) mode, a centrally stopped aperture (ring aperture) excludes direct backscattered light. As infrared laser light can reach deeper layers, it is used in retro-mode imaging, a modified form of indirect imaging. The retro mode only utilizes a portion of the annular aperture, not the entire ring aperture used in the indirect mode. The confocal aperture allows the passage of backscattered light from a particular direction and prevents its passage from other directions, thereby creating a pseudo-three-dimensional image by casting a shadow on the side of the aberrant feature. The scattered light that enters the deviated aperture improves contrast and delineation by casting a shadow on aberrant features. The laterality of the annular aperture affects how the lesions' shadows are visible and can be either right-deviated or left-deviated. To identify subretinal and RPE changes, retro-mode imaging offers several advantages. It is a quick, easy, and non-invasive imaging method. The imaging procedure resembles fundus photography. Contrary to FA and ICG angiography, retro-mode imaging does not require an extended capture time or intravenous dye infusion. Owing to the long wavelength of the infrared laser, the examination can be done even in the presence of lens opacity or undilated pupils. Since infrared light is invisible, people are more comfortable during the examination [19].

25.5 Techniques

The patient should sit comfortably at a well-matched table height. The table height should be matched according to each patient so that the patient leans forward into the fundus camera; this reduces the chances of the patient pulling the head back during the procedure. The patient should be asked to place his/her chin on the chin rest with the forehead well approximated to the head bar (Fig. 25.3). The photographer should align the camera using the joystick to move back and forth and upward and downward, directing it toward the patient's fundus through the pupil using the fundus camera. The image should be focused before capturing the picture to eliminate unwanted reflexes or artifacts. The crosshairs should be kept in sharp focus for good focusing, and the camera dial can be used for finer focusing. Patients should be asked to blink before capturing the fundus image as this gives a better lubricated corneal surface, thereby improving image quality and preventing patients from blinking during fundus image capture.

25.5.1 Stereophotography

Stereophotography gives important diagnostic information by imparting a sense of depth. It was used as early as 1909 but was popularized by Lee Allen in the 1960s, who described a practical sequential stereo fundus photography technique [20]. It allows in-depth interpretation of both eyes' images simultaneously taken from slightly different angles. The angiogram is read from right to left; therefore, this order is important as

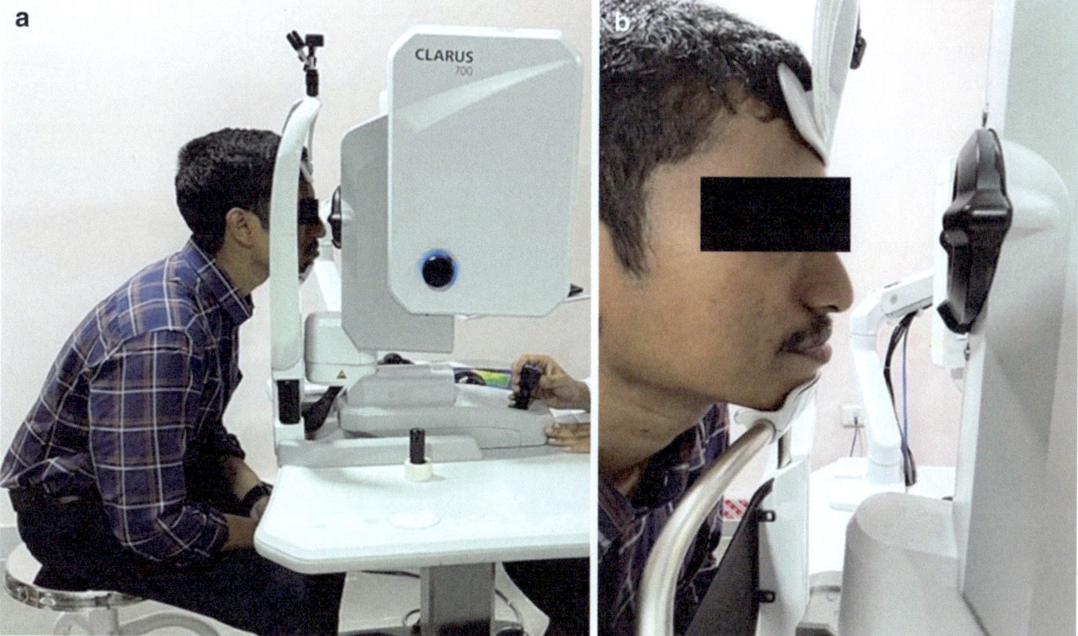

Fig. 25.3 Fundus photography on the fundus camera. (**a**) Patient positioning. (**b**) Optimal position of the head

the photographs are taken and positioned on the film accordingly. The lateral shifting of the fundus camera by a few millimeters between two consecutive photographs causes cornea-induced parallax as the illuminating beam of the fundus camera passes through the opposite slopes of the cornea. This cornea-induced parallax gives a hyper-stereoscopic effect which is appreciated on viewing the sequential pair of photographs together [16]. Specially-made stereo viewers are available to read the stereo images [21, 22].

25.6 Clinical Application and Interpretation

25.6.1 Age-Related Macular Degeneration

Age-related macular degeneration (AMD) is a common macular condition affecting older persons characterized by the development of drusen in the macula, followed by geographic atrophy (GA) or MNV.

Drusen appear differently on FAF according to the size, composition, and condition of the ellipsoid and retinal pigment epithelium (RPE) layer (Figs. 25.4 and 25.5b, e). Cuticular drusen exhibit hypo-autofluorescence on FAF.

Geographic atrophy: Depigmented, hypo-autofluorescent regions corresponding to RPE loss in dry AMD may indicate early GA (Fig. 25.6a). Loss of intrinsic fluorophores is seen in RPE atrophy, leading to negligible/nil FAF signal with clearly defined borders. Perilesional hyper-autofluorescence, which indicates functional disturbances in RPE, is occasionally seen around GA and suggests progression (Fig. 25.6b) [23].

Initially, the FAM (Fundus autofluorescence in age-related macular degeneration) investigation identified eight patterns of FAF in the junction zone of GA [24], which were subsequently updated to include a ninth pattern [25]. Eyes are categorized as "none" (when there is no evidence of enhanced autofluorescence signal at the outer margins of the GA), "localized" (focal, patchy, and banded autofluorescence is detected), and "diffuse" (branching, fine granular, fine granular with punctuated spots, trickling, and reticular autofluorescence is detected) in the junction zone of atrophy [26]. The significance of these patterns lies in the possibility that they correspond to various phenotypic forms of the illness. Analysis of natural history showed that different subtypes of FAF grow at different rates and that the progression of atrophy in GA and the FAF pattern are strongly correlated [25, 26].

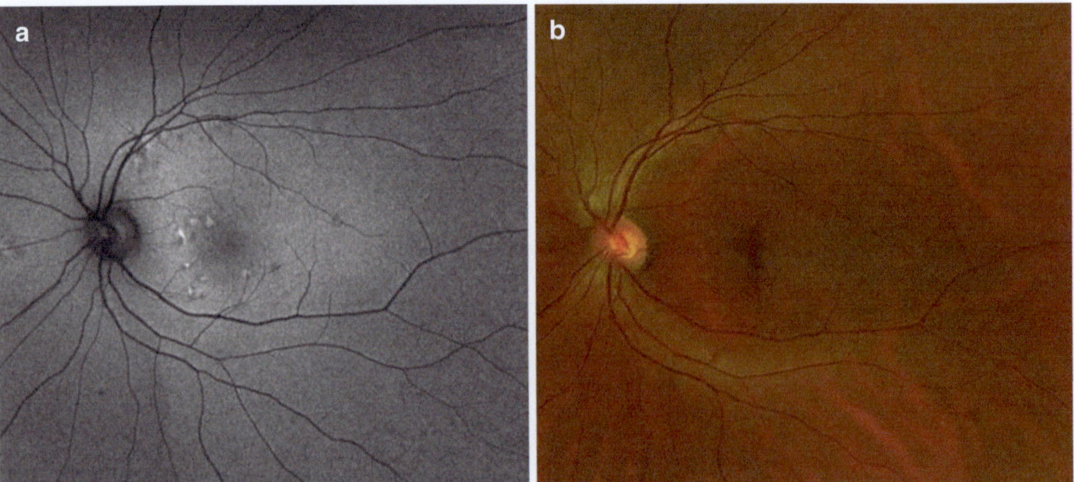

Fig. 25.4 Drusen seen as (**a**) a hyper-autofluorescent lesion on autofluorescence imaging, and a yellowish lesion on (**b**) a multi-color fundus image. (Image courtesy: Rajeev K Reddy Pappuru, MD)

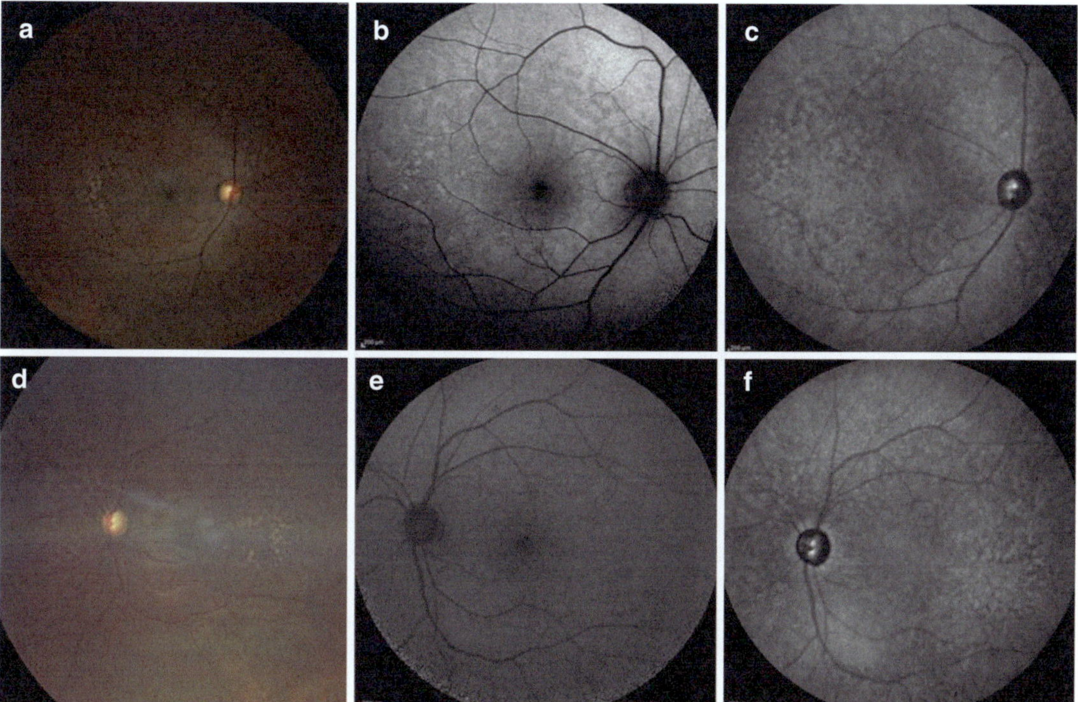

Fig. 25.5 Familial dominant drusen. Color fundus photographs (**a** and **d**) showing drusen which are seen as hyperfluorescent lesions on autofluorescence imaging (**b** and **e**) and hyper-reflective lesions on IR (**c** and **f**). (Image courtesy: Deepika C Parameswarappa, MD)

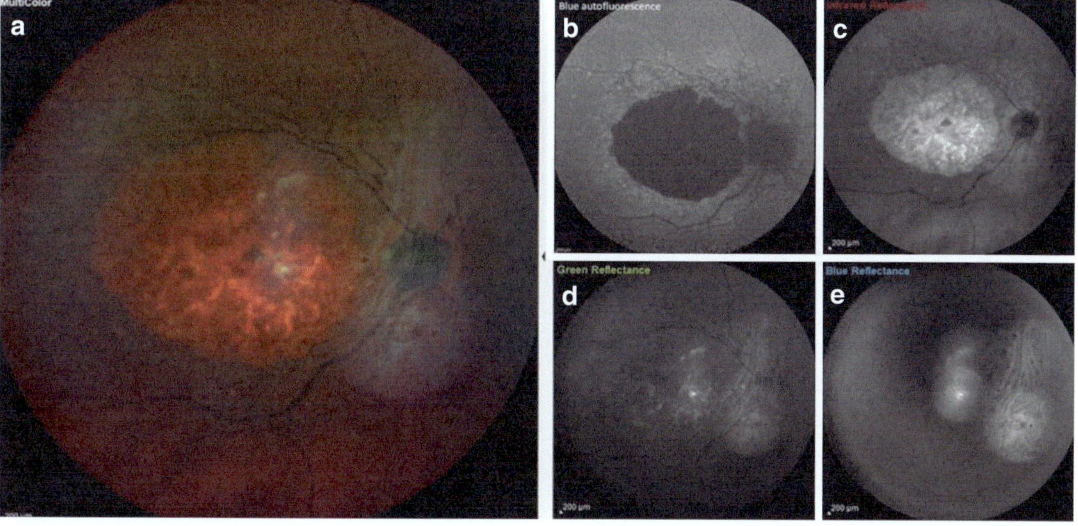

Fig. 25.6 Geographic atrophy in dry AMD. (**a**) Multicolor fundus image. (**b**) Blue autofluorescence (white arrow shows the perilesional hyper-autofluorescence) (**c**) Infrared reflectance: delineating the extent of GA. (**d**) Green reflectance image and (**e**) Blue reflectance image. Central macula and disc details appeared as hazy due to artifact. (Image courtesy: Mudit Tyagi, MD)

Multi-color imaging is a good tool for determining the size and extent of GA and assessing the extent of fovea sparing. IR pictures are best for visualizing GA (Fig. 25.6c). Refractile drusen are a common complication of AMD and are considered a key predictive biomarker for the emergence of central GA. Soft drusen are seen as green structures with orange borders in the multi-color composite image; the reticular drusen are distinguished as shiny, light-yellow structures. In GR and BR, refractile drusen are hyper-reflectant, but soft drusen only appear slightly hyper-reflectant (Fig. 25.4c, f) [27].

Drusen has a pseudo-3D appearance on retromode imaging, consistent with OCT (optical coherence tomography) imaging. Retro-mode imaging identifies more drusen than conventional color fundus photography and cSLO. Retromode imaging is most sensitive in identifying subtle drusen and can efficiently distinguish between various types of drusen. It can accurately determine the extent of GA and detect retinal changes related to exudative AMD, such as choroidal neovascularization (CNV) and cystoid macular edema (CME) [19].

RPE tears: Hypo-autofluorescence with well-defined borders is seen in areas with absent RPE, and the adjacent rolled-over RPE appears hyper-autofluorescent.

25.6.2 Polypoidal Choroidal Vasculopathy (PCV)

Massive submacular hemorrhage or orange subretinal nodules are strong indicators of PCV and appear hypo-autofluorescent due to the blockage of the underlying fluorescence by the hemorrhage (Fig. 25.7). In most PCV patients, polypoidal lesions can be found with multi-color imaging. Since the lesions are below the RPE, it is best to visualize the polypoidal lesions and branching neovascular network (BNN) using a multi-color composite or infrared reflectance imaging. On multi-color imaging, polypoidal lesions appear as dark-green oval lesions, while BNN is seen as a stippled gray area on IR. Details of pigment epithelial detachment (PED) and subretinal hemorrhage are also clearly discernible [27]. The physical characteristics of PCV, such as polypoidal lesions and branching vascular networks, can be easily seen with retro-mode imaging [19].

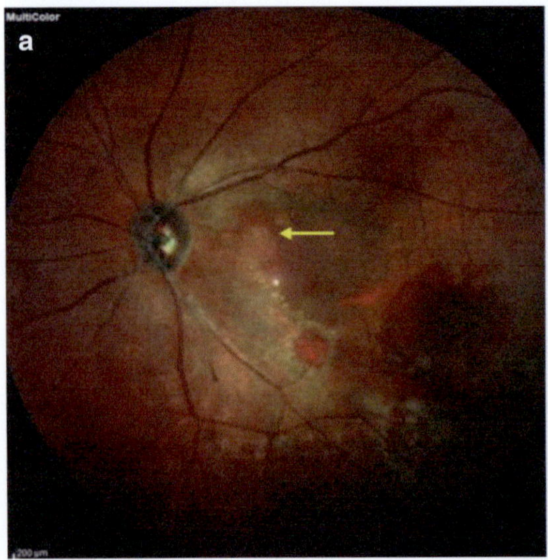

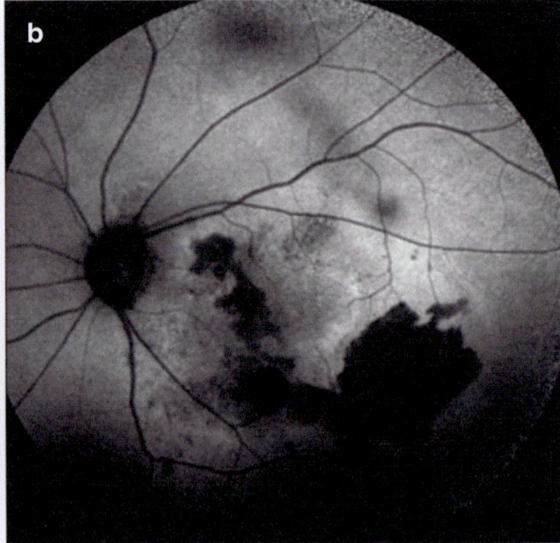

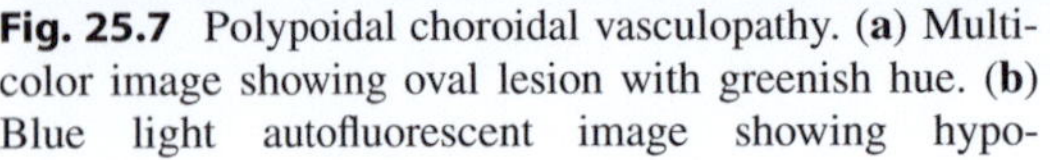

Fig. 25.7 Polypoidal choroidal vasculopathy. (**a**) Multi-color image showing oval lesion with greenish hue. (**b**) Blue light autofluorescent image showing hypo-autofluorescent lesion due to blockage of underlying autofluorescence by hemorrhage. (Image courtesy: Mukesh Jain, MD)

25.6.3 Central Serous Chorioretinopathy

Central serous chorioretinopathy (CSC) occurs due to choroidal dysfunction and idiopathic leak through the RPE leading to serous retinal detachment. Granular hyper-autofluorescence is seen on FAF, corresponding to subretinal precipitates on OCT. These precipitates occur due to the separation of the neurosensory retina from the RPE layer and are believed to be debris from the photoreceptor layer along with macrophages. In chronic CSC (longer than 6 months), gravitational tracts are seen as granular hyper-autofluorescent/hypo-autofluorescent areas, based on the disease duration, due to long-standing subretinal fluid (Fig. 25.8). NIRAF gives better details than BAF in CSC and is preferred for diagnosis and monitoring [27].

Multi-color imaging detects pigment epithelial detachment (PED) and RPE atrophy; sub retinal fluid (SRF) is best demonstrated with GR. Since PED is located at a deeper level than SRF, multi-color imaging recognizes it as an elevation of the retinal contour and gives it a greenish hue that is darker than SRF. PED has smaller, well-circumscribed sizes and pink rings around it, distinguishing it from SRF on multi-color imaging. PED is best detected on infrared images due to its deep location. Infrared imaging provides a superior view of RPE atrophy compared to BR or GR imaging. On multi-color imaging, focal leaks are seen as orange spots [27].

25.6.4 Macular Dystrophies

25.6.4.1 Stargardt Disease

The initial stages have increased lipofuscin production and a corresponding rise in autofluorescence. Eventually, chorioretinal atrophy occurs, causing macular hypo-autofluorescence outlined by hyper-autofluorescent flecks (Fig. 25.9) [27]. On multi-color imaging, the delineation of the central area of atrophy is clearer [27]. Any material deposition in the retina is seen as a raised area with various sizes and shapes, uneven borders, and darker hues on retro-mode imaging [19].

25.6.4.2 Best Disease

The vitelliform stage has well-defined, uniform hyper-autofluorescence at the macula. A hyper-autofluorescent layer is seen settled beneath iso-autofluorescent fluid due to gravity in the

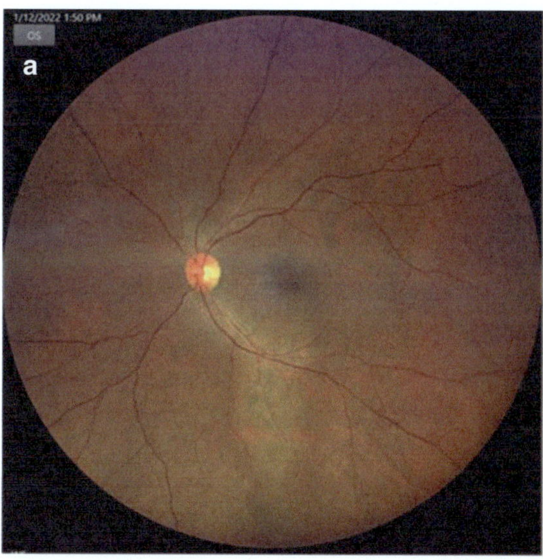

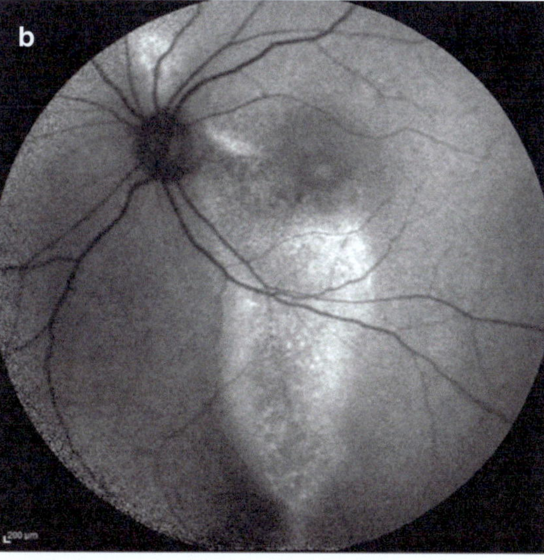

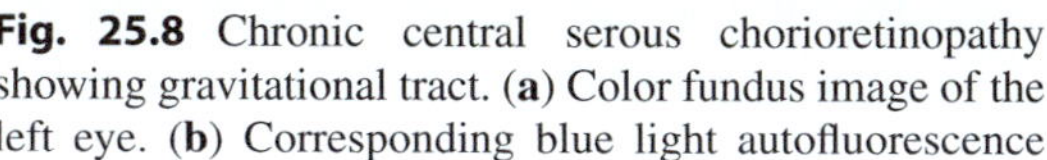

Fig. 25.8 Chronic central serous chorioretinopathy showing gravitational tract. (**a**) Color fundus image of the left eye. (**b**) Corresponding blue light autofluorescence image showing hypo-autofluorescent gravitational tract with hyper-autofluorescent border. (Image courtesy: Vivek Pravin Dave, MD)

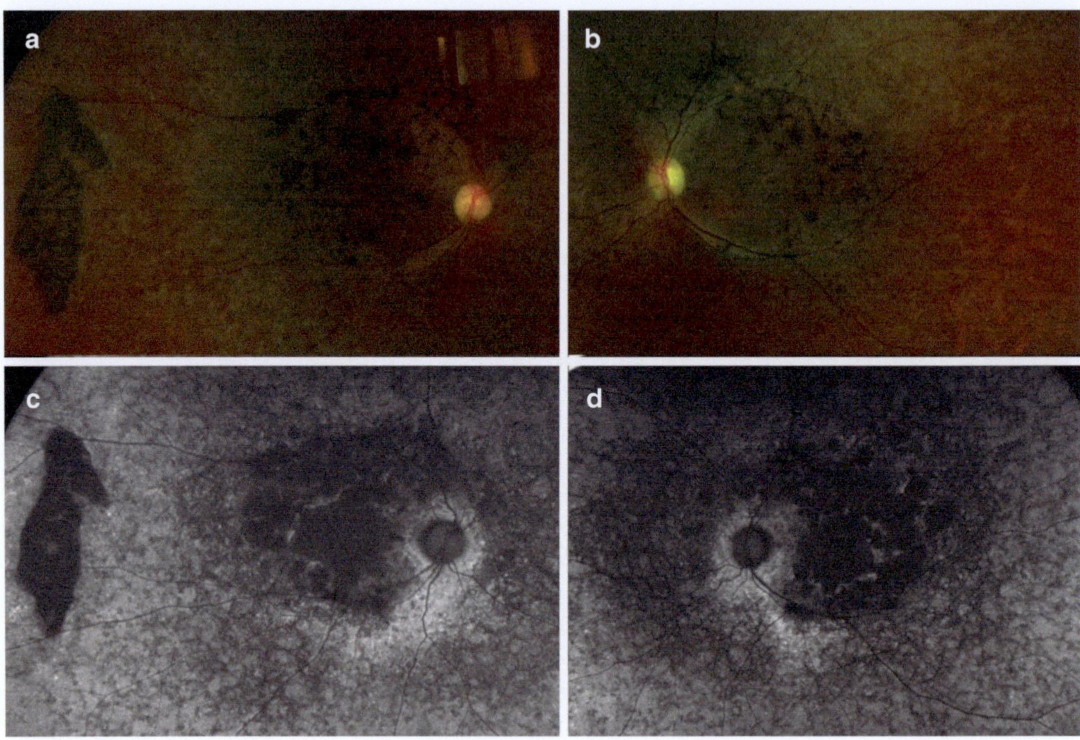

Fig. 25.9 Stargardt's disease. (**a**, **b**). Multi-color image of left and right eye, respectively; (**c**, **d**). Autofluorescence image showing distinctly demarcated central macular atrophy in both eyes. (Courtesy: Subhadra Jalali, MD)

pseudohypopyon stage. A dark lesion surrounded by hyper-autofluorescent deposits is seen in the vitelliruptive stage. Chorioretinal atrophy occurs in the atrophic stage, resulting in hypo-autofluorescence [27]. Retinal elevation during the pseudohypopyon stage is defined more clearly on composite multi-color and blue reflectance imaging. Subretinal lipofuscin is seen better in GR images. The multi-color image shows several orange dots corresponding to yellow lesions and a greenish hue over the macula, suggesting increased retinal thickness. Numerous white hyper-reflective spots in the infrared images indicate RPE level changes [27].

25.6.4.3 Retinitis Pigmentosa (RP)

The inner/outer-segment junction disruption edge seen on OCT corresponds to the hyper-autofluorescent "Robson-Holder ring" (Fig. 25.10). Also, kinetic and automated perimetry show a correlation between the size of the ring and visual function; the more central the ring, the smaller the visual field. Other retinal dystrophies exhibit similar hyper-autofluorescent rings, such as Best macular dystrophy, Leber congenital amaurosis (LCA), X-linked retinoschisis, bull's eye maculopathy, and cone dystrophy [27]. Multi-color imaging is better at identifying macular changes and complications in patients with RP.

25.6.4.4 Fundus Albipunctatus

FAF shows hyper-autofluorescence foci correlating to the white dots; however, not all the lesions show hyper-fluorescence [27].

25.6.4.5 Choroideremia

Multi-color imaging shows the surrounding chorioretinal atrophy and RPE tissue at the macula significantly better than the color fundus photo. In contrast to GR and BR, the remnant RPE tissue is seen in infrared. In individuals with choroi-

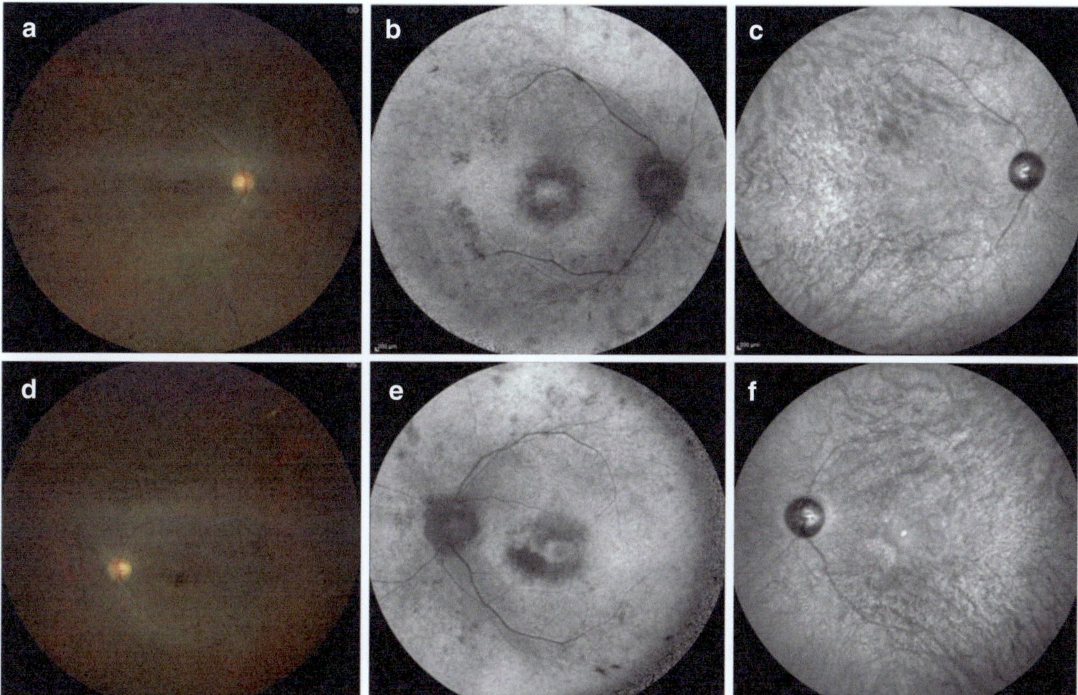

Fig. 25.10 Retinitis pigmentosa. (**a** and **d**) Color fundus photograph. (**b** and **e**) Blue light autofluorescence images (BAF). (**c** and **f**) IR images. (Image courtesy: Deepika C Parameswarappa, MD)

deremia, multi-color imaging can be used to assess the viability of the retina and monitor disease progression [27].

25.6.5 White Dot Syndromes

25.6.5.1 Multiple Evanescent White Dot Syndrome (MEWDS)

On FAF, hyperfluorescent lesions are seen, as photoreceptor loss unmasks the autofluorescence of the underlying RPE [27].

25.6.5.2 Punctate Inner Choroidopathy (PIC)

Active PIC lesions manifest as chorioretinal nodules at the sub-RPE level, which show faint hyper-autofluorescence initially or change into hypo-autofluorescent patches when the nodules breach through the RPE. A hyper-autofluorescent border that is seen around these hypo-autofluorescent lesions correlates with photoreceptor loss on SD-OCT [27].

25.6.6 Drug Toxicity

A hyper-autofluorescent parafoveal ring corresponding to photoreceptor damage is seen on FAF that diminishes over time due to RPE atrophy. Bilateral bull's eye maculopathy is seen in the late stage of the disease. An arcuate band of hypo-reflectance surrounds the speckled hyper-reflectance at the macula, best seen on infrared images. Multi-color imaging detects a greater extent of retinal involvement than color fundus photos [27].

25.6.7 Vascular Retinopathy

25.6.7.1 Diabetic Retinopathy (DR)

Microaneurysms appear as dark red dots on multi-color imaging, hard exudates as greenish-yellow, and cotton wool spots appear greenish-white. Multi-color imaging can rapidly detect early subtle neovascularization in proliferative

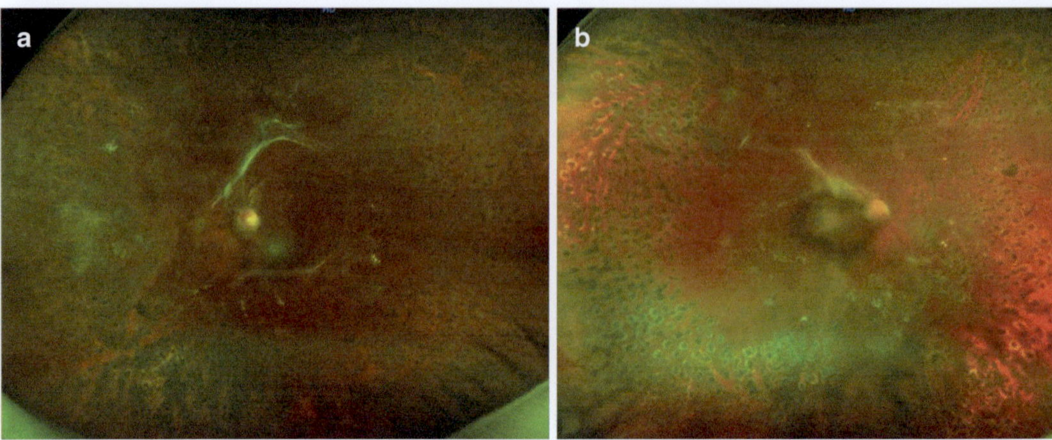

Fig. 25.11 Ultra-wide field multi-color image of right (**a**) and left (**b**) eyes of a case of proliferative diabetic retinopathy after panretinal photocoagulation. Regressing new vessels can be appreciated in both eyes. (Image courtesy: Brijesh Takkar, MD)

diabetic retinopathy that may be undetected on color fundus photos. (Fig. 25.11) [27].

25.6.7.2 Retinal Vascular Occlusion

Multi-color imaging can identify mild retinal thickening and macular edema. Macular edema appears as a green hue over the affected retina. Multi-color imaging enables the diagnosis and monitors the progression of the disease and its response to treatment. It aids in deciding treatment and prognostication [27].

25.6.8 Miscellaneous Retinal Lesions

25.6.8.1 Macular Hole

The macular hole margin, SRF, and RPE atrophy are visualized better through multi-color imaging than in color fundus photos. Multi-color imaging can also identify inner retinal changes in patients who had undergone internal limiting membrane (ILM) peeling. Spectral-domain optical coherence tomography (SD-OCT) is typically used to diagnose dissociated optic nerve fiber layers resulting from ILM peeling in macular hole repair. The dissociated optic nerve fiber layer appears as darker arcuate areas on multi-color imaging. BR is better than GR for assessing the dissociated optic nerve fiber layer [27].

25.6.8.2 Macular Telangiectasia Type 2

BR imaging reveals a distinctive oval parafoveal area with enhanced reflectance. It is a reliable; quick, and non-invasive diagnostic method for detecting macular telangiectasia [27].

25.6.8.3 Epiretinal Membrane

The best way to visualize the hyper-reflective surface folds of the epiretinal membrane are with GR imaging. The ERM is visible in multi-color imaging as greenish retinal membranes [27].

25.6.8.4 Angioid Streaks

Angioid streaks are highlighted as dark orange in multi-color imaging (Fig. 25.12). In contrast to GR and BR, these are better seen in infrared. Complications like CNV can be better detected through multi-color imaging [27].

25.6.8.5 Retinochoroidal Colobomas

The neurosensory retina located within the coloboma (also known as the intercalary membrane) is the most frequent location for retinal breaks and retinal detachments (Fig. 25.13) [28]. Goel et al. have reported the efficacy of multi color imaging (MCI) in detecting intercalary membrane detachment [29].

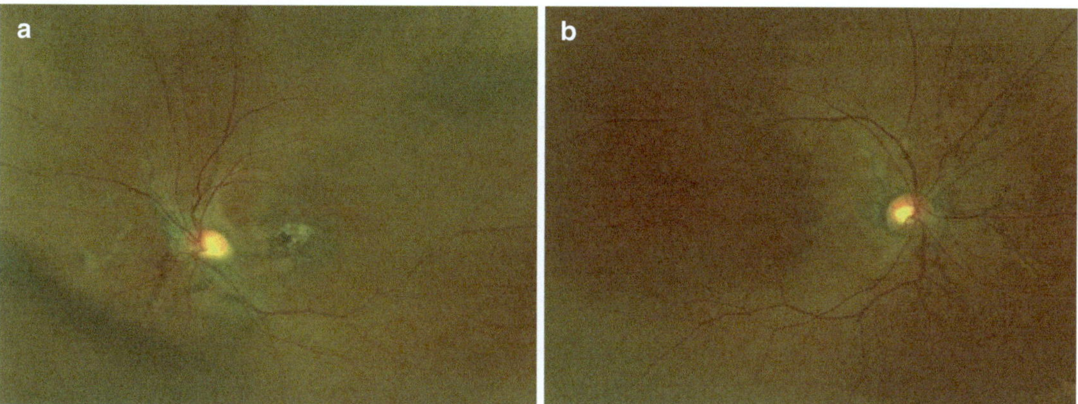

Fig. 25.12 Multi-color fundus image in the right (**a**) and left eye (**b**) in a case of angioid streaks. (Image courtesy: Vivek Pravin Dave, MD)

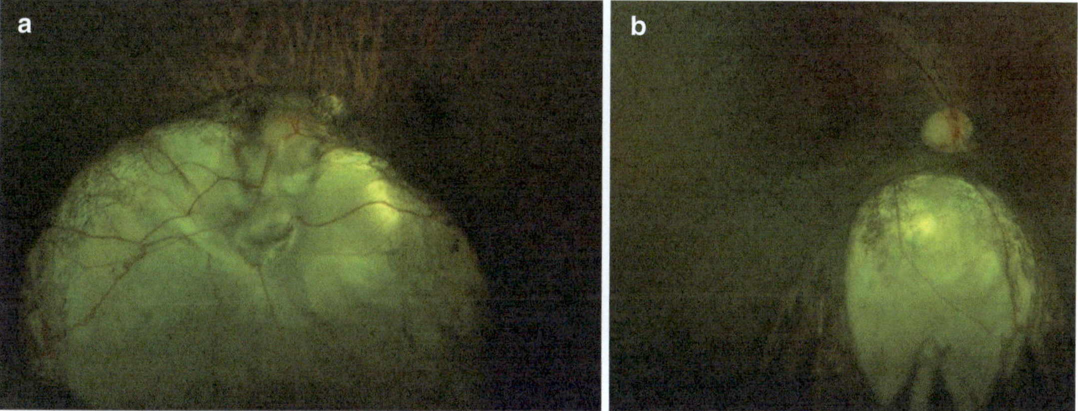

Fig. 25.13 Multi-color image of right (**a**) and left (**b**) eye in a case of retinochoroidal coloboma. (Image courtesy: Mukesh Jain, MD)

25.6.8.6 Myelinated Nerve Fibers (MNF)

The MNF appears greenish or greenish-orange on a multi-color image according to the retinal thickness. Infrared is best for detecting retinal thickening due to the high melanin content of MNF. Multi-color images and infrared images demarcate disc margins better than CFP [27].

25.6.8.7 Choroidal Disorders

The characteristics of choroidal and retinal pigmentary lesions, such as choroidal nevus, choroidal melanoma, and choroidal hemangioma, including margin, extent, and halo, can be detected using multi-color imaging, especially when combined with infrared imaging.

25.6.9 Optic Nerve Head Disorders

Retinal nerve fiber layer (RNFL) defects are highlighted by multi-color imaging as wedge defects without a greenish hue in glaucoma, as opposed to the greenish hue apparent in healthy RNFL. Due to the wide, shallow, and slanted disc, myopic crescent, and macular degeneration in myopic eyes, it can be challenging to interpret the cupping of the optic disc and the health of the neuroretinal rim. Unlike color and red-free optic disc photography, multi-color imaging can distinguish between the neuroretinal rim and optic cup. The use of multi-color imaging helps diagnose the optic disc pit [30]. Retinoschisis, serous macular detachment, and retinal atrophy are some of the signs of optic disc pit maculopathy [27].

25.6.10 Pathologic Myopia

Myopic maculopathy lesions are categorized into five categories, ranging from 0 to 4, according to the META-PM (meta-analysis of pathological myopia) classification system (Table 25.3), developed using fundus photographs. Lacquer cracks, myopic CNV, and Fuchs' spots were added as plus signs since they can arise from or coexist in the eyes with any of the myopic maculopathy categories and cause central vision loss. Myopic CNV (Fig. 25.14a) usually appears on fundoscopy as a small, flat, grayish subretinal lesion underneath or near the fovea, with or without hemorrhage [31]. Lacquer cracks may often be difficult to identify due to a lack of contrast in the myopic fundus. Fundus autofluorescence imaging only detects 12.5% of lacquer cracks, which appear as linear hypo-autofluorescence, whereas infrared has a comparatively high sensitivity (92.9%); lacquer cracks are seen as hyper-reflective lines (Fig. 25.14b) [32]. UWF fundus imaging can help identify peripheral retinal lesions like lattice degeneration, which is common in high myopia (Fig. 25.14c).

Table 25.3 Classification of Myopic Maculopathy according to META-PM study [32]

META-PM classification	Myopic retinal changes	Fundus appearance
Category 0	No myopic retinal changes	
Category 1	Tessellated fundus	Well-defined choroidal vessels can be observed clearly around the fovea and arcade vessels
Category 2	Diffuse chorioretinal atrophy	The posterior pole appears yellowish-white, the extent of which is variable
Category 3	Patchy chorioretinal atrophy	Well-defined, grayish-white lesions of variable size; between one and several choroidal lobules
Category 4	Macular atrophy	Well-defined, round chorioretinal atrophic lesion is grayish-white or whitish around a regressed fibrovascular membrane that enlarges with time. Generally, macular atrophy is centered on the central fovea and has a round shape
+Lc	Lacquer cracks	Yellowish thick linear pattern
+CNV	Choroidal neovascularization	Active CNV should be accompanied by exudative activity or hemorrhage. Serous retinal detachments can be present
+Fs	Fuchs spot	Pigmented spot representing the dry fibrovascular scar of myopic CNV
–	Posterior staphyloma	Local bulging of the sclera at the posterior pole that has a radius that is less than the surrounding curvature of the wall of the eye

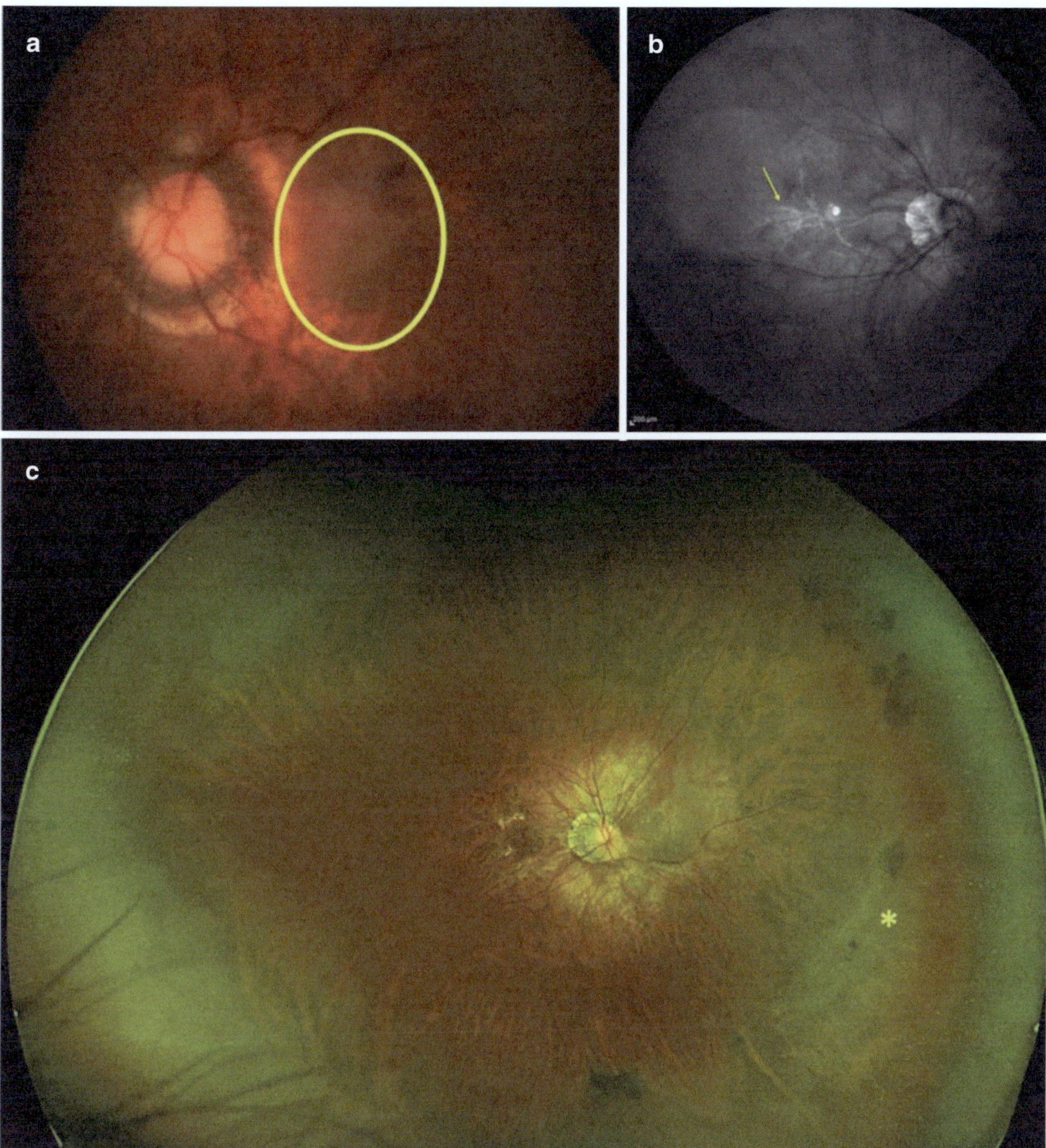

Fig. 25.14 Pathological myopia. (**a**) Myopic CNVM (yellow circle) is seen as a grayish lesion at the macula. (**b**) Lacquer cracks (yellow arrow) are seen as hyper-reflective lines on IR imaging. (**c**) The ultra-wide field image shows lattice degeneration (asterisk)

25.7 Conclusion

Fundus photography is useful for documenting and monitoring progress during treatment and telemedicine, patient education, and academic purposes. However, it requires good judgment to use the correct imaging mode and FOV; this varies according to the clinical condition of the patient and the requirements for the enhanced visualization of the pathology. It is an essential and indispensable tool for an ophthalmologist if used wisely.

Funding Hyderabad Eye Research Foundation, Hyderabad, India.

Disclosure TYYL: Consultant: Allergan, Bayer, Boehringer Ingelheim, Iveric Bio, Novartis, Oculis, Roche; Speaker: Alcon, Bayer, Chendu Kanghong Biotech, Novartis, Roche. Other authors: Nil

References

1. Jackman WT, Webster JD. On photographing the retina of the living human eye. Philadel Photogr. 1886;23(275):275–6.
2. Ciardella A, Brown D. Wide-field imaging. In: Agarwal A, editor. Fundus fluorescein and Indocyanine green angiography: a textbook and atlas. 1st ed. Thorofare: Slack Inc.; 2007. p. 79–84.
3. Hansell P, Beeson EJG. Retinal photography in color. Br J Ophthalmol. 1953;37(2):65.
4. Donaldson DD. A new camera for stereoscopic fundus photography. Trans Am Ophthalmol Soc. 1964;62:429–58.
5. Panwar N, Huang P, Lee J, Keane PA, Chuan TS, Richhariya A, Teoh S, Lim TH, Agrawal R. Fundus photography in the 21st century—a review of recent technological advances and their implications for worldwide healthcare. Telemed J E Health. 2016;22(3):198–208.
6. Fundus photography overview—ophthalmic photographers' society. 2023. https://www.opsweb.org/page/fundusphotography.
7. Bennett TJ. Scanning laser ophthalmoscopy. The Ophthalmic Photographers' Society Inc; 2023. https://www.opsweb.org/page/SLO.
8. Choudhry N, Duker JS, Freund KB, et al. Classification and guidelines for wide-field imaging: recommendations from the International Wide-Field Imaging Study Group. Ophthalmol Retina. 2019;3(10):843–9.
9. Jain AB, Prakash VJ, Bhende M. Techniques of fundus imaging. Med Vis Res Found. 2015;33:100.
10. Klufas MA, Kiss S. Widefield Imaging. In: Sadda SR, Schachat AP, Wilkinson CP, Hinton DR, Wiedemann P, Freund KB, Sarraf D, editors. Ryan's Retina. 7th ed. Elsevier Health Sciences; 2022. p. 170-202.
11. Nagpal M, Mohan G, Soni A, Talati S, Mehrotra N. Wide-field Multimodal Imaging. Retina Today. 2020. https://retinatoday.com/articles/2020-jan-feb/widefield-multimodal-imaging.
12. Agarwal K, Vinekar A, Chandra P, Padhi TR, Nayak S, Jayanna S, Panchal B, Jalali S, Das T. Imaging the pediatric retina: an overview. Indian J Ophthalmol. 2021;69(4):812.
13. Chhablani J, Kozak I, Barteselli G, El-Emam S. A novel navigated laser system brings new efficacy to the treatment of retinovascular disorders. Oman J Ophthalmol. 2013;6(1):18.
14. Iqbal U. Smartphone fundus photography: a narrative review. Int J Retina Vitreous. 2021;7(1):44.
15. Bennett TJ, Barry CJ. Ophthalmic imaging today: an ophthalmic photographer's viewpoint—a review. Clin Experiment Ophthalmol. 2009;37(1):2–13.
16. Bennett TJ. Monochromatic fundus photography. The Ophthalmic Photographers' Society Inc; 2023. https://www.opsweb.org/page/Monochromatic.
17. Mishra C, Tripathy K. Fundus camera. In: StatPearls. Treasure Island, FL: StatPearls Publishing; 2023. http://www.ncbi.nlm.nih.gov/books/NBK585111/.
18. Bittencourt MG, Hassan M, Halim MS, Afridi R, Nguyen NV, Plaza C, Tran AN, Ahmed MI, Nguyen QD, Sepah YJ. Blue light versus green light fundus autofluorescence in normal subjects and in patients with retinochoroidopathy secondary to retinal and uveitic diseases. J Ophthal Inflamm Infect. 2019;9:1–9.
19. Lee WJ, Lee BR, Shin YU. Retromode imaging: review and perspectives. Saudi J Ophthalmol. 2014;28(2):88–94.
20. Allen L. Ocular fundus photography: suggestions for achieving consistently good pictures and instructions for stereoscopic photography. Am J Ophthalmol. 1964;57(1):13–28.
21. Nema HV, Nema N. Diagnostic procedures in ophthalmology. JP Medical Ltd; 2014.
22. Bennet TJ. Stereo photography-rotational stereo imaging. The Ophthalmic Photographers' Society Inc; 2013. https://www.opsweb.org/blogpost/777793/Stereo-Photography?tag=3D.
23. Yung M, Klufas MA, Sarraf D. Clinical applications of fundus autofluorescence in retinal disease. Int J Retin Vitr. 2016;2:1–25.
24. Bindewald A, Schmitz-Valckenberg S, Jorzik JJ, Dolar-Szczasny J, Sieber H, Keilhauer C, Weinberger AW, Dithmar S, Pauleikhoff D, Mansmann U, Wolf S. Classification of abnormal fundus autofluorescence patterns in the junctional zone of geographic atrophy in patients with age related macular degeneration. Br J Ophthalmol. 2005;89(7):874–8.
25. Holz FG, Bindewald-Wittich A, Fleckenstein M, Dreyhaupt J, Scholl HP, Schmitz-Valckenberg S, FAM-Study Group. Progression of geographic atrophy and impact of fundus autofluorescence patterns in age-related macular degeneration. Am J Ophthalmol. 2007;143(3):463–72.
26. Schmitz-Valckenberg S, Bindewald-Wittich A, Dolar-Szczasny J, Dreyhaupt J, Wolf S, Scholl HP, Holz FG. Correlation between the area of increased autofluorescence surrounding geographic atrophy and disease progression in patients with AMD. Invest Ophthalmol Vis Sci. 2006;47(6):2648–54.
27. Tan A, Fleckenstein M, Schmitz-Valckenberg S, Holz FG. Clinical application of multi-color imaging technology. Ophthalmologica. 2016;236(1):8–18.
28. Gopal L, Badrinath SS, Sharma T, Parikh SN, Biswas J. Pattern of retinal breaks and retinal detachments

in eyes with choroidal coloboma. Ophthalmology. 1995;102(8):1212–7.
29. Goel S, Saurabh K, Roy R. Multicolour imaging in retinochoroidal coloboma. Clin Exp Optom. 2020;103(5):710–1.
30. Saurabh K, Roy R, Shah D, Sinha RS. Multicolour imaging in a patient with optic disc pit maculopathy. Clin Exp Optom. 2018;101(6):805–6.
31. Ohno-Matsui K, Ikuno Y, Lai TY, Cheung CM. Diagnosis and treatment guideline for myopic choroidal neovascularization due to pathologic myopia. Prog Retin Eye Res. 2018;63:92–106.
32. Ohno-Matsui K, Lai TY, Lai CC, Cheung CM. Updates of pathologic myopia Prog. Retin Eye Res. 2016;52:156–87.

26 Dye-Based Angiography

Ashwini Kulkarni, Timothy Y. Y. Lai, Simon K. H. Szeto, and Niroj Kumar Sahoo

26.1 Introduction

The evaluation of retinal disorders and retinal imaging has evolved from using crude instruments in fundoscopy to dye-based imaging techniques. At present, high-resolution imaging of retinal and choroidal vessels is possible with modern, high-quality fundus cameras, digital imaging, and photographic filters. Fluorescein angiography (FA) is an efficient tool for evaluating retinal circulation, and indocyanine green angiography (ICGA) offers a more precise resolution of the choroidal circulation. In this chapter, we will highlight the basics of retinal imaging, equipment, techniques of FA and ICGA, image analysis, and their clinical implications.

A. Kulkarni
Kode Venkatadri Chowdary Campus, LV Prasad Eye Institute, Vijayawada, India

T. Y. Y. Lai · S. K. H. Szeto
Department of Ophthalmology and Visual Science, The Chinese University of Hong Kong, Faculty of Medicine, Pok Fu Lam, Hong Kong
e-mail: tyylai@cuhk.edu.hk

N. K. Sahoo (✉)
Anant Bajaj Retina Institute, Kode Venkatadri Chowdary Campus, L V Prasad Eye Institute, Vijayawada, India

26.2 Fundus Fluorescein Angiography

26.2.1 History

In 1954, Edward Maumenee used fluorescein dye intravenously to study ocular vasculature in choroidal hemangiomas with a Goldmann slit lamp, contact lens, and a cobalt blue filter. Later, Chao and Flocks gave the earliest description of fluorescein angiography (FA) in 1958 by studying its circulation time in cats [1]. Novotny and Alvis (1961) gave a detailed description of the fundus camera used for FA with the filter details and technique of FA that remains relatively unchanged to date [2]. Indocyanine green angiography (ICGA) was initially developed for cardiologists for the measurement of cardiac output accurately (Kodak Research Laboratories) [3], and in 1972, Flower and Hochheimer were the first to use intravenous ICGA to visualize the human choroid [4]. Yannuzzi and colleagues demonstrated a 1024-line resolution system that was synthesized with the proper flash synchronization and image-storing capability for high-resolution, long-duration ICGA [5]. Advances in developing high-quality photography equipment, photographic filters, newer printing techniques, and digital imaging can now generate high-resolution retina and choroid angiography.

T. Das, P. Satgunam (eds.), *Ophthalmic Diagnostics*, https://doi.org/10.1007/978-981-97-0138-4_26

26.2.2 Technology

26.2.2.1 Basic Principle

The emission of light from any source other than a high-temperature source is called luminescence. When a luminescent material absorbs light energy, a few electrons are elevated into a higher energy state. These electrons decay spontaneously into lower energy states by emitting an equivalent amount of energy as light. When this emitted energy is within the visible light spectrum (400–700 nm), it is called luminescence. Fluorescence is a type of luminescence that is maintained only by continuous excitation. Phosphorescence is a type of luminescence that emits light even after the excitation is stopped. In fluorescence, excitation occurs at one wavelength, and emission occurs through a longer wavelength [6, 7].

26.2.2.2 Sodium Fluorescein

Sodium fluorescein is an orange-red crystalline hydrocarbon with a molecular weight of 376.27 Daltons. It is a water-soluble dye; the liver and kidney eliminate it within 24–36 h [7]. During FA, intravenously injected Sodium fluorescein (Na Fl) remains 80% bound to proteins, and the remaining 20% circulates freely in the bloodstream. The unbound dye has an excitation peak in the blue range of the visible spectrum with peak absorption at 465–490 nm. In a flash-based fundus camera, a blue excitation filter allows only the blue light to enter the retina and absorbs all other light. Fluorescein in the bloodstream, excited by blue light, emits green-yellow light at 520–530 nm. A barrier filter placed in front of the film allows only green-yellow light to be captured electronically as a digital image and filters out the blue excitation light [6].

26.2.2.3 Imaging

Digital imaging has replaced traditional film-based imaging and is commonly used in FA. It offers multiple advantages, such as higher image resolution, ease of analysis, better storage, and instant access to images. It also aids in image reproducibility, image export for telemedicine, and better patient education. Digital imaging also has a shorter learning curve. A digital camera captures a single image of the retina using flashlight illumination and captures true-color images of the retina.

26.2.2.4 Stereo Photography

Stereo photography allows in-depth stereoscopic interpretation of images of both eyes simultaneously taken from slightly different angles [8]. A slight change in angle causes the illuminating beam of the fundus camera to pass through the opposite slopes of the cornea. This results in cornea-induced parallax that gives a hyper-stereoscopic effect (see Chap. 25 for further details) [9].

26.2.2.5 Camera and Ancillary Equipment

Filters: The exciter filter transmits blue light at 465–490 nm (absorption peak of fluorescein), and the barrier filter transmits light at 525–530 nm (emitted peak of fluorescein) (Fig. 26.1). Newer digital fundus cameras use high-sensitivity monochrome sensors with excitation (580 nm) and barrier filters (695 nm) of longer wavelengths to overcome lens autofluorescence [7, 10].

The field of view in wide field imaging (WFI) is beyond 60–100°. The field of view in ultra-wide field imaging (UWFI) is up to 200° and can image over 80% of the retinal surface (see Chap. 25 for further details).

26.2.2.6 Confocal Scanning Laser Ophthalmoscope

The confocal scanning laser ophthalmoscope (cSLO) can be used for several retinal imaging modalities, such as FA, ICGA, and fundus autofluorescence (FAF). Refer to Chap. 25 for further details.

26.2.3 Techniques

26.2.3.1 Fundus Fluorescein Angiography

Written informed consent is taken after the procedure is explained to the patient. The patient's pupils are dilated to facilitate imaging of the

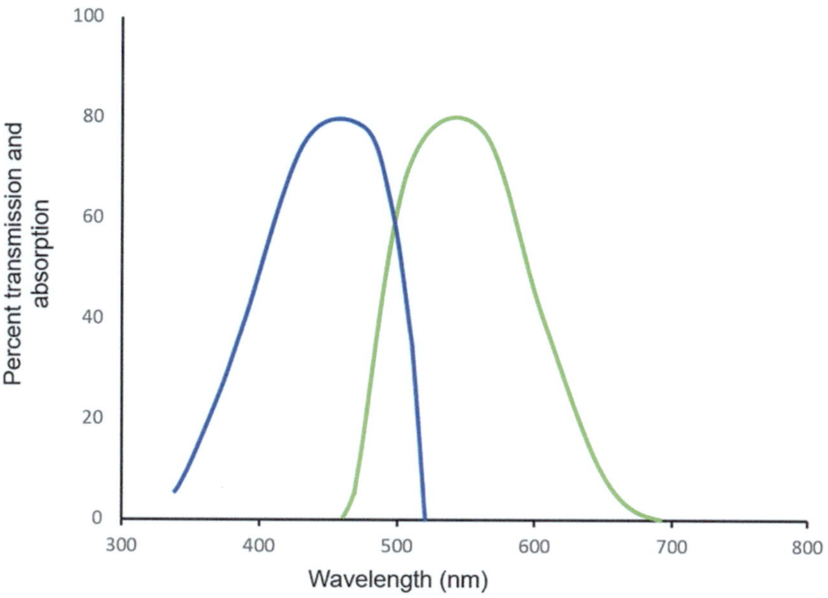

Fig. 26.1 The absorption (465–490 nm) and emission (at 525–530 nm) spectrum of fluorescein dye

Table 26.1 Essential supplies for fluorescein angiography

Supply	Description	Purpose
Catheter	23 g scalp vein needle or 22 g intravenous catheter	For intravenous dye administration
Syringe	5 mL disposable	To administer dye
Dye (Na Fl)	10 mL of 5% (500 mg) or 5 mL of 10% (500 mg) or 3 mL of 25% (750 mg)	To visualize retinochoroidal vasculature
Needle	20 g, 1 ½ inch needle	To withdraw the dye
Tourniquet	Stretchy latex-free/latex-based/ with velcro closure	To help localize peripheral veins to achieve successful venipuncture
Alcohol swab	60–70% isopropyl alcohol or ethanol, single-use swab, or cotton wool ball	To disinfect the skin surface before IV cannulation
Adhesive tape	Nonsterile micropore paper tape/ transpore polyethylene tape	For securing the IV cannula
Gloves	Latex/nitrile/vinyl	To maintain asepsis
Emergency medicine	Antihistamines, atropine, adrenaline, corticosteroids, etc.	For quick administration of drugs in case of adverse reactions

peripheral retina. The primary eye to be examined should be correctly identified and positioned for proper alignment, focus, and comfort. The FA tray (Table 26.1) should be kept ready. Color fundus photographs and monochromatic red-free filter images are obtained before the dye is administered. Before injecting the dye, the angiographer should pre-focus the area of interest. A bolus injection of the dye is administered into the upper limb vein via a small gauge scalp vein needle or intravenous catheter (Fig. 26.2). The angiographer should start the timer as soon as the dye is injected and begin capturing images immediately thereafter to capture the choroidal flush and early arteriovenous phase (every 1–2 s in the early phase). The arm-to-retina circulation time is usually 10–12 s in normal individuals and up to 20 s in older individuals. During the early phase,

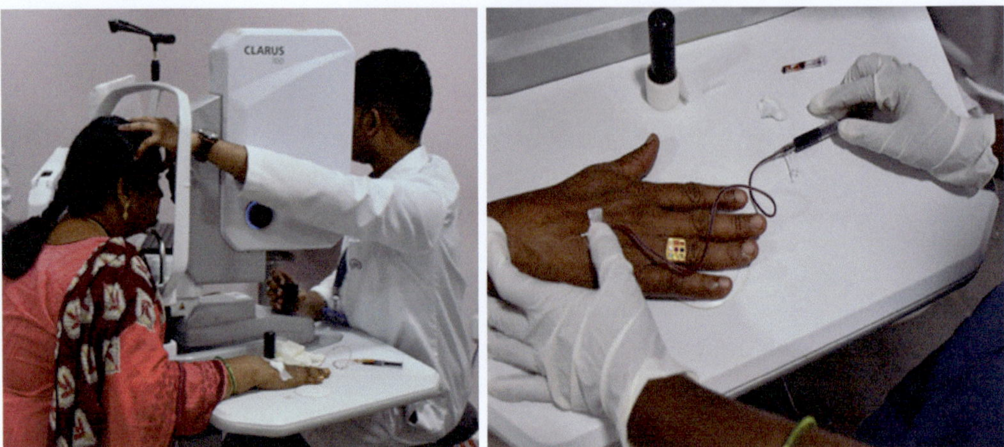

Fig. 26.2 (Left) Patient positioning during the FFA procedure. (Right) Butterfly needle with fluorescein dye

images of only one eye can be captured. Photographs of other parts of the retina in the primary and fellow eyes are obtained as soon as the early phase is complete. The examiner should use his/her judgment to follow a particular order in capturing various areas of interest as required in the specific case. At the end of the procedure, the patient should be re-informed that his/her urine and skin may have orange discoloration due to the dye. Na Fl may be administered orally at 25 mg/kg body weight in children with difficult IV access. Fundus images are captured 40–60 min after dye ingestion, but the quality of images is generally suboptimal [11].

26.2.3.2 Side Effects and Complications

Mild side effects of Na Fl dye usage are nausea, vomiting, and minimal extravasation of the dye; generally, these subside with time without any specific treatment. Moderate side effects include pruritis, urticaria, syncope, thrombophlebitis, pyrexia, and local tissue necrosis; these require medical intervention, and patients usually recover well. Severe adverse reactions include anaphylaxis, shock, laryngeal edema, bronchospasm, myocardial infarction, and convulsions; these require intensive treatment. Very few cases of death have been reported, with an estimated risk of death of less than 1 in 220,000 [12].

26.2.3.3 Contraindications

An absolute contraindication for FA is a known allergy or a history of severe adverse reactions during previous fluorescein dye injection. The dye can be used cautiously in advanced renal failure patients on regular dialysis, and the dose of fluorescein injection can be reduced to half. Intradermal testing of diluted Na Fl can be done in selected cases [7]. The presence of heart disease, arrhythmias, or cardiac pacemakers are not contraindications. No fetal complications from fluorescein injection during pregnancy have been reported yet. However, it is generally best to avoid angiography in pregnant women, especially in the first trimester. Fluorescein dye has been detected for up to 72 h in breastmilk after IV administration. To limit neonatal exposure, the US Food and Drug Administration suggests that nursing mothers should "pump-and-dump" the breastmilk for at least 96 h after fluorescein dye injection [13].

26.2.4 Clinical Application and Interpretation

26.2.4.1 Basic Anatomical Considerations

The ophthalmic artery divides into two main branches of posterior ciliary arteries: the lateral and medial, which supply the lateral and medial portions of the disc and choroid. A vertical zone of slightly delayed filling may be seen during angiography, which traverses the disc and the papillomacular area. This zone demarcates the border between the two main posterior ciliary arteries. It is called the "watershed zone," and patchy choroidal filling is often seen during FA within this zone. The ciliary arteries supply most of the disc; thus, fluorescein is first seen at the optic nerve head and the choroid before it is seen in the retinal artery system. The choriocapillaris has a lobular arrangement and demonstrates patchy filling in a transverse manner, with one lobule spilling over into the other. The foveal avascular zone (FAZ) is 400–500 µm in diameter and represents the area of the macula devoid of any retinal capillaries.

26.2.4.2 Normal Fluorescein Angiography

FA is a serial analysis of the vascular structure of the choroid and retina over specific time intervals. Fluorescein dye enters the ocular circulation through the short posterior ciliary arteries, which supply the choroid, and the central retinal artery that supplies the retina.

The six phases of FA are listed in Table 26.2.

26.2.4.3 Abnormal Fluorescence Angiography

Abnormal fluorescence [7, 14] is primarily of two types: hypofluorescence and hyperfluorescence. Hypofluorescence is a reduction/absence of normal fluorescence, and hyperfluorescence means increased fluorescence.

Table 26.2 Fluorescein angiography phases and their appearances

FA phases	Time (normal eye)	Appearance
Prearterial (choroidal flush)		Choriocapillaris and the bigger choroidal vessels start to fill with dye. Fluorescein is seen in the choroidal circulation around 1 s earlier than in the retinal circulation
Arterial	10 s	1–2 s after the choroidal flush, the central retinal artery fills, and the dye flows into the retinal arterioles (Fig. 26.3a). The avascular zone of the fovea is generally hypofluorescent due to the presence of taller, more pigmented RPE cells, xanthophyll pigment, and the absence of retinal capillaries in the center of the fovea
Arteriovenous		Complete filling of the arteries and capillaries is followed by an initial laminar flow in the vein (Fig. 26.3b). The plasma that contains unbound fluorescein flows along the vessel wall. The blood flow is faster in the center of the lumen. This differential flow rate of the different blood components creates the laminar venous flow pattern
Venous phase		Fluorescein filling in the veins increases; the two parallel laminae along the wall steadily get thicker and eventually meet to form a broad fluorescein dye column in the retinal veins (Fig. 26.3c). The dye in the posterior ciliary vascular system fluoresces both from the edge of the disc and the tissue between the center and circumference of the disc. Numerous capillaries of the central retinal artery on the surface of the disc fill up, making the disc hyperfluorescent on the angiogram
Transit phase		The transit phase is the first complete passage of blood containing fluorescein through the choroid and retina. The macula has the quickest transit time, and the peripheral retina has a longer transit time
Recirculation phase or late phase	10 min	The fluorescein is gradually emptied from the choroidal and retinal vasculature, and the vessels turn gray 3–5 min after the injection (Fig. 26.3d)

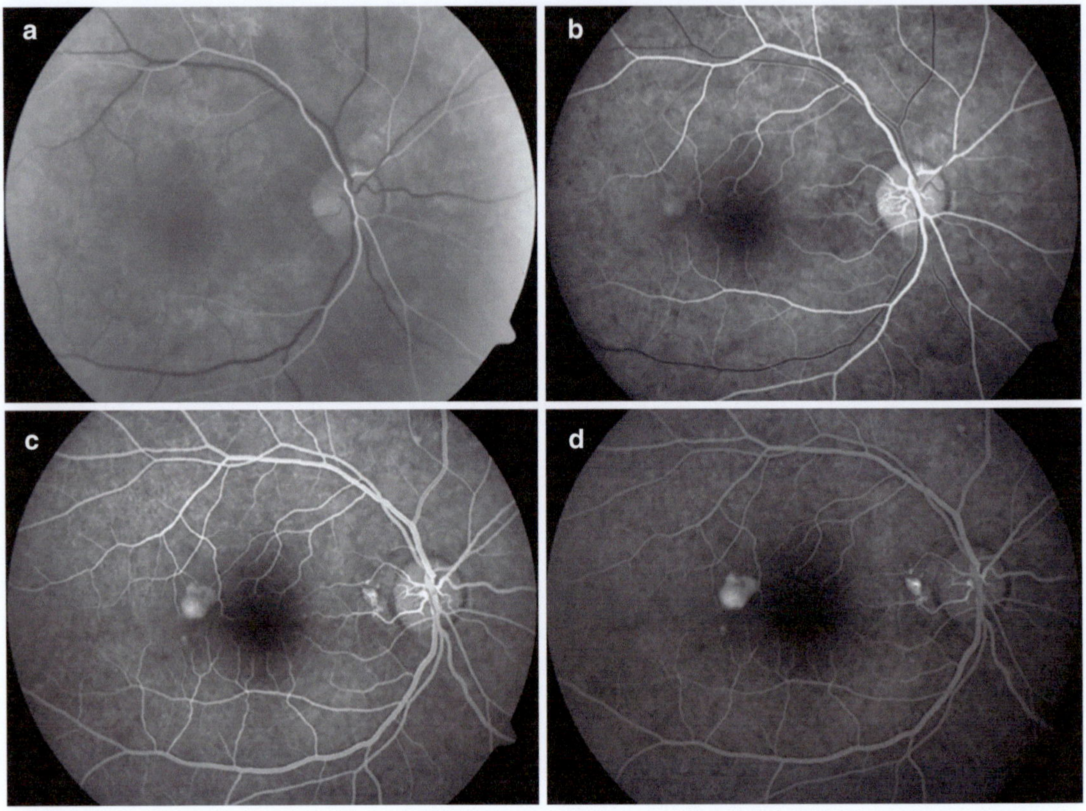

Fig. 26.3 Normal phases of FA. (**a**) Arterial phase with background choroidal flush. (**b**) Arteriovenous phase. (**c**) Venous phase. (**d**) Late phase: the retinal arteries are beginning to empty. Pooling can be seen temporal to the macula due to a pigment epithelial detachment

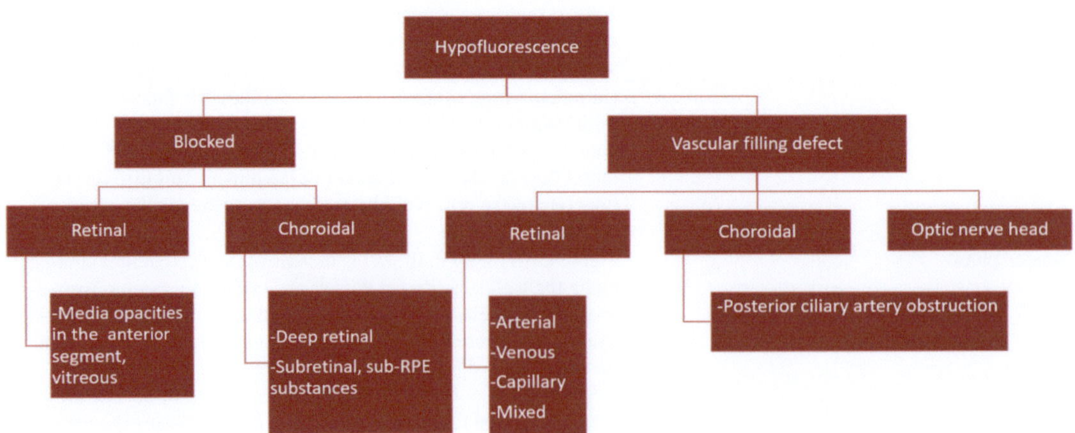

Fig. 26.4 Causes of hypofluorescence

A. **Hypofluorescence**

   Hypofluorescence refers to an abnormally dark area on the angiogram. It can be caused by blocked fluorescence or a vascular filling defect (Figs. 26.4 and 26.5; Table 26.3).

B. **Hyperfluorescence** (Figs. 26.6 and 26.7; Table 26.3)

Hyperfluorescence is the abnormal increase in fluorescence and can be classified as [1] pre-injection fluorescence, [2] transmitted fluorescence, [3] abnormal vessels, [4] leakage, and [5] staining (Fig. 26.6).

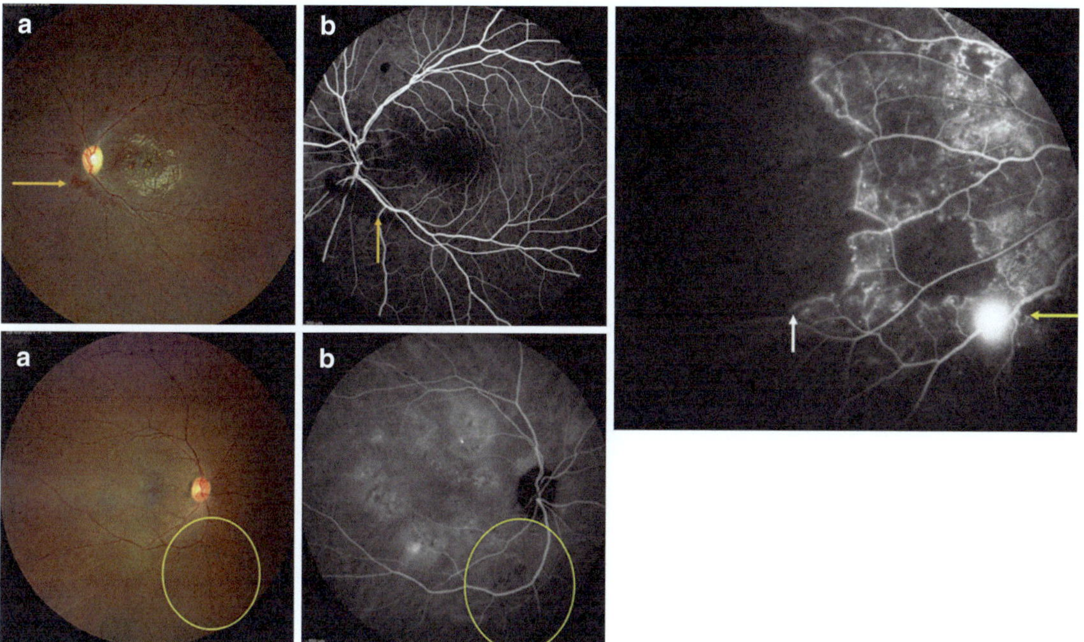

Fig. 26.5 Left upper panel: Blocked retinal fluorescence due to retinal hemorrhage (the yellow arrow in the color fundus image (left) and FA (right)) (Image courtesy: Navya Cherukuri, MD). Left lower panel: Blocked choroidal fluorescence (yellow circle) due to congenital hypertrophy of retinal pigment epithelium (CHRPE in the color fundus image (left) and FA (right)) (Image courtesy: Rajeev K Reddy Pappuru, MD). Right panel: Hypofluorescent capillary non-perfusion area (white arrow) with hyperfluorescence due to leakage from retinal neovascularization (yellow arrow). (Image courtesy: Hitesh Agrawal, MD)

Table 26.3 Interpretation and clinical application of fluorescein angiography

FA appearance	Category	Mechanism	Common examples
Hypofluorescence	Vascular filling defects	Vascular obstruction, absence of vessels	Retina: Central or branch artery occlusion, capillary non-perfusion in DR (diabetic retinopathy), RVO (retinal vein occlusion). Choroid: Malignant hypertension, toxemia, lupus choroidopathy
	Blocked fluorescence	Reduction/absence of normal retinal or choroidal fluorescence due to tissue, blood, or fluid barrier located anterior to it	Retina: Vitreous hemorrhage, inflammatory debris, vitreous membranes, retinal hemorrhage. Choroid: Any fluid, exudate, hemorrhage, or scar present deep to the retina and in front of the choroidal vasculature result in blocked choroidal fluorescence

(continued)

Table 26.3 (continued)

FA appearance	Category	Mechanism	Common examples
Hyperfluorescence	Pre-injection fluorescence	Mismatched monochromatic filters	It is the continuous emission of fluorescent light in the abscence of fluorescein dye in the ocular structures. Eg: Astrocytic hamartomas Drusen of the optic nerve head
	Transmitted fluorescence, window defect	Absent, atrophic, or attenuated RPE, lack of pigment in RPE	Geographic atrophy RPE (retinal pigment epithelium) rip
	Abnormal vessels	Fluorescence of the vessel course	Tortuosity and dilatation; anastomosis, neovascularization, aneurysms, telangiectatic vessels, tumor vessels
	Leakage	Fluorescein in the extravascular space	Physiological: Choriocapillaris around disc margins, lamina cribrosa, peripapillary atrophy Pathological: Retinal or disc neovascularization, intraocular inflammation, intraocular tumors, cystoid retinal edema, non-cystoid retinal edema Pooling: Central serous chorioretinopathy, serous pigment epithelial detachment
	Staining		Physiological: Disc, sclera Pathological: Fibrotic tissues, chorioretinal scars, staphyloma, drusen

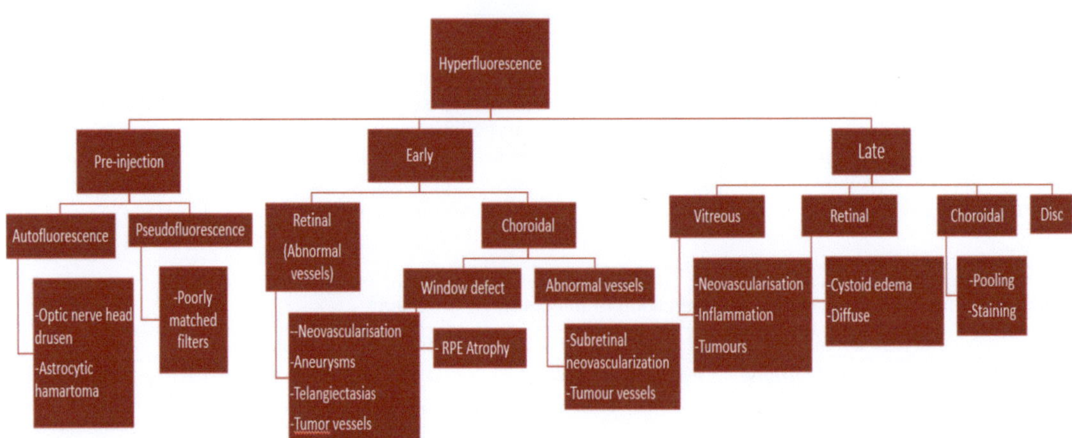

Fig. 26.6 Causes of hyperfluorescence

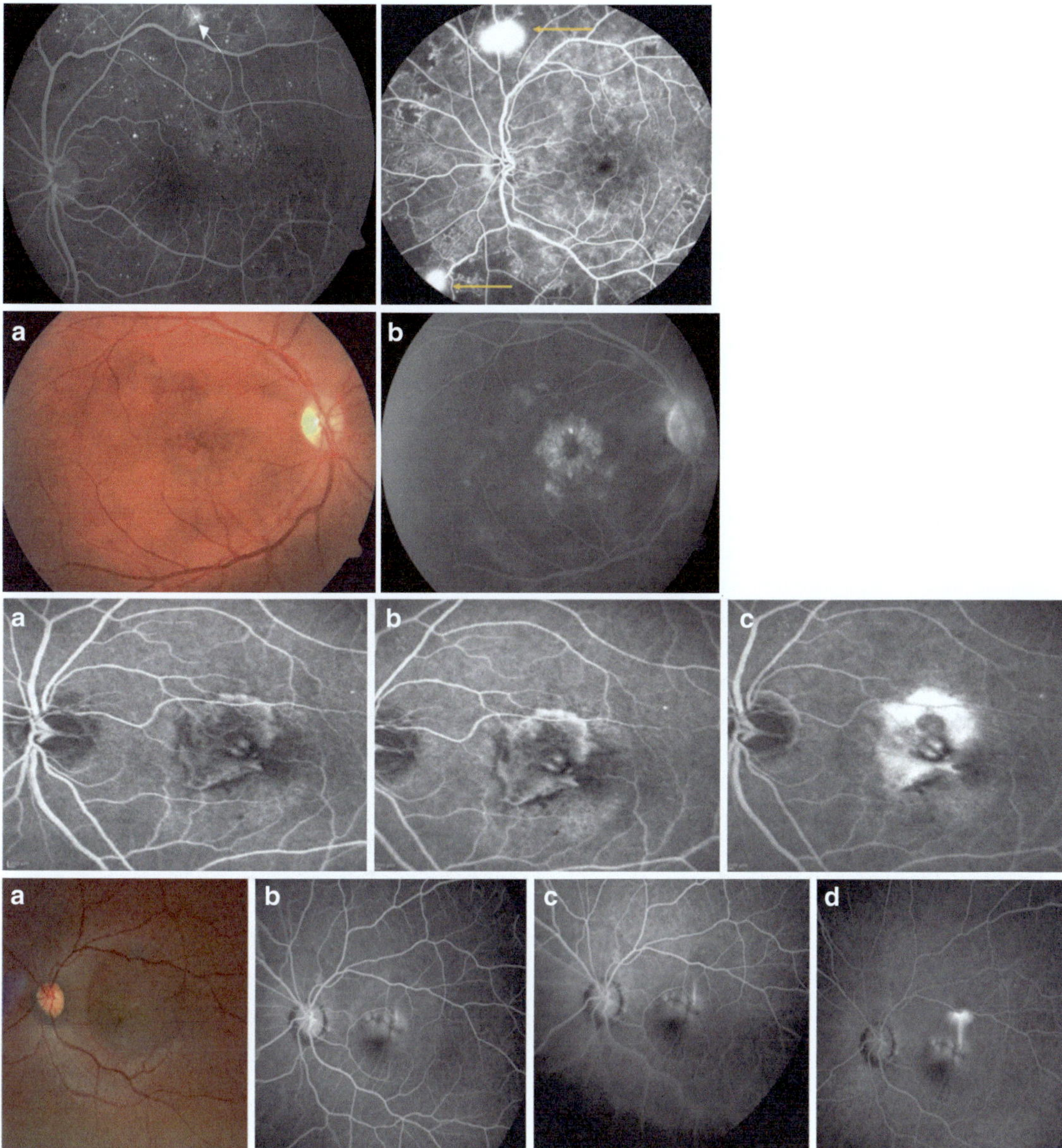

Fig. 26.7 *Row 1*. Proliferative diabetic retinopathy: multiple microaneurysms and neo vessels elsewhere (NVE) (arrow) (Right-side image courtesy: Hitesh Agrawal, MD). *Row 2*. (**a**) Right eye fundus photograph showing microaneurysms, dot hemorrhage, and cystoid macular edema in a patient with non-proliferative diabetic retinopathy with intermediate uveitis. (**b**) FA shows a petaloid appearance corresponding to the cystoid edema. *Row 3*. Classic macular new vessels (MNV): (**a**) Lacy pattern of MNV in the early phase, (**b**) mid-phase, and (**c**) late phase showing the lacy pattern increasing in size and intensity with progressive leakage. *Row 4*. Acute central serous chorioretinopathy (CSC): smokestack appearance on progressive phases of the angiogram (Image courtesy: Udit Ajmani, MD, and Sameera Nayak, MD)

26.3 Indocyanine Green Angiography

26.3.1 Technology

26.3.1.1 Properties of Indocyanine Green

Indocyanine green (ICG) has a molecular weight of 774.96 Daltons and is an anionic tricarbocyanine dye [15]. To avoid recrystallization, the finished product contains 5–9.5% sodium iodide [16]. Near-infrared light is absorbed by ICG. The maximum absorption occurs at 790 nm, and the maximum emission occurs at 835 nm (Fig. 26.8) [17]. These optical characteristics enable ICG imaging through melanin, macular pigment, and blood. ICG is mostly attached to plasma proteins, especially to globulins like A1-lipoproteins. The liver metabolizes the dye actively and depends on hepatocellular function and liver blood flow. ICG is excreted into the bile [3]. The kidneys, lungs, and placenta do not show dye uptake [20]. The amount of dye that leaks out of the fenestrations in the choroidal arteries is low due to the high molecular weight of ICG and because the dye usually remains bound to plasma proteins. These properties make ICG ideal for studying the choroidal vascular network.

26.3.1.2 Toxicity

ICG is a well-tolerated and safe dye. Furthermore, subcutaneous extravasation of the dye has no significant local effects [18, 21]. The incidence of side effects is usually low, ranging from 0.15% for mild events (such as nausea, vomiting, sneezing, and itching) to 0.2% for moderate events (such as urticaria, syncope, pyrexia, and nerve palsy) to 0.05% for severe events (such as bronchospasm, laryngospasm, and anaphylaxis) [7, 21]. Although the dye has no obvious association with iodide or shellfish sensitivity, a dose-dependent pseudoallergic mechanism may occur in some people allergic to iodine and shellfish [16]. However, due to concerns about potential anaphylaxis, the dye should not be administered to patients with a history of confirmed iodine allergy [21]. Since the incidence of adverse events is 9.3% in dialysis patients, caution is necessary; in patients with kidney comorbidities [16] and liver diseases [19]. ICG is a pregnancy category C drug per the US Food and Drug Administration (FDA) classification, which means that optimal safety studies for the dye on pregnant women have not been carried out [20].

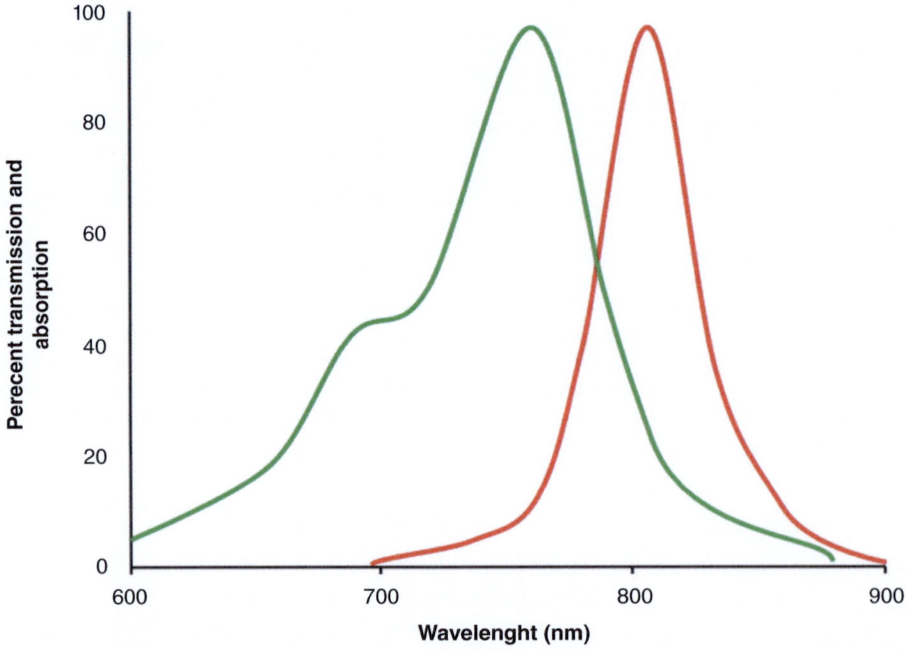

Fig. 26.8 Absorption (790 nm) and emission (835 nm) spectrum of ICG

26.3.1.3 Instrument

White light with excitation and barrier filters (640–780 nm and 820–900 nm, respectively) serves as the light source for digital cameras. In a cSLO system, a laser monochromatic light is utilized for excitation (785–790 nm), and the barrier filter is set at 805 nm.

26.3.2 Techniques

26.3.2.1 Injection Technique

ICG (25 mg) is dissolved in 5 mL of solvent (for flash-based fundus cameras) or 3 mL (for cSLOs cameras). For combined FA and ICG angiography, the solvent can be saline or a Sodium fluorescein solution at 10, 20, or 25% concentrations. A 5 mL saline flush should follow the rapid injection of intravenous ICG. Infracyanine green, the iodine-free version of ICG, is available for people with iodine allergies. The injection technique is identical, but a glucose-based solvent is required to prepare the bolus. Thus, combined FA and infracyanine green angiography may not be feasible [7].

26.3.2.2 Normal Phases of ICGA

The ICG filling of the choroid at the posterior pole shows the following stages, depending on the passage of time (Table 26.4, Fig. 26.9) [22].

Dynamic ICGA refers to the simultaneous videography of choroidal and retinal vessel-filling patterns as the ICG dye is injected. It is possible with cSLO.

Table 26.4 Phases of indocyanine green angiography

ICG phases	Time (normal eye)	Appearance
Early phase Prearterial and arterial-1 (Fig 26.9a)	First 2 s	The ICG dye enters the eye, filling the choriocapillaris rapidly; the filling is completed in 2 s. The choroidal veins commence to fill concurrently with the choriocapillaris. The major retinal vessels appear dark and block the choroidal fluorescence underneath them
Early phase Prearterial and arterial-2	3–5 s	The choroidal veins are more noticeable. The retinal arterioles begin to fill with ICG dye
Early phase Prearterial and arterial-3	6 s–3 min	The watershed zone begins to get filled, and the larger choroidal arteries and veins begin to fade
Middle phase (Fig. 26.9b)	3–15 min	The fluorescence in the choroidal vein fades; thus, the choroidal vascular characteristics are less distinct as they travel parallel to the periphery. Large choroidal veins in myopic eyes occasionally exhibit laminar flow, a layered blood flow pattern created by the slower, nonturbulent travel of blood along the vessel wall
Late phase (Fig. 26.9c)	15–60 min	The optic disc becomes dark. The major choroidal and retinal arteries are seen as dark structures on a homogeneous, faintly fluorescent background

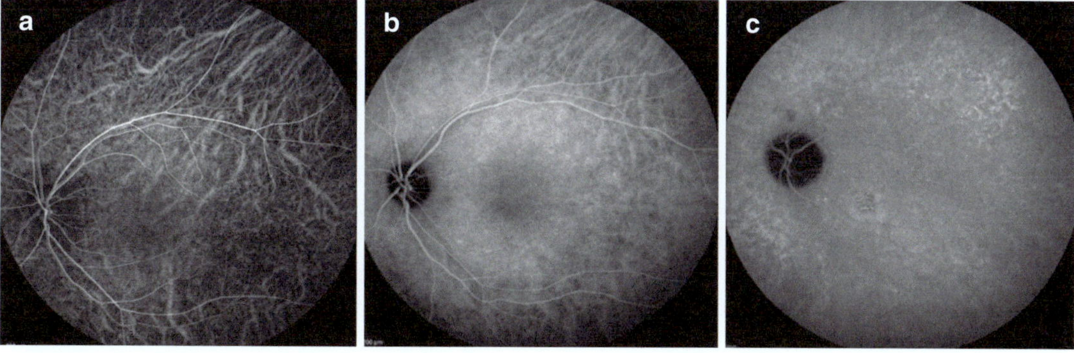

Fig. 26.9 Normal phases of ICGA. (**a**) Early phase: shows greater prominence of vessels. (**b**) Mid phase: shows fading of choroidal vessels, but retinal vessels are still visible; diffuse tissue staining is also present. (**c**) Late phase

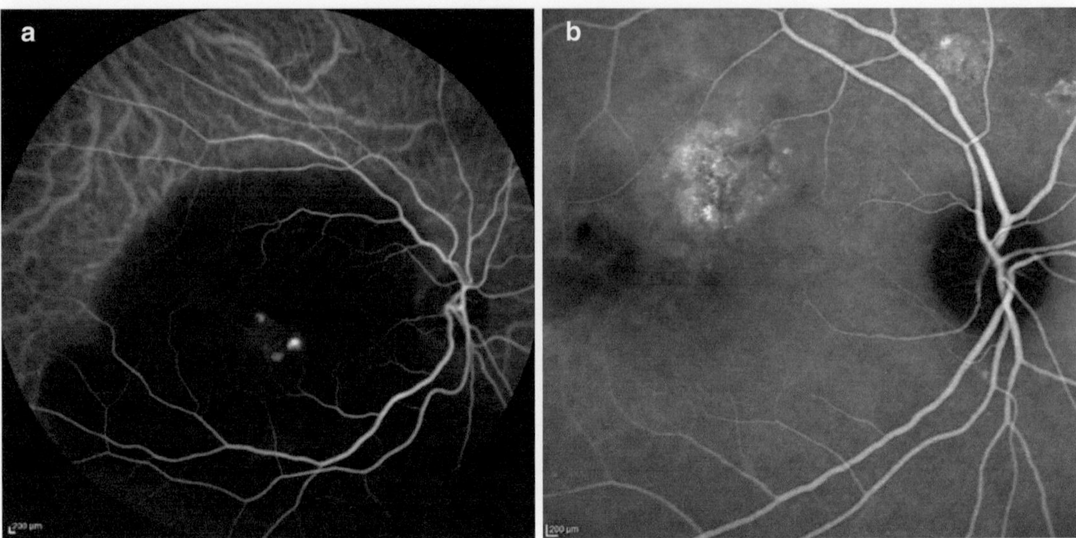

Fig. 26.10 A hotspot (**a**) and a plaque (**b**) as seen on ICG angiography. (Image courtesy: Hardik Kiri, MD)

Hyperfluorescence in ICGA: Generally, there are two patterns of hyperfluorescence in ICGA: hot spot and plaque.

A Hotspot (Fig. 26.10a) is an area of abnormal intense hyperfluorescence of more than 1-disc diameter seen during the mid to late phases of ICGA. It is usually seen in retinal angiomatous proliferation (RAP) and polypoidal chorial vasculopathy (PCV).

A Plaque (Fig. 26.10b) is an area of abnormal intense hyperfluorescence of more than 1-disc diameter in size seen during the mid to late phases of ICGA. It is seen in occult macular neovascularization (MNV) and central serous chorioretinopathy (CSC).

26.3.3 Clinical Application and Interpretation of Indocyanine Green Angiography

26.3.3.1 Age-Related Macular Degeneration (AMD)

This section will use the "Consensus on Neovascular Age-Related Macular Degeneration Nomenclature (CONAN)" study group-recommended new consensus nomenclature [23]. According to the Macular Photocoagulation Study, type 1 MNV tends to correlate with "occult" CNV on FA, and type 2 MNV is typically seen to correspond with "classic" CNV [24].

Type 1 MNV. A dynamic ICGA can identify the neovascular network (Fig. 26.11) in fibrovascular PED (pigment epithelial detachment) type of occult MNV, feeder vessels, and distinguish between a type 1 MNV and a type 3 MNV [5, 7, 26].

Type 2 MNV. ICGA shows a discrete hyperfluorescent neovascular network in the early phase and a dark rim at the MNV boundary that correlates to a hyperreflective ring on near-infrared reflectance imaging [27].

Type 3 MNV. ICGA demonstrates the vascularity of the fibrovascular PED or late leakage of an undetermined source (LLUS). When the PED is present, type 3 MNV is typically seen within the PED area rather than at the margin. These lesions also exhibit increasing leakage in the late stage; this is not seen in the other MNV lesions. Dynamic ICGA can capture the progressive filling of the lesion, enabling the location of very small type 3 MNV lesions of recent onset [25, 27]. The diagnosis of type 3 MNV has been typically based on the temporal evidence of the dye filling into at least one retinal arteriole that descends into the deep retinal space to a vascular

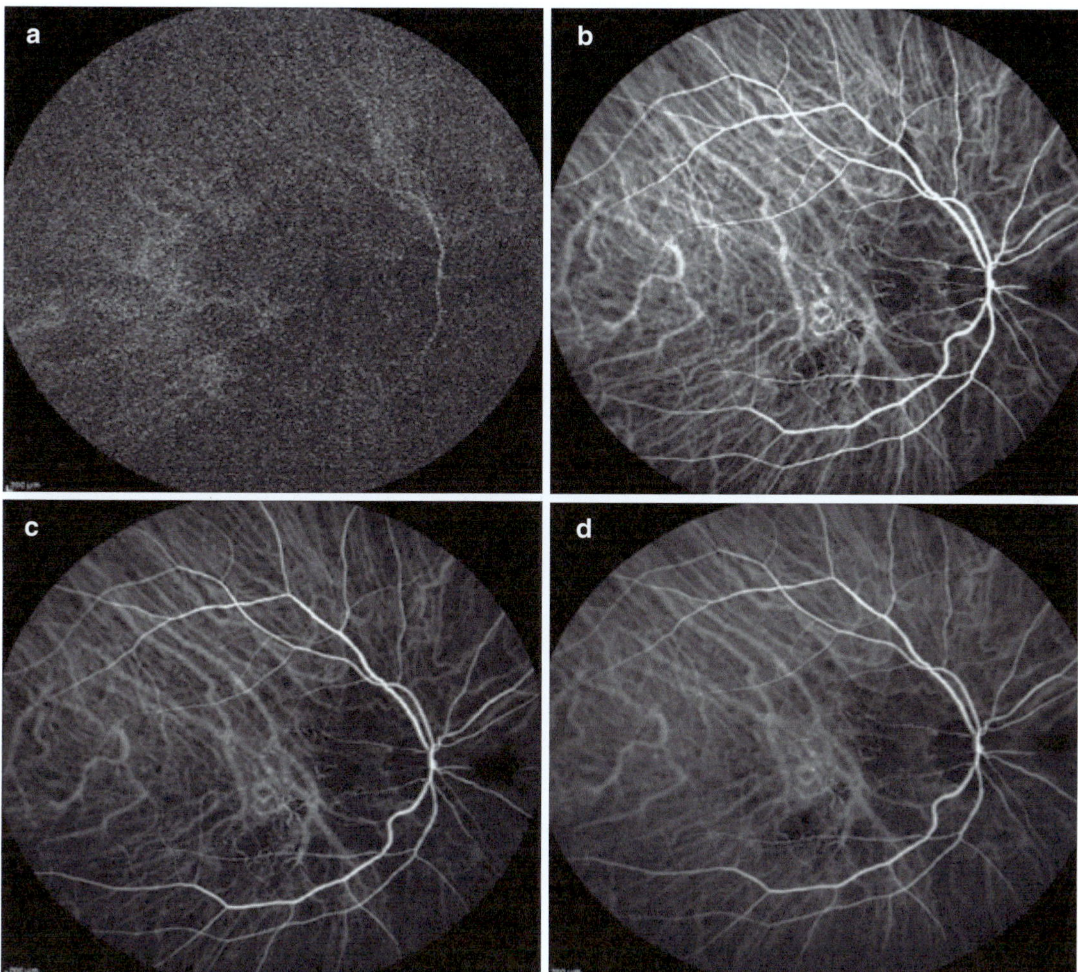

Fig. 26.11 ICGA showing the vascular network in the early phases. (**a**) Choroidal vessels are beginning to fill, but no network is seen in the early phase. (**b**) The neovascular network can be discerned, mixed in a background of hyperfluorescent choroidal vessels. (**c**) Choroidal vessels are beginning to empty, and the network is becoming more well defined. (**d**) Choroidal vessels become less distinct, but the neovascular network is visible. (Image courtesy: Rajeev K Reddy Pappuru, MD)

connection and with at least one draining retinal vein, as visualized on dynamic ICG [7].

26.3.3.2 Polypoidal Choroidal Vasculopathy (PCV) or Aneurysmal Type 1 MNV

Polypoidal choroidal vasculopathy (PCV) or aneurysmal type 1 MNV can be identified and characterized with improved sensitivity and specificity using ICGA [15]. In the initial stages of the ICGA, the various morphological traits of the vascular lesion are apparent. Branched neovascular networks (BNNs), a form of aberrant vascular networks (AVNs), can be detected in the first 30 s, especially in the feeder vessels. In the first minute, interconnecting channels, a type of AVN, can be detected, which show a lack of feeder vessels. Early hyperfluorescence originating from the choroid (observed in the first 6 min) can be used to identify polypoidal lesions (Fig. 26.12). Additional features include pulsatile filling of the polypoidal lesion (seen on dynamic ICGA) and a hypofluorescent halo surrounding the hyperfluorescent nodule. After

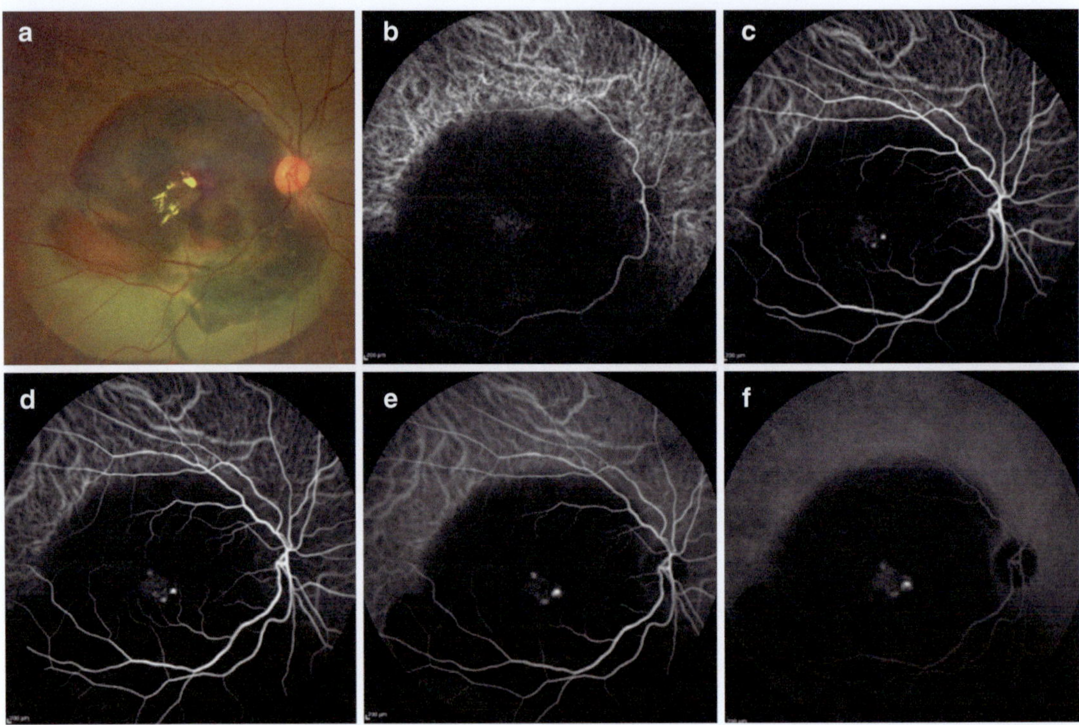

Fig. 26.12 (**a**) Right eye color fundus photo showing massive macular hemorrhage. (**b**) Blocked hypofluorescence due to subretinal hemorrhage in early phase ICGA. (**c–e**) Polypoidal lesion filling up progressively on ICGA images. (**f**) Late phase ICGA: empty choroidal and retinal vessels are seen, and polypoidal hyperfluorescence is seen to be reduced. (Image courtesy: Hardik Kiri, MD)

10 min of ICG dye injection, late geographic hyperfluorescence (LGH) is visible as a hyperfluorescent, well-delineated lesion with a rosette pattern [28]. After 20 min of ICG dye injection, i.e., in the late phase, dye washout is seen from these bulging dilated lesions [7].

26.3.3.3 Pachychoroid Disease Spectrum

In ICG, pachychoroid spectrum disease is characterized by dilated submacular vessels (pachyvessels). The pachyvessels are dilated and relatively straight choroidal vessels without attenuation. This contrasts with normal choroidal vessels that typically taper in caliber as they approach the macula. Central serous chorioretinopathy (CSC) is one of the pachychoroid diseases. In the mid to late phases of ICGA, CSC shows multiple areas of choroidal hyperpermeability (Fig. 26.13) [29]. The localized RPE leak evident on FA may have an underlying region of choroidal hyperpermeability. In conditions caused by severe and chronic CSC, areas of choroidal hyperpermeability often persist and help differentiate CSC from AMD in elderly people with signs of type 1 MNV detected by OCT (optical coherence tomography). The management of CSC relies on identifying choroidal hyperpermeability on ICGA, as the verteporfin photodynamic therapy (PDT) is targeted to these regions [7].

Numerous serous PED, choroidal filling defects, focal or punctate hyperfluorescent areas that may indicate choroidal ischemia, punctate hyperfluorescent spots, delays in the arterial filling of the choroidal arteries and choriocapillaris, and venous congestion are other ICGA findings in the pachychoroid disease spectrum [21].

Pachychoroid neovascularization exhibits type 1 MNV without aneurysmal dilations (polypoidal lesions). In eyes with pachychoroid neovascularization, type 1 MNV fluorescence may

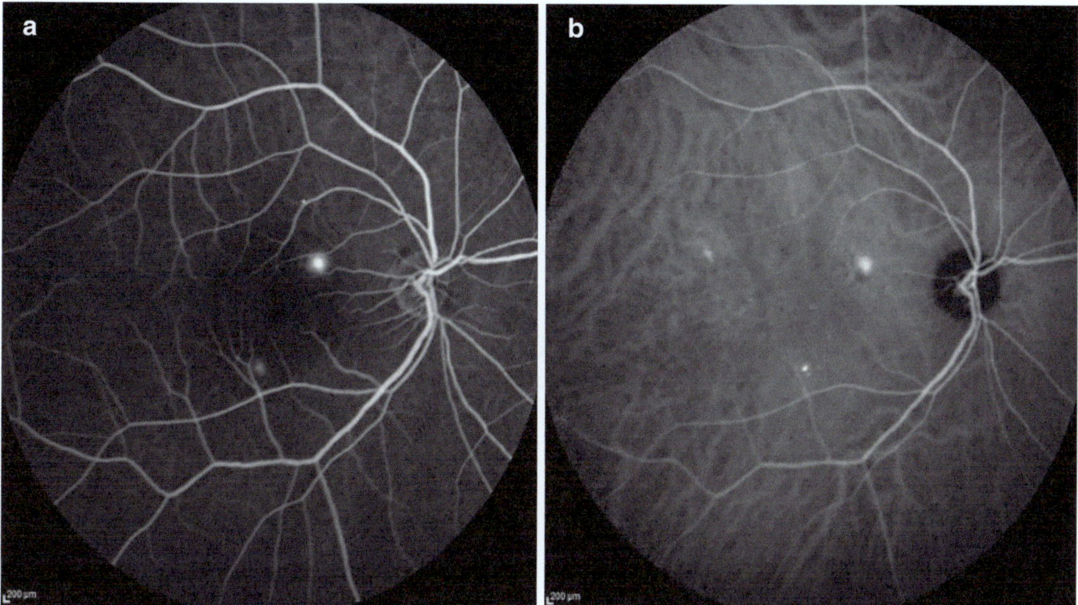

Fig. 26.13 Focal leaking points on FFA (**a**) and choroidal vessel hyperpermeability and hot spots on ICG (**b**) in CSC

be masked by diffuse leakage from underlying dilated choroidal vessels during ICG angiography. These type 1 MNV lesions are detected better with OCT angiography, which frequently demonstrates a well-defined "tangled network" of flow signals [7].

26.3.3.4 Choroidal Tumors

FA and ICGA are used to evaluate tumor size, location, and proximity to surrounding anatomical structures and to establish a baseline for assessing treatment response and adverse effects. It is a useful tool for identifying the nature of choroidal tumors [7].

(a) Choroidal hemangioma: FA for choroidal hemangioma is barely useful as it appears normal if the lesions do not have exudative complications. The ICGA findings of choroidal hemangioma are distinct and pathognomonic; a lobular, uniform, and well-defined pattern of hyperfluorescence is seen soon after dye administration. Intrinsic vascular patterns in the tumor are visible within 30 s of dye injection, and by 1 min, choroidal hemangiomas appear well-defined and hyperfluorescent as they fill completely with dye. A late "washout" phenomenon is seen as the dye fades out, and the tumor appears hypofluorescent with a hyperfluorescent rim (Fig. 26.14). This washout pattern occurs due to the tumor's high flow and low-resistance properties, leading to the rapid outflow of dye and tumor emptying earlier than the surrounding choroidal tissue [30, 31].
(b) Choroidal melanoma: When outer retinal atrophy is present, along with the filling of the choroidal capillaries, an irregular hyperfluorescence in the tumor may be seen in the early transit phase of FA [5]. In the late phases, varying amounts of leakage can be seen. Clumps of orange pigment appear hypofluorescent. The near-infrared light used in ICGA offers better penetration of the pigmented layers of the fundus than the short-wavelength light used for FA. Therefore, ICGA reveals the intrinsic microvascular structures of the tumor, which are seen as hyperfluorescent vessels on a hypofluorescent background (Fig. 26.15) [7].
(c) Choroidal metastases: In the early stages, blocking of the background fluorescence is seen on FA with mottled hyperfluorescence

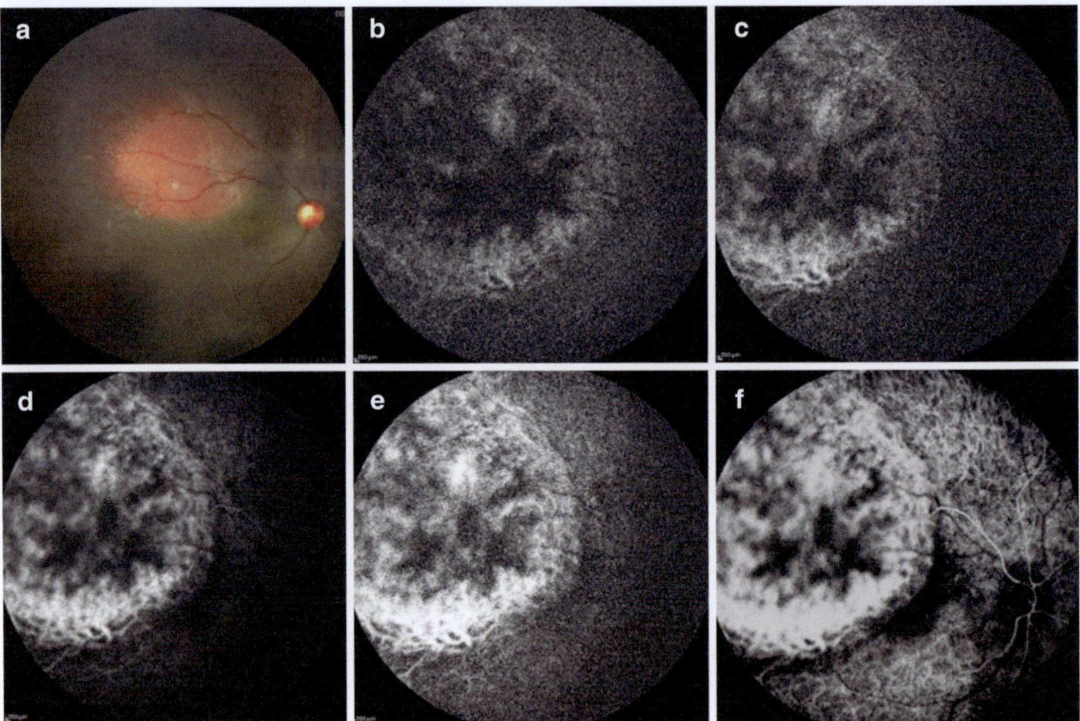

Fig. 26.14 Choroidal hemangioma. (**a**) Right eye color fundus photo showing a reddish, well-circumscribed choroidal mass. (**b**–**e**) A lobular, uniform, and well-defined pattern of hyperfluorescence is seen soon after dye administration. (**f**) Choroidal hemangiomas appear well-defined and hyperfluorescent in 1 min. (Image courtesy: Vishal Ramesh Raval, MD)

due to the RPE defects. Irregular areas of hyperfluorescence are seen in the late phases of FA corresponding with the tumor, a variable amount of hyperfluorescent leakage, and pooling in the subretinal space. Choroidal metastases can be seen with ICGA as clearly defined patches of hypofluorescence without any intrinsic microvascular networks. Hypofluorescence is typically noted throughout all the phases of the ICGA, with progressive attenuation in the late stages that lead to a giraffe or leopard skin pattern [32].

26.3.3.5 Varix of the Vortex Vein Ampulla

A varix of the vortex vein ampulla is an exceptionally large dilation of the vortex vein seen as a single, smooth, red-brown elevation [33]. ICG angiography exhibits the typical early and consistent fluorescence with uniform filling [34].

26.3.3.6 Choroidal Inflammation

(a) Multiple evanescent white dot syndrome (MEWDS): At the posterior pole and peripheral retina, ICGA reveals a pattern of many hypofluorescent regions with a distinctive lobulated form. These spots are larger on ICGA images than on fundus examination and FA [15], become detectable in the mid-to late phases, and range in size from 50 to 1000 μm. Additionally, hypofluorescence can be seen in the peripapillary region [35]. The hypofluorescent patches in the ICGA vanish over time when the inflammation subsides [7].

(b) Multifocal choroiditis: Active lesions are visible as uniform hypofluorescent patches on ICGA [36]. These lesions could disappear or, more often, turn into chorioretinal scarring. After successful therapy, the hypofluorescent patches are smaller and fewer in number. On

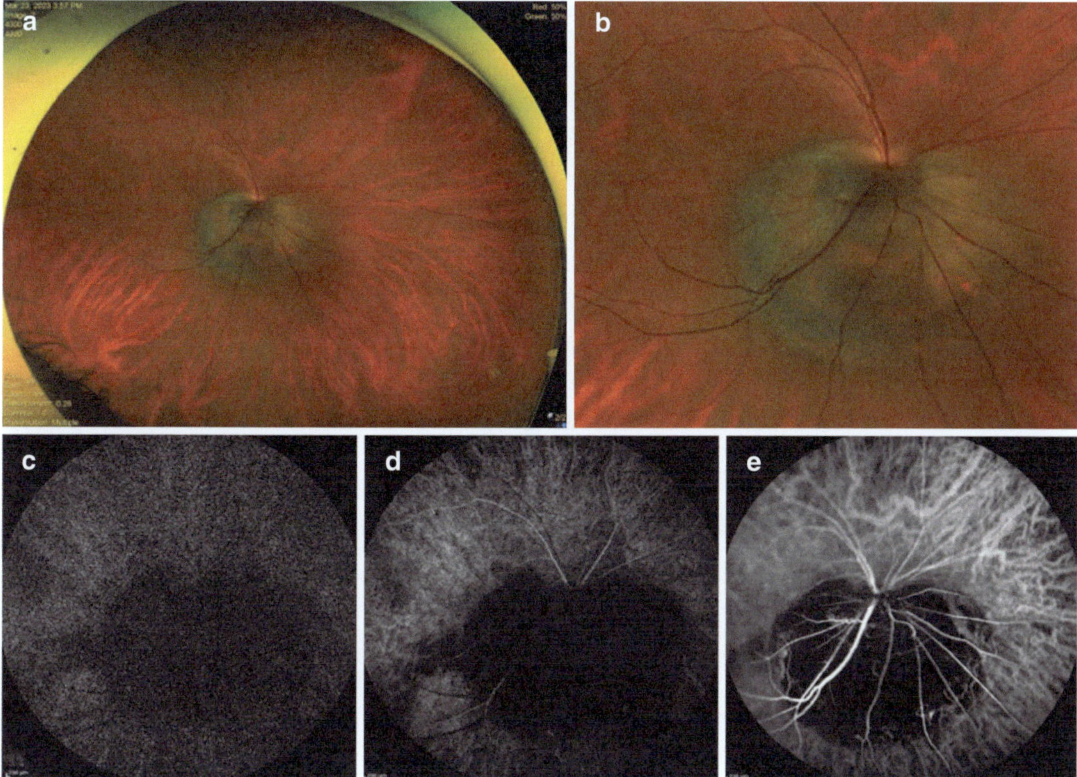

Fig. 26.15 Choroidal melanoma: (**a**) right eye wide field color fundus photograph showing a well-defined, optic disc mass; (**b**) enlarged view. (**c**, **d**) Early phase ICGA: blocked fluorescence due to the tumor is seen as the retinal vessels are filling gradually. (**e**) In the mid-phase, fine vessels are seen within the tumor- "double circulation." (Image courtesy: Vishal Ramesh Raval, MD)

ICGA, the scars appear more hypofluorescent than the surrounding tissue, and a window defect enables one to see the massive choroidal vessels [7].

(c) Birdshot chorioretinopathy: On ICGA, these lesions appear as round or oval hypofluorescent spots of similar size dispersed across the fundus, predominantly in the nasal quadrant, followed by dye leakage in the late phases, making the choroidal vessels appear hazy [37]. ICGA angiography is the gold standard for diagnosing and monitoring the activity of birdshot lesions as this method allows these lesions to be better visualized than on FA. In the chronic phase of the disease, the hypofluorescent spots corresponding to chorioretinal scars are evident in the late stages of the angiography [7, 15].

(d) Acute posterior multifocal placoid pigment epitheliopathy (APMPPE). In the early stages of ICGA, APMPPE lesions appear as numerous placoid/ameboid hypofluorescent patches larger than those observed clinically or with FA. The lesions are progressively more prominent and darker than the surrounding unaffected areas in the late stages of ICGA. Some of these lesions are gone after therapy and become barely detectable during clinical examinations and with ICGA. Other lesions may turn into scars with the loss of RPE, the choriocapillaris, and the outer retinal layer [7]. On ICGA, these inactive lesions generally exhibit a window defect. ICGA is also helpful in monitoring the course of the disease and response to treatment [38].

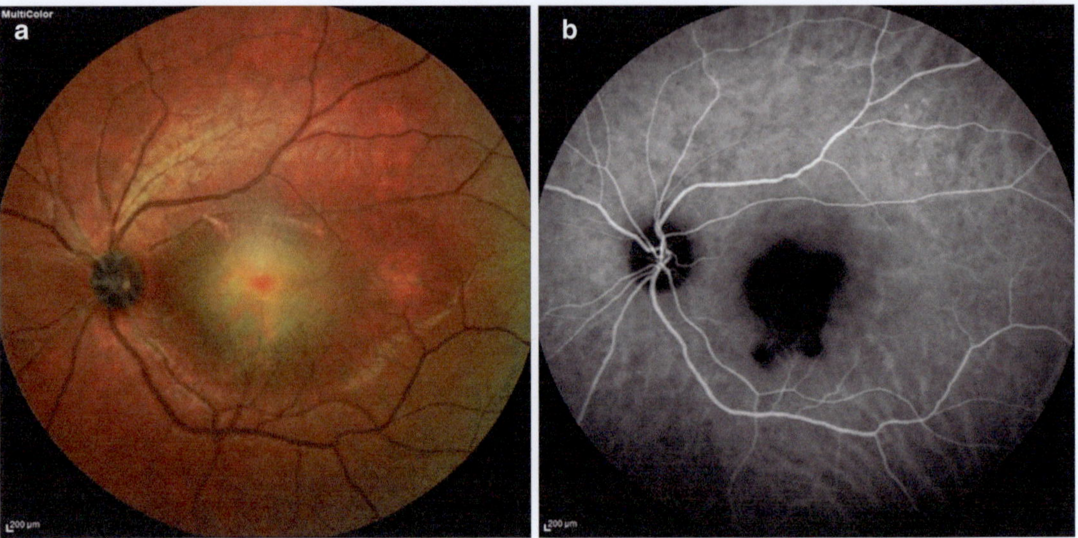

Fig. 26.16 Tubercular choroidal granuloma: hypofluorescence seen corresponding to the lesion in mid-phase ICGA

(e) Serpiginous choroidopathy: On ICGA, the active edges of the lesion appear hypofluorescent [39]. Late hyperfluorescence is a marker of choroidal hyperpermeability and may indicate a more rapid progression of the illness. The boundaries of the healed lesions are clearly defined and appear hypofluorescent. The pigmentation of the lesion edges often appears dark on ICGA due to blocked fluorescence. At the same time, the atrophy of the RPE and choriocapillaris enables the visualization of the underlying large- and medium-sized choroidal arteries [7].

(f) Choroidal granulomas: Choroidal granulomas can be seen in both primary and secondary stromal choroiditis like Vogt-Koyanagi-Harada disease and tubercular and sarcoid uveitis. Choroidal granulomas displace choroidal vessels and block ICG dye from filling the area of the choroidal stroma occupied by the choroidal granulomas (Fig. 26.16). As a result, during the early and middle phases of ICGA, they present as hypofluorescent round lesions. The granulomas gradually get surrounded by the dye in the late phases, making them less prominent [7]. After therapy, these gradually shrink and eventually disappear, which can be better identified and monitored by ICGA [40].

26.4 Conclusions

Dye-based angiography can give detailed information about the shape, extent, and vascularity of most retinochoroidal pathologies effectively and affordably. It is invaluable in establishing diagnosis, prognosticating, and managing several diseases, making it one of the most commonly used tools in an ophthalmologist's armamentarium.

Funding Hyderabad Eye Research Foundation, Hyderabad, India.

Disclosure TYYL: Consultant: Allergan, Bayer, Boehringer Ingelheim, Iveric Bio, Novartis, Oculis, Roche; Speaker: Alcon, Bayer, Chendu Kanghong Biotech, Novartis, Roche.

References

1. Flocks M, Miller J, Chao P. Retinal circulation time with the aid of fundus cinephotography. Am J Ophthalmol. 1959;48(1):3–6.
2. Novotny HR, Alvis D. A method of photographing fluorescence in circulating blood of the human eye. Tech Doc Rep SAMTDR USAF Sch Aerosp Med. 1960;60:1–4.
3. Ott P. Hepatic elimination of indocyanine green with special reference to distribution kinetics and the influ-

ence of plasma protein binding. Pharmacol Toxicol. 1998;83:1–48.
4. Flower RW, Hochheimer BF. Clinical infrared absorption angiography of the choroid. Am J Ophthalmol. 1972;73:458–9.
5. Yannuzzi LA, Slakter JS, Sorenson JA, et al. Digital indocyanine green videoangiography and choroidal neovascularization. Retina. 1992;12:191–223.
6. Berkow JW, Flower RW, Orth DH, Kelley JS. Fluorescein and Indocyanine green angiography—technique and interpretation. San Francisco: American Academy of Ophthalmology; 1997.
7. Sadda SR, Schachat AP, Wilkinson CP, Hinton DR, Wiedemann P, Freund KB, et al. Ryan's Retina E-Book. Elsevier Health Sciences; 2022. p. 2949.
8. Allen L. Ocular fundus photography: suggestions for achieving consistently good pictures and instructions for stereoscopic photography. Am J Ophthalmol. 1964;57(1):13–28.
9. Bennet TJ. Stereo photography—rotational stereo imaging. The Ophthalmic Photographers' Society Inc; 2013. https://www.opsweb.org/blogpost/777793/Stereo-Photography?tag=3D.
10. Spaide RF. Fundus autofluorescence and age-related macular degeneration. Ophthalmology. 2003;110(2):392–9.
11. Watson AP, Rosen ES. Oral fluorescein angiography: reassessment of its relative safety and evaluation of optimum conditions with use of capsules. Br J Ophthalmol. 1990;74(8):458–61.
12. Lipson BK, Yannuzzi LA. Complications of intravenous fluorescein injections. Int Ophthalmol Clin. 1989;29(3):200–5.
13. Alcon Laboratories, Inc. Fluorescite (fluorescein injection, USP) 10% intravenous injection [package insert]. US Food and Drug Administration. https://www.accessdata.fda.gov/drugsatfda_docs/label/2006/021980s000lbl.pdf.
14. Rabb MF, Burton TC, Schatz H, Yannuzzi LA. Fluorescein angiography of the fundus: a schematic approach to interpretation. Surv Ophthalmol. 1978;22(6):387–403.
15. Cohen SY, Dubois L, Quentel G, et al. Is indocyanine green angiography still relevant? Retina. 2011;31:209–21.
16. Benya R, Quintana J, Brundage B. Adverse reactions to indocyanine green: a case report and a review of the literature. Catheter Cardiovasc Diagn. 1989;17:231–3.
17. Flower RW, Hochheimer BF. Indocyanine green dye fluorescence and infrared absorption choroidal angiography performed simultaneously with fluorescein angiography. Johns Hopkins Med J. 1976;138:33–42.
18. Cherrick GR, Stein SW, Leevy CM, et al. Indocyanine green: observations on its physical properties, plasma decay, and hepatic extraction. J Clin Invest. 1960;39:592–600.
19. Costa DL, Huang SJ, Orlock DA, et al. Retinal-choroidal indocyanine green dye clearance and liver dysfunction. Retina. 2003;23:557–61.
20. Fineman MS, Maguire JI, Fineman SW, et al. Safety of indocyanine green angiography during pregnancy: a survey of the retina, macula, and vitreous societies. Arch Ophthalmol. 2001;119:353–5.
21. Hope-Ross M, Yannuzzi LA, Gragoudas ES, et al. Adverse reactions due to indocyanine green. Ophthalmology. 1994;101:529–33.
22. Yannuzzi LA, Flower RW, Slakter JS. Indocyanine green angiography. Mosby Incorporated; 1997.
23. Spaide RF, Jaffe GJ, Sarraf D, et al. Consensus nomenclature for reporting neovascular age-related macular degeneration data: consensus on neovascular age-related macular degeneration nomenclature study group. Ophthalmology. 2020;127(5):616–36.
24. Macular Photocoagulation Study Group. Subfoveal neovascular lesions in age-related macular degeneration. Guidelines for evaluation and treatment in the macular photocoagulation study. Arch Ophthalmol. 1991;109:1242–57.
25. Freund KB, Ho IV, Barbazetto IA, et al. Type 3 neovascularization: the expanded spectrum of retinal angiomatous proliferation. Retina. 2008;28:201–11.
26. Schmidt-Erfurth U, Kriechbaum K, Oldag A. Three-dimensional angiography of classic and occult lesion types in choroidal neovascularization. Invest Ophthalmol Vis Sci. 2007;48:1751–60.
27. Yannuzzi LA, Negrao S, Iida T, et al. Retinal angiomatous proliferation in age-related macular degeneration. Retina. 2001;21:416–34.
28. Anantharaman G, Sheth J, Bhende M, Narayanan R, Natarajan S, Rajendran A, Manayath G, Sen P, Biswas R, Banker A, Gupta C. Polypoidal choroidal vasculopathy: pearls in diagnosis and management. Indian J Ophthalmol. 2018;66(7):896.
29. Cheung CMG, Lee WK, Koizumi H, et al. Pachychoroid disease. Eye (Lond). 2019;33(1):14–33.
30. Shields CL, Honavar SG, Shields JA, et al. Circumscribed choroidal hemangioma: clinical manifestations and factors predictive of visual outcome in 200 consecutive cases. Ophthalmology. 2001;108:2237–48.
31. Arevalo JF, Shields CL, Shields JA, et al. Circumscribed choroidal hemangioma: characteristic features with indocyanine green video-angiography. Ophthalmology. 2000;107:344–50.
32. Krause L, Bechrakis NE, Kreusel KM, et al. Indocyanine green angiography in choroid metastases. Ophthalmologe. 2002;99(8):617–9.
33. Osher RH, Abrams GW, Yarian D, et al. Varix of the vortex ampulla. Am J Ophthalmol. 1981;92:653–60.
34. Singh AD, De Potter P, Shields CL, et al. Indocyanine green angiography and ultrasonography of a varix of vortex vein. Arch Ophthalmol. 1993;111:1283–4.
35. Gross NE, Yannuzzi LA, Freund KB, et al. Multiple evanescent white dot syndrome. Arch Ophthalmol. 2006;124:493–500.
36. Slakter JS, Giovannini A, Yannuzzi LA, et al. Indocyanine green angiography of multifocal choroiditis. Ophthalmology. 1997;104:1813–9.

37. Fardeau C, Herbort CP, Kullmann N, et al. Indocyanine green angiography in birdshot chorioretinopathy. Ophthalmology. 1999;106:1928–34.
38. Schneider U, Inhoffen W, Gelisken F. Indocyanine green angiography in a case of unilateral recurrent posterior acute multifocal placoid pigment epitheliopathy. Acta Ophthalmol Scand. 2003;81:72–5.
39. Giovannini A, Mariotti C, Ripa E, et al. Indocyanine green angiographic findings in serpiginous choroidopathy. Br J Ophthalmol. 1996;80:536–40.
40. Invernizzi A, Agarwal A, Mapelli C, et al. Longitudinal follow-up of choroidal granulomas using enhanced depth imaging optical coherence tomography. Retina. 2017;37(1):144–53.

Paediatric Wide-Field Retinal Imaging

27

Sourav Pal

27.1 Introduction

The use of wide-field imaging on paediatric subjects is primarily targeted at but is not restricted to the detection of retinopathy of prematurity (ROP). Early detection of the disease at stage-1, which appears as a thin demarcation line on the retina between the vascular and avascular region, can largely reduce the risk of severe vision loss. Therefore, for finding signatures of ROP at its early stage, imaging of the extreme peripheral regions around the *ora serrata* becomes far more important than imaging the central part of the retina.

27.2 History and Stages of ROP

The disease was more apparent with the invention of incubators in the early 1940s. ROP was first reported in 1942 and identified as a cause of excess oxygen concentration inside incubators. In 1949, Owens and Owens [1] described the early stages of ROP and its progression. With the advancement of incubators and the increased number of premature survivals, cases of vision loss due to ROP significantly increased by the 1950s. The first attempt to deal with this problem universally was made by Reese et al. [2] by classifying the disease in 1953. More than 30 years went by, and many such attempts were made [3–6] before a group of 23 ophthalmologists from 11 different counties collaborated to propose the International Classification of Retinopathy of Prematurity (ICROP) in 1984 [7] to define protocols for ROP studies. The third edition, published in 2021, is currently used for ROP screening [8]. In all practical cases, the state of vascularization is investigated, classified, and recorded in multiple circular zones with the optic disc at the centre.

The central zone or Zone-I is the circular area around the optic disc with a radius twice the distance between the optic disc and macula (*d*). (Fig. 27.1). Zone-I boundary makes an angle of approximately 45° at the centre of the eyeball [9] (Fig. 27.2). This slightly varies for premature babies with postmenstrual age (PMA) due to rapid changes in the eyeball size [9].

Zone-II is the annular region concentric to Zone-I and adjacent to it with an extension till nasal ora serrata. The boundary of Zone-II closely matches the equator [10] (Fig. 27.2), at least on the nasal side. The Zone-II boundary makes an angle between 180 ° and 200° at the centre of the eyeball. Additionally, ICROP defines a narrow annular zone inside Zone-II. This is named Posterior *Zone*-II, adjacent to Zone-I, and has a thickness twice the diameter of the optic disc. In ICROP, this is marked as an area prone to more severe disease than ROP.

S. Pal (✉)
Forus Health Pvt. Ltd., Bengaluru, India
e-mail: sourav@forushealth.com

T. Das, P. Satgunam (eds.), *Ophthalmic Diagnostics*, https://doi.org/10.1007/978-981-97-0138-4_27

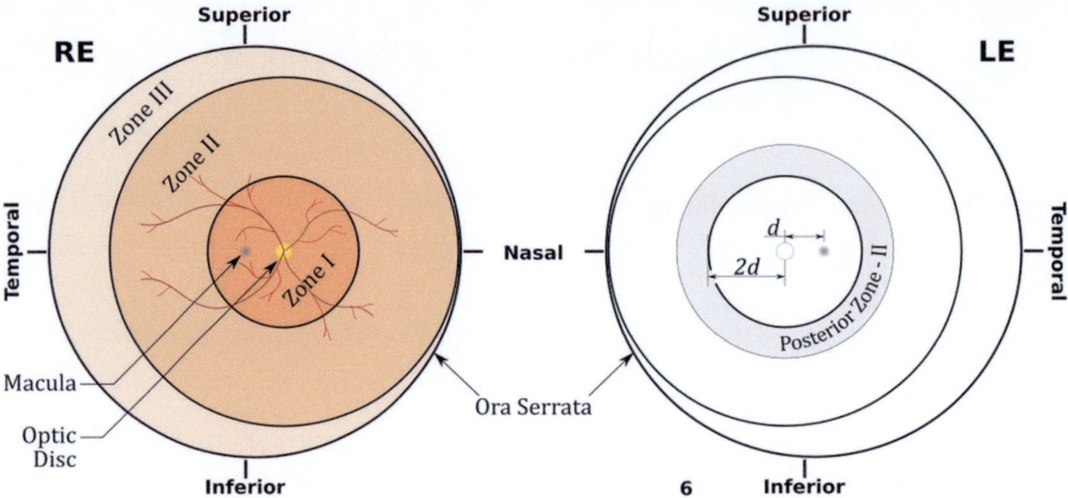

Fig. 27.1 Schematic representation of three zones and other features of the left (LE) and right (RE) eyes

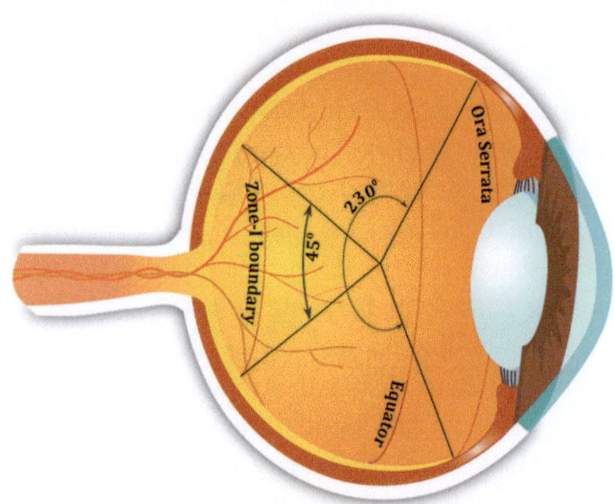

Fig. 27.2 Different zones and FoV at the centre of the eye

Zone-III is the crescent-shaped retinal area on the temporal side of Zone-II. By Toslak et al. [10] and Atkinson [11], the far extent of Zone-III makes an angle of 230° at the centre of the eyeball.

Therefore, it is evident that a conventional fundus camera system with a field of view (FoV) between 40 ° and 50° can image up to Zone-I normally. An odd tilt in the device is needed to cover Zone-III and image ora serrata. A similar attempt was made with the Pictor imaging system (Volk Optical Inc., Mentor, USA), a portable non-contact digital fundus camera with an FoV of 45 ° . In a study, Prakalapakorn et al. [12] could image only Zone-I and little beyond that. Results show the possibility of detecting *pre-plus* or *plus* diseases [13], characterized by dilated and tortuous arterioles near the posterior pole. But it failed to capture signatures of an early stage of ROP. Hence, a wide-field imaging system, which gives flexibility to the user and allows imaging up to the ora serrata with no or little tilt in the device, remained the first preference over the years.

27.3 Wide-Angle Imaging Technology

A binocular indirect ophthalmoscope (BIO) is the gold standard for ROP screening. But it necessitates an experienced ophthalmologist. Screening using BIO is generally time-consuming. Thus, ROP screening with BIO is less practical for developing countries with poor patient-to-physician ratios; therefore, there is a need for wide-angle digital cameras. The wide-angle camera facilitates photo-document a larger area of the retina in a lesser time for future reference. Additionally, a minimally trained technician with a wide-angle camera can participate in an ROP screening programme. Telemedicine-based ROP screening is effective too [14–16]. It overcomes the barrier of poor patient-to-physician ratio and reaches out to larger populations to ensure timely screening and treatment wherever necessary. Wide-angle imaging system with digital image recorder is an inseparable part of the programmes.

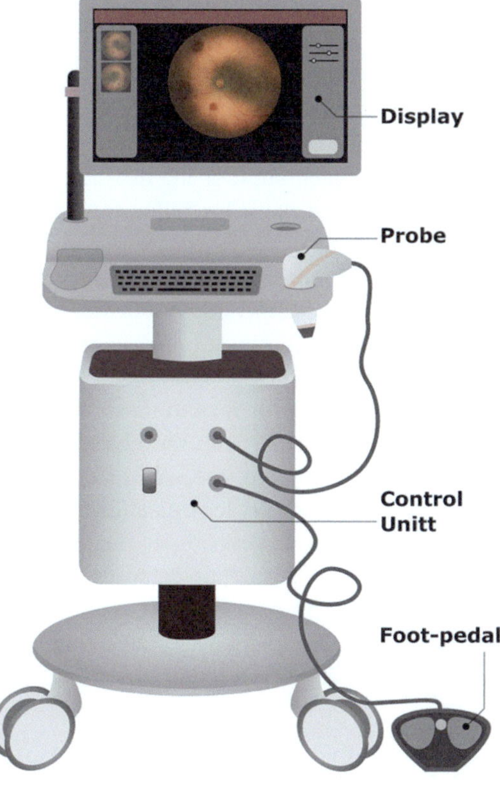

Fig. 27.3 System architecture adopted by RetCam, PanoCam, and Icon

27.3.1 Currently Available Wide-Angle Cameras

RetCam by Natus Medical Inc. (Middleton, USA), previously known as Clarity Medical System Inc., is the first paediatric retinal camera with FoV from 30 to 130° through changeable front attachments. Many other manufacturers, like Forus Health Pvt. Ltd. (Bangalore, India), Phoenix (Pleasanton, USA), and Visunex Medical Systems (Fremont, USA) subsequently introduced wide-field imaging devices, named 3nethra neo, Icon and PanoCam, respectively. Devices like RetCam, PanoCam and Icon build on a trolley, as shown in Fig. 27.3. Probe consists of imaging and illumination optics along with an imaging sensor. All of them has integrated display and computing system. Control unit generally holds light sources and other control circuits that establish a communication between software and imaging system. All of them uses a foot-pedal to control light intensity and focus on the retina as and when needed. PanoCam probe has the distinctive quality of operating wirelessly. Conversely, 3nethra neo has a compact control unit that holds the probe, which contains light source, illumination, and imaging optics. It gets connected to and uses a laptop/PC as display and computing system. Figure 27.4 shows an upgraded version of 3nethra neo, which facilitates fluorescein imaging is named as 3nethra neo-HD FA.

Table 27.1 presents various models offered by the above four manufacturers and their comparison. Despite diversified features, many similarities in basic structure exist. All systems use white

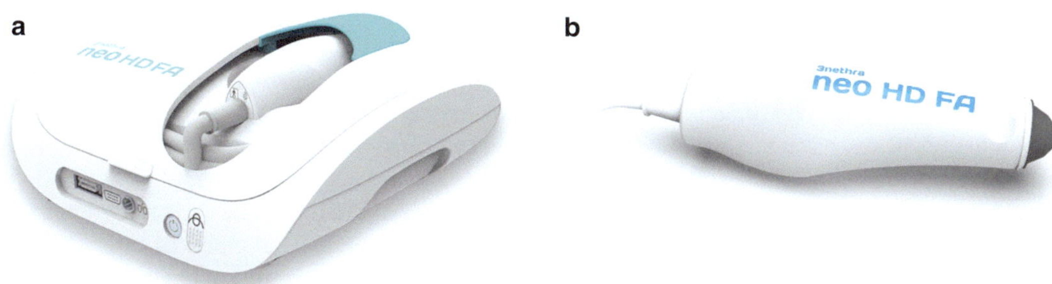

Fig. 27.4 3nethra neo-HD FA by Forus Health Pvt. Ltd.; (**a**) probe and its control unit, (**b**) imaging unit/probe

Table 27.1 Presents various models offered by the above four manufacturers and their comparison

Device	Manufacturer	FoV	Imagesize	Portability	FA
RetCam shuttle	Natus Medical	130°	VGA	Heavy	No
RetCam 3		130°	2 MP	Heavy	Yes
RetCam envision		130°	1.5 MP	Heavy	Yes
3nethra neo	Forus Health	120°	4 MP	Compact	No
3nethra neo-HD FA		150°	20 MP	Compact	Yes
Panocam LT	Visunex Medical Systems	130°	8 MP	Heavy	–
Panocam Pro		130°	13 MP	Heavy	–
Icon	Phoenix	100°	–	Heavy	–

MP megapixel; *VGA* video graphics array

ring-shaped light to illuminate the retina, operate in contact with the cornea, and obtain true colour images.

27.4 Technology

We describe the technology using a camera system made in India. But basically, the technology is similar across currently available cameras.

27.4.1 Optical Design of Imaging System

Most of the wide-angle fundus cameras in paediatric imaging works in contact with the cornea to avoid an increase in lens diameter abnormally. Generally, a meniscus lens is selected as the contact lens. The radius of the contact surface is generally selected between 6 and 7 mm to match it with the corneal curvature of the baby. Optical components that follow contact lens act like a relay system; these generally form an intermediate real image of the retina before carrying it forward and shaping it appropriately for the selected sensor. The imaging system of the 3nethra neo-HD FA (Forus Health, Bangalore, India) is schematically shown in Fig. 27.5. Imaging systems of wide-angle cameras have strategically similar designs but differ in how they distribute the optical power.

There are two groups of relay lenses.

Relay lens Group-1 forms an intermediate image and guides rays towards the aperture of the system. The 3nethra neo-HD FA uses a trans-pupillary illumination scheme. The aperture is placed at a plane conjugate to the pupil of the eye so that the entrance pupil of the imaging system coincides with the pupil for reflex-free imaging (see Sect. 27.4.3.1).

Relay lens Group-2 determines the final image size suitable for the camera/sensor in use. Another job of it is balancing residual aberration from the previous group of lenses. The 3nethra neo-HD FA uses a tunable focus lens to make the necessary correction aligned with the changes in the refractive power of the eye. An electronically controlled tunable focus lens enables a smooth, vibration-free operation. Without such lenses, a physical movement of Group-2 lenses is needed for focus. Although contact and Group-1 lenses decide the FoV, Group-2 lenses play an important role in image formation without vignetting.

27.4.2 Understanding of Field of View

Understanding and expressing the FoV correctly is critical when working with wide-angle fundus cameras. Historically, the FoV is defined as the angle subtended by the front optics of any imaging system at the pupil of the eye (Fig. 27.6a). This is usually named as external angle, θ_{ex} [11]. An oversimplified expression, $\theta_{in} = \theta_{ex}/1.33$ for calculation of internal angle θ_{in} is sometimes useful but not accurate in all practical cases. A ray of light from the retina follows a multifold path through the vitreous humour, crystalline lens, and

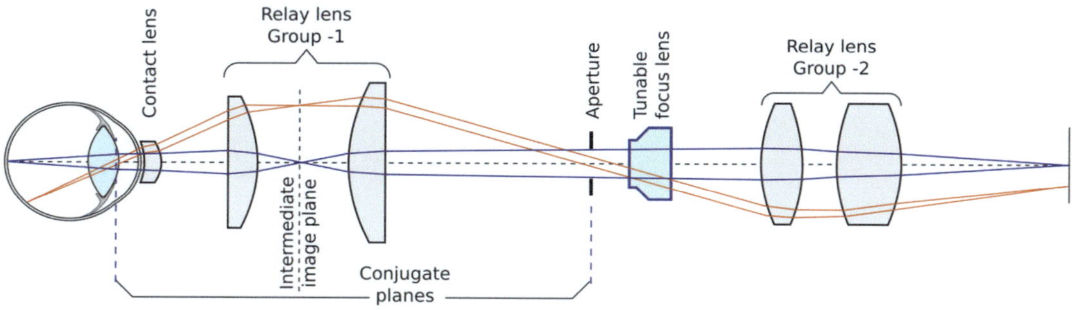

Fig. 27.5 Schematic of 3nethra neo-HD FA imaging system

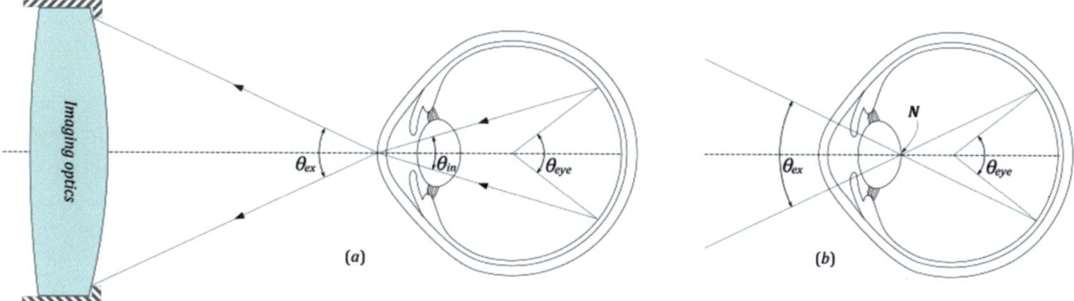

Fig. 27.6 Illustration of external angle, internal angle, and eye angle

aqueous humour, having refractive indices of 1.33, 1.42, and 1.33, respectively, before exiting the eye. Finding the nodal point of the eye and mapping the external angles in relation to it is, therefore, beneficial for greater precision. The eye angle ,θ_e, is the angle subtended by the retinal area being imaged at the centre of the eyeball. Modern-day wide-angle cameras use θ_e to specify the FoV of the system.

Figure 27.6b schematically presents θ_{ex} and θ_e, in reference to the nodal point of the eye *N*, which is very close to the posterior surface of the crystalline lens [17]. With these factors considered, Yao et al. [18] arrived at the following relationship between the two angles.

$$\theta_e = \theta_{ex} + 2\sin^{-1}\left(0.51\sin\left(\theta_{ex}/2\right)\right)$$

As per the above expression, an external angle of 50° is equivalent to an eye angle of 74.89 ° , which closely matches the result presented by Atkinson [11]. As per Atkinson and Mazo, $\theta_e = 1.48\,\theta_{ex}$, which is also effective in many practical cases.

27.4.3 Illumination System of Wide-Angle Cameras

Fundamentally, there are two types of illumination systems: (1) *trans-pupillary*—uses a clear window of the pupil of the eye to throw light onto the retina, and (2) *trans-scleral*—utilizes sections of the sclera to deliver light to the retina.

27.4.3.1 Trans-pupillary Illumination System

A trans-pupillary illumination system is the most widely used illumination scheme for retinal imaging [19] (Table 27.1). It complies with the Gullstrand principle [20–22], which states that the lighting and imaging channels must be separated near the pupil, from the corneal surface to the crystalline lens, for glare-free retinal imaging. In general, the illumination beam enters through an annular zone near the margin of the pupil, and the light scattered back from the retina is collected through the central part of the pupil (Fig. 27.7) [19, 22]. Fig. 27.7(b) shows the

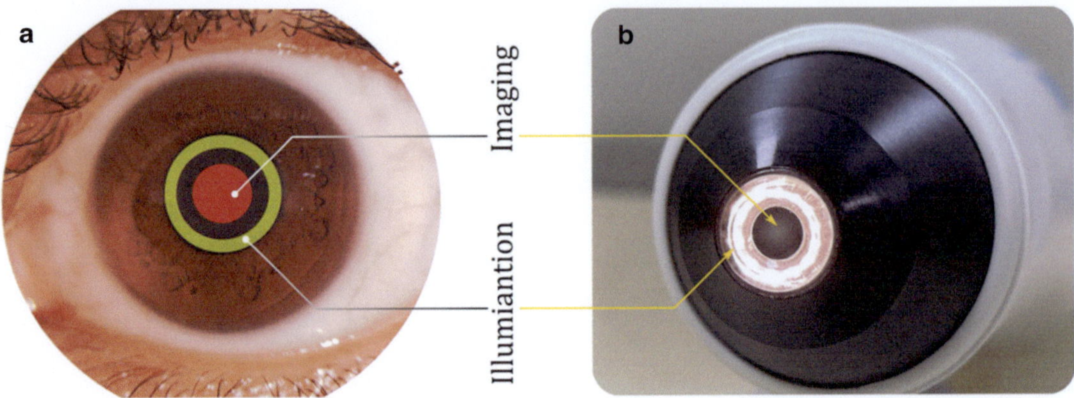

Fig. 27.7 A schematic of trans-pupillary illumination that follows the Gullstrand principle. (**a**) The illumination beam enters through an annular zone near the margin of the pupil; the light scattered back from the retina is collected through the central part of the pupil. (**b**) The tip of the imaging probe in 3nethra neo-HD FA

arrangement in the 3nethra neo-HD FA. A smaller diameter of the ring illumination system leaves little space for the imaging beam, which can severely affect the optical resolution and light throughput. Given that a larger ring diameter will require a larger pupil for better imaging, a judicial selection of ring diameter is very important. To make the system suitable for a wider age group, it must be designed considering the rapid structural changes in the eye, and hence the nature of light reflex, from premature to infants.

RetCam uses a bundle of optical fibre arranged in the shape of a ring to generate a ring light. The other end of the fibre bundle is fused and is used as a light collector from a halogen source. In contrast, 3nethra neo or 3nethra neo-HD FA uses a waveguide structure made of acrylic material to shape desired ring light. It uses an array of LEDs arranged on an annular PCB (printed circuit board) as a light source, placed near the base of the waveguide structure. Light gets coupled into the waveguide, bounces back from the walls due to total internal reflection, and propagates towards the circular output end of it.

27.4.3.2 Trans-scleral Illumination

Trans-scleral illumination is an alternative to the trans-pupillary illumination scheme that utilizes the pupillary area fully for imaging [10, 23–28]. The history of trans-scleral illumination can be traced back to the early 1970s when Pomerantzeff et al. [29, 30] imaged the retina by delivering light through the palpebral region of the sclera. Named, *Equator-plus*, it had an extended FoV to capture the retina from anterior to the equator, nearly 148°.

In 2002 Panoret–1000, a trans-scleral illumination-based system, was introduced. It could obtain images of the optic disc and ora serrata together in a single frame. But the clinical deployment of this device was not successful. Unlike the Equator-plus camera that delivers light through the eyelid, the illumination system of Panoret–1000 requires scleral contact increasing the risk of contamination, inflammation, and abrasion to the sclera and cornea. Currently, Panoret–1000 is commercially not available.

Pars-plana (a Latin phrase for *Flat area*) is a flat portion of sclera 3–4 mm posterior to the limbus with a width of ~4 mm. Pars-plana region has a comparatively lower density of muscle, blood vessels, pigmentation, and consequently more transparent than other parts of the sclera. Therefore, scleral illumination through the pars-plana region is of utmost interest to recent investigators. Figure 27.8 schematically represents a trans-pars-scleral illumination scheme, where generally, a fibre-optics illumination probe is placed over the sclera on the pars-plana region to produce a diffuse illumination over the retina. Thus, the entire pupil area is available for imaging without any possibility of crosstalk with the illumination beam. The transitive pars-plana area reduces the risk of any physical hazard by enabling suitable light levels on the retina with little input energy.

The primary benefit of trans-scleral lighting is the ability to use the entire pupil area for imaging. This allows for some degree of wide-angle imaging even without pupil dilation. Additionally, it gives freedom to the designer to plan optical systems with higher resolution. Wide-angle cameras of Table 27.1, having a field of view around 130° offer an optical resolution ranging between 20 and 35 lp/mm at the centre of the field.

The biggest disadvantage of trans-scleral illumination is its usability and, in some cases, associated safety issues. This type of illumination

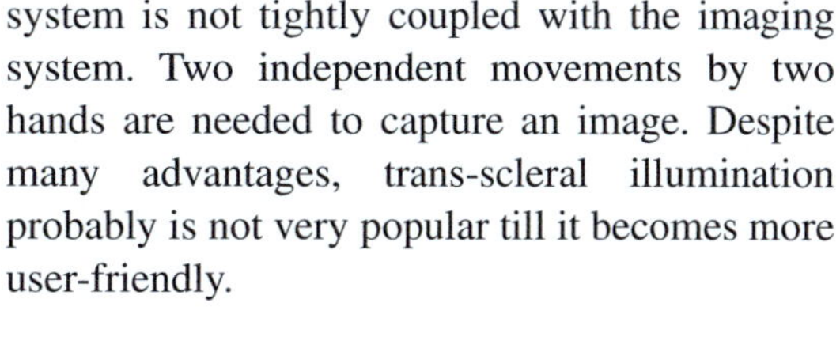

system is not tightly coupled with the imaging system. Two independent movements by two hands are needed to capture an image. Despite many advantages, trans-scleral illumination probably is not very popular till it becomes more user-friendly.

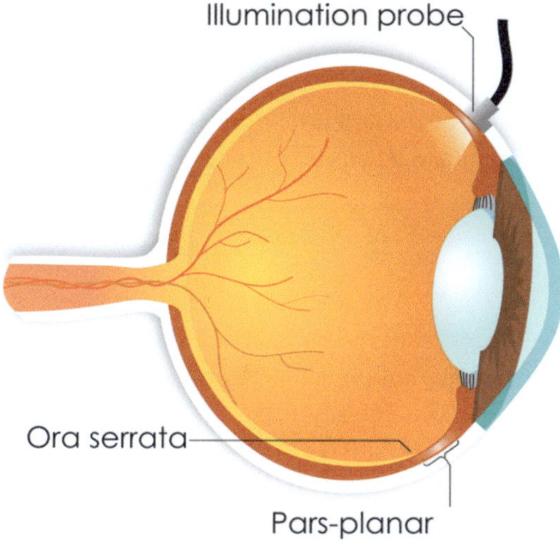

Fig. 27.8 Schematic representation of trans-pars-planar illumination scheme

27.4.4 Fluorescein Angiography

Most state-of-the-art wide-angle fundus cameras can perform fundus fluorescein angiography (FA). FA is a tool for investigating vascular changes not evident in a colour fundus image. The development of digital imaging in the late twentieth century made FA easier and more practical, and it has become an indispensable part of ROP treatment [31]. Currently, FA is invariably performed before laser photocoagulation to map the retinal vascularization more precisely.

In FA, retinal images are captured with the time of acquisition offset from the injection of Sodium fluorescein (NaFl) dye. NaFl absorbs energy in the blue and emits it in the green region of the visible spectrum [32]. A typical absorption and emission spectrum of the NaFl is shown in Fig. 27.9. It has peak absorption at 495 nm, which is pH dependent and slightly shifts towards the left when injected into blood [33]. NaFl emits light in the approximate range of 515–600 nm, with a peak at 540 nm.

The source is typically selected with a peak around 480 nm. A typical spectrum of the source

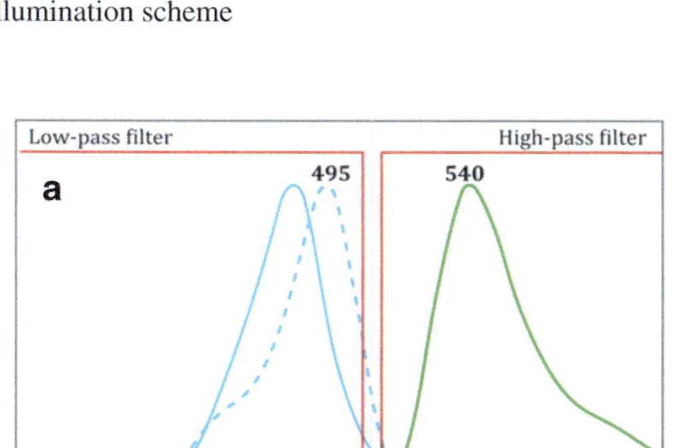

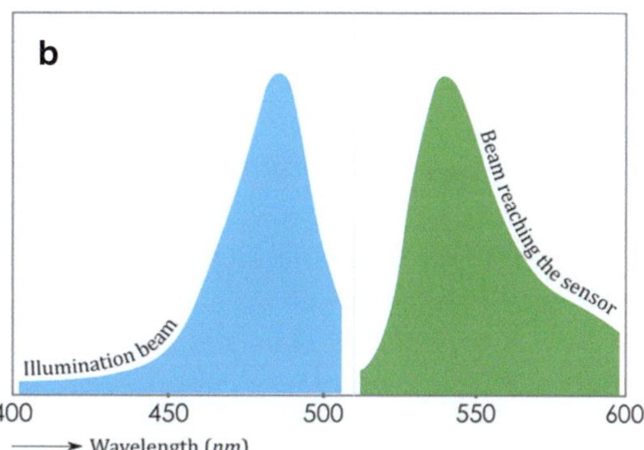

Fig. 27.9 Spectrum associated with fluorescein angiography (**a**) absorption and emission spectrum of sodium fluorescein; (**b**) spectrum of illumination and imaging beam after going through optical filters

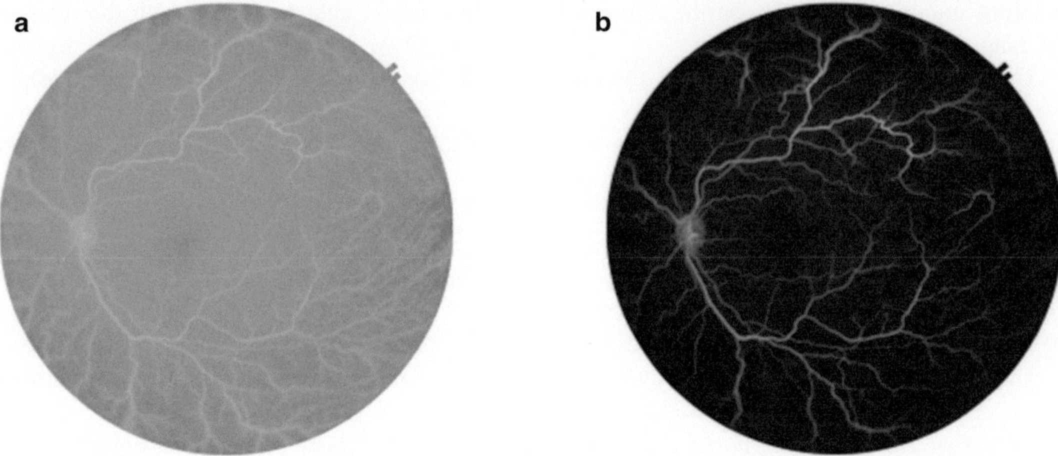

Fig. 27.10 Images of the retina captured under blue light and Sodium fluorescein injected into blood (**a**) without and (**b**) with a barrier filter into the imaging path

is presented by a continuous blue line in Fig. 27.9a. It is filtered further with a low-pass filter, known as an excitation filter, with a cut-on wavelength of around 500 nm (blue dotted line in Fig. 27.9a). Some system uses an excitation filter in conjunction with a powerful white light source, such as a halogen lamp, to produce the necessary blue light beam for FA. Light scattered back from the retina is filtered just before the sensor with a long-pass filter, commonly known as a barrier filter, with a cut-off wavelength near 515 nm. A bandpass filter can alternatively be used for this purpose. Once illuminated with blue light, all parts of the retina reflect blue light towards imaging optics. Only the parts of the retina containing blood (blood vessels or areas of blood spillage) absorb blue and emit in the green region. Without a barrier filter, the camera detects both green and blue light returning from all parts of the retina and captures a picture like Fig. 27.10a. Fluorescein angiograph (Fig. 27.10b) is then captured by blocking blue rays with a barrier filter.

Edmund Optics [34] offers a pair of excitation and barrier filters, where an excitation filter has a cut-on wavelength at 506 nm, and a barrier filter (a bandpass filter) has a lower cut-off at 513 nm. To prevent spillover, which could reduce image contrast, it is required that the boundaries of the excitation and barrier filters are well separated.

27.4.5 Image Sensors

The image sensor is the last but not the least important part of the retinal camera. Two types of sensors are commonly used; (1) charged couple device (CCD) and (2) complementary metal-oxide semiconductor (CMOS). Until the first decade of this century, CCDs were the preferred digital sensor for retinal imaging and many other scientific experiments. CCDs are generally sensors having larger pixel sizes, excellent sensitivity, higher dynamic range, and low noise characteristics [35]. Higher sensitivity with lower noise allows imaging at a lower light level suitable for fundus imaging. More importantly, higher dynamic range facilitates imaging of the bright optic disc and comparatively darker peripheral region simultaneously with satisfactory details.

CMOS sensors remained far behind CCDs in three qualities, as mentioned earlier, for many years [36]. In the previous decade, COMOS was increasingly recognized and used in many imaging products, including medical devices and scientific experiments. (For example, in 2015, SONY decided to discontinue CCD manufacturing and focus on CMOS technology).

Recent developments in the semiconductor industry helped significantly to improve the sensitivity, noise quality, and dynamic range of CMOS sensors, which are now at par with CCD. Additionally, CMOS consumes much lower power than a CCD, which makes it suitable for handheld, portable, and battery-operated systems. In CMOS, a pixel size of a few degrees smaller than that of CCDs can be achieved, and therefore a much higher megapixel sensor can be produced in smaller sized devices. But one must be careful about selecting cameras with very small pixel sizes as this can increase the risk of crosstalk. The possibility of erecting an ON-chip processing unit with CMOS technology makes the overall size of CMOS cameras much smaller than a CCD camera. It also facilitates high-speed readout and, subsequently faster frame rate.

The performance of any camera system depends mainly on the judicial selection of the sensor. A frame rate of at least 15 frames per second (FPS) is essential for handheld imaging of the paediatric subject. A dynamic range close to 70 dB or more is suitable for capturing bright optic disc and darker periphery with useful details. Cameras with a signal-to-noise ratio (SNR) higher than 40 dB are desirable. Compared to colour fundus imaging, FA requires greater quantum efficiency to capture generally weak fluorescence.

27.5 Imaging Technique

Primary challenges in premature/infant screening are accessibility, poor cooperation, and a shorter time window for imaging. It is practically impossible to image a baby's eyes in a supine position with conventional tabletop devices. Conversely, it is too early to make the newborn sit upright and place the chin over the chinrest. A portable handheld device is very much necessary for paediatric screening. A contact base operation is preferable for non-cooperative subjects, despite potential health risks like contamination or cornea scarring on rare occasions. Moreover, a wide-angle camera facilitates capturing a larger portion of the retina in a single image, reducing the screening time. This section will mainly focus on imaging techniques associated with the devices presented in Table 27.1.

Contact devices use sterile lubricant gel between the contact lens and cornea to ensure smooth movement while manoeuvring the probe during the operation. Eye gel also creates a continuous medium of refractive index close to 1.4, which is between the corneal refractive index of 1.33 and the refractive index of a glass, commonly 1.5. It reduces Snell's reflection of light at the corneal surface, which can create glare/artefact on the final image. A uniform contact of the imager with the cornea ensures continuity in the medium, reducing the risk of air pocket formation and unwanted artefacts due to reflection.

It is comparatively easier to capture a macula-centric image. The main challenge is to capture ora serrata that needs a tilt even with the device having FoV as large as 150 ° . In imaging premature babies, it is advisable to use an eyelid speculum to create space for easy manoeuvring of the imaging device, and occasionally, a depressor is used to improve the visibility of the peripheral region further (Fig. 27.11).

Proper dilation of the pupil is essential for a uniformly illuminated retinal image. An inappropriate dilation can lead to a central shadow on the captured image by blocking the light rays near the outer edge of the ring light (Fig. 27.12).

FA is an invasive procedure and demands special attention. It is highly advisable to perform FA near a life support system to tackle the rare adverse effect of NaFl on the human body. Before starting the procedure for FA, a colour fundus image is generally taken to set an appropriate

Fig. 27.11 (**a**) Speculum (**b**) depressor occasionally used for ROP screening

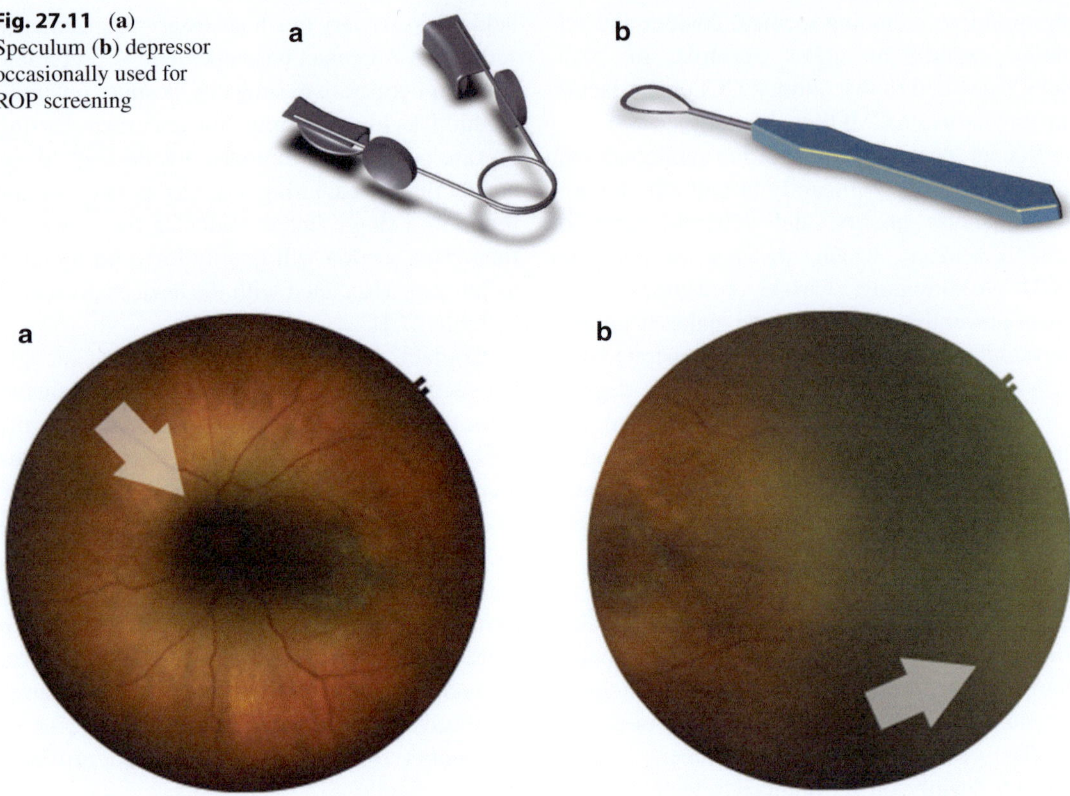

Fig. 27.12 Possible image artefacts in ROP images; (**a**) shadow due to undilated pupil and (**b**) reflection observed due to formation of air pockets inside lubricant gel (white arrow; images captured with the 3nethra neo-HD FA)

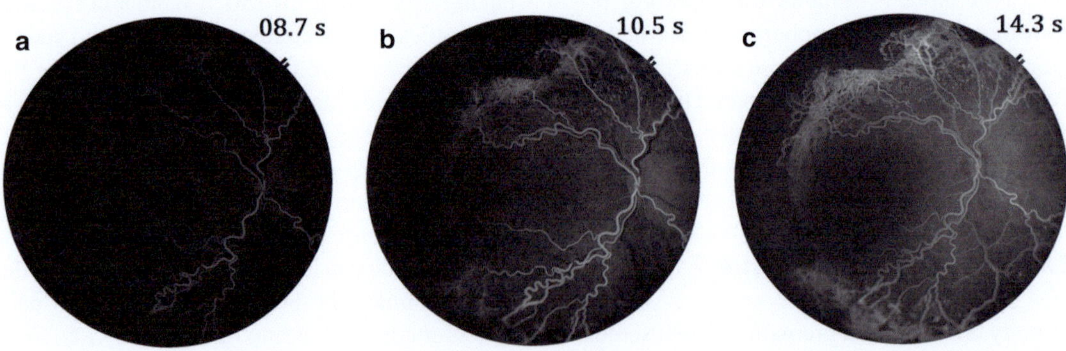

Fig. 27.13 Progress dye into the blood after (**a**) 8.7 s, (**b**) 10.5 s, and (**c**) 14.3 s after injecting the dye. (Camera: 3nethra neo-HD FA)

focus for the subject. A 10% solution of Sodium fluorescein dye at 0.1 ml per *kg* of baby's weight is generally injected intravenously, followed by an isotonic saline flush [31]. In some situations, oral NaFl dosing is used as an alternative. A timer is started at the time of injection of the dye. Software associated with the device attaches a time stamp from the timer running at the time of the image capture and saves it with the image. Time stamps carry vital information as the contrast and characteristic of the image primarily depends on the offset from the time of the shot. The image in Fig. 27.13a is captured when the dye reaches retinal blood vessels, and as a result, arteries are lighter compared to other parts of the retina. As time progresses, dye reaches other capillaries, and an image similar to Fig. 27.13c is captured.

27.6 Clinical Application

Wide-field imaging in the paediatric sector is predominantly used for ROP screening. The retina is imaged up to 100–130° in a single click. The FoV can also be increased by montaging the images or using ultra-wide field imaging system. These help in documentation, compare the retinopathy status between different follow-up visits, monitor the response to treatment, training, and telescreening. Besides better parental understanding of the disease's progression and consequently better cooperation, image-based counselling allows parents to make decisions about their course of treatment and supports that course of action in the event of a medicolegal dispute. The imaging devices can pick of subtle vascular changes which a busy practitioner might miss while screening a large number of patients with indirect ophthalmoscope. Image of mature retina without any signature of ROP are presented in Panel-1(a, b) of Fig. 27.15. Whereas as mild tortuosity in the blood vessels is noticed on the image presented in Panel-1(c) of Fig. 27.14, as an indication of plus disease. Figure 27.14 also describes the various states of ROP [8].

Stage-1 ROP (Fig. 27.14, Panel 2a). A thin demarcation, relatively flat, at the junction of vascular and avascular regions is seen.

Stage-2 ROP (Fig. 27.14, Panel 2b). The demarcation line changes into a wider elevated ridge. Isolated tufts of neovascular tissue on the retinal surface, commonly known as *popcorn*, may be seen posterior to the ridge in Stage-2 (white arrow, Panel 2c).

Stage-3 ROP (Fig. 27.14, Panel 3a). Extra-retinal neovascular proliferation extends from the ridge into the vitreous and is continuous, with the posterior aspect of the ridge producing a ragged appearance as proliferation progresses.

Stage-4 ROP (Fig. 27.14, Panel 3b and c). It is characterized by a partial retinal detachment that spares or includes the fovea. Clinical signs of retinal detachment include loss of fine detail in the choroidal vasculature or the granular pigment epithelium, a ground glass appearance compared to the neighbouring connected retina, or both (Fig. 27.14, Panel 4a).

Stage-5 ROP (Fig. 27.14, Panel 4b). A total detachment is a rule.

Field of view is sometime extended beyond the limit set by the imaging system by stitching multiple images together, as presented in Fig. 27.15. Figure 27.15a shows a montage of four different colour fundus images having area of overlapping. Three angiographs, with similar time stamp, are stitched together and presented in Fig. 27.15b.

Besides ROP screening, wide-angle imaging is also used to study retinoblastoma in infants (Fig. 27.16).

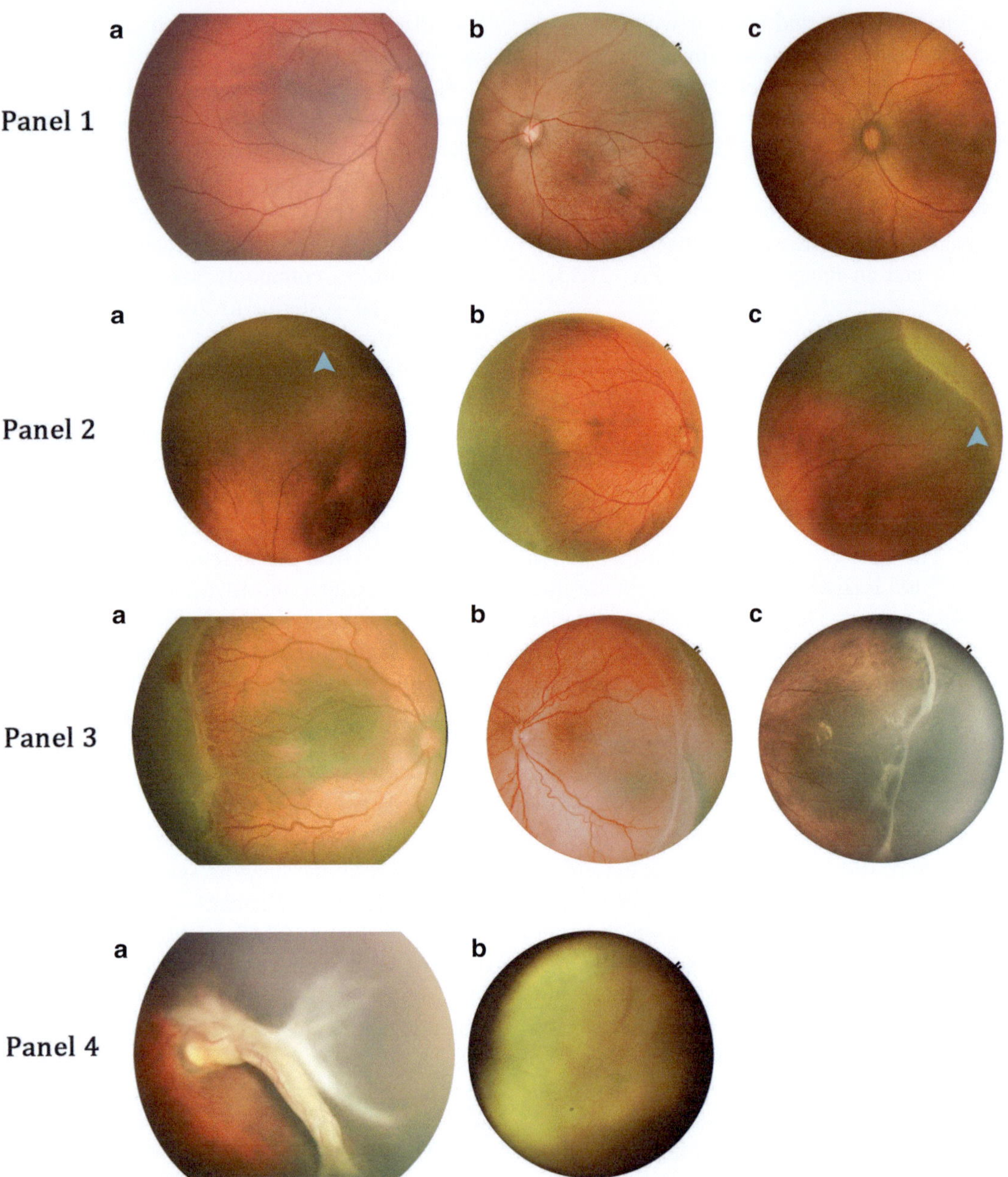

Fig. 27.14 Panel 1. (**a**)†, (**b**) Mature retina without ROP; dichotomously branching of retinal blood vessels seen up to the end of the retina imaged, and (**c**) plus disease, showing tortuosity in the blood vessels in Zone-II. Panel 2. (**a**) Stage-1 with thin demarcation line in Zone-III. (**b**)† Stage-2 Zone-II ROP showing a ridge, hyperacutely branching retinal blood vessels, mild dilatation, and tortuosity. (**c**) Stage-2 ROP shows a thick and elevated demarcation line in Zone-III with popcorn lesion. Panel 3. (**a**)† The right eye shows Stage-3 Zone-II ROP with plus; note the finger like extensions from the posterior aspect of the ridge representative of extra-retinal fibrovascular proliferation. (**b**)† The left eye showing Stage-4A with plus and narrowing of the angle between the temporal retinal vascular arcades. There was a fractional retinal detachment along the fibrovascular proliferation temporally, and (**b**) Stage-4A in Zone-III on the temporal side of the left eye with loss of choroidal detail on the extreme right of the image. Panel 4. (**a**)† The left eye Stage-4B Cicatricle ROP showing a retinal fold extending temporally from the optic disc. The macula and temporal vascular arcades are dragged within the retinal fold. (**b**)† Stage-5 ROP with total closed funnel retinal detachment. †Captured at LV Prasad Eye Institute, Bhubaneswar, India. (© Tapas R Padhi, MD, with permission)

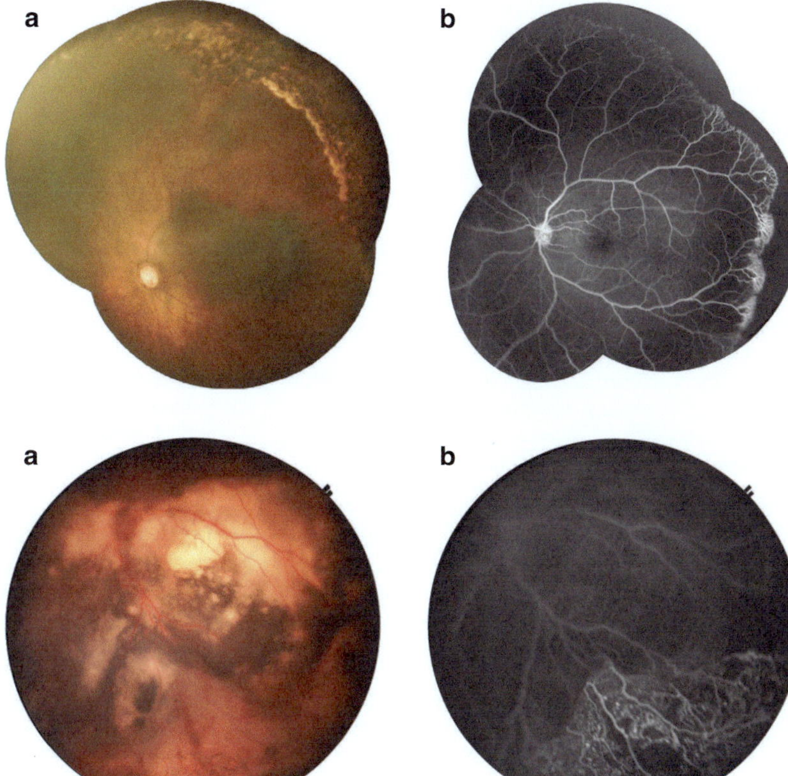

Fig. 27.15 Montage of (**a**) colour fundus images and (**b**) fluorescein angiographs. (**a**) shows structure created by photocoagulation at the top of the image

Fig. 27.16 (**a**) Colour fundus image (**b**) angiograph of a subject suffering from retinoblastoma

27.7 Conclusion

Wide-angle cameras with trans-pupillary illumination are the preferred tools for paediatric screening. The study on trans-pars-planar illumination will continue to search for a potential alternative which frees the pupil for imaging and helps extend FoV beyond the current standard. Trans-pars-planar illumination, as far as the author is aware, has not yet been demonstrated for FA and may be an area to explore. However, it may encounter difficulties due to the shorter penetration depth of blue light. A transition from trans-pupillary lighting to a trans-pars-planar illumination system may occur soon, whereas the imaging system may continue with its current structure. The use of CMOS sensors for retinal imaging is expected to increase after the recent advancement in the respective field.

Funding Nil.

Disclosure Forus Employee.

References

1. Owens WC, Owens EU. Retrolental fibroplasia in premature infants. Am J Ophthalmol. 1949;32:1–21.
2. Reese AB, King MJ, Owens WC. Classification of retrolental fibroplasia. Am J Ophthalmol. 1953;36(10):1333–5.
3. Patz A. Retrolental fibroplasia. Surv Ophthalmol. 1969;14(1):1–29.
4. Flynn JT, O'Grady GE, Herrera J, et al. Retrolental fibroplasia: I. Clinical observations. Arch Ophthalmol. 1977;95(2):217–23.
5. Kushner BJ, Essner D, Cohen IJ, Flynn JT. Retrolental fibroplasia. II. Pathologic correlation. Arch Ophthalmol. 1977;95(1):29–38.
6. Kingham JD. Acute retrolental fibroplasia. Arch Ophthalmol. 1977;95(1):39–47.
7. The Committee for the Classification of Retinopathy of Prematurity. An international classification of retinopathy of prematurity. Arch Ophthalmol. 1984;102(8):1130–4.
8. The Committee for the Classification of Retinopathy of Prematurity. An international classification of retinopathy of prematurity, Third edition. Arch Ophthalmol. 2021;128(10):51–68.
9. Wang SK, Korot E, Zaidi M, et al. Modeling absolute zone size in retinopathy of prematurity in relation

to axial length. Sci Rep. 2022;12:4717. https://doi.org/10.1038/s41598-022-08680-5.
10. Toslak D, Chau F, Erol MK, et al. Trans-pars-planar illumination enables a 200° ultra-wide field pediatric fundus camera for easy examination of the retina. Biomed Opt Express. 2020;11:68–76.
11. Atkinson A, Mazo C. Imaged area of the retina. https://www.freelists.org/archives/optimal/02-2017/pdf91WmMGLh6Q.pdf.
12. Prakalapakorn SG, Wallace DK, Freedman SF. Retinal imaging in premature infants using the Pictor noncontact digital camera. J AAPOS. 2014;18(4):321–6.
13. Davitt BV, Wallace DK. Plus disease. Surv Ophthalmol. 2009;54(6):663–70.
14. Vinekar A, Gilbert C, Dogra M, et al. The KIDROP model of combining strategies for providing retinopathy of prematurity screening in underserved areas in India using wide-field imaging, tele-medicine, non-physician graders and smart phone reporting. Indian J Ophthalmol. 2014;62(1):41–9.
15. Vinekar A, Jayadev C, Mangalesh S, et al. Role of tele-medicine in retinopathy of prematurity screening in rural outreach centers in India—a report of 20,214 imaging sessions in the KIDROP program. Semin Fetal Neonatal Med. 2015;20(5):335–45.
16. Ji MH, Zaidi M, Bodnar Z, et al. Effective field of view of wide-field fundus photography in the Stanford University Network for Diagnosis of Retinopathy of Prematurity (SUNDROP). Sci Rep. 2022;12:19276. https://doi.org/10.1038/s41598-022-22964-w.
17. Harris WF. Nodes and nodal points and lines in eyes and other optical systems. Ophthalmic Physiol Opt. 2009;30(1):24–42.
18. Yao X, Toslak D, Son T, Ma J. Understanding the relationship between visual-angle and eye-angle for reliable determination of the field-of-view in ultra-wide field fundus photography. Biomed Opt Express. 2021;12:6651–9.
19. DeHoog E, Schwiegerling J. Fundus camera systems: a comparative analysis. Appl Opt. 2009;48:221–8.
20. Gullstrand A. New methods of reflexless ophthalmoscopy. Berichte Deutsche Ophthalmologische Gesellschaft. 1910;36:326.
21. Keeler R, Singh AD, Dua HS. Reflecting on reflections: Gullstrand's large reflex-free ophthalmoscope. Br J Ophthalmol. 2010;94:826.
22. Kaschke M, Kaschke KH, Rill MS. Optical devices in ophthalmology and optometry. Wiley-VCH; 2013.
23. Toslak D, Thapa D, Chen Y, et al. Trans-palpebral illumination: an approach for wide-angle fundus photography without the need for pupil dilation. Opt Lett. 2016;41(12):2688–91.
24. Toslak D, Thapa D, Chen Y, et al. Wide-field fundus imaging with trans-palpebral illumination. Proc SPIE Int Soc Opt Eng. 2017;10045:100451X. https://doi.org/10.1117/12.2252491.
25. Wang B, Toslak D, Alam MN, et al. Contact-free trans-pars-planar illumination enables snapshot fundus camera for nonmydriatic wide field photography. Sci Rep. 2018;8:8768. https://doi.org/10.1038/s41598-018-27112-x.
26. Laforest T, Künzi M, Kowalczuk L, et al. Transscleral optical phase imaging of the human retina. Nat Photonics. 2020;14(7):439–45.
27. Lingenfelder C, Koch F, Koelbl P, et al. Transscleral LED illumination pen. Biomed Eng Lett. 2017;7:311–5.
28. Kölbl PS, Lindner C, Lingenfelder C, et al. An extra-ocular non-invasive transscleral LED-endoilluminator for eye speculum integration. Graefes Arch Clin Exp Ophthalmol. 2015;253:1529–35.
29. Pomerantzeff O, Govignon J. Design of wide-angle ophthalmoscope. Arch Ophthalmol. 1971;80:420–4.
30. Pomerantzeff O. Equator-plus camera. Invest Ophthalmol Vis Sc. 1975;14:401–6.
31. Lepore D, Molle F, Pagliara MM, et al. Atlas of fluorescein angiographic findings in eyes undergoing laser for retinopathy of prematurity. Ophthalmology. 2011;118(1):168–75.
32. Chopdar A. Fundus fluorescein angiography. Elsevier Health Service; 1996.
33. Doughty MJ. pH dependent spectral properties of sodium fluorescein ophthalmic solutions revisited. Ophthalmic Physiol Opt. 2010;30:167. https://doi.org/10.1111/j.1475-1313.2009.00703.x.
34. Fluorescence Filter Set. https://www.edmundoptics.in/p/fluorescence-filter-set-for-fitc-fluorescein/21528/.
35. Durini D. High performance silicon imaging: fundamentals and applications of CMOS and CCD sensors. Elsevier Science; 2019.
36. Bigas M, Cabruja E, Forest J, Salvi J. Review of CMOS imagers. Microelectron J. 2006;37(5):433–51.

28 Optical Coherence Tomography and Optical Coherence Tomography-Angiography

Niroj Kumar Sahoo, Priya R. Chandrasekaran, Ninan Jacob, and Gemmy Cheung

28.1 Introduction

28.1.1 Principles of Optical Coherence Tomography (OCT)

The fundamental principle behind OCT imaging is light interference. The basic mechanism of an OCT can be described with the help of a Michelson interferometer, as described below. The light from a low coherence (high bandwidth) source is split into two paths by a coupler, directing it along two separate arms of the interferometer, the sample arm, and the reference arm. As the light exits either arm, it is passed through lenses and mirrors to control its shape, depth of focus, intensity, etc. A reference mirror reflects the light back into the reference arm, and it returns along the same path it came on, whereas the light in the sample arm is backscattered by the sample of interest. The returning light from both arms recombines at the coupler and generates an interference pattern recorded by the detector. The sample beam has to be moved across the sample to record an A scan at each point, which can be combined to generate an OCT image or a B scan. For a given wavelength, the axial resolution is based on the bandwidth, whereas the lateral resolution is limited by the diffraction caused by the pupil and the minimum spot size of the focused probing beam. [1].

28.1.2 OCT Systems (Table 28.1)

The early time-domain (TD)-OCT technology is based on scanning reference delay. This setup is limited by the time constraints and mechanical inertia imposed by the moving reference mirror, limiting the number of A scans to a few thousand per second. Most systems in clinical use now are Fourier-domain (FD)-OCT [Fig. 28.1]. The key difference between the two is that the FD-OCT uses a static reference mirror, which facilitates higher data acquisition speeds. By performing an inverse Fourier transform, the acquired wavenumber-dependent data is transformed into axial scan information. FD-OCT imaging includes spectral-domain OCT (SD-OCT) and swept-source OCT (SS-OCT). [1].

28.1.2.1 SD-OCT

Spectrometer-based FD-OCT uses a diffraction grating element to spatially separate the different wavelength contributions into a line image recorded by a high-speed charge-coupled device (CCD) line camera. A Fourier transform is

N. K. Sahoo
Kode Venkatadri Chowdary Campus, LV Prasad Eye Institute, Vijayawada, India

P. R. Chandrasekaran · G. Cheung (✉)
Singapore National Eye Centre, Singapore Eye Research Institute, Singapore, Singapore
e-mail: Gemmy.cheung.c.m@singhealth.com.sg

N. Jacob
Anant Bajaj Retina Institute, Kode Venkatadri Chowdary Campus, L V Prasad Eye Institute, Vijayawada, India

T. Das, P. Satgunam (eds.), *Ophthalmic Diagnostics*, https://doi.org/10.1007/978-981-97-0138-4_28

Table 28.1 Comparison of various OCT systems

Features	TD-OCT Movable reference mirror	SD-OCT Fixed reference mirror Spectrometer	SS-OCT Tunable laser light source
Wavelength	810 nm	840 nm	1052 nm
A scan/s	512 scans/s	50,000 scans/s	100,000 scans/s
Axial resolution	10 μm	8 μm	6 μm
Lateral resolution	20 μm	20 μm	20 μm
Artifacts	More	Less	Less
Length of line scan	6 mm	Up to 9 mm	Up to 12 mm
Range of imaging	Vitreoretinal interface to retinal pigment epithelium	Posterior cortical vitreous to sclera using enhanced depth imaging mode	Posterior cortical vitreous to sclera

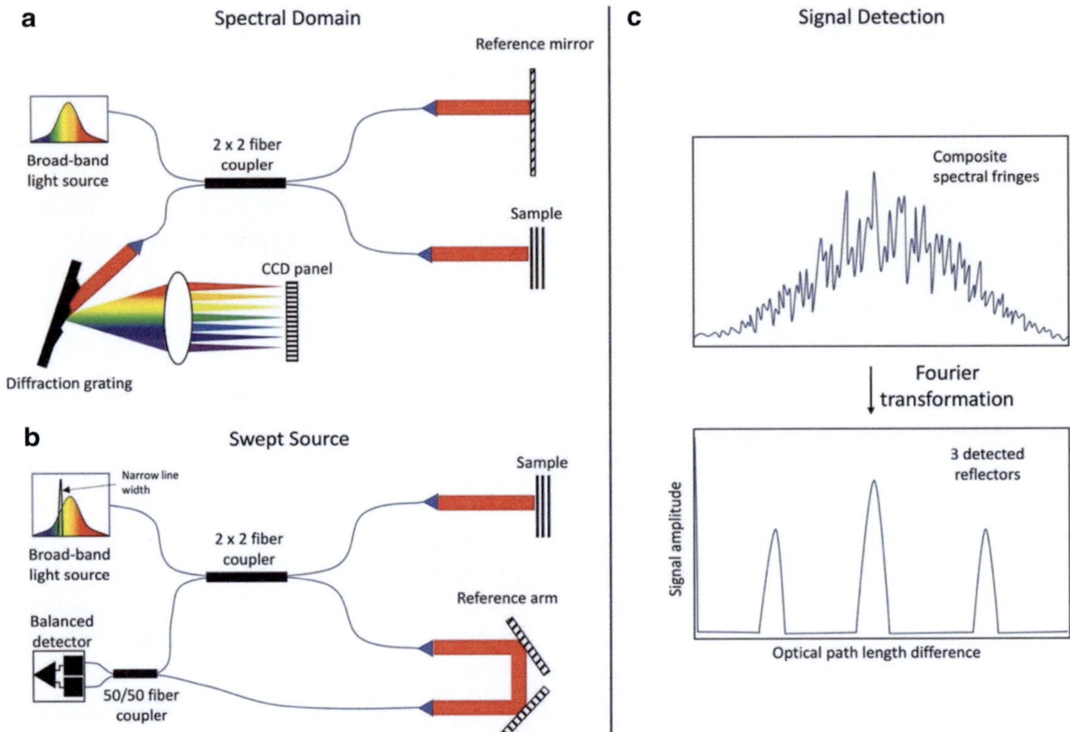

Fig. 28.1 Fourier-domain optical coherence tomography (OCT). (**a**) Schematic diagram of a spectral-domain OCT. It uses a spectrometer for the detection of interference signals. (**b**) Schematic diagram of a swept-source OCT. It uses a rapid wavelength-swept light source and balanced detection to detect interference signals. (**c**) Example of signal detection for the three partial reflectors. Fourier transformation results in the production of three images corresponding to the reflectors. [*CCD charge-coupled device*]

performed on the spectrally resolved interference pattern detected by the camera array to obtain the A scan [1, 2].

28.1.2.2 SS-OCT

The broadband light source is replaced by a tunable laser rapidly sweeping a narrow line width over a broad range of wavelengths [1, 2]. In contrast to SD-OCT, SS-OCT uses a high-speed complementary metal oxide semiconductor (CMOS) camera and two parallel photodetectors. A long imaging range of nearly 7.5 mm allows a better view of the vitreoretinal interface and the choroid in a single frame [1, 2].

28.1.3 Scanning Protocols and Quantitative Measures: (Tables 28.2 and 28.3)

Various pre-set acquisition protocols are available on most commercial OCT instruments. These differ in the area covered, the distance between adjacent scans, the number of scans averaged at each location, and the orientation of scans. Understanding these will ensure that the most appropriate protocol is used for the pathology being evaluated. Most commercial instruments also provide the user with basic software which supports retinal layer segmentation and quantitative assessments such as retinal thickness. Since the boundaries used for quantification differ between instruments, quantitative values such as central retinal thickness must be converted before comparing the instruments. As scan speed increases, dense volume scans can be acquired, which can, in turn, be used to generate en face images. In enhanced depth imaging (EDI)-mode, the instrument is purposefully displaced to image the deeper layers. Since the

Table 28.2 OCT scanning protocols and measurements

1. *Macular cube scan*	
A macular cube scan or a three-dimensional (3D) scan consists of a number of horizontal line scans composed of a 6 mm x 6 mm, 7 mm x 7 mm square grid, or a 12 mm x 9 mm rectangular grid. It generates a 3D view of the image, which can be subject to complex analysis	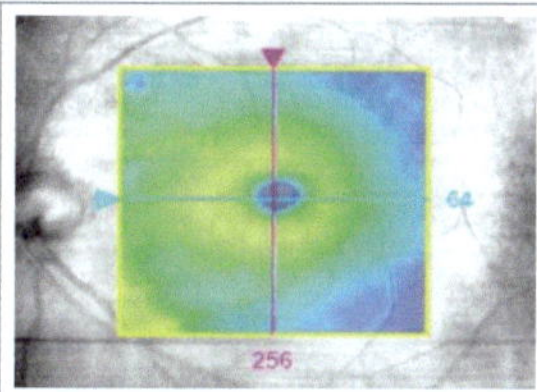
2. *Radial scan*	
The radial scan consists of 6–12 line scans arranged at equal angles with a common axis. By coinciding with the common axis with the fovea, the relationship of the lesion with the fovea can be ascertained	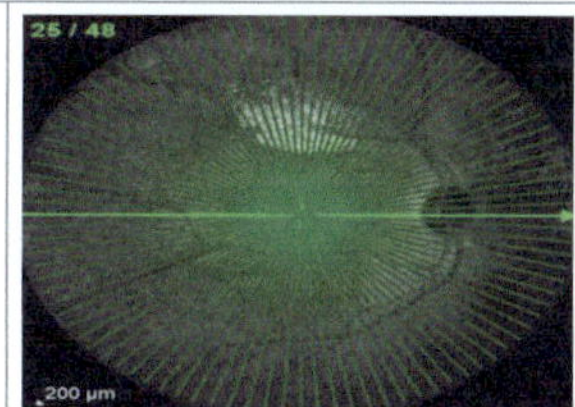
3. *Raster scan*	
A raster scan consists of a series of parallel line scans that can be oriented at any angle and has a high resolution. The length, angle, and spacing between the lines can be adjusted to acquire the best view of the area of interest	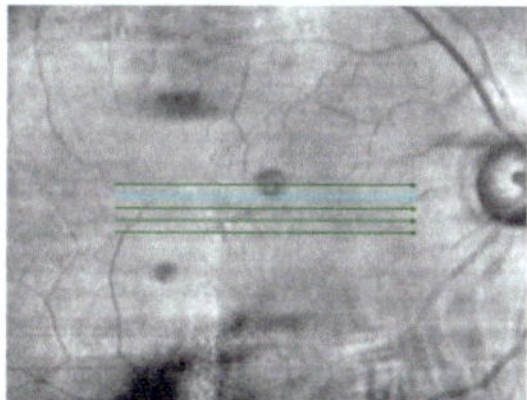
Center point	The intersection of the six radial scans of the fast macular thickness protocol of the OCT
Central subfield	Circular area of diameter 1 mm centered around the center point. A total of 128 thickness measurements are made in this circular area in the fast macula protocol
Center point thickness	The average thickness values for the six radial scans at their point of intersection
Central subfield mean thickness	The mean value of the 128 thickness values obtained in the central subfield
Retinal thickness	Value in µm of the distance between the OCT layers assumed to be the RPE and the internal limiting membrane
Subfoveal choroidal thickness	Value in µm of the distance from the outer edge of the hyperreflective line corresponding to the retinal pigment epithelium to the inner surface of the sclera

Table 28.3 Commercially available wide-field OCT machines

NIDEK Mirante (NIDEK Co. Ltd., Gamagori, Japan)	SLO/HD-OCT	160° FOV
Heidelberg Spectralis OCT (Heidelberg Engineering, Heidelberg, Germany)	Confocal SLO/SD-OCT Combination with ocular Staurenghi 230 SLO retina lens	55° FOV 150° FOV
Optos Silverstone (Optos PLC, Dunfermline, UK)	cSLO/SS-OCT	200° FOV
Optos Monaco (Optos PLC, Dunfermline, UK)	cSLO/SD-OCT	200° FOV

FOV field of vision, *HD* high definition, *OCT* optical coherence tomography, *SLO* scanning laser ophthalmoscope, *cSLO* confocal scanning laser ophthalmoscope

deeper portions of the choroid are now closer to the zero-delay line, there is enhanced imaging of these structures.

28.1.4 OCT Artifacts

Some common artifacts include misidentification of the inner and outer retinal layers, and issues with mirrors, being out-of-register, degraded images, cut edges, off-center images, and motion and blink artifacts [3].

28.1.5 Principles of OCTA

Optical coherence tomography angiography (OCTA) is a noninvasive imaging modality that evaluates the retinal and choroidal vasculature. The OCTA images are generated using an OCT-based system. Flow signals from the OCTA arise from detecting changes in the reflectivity of light when the same location is scanned over time, which is attributed to the movement of red blood cells. A threshold masking strategy can be used to block OCTA signals from tissues below a threshold OCT signal. If the threshold level is too low, areas of low signal strength without true blood flow, like the sclera and vitreous, can be incorrectly displayed as having flow. Conversely, if the threshold level is too high, areas of low flow will be incorrectly displayed as having no flow. While manufacturers set threshold values, it is good practice to analyze OCTA data in conjunction with structural OCT to confirm the validity of the OCTA signal [4].

Table 28.4 Commercially available OCTA machines

Manufacturer	Device name	OCT modality	Algorithm
Carl-Zeiss Meditech	Cirrus HD-OCT Angioplex PLEX elite 9000	Spectral-domain Swept-source	OMAG OMAG
Topcon	DRI OCT triton	Swept-source	OCTARA
Optovue	RTVue XR Avanti Angiovue	Spectral-domain	SSADA
Heidelberg Engineering	Spectralis OCT angiography	Spectral-domain	FSADA
Canon	OCT-HS 100	Spectral-domain	Modified FSADA
Nidek	RS-3000 advance Angioscan	Spectral-domain	CODAA
OPTOPOL	REVO NX OCTA	Spectral-domain	SOA

CODAA complex optical coherence tomography difference analysis angiography, *SADA* full-spectrum amplitude-decorrelation angiography, *OCTARA* optical coherence tomography angiography ratio analysis, *OMAG* optical microangiography, *SOA* spectral domain optical coherence tomography angiography, *SSADA* split-spectrum amplitude-decorrelation angiography

28.1.5.1 OCTA Algorithms (Table 28.4)

Several strategies have been developed to analyze information related to both phase and intensity of the reflected light. Most commercially available instruments utilize complex signal-based algorithms based on both phase and intensity. These include optical microangiography (OMAG), split-spectrum amplitude-decorrelation angiography (SSADA),

OCTA ratio analysis (OCTARA), and probabilistic algorithms [4].

28.1.5.2 Scanning Protocols and Quantitative Measures: (Tables 28.5 and 28.6)

Similar to OCT, commercial OCTA instruments generally come with pre-set acquisition algorithms according to scan area, for example, 3 × 3 mm, 6 × 6 mm, 9 × 9 mm, and 12 × 12 mm. It is also possible to produce montage images by stitching together images to provide a wider field of view. In addition, pre-set segmentation strategies are also commonly available, with most instruments being able to generate the superficial and deep retinal plexus. There are some variations in the pre-set segmentations for the outer retina (e.g., the outer retina and choriocapillaris (ORCC) slab, the outer retina slab). It is also important to understand that differences in the boundaries exist between instruments, even for the same slab. Several quantitative measures of the presence and absence of flow (non-perfusion) can be derived from OCTA. Metrics describing the presence of flow include vessel density, perfusion density, and vessel length density. Various metrics have been used to describe the properties of the foveal avascular zone (FAZ), including FAZ area, circularity and acircularity index, and axis ratio [5].

28.1.5.3 OCTA Artifacts

Accurate interpretation of OCTA requires a good understanding of potential artifacts, including those arising from motion, blink, projection, seg-

Table 28.5 Common terminology used in OCTA

Field of view	3 × 3 mm, 6 × 6 mm, 8 × 8 mm, 9 × 9 mm, 12 × 12 mm, 15 × 9 mm The sampling density may or may not change for different fields of view, depending on the machine
Montage	Enables fields of view of up to 100° by stitching together smaller fields of view without sacrificing image resolution
Vitreous slab	Above the ILM; normally avascular
Superficial retinal plexus	Superficial portion of the inner retina; ILM to the outer border of IPL
Deep retinal plexus	Deep portion of the inner retina; outer border of IPL to the outer border of OPL
Inner retina	Combination of superficial and deep retinal plexus
Outer retina	Outer border of OPL to RPE; normally avascular
Choriocapillaris	Bruch's membrane to 10–20 μm below
Deeper choroid	Larger choroidal vessels, >20 μm below the Bruch's membrane
Choroid	Combination of the choriocapillaris and deeper choroid

ILM internal limiting membrane, *IPL* inner plexiform layer, *OPL* outer plexiform layer, *RPE* retinal pigment epithelium

Table 28.6 OCTA measurements

Foveal avascular zone	The central area of the macula devoid of retinal capillaries
Acircularity index	Ratio of the perimeter of the FAZ to the perimeter of a circle with an equal area. Irregular FAZ perimeters have a higher acircularity index
Circularity index	Ratio of the area of FAZ to the area of a circle with an equal perimeter. Irregular FAZ is associated with a decreased circularity index
Axis ratio	Ratio between an ellipse's major and minor axes fits with second-order moments. An elongated FAZ has a greater axis ratio
Vessel density	The proportion of blood vessel area over the total measured area based on the binarized image for indicating the perfusion of the retinal microvasculature
Vessel length density/ skeleton density	Modification of VD which quantifies the vessel density by performing an additional skeletonizing process which reduces the width of each blood vessel to 1 pixel, regardless of the vessel diameter
Vessel diameter index	Measure of the vessel caliber. Calculated by dividing the area occupied by blood vessels in the binarized image by the length of blood vessels in the skeletonized image
Fractal dimension	Measures the complexity of a vasculature branching pattern
Vessel tortuosity	Compares the length of a vessel's flow path to a straight line between its path's starting and ending points

FAZ foveal avascular zone, *VD* vessel density

mentation, and shadow. Furthermore, the accuracy of quantitative measures such as vessel density may be affected by vessel doubling, media opacity, and stretch [4].

28.2 Applications of OCT and OCTA in Retinal Conditions

28.2.1 Diabetic Retinopathy

28.2.1.1 Non-proliferative Diabetic Retinopathy (NPDR)

Common features in DR include microaneurysms (MA), dot and blot hemorrhages, cotton wool spots (CWS), and hard exudates (HE); MAs typically appear as small, medium to high echoes with minimal back-shadowing in the INL (inner nuclear layer) and NFL (nerve fiber layer). On en face OCTA, they appear as focally dilated saccular and fusiform capillaries and may arise from different layers of the choroidal plexus. Retinal hemorrhages appear as areas of hyperreflectivity within the retina. Sub-hyaloid hemorrhage is seen as a highly reflective lesion above the ILM (internal limiting membrane), causing the shadowing of the underlying retinal layers. HEs are hyperreflective spots, larger than 30 μm, seen in the outer retinal layers, most commonly the OPL (outer plexiform layer), with associated back-shadowing and a reflectivity similar to the RPE–BM (retinal pigment epithelium–Bruch's membrane) complex. Cotton wool spots appear as hyperreflective, nodular, or elongated lesions in the NFL, which may also involve the GCL (ganglion cell layer), with associated back-shadowing [6]. OCTA may detect areas of non-perfusion within the retina. Quantitative measures may demonstrate a reduction in vessel density or perfusion density in eyes with NPDR compared to eyes without DR.

28.2.1.2 Proliferative Diabetic Retinopathy (PDR)

Extensive areas of non-perfusion can often be seen on OCTA [Fig. 28.2]. On OCT, NVD (new vessels on disc) is seen as hyperreflective tissue on the disc (attached posterior hyaloid) or protruding from the disc into the vitreous (detached posterior hyaloid). The NVE (new vessels elsewhere) are seen as homogenous hyperreflective loops breaching the ILM and breaching the vitreous with posterior retinal shadowing [7]. On OCTA, the flow signal can be detected by segmenting above the disc or peripapillary retinal surface (NVD) and above the ILM (NVE) [7]. Accurate segmentation is critical because this helps to differentiate it from intraretinal microvascular abnormalities (IRMA), which do not show flow signals above the vitreoretinal interface slab. Exuberant vascular proliferation (EVP) is seen as the proliferation of irregular, fine, small-caliber vessels at the margin of new vessels, which is a sign of more active disease.

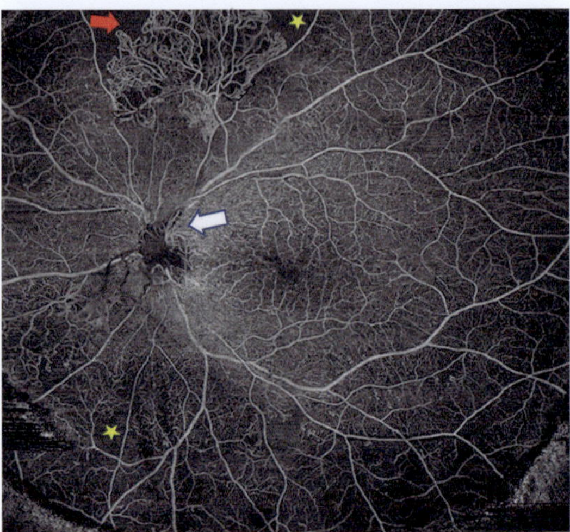

Fig. 28.2 Wide-field OCTA of a patient with proliferative diabetic retinopathy showing neovascularization of the disc (white arrow), neovascularization elsewhere (red arrow), and extensive areas of capillary non-perfusion areas (*yellow stars*)

28.2.1.3 Diabetic Maculopathy and Diabetic Macular Edema

Diabetic macular edema (DME) is the accumulation of excess fluid in the extracellular space within the retina in the macular area and the subretinal space [Fig. 28.3]. With OCT, DME can be assessed quantitatively, and the location with regard to the center of the fovea can be defined more precisely. The International Council of

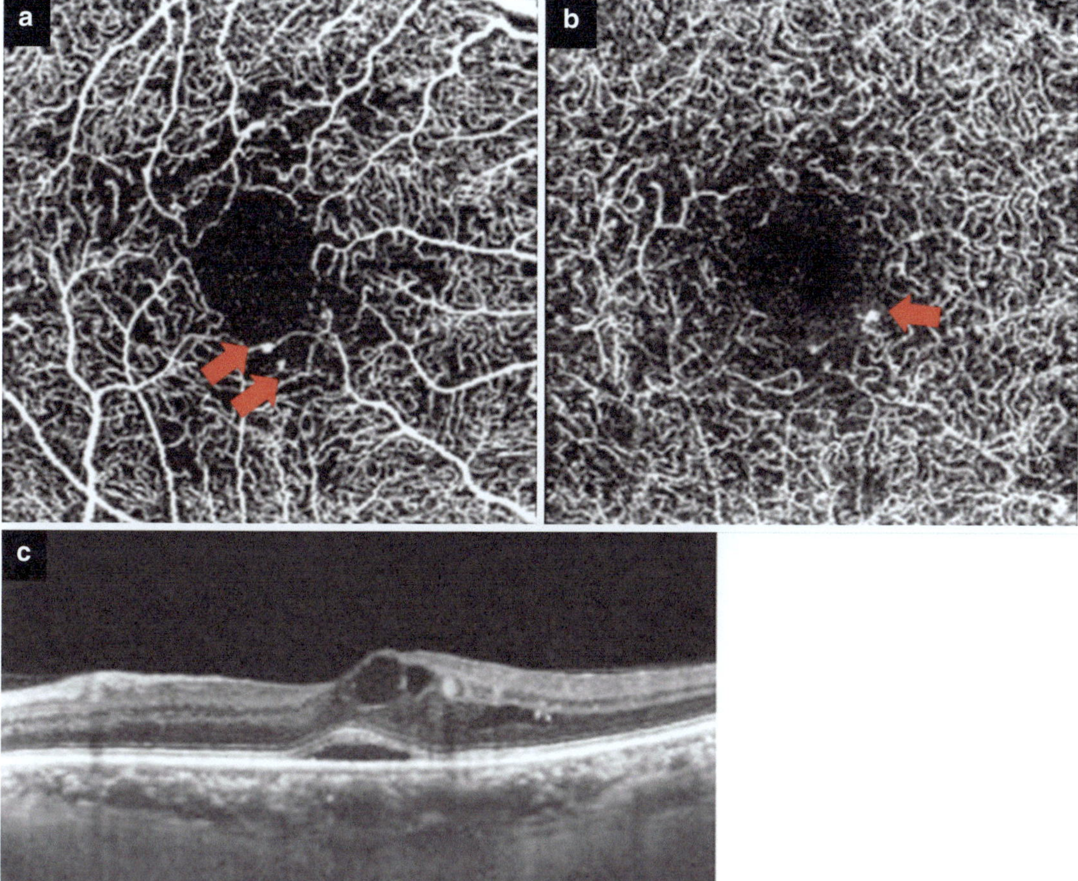

Fig. 28.3 OCTA of an irregular foveal avascular zone and reduced vessel density in the superficial plexus (**a**) and the deep plexus (**b**). Microaneurysms (red arrows) can be seen. (**c**) OCT shows intraretinal cysts and subretinal fluid in an eye with diabetic macular edema

Ophthalmology has classified DME into non-center-involved DME, when the retinal thickening in the macula does not involve the central subfield zone (1 mm in diameter), and center-involved DME, when the retinal thickening in the macula involves the central subfield zone. Most clinical trials for DME have used a quantitative threshold for central retinal thickness (CRT) or central subfield thickness (CSFT) with Protocol I and Protocol T studies, including eyes where the CSFT is above 320 μm. In addition, various morphological forms of DME (e.g., cystoid, serous) have been reported, but there is a lack of standardization for their definition. Identifying vitreomacular interface abnormalities in eyes with DME may impact the management options.

In addition to macular edema, OCT is also useful for assessing the integrity of the retinal layers. Disorganization of retinal inner layers (DRIL) may be seen in some eyes of diabetic patients and has been associated with ischemia. On OCT, DRIL is defined as the inability to distinguish between the GCL-IPL complex, INL, and OPL. DRIL is assessed on OCT B scans by looking at the central 1 mm retinal zone. Disorganization of more than 50% or > 500 μm of this area is considered significant and is associated with a worse visual prognosis. The integrity of the ELM and EZ is regarded as a good prognostic indicator in eyes with DME; however, their assessment might be difficult [8].

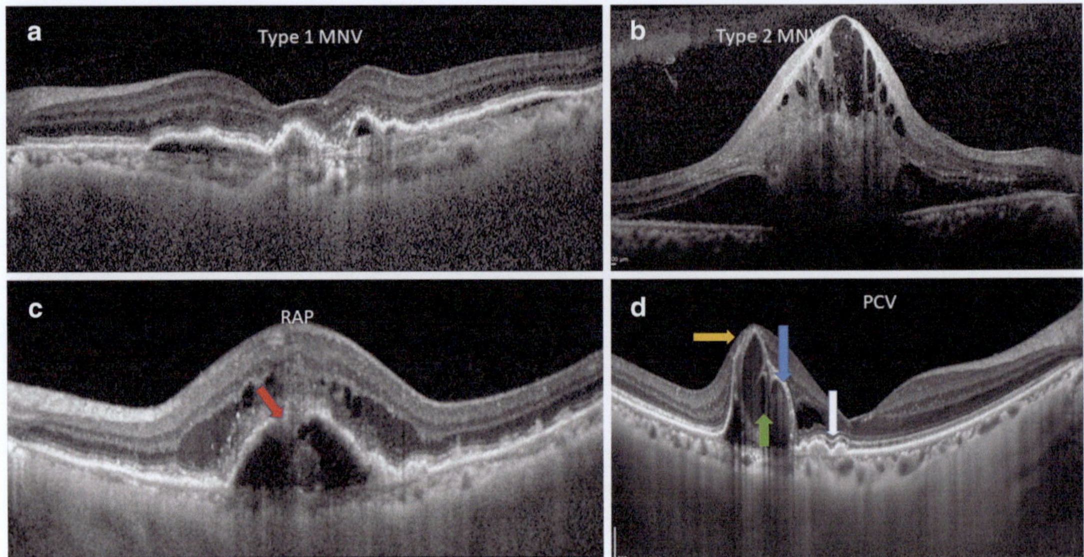

Fig. 28.4 (**a**) Horizontal OCT scan of a patient with Type 1 (occult) MNV showing a double layer sign, PED, and intact RPE. (**b**) Horizontal OCT scan of a patient with Type 2 (classic) MNV showing hyperreflective material above the RPE with subretinal fluid and intraretinal fluid. (**c**) Horizontal OCT scan of a patient with Type 3 (RAP) MNV showing PED with intraretinal anastomosis (red arrow) and intraretinal fluid. (**d**) Horizontal OCT scan of a patient with PCV showing tall-peaked PED (yellow arrow), notched PED (blue arrow), sub-RPE ring (green arrow), and a double layer sign (white arrow)

On OCTA, it has been shown that vessel density and perfusion density are lower in eyes with DME. Also, there is an increase in FAZ area and acircularity index and a decrease in circularity index in eyes with DME. The fractal dimension is also lower in eyes with DME [9].

28.2.2 Age-Related Macular Degeneration (AMD)

28.2.2.1 Early and Intermediate AMD

Drusen are hallmarks of AMD and can be observed with clinical examination. However, the depth of these extracellular deposits can be more precisely assessed using OCT. In cross-sectional OCT, soft drusen appear as reflecting basal-laminar deposits between the RPE and BM; the reticular pseudodrusen appear as subretinal drusenoid deposits (SDD) above the RPE. SDD may be associated with extensive disruption of the ellipsoid zone [10]. Confluent drusen may coalesce and form drusenoid PED, which has a smooth contour because of the detachment of the hyperreflective RPE with homogenous moderate to high reflectivity content. Pigment clumping on top of the PED can be seen as hyperreflective foci.

28.2.2.2 Neovascular AMD

OCT and OCTA can detect the presence of new vessels and determine the subtype based on its relationship to the RPE (Fig. 28.4). Type 1 macular neovascularization (MNV) typically appears as a detachment of the RPE from the underlying BM, and the sub-RPE space shows heterogeneous reflectivity. Type 2 MNVs above the RPE typically appear as subretinal hyperreflective material [11]. Type 3 MNV appears as a hyperreflective lesion between the sub-RPE compartment and the neurosensory retina [12]. Type 3 MNV can be further classified into three stages. Stage 1 is the stage of intraretinal neovascularization (IRN), wherein capillaries originate from

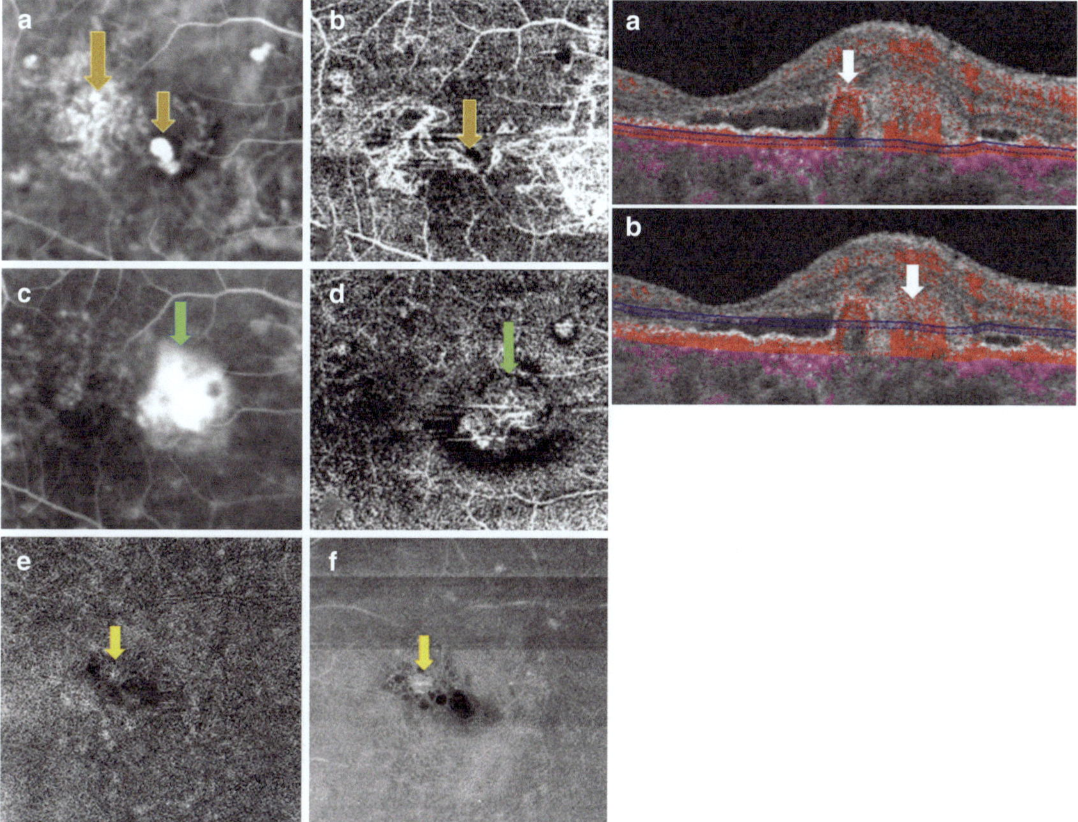

Fig. 28.5 Left Panel. (**a**) ICGA of a patient with PCV showing polyp with branching vascular network (yellow arrows) corresponding to the thumb-shaped PED on horizontal OCT in Fig. Right panel **a** (**b**) OCTA of the same patient through the thumb-shaped PED (white arrow in Fig. Right panel **a**) showing flow within the polyp along with branching vascular network (yellow arrow). (**c**) ICGA of the same patient showing a plaque suggestive of classic MNV (green arrow) corresponding to the area of subretinal hyperreflective material on horizontal OCT in Fig. Right panel **b** (**d**) OCTA of the same patient through the subretinal hyperreflective material (white arrow in Fig. Right panel **b**) showing a corresponding large network (green arrow). (**e**) OCTA of a patient with RAP lesion in the deep retinal plexus (yellow arrow). (**f**) En face image of the same patient with RAP showing patchy vessel atrophy (yellow arrow)

the deep retinal capillary plexus; stage 2 is the stage of subretinal neovascularization where the IRN extends into the subretinal space, and stage 3 is the stage of choroidal neovascularization. Finally, PCV (polypoidal choroidal vasculopathy) is considered a variant of type 1 MNV. The branching neovascular network (BVN) has a similar OCT appearance as a type 1 MNV, while the polypoidal lesion(s) are associated with the appearance of a sharp-peaked PED with a hyporeflective sub-RPE ring. Based on the APOIS (Asia Pacific Ocular Imaging Society) workgroup recommendations, the combination of sub-RPE ring-like lesion, en face OCT complex RPE elevation, and sharp-peaked PED can differentiate PCV from typical neovascular AMD with high sensitivity and specificity. OCTA can detect flow signals within the MNV. By carefully selecting the segmentation in relation to the RPE in cross-sectional scans, OCTA can complement OCT in determining the subtype of MNV (Fig. 28.5). The en face OCTA provides further information related to the size and morphology of the MNV. In PCV, however, reports have found variable flow signals within the polypoidal lesions; these have been attributed to turbulent or slow flow.

The level of activity from the MNV can be assessed with OCT based on intraretinal fluid, subretinal fluid (SRF), and subretinal hyperreflective material. The presence of SRF and IRF (intraretinal fluid) on OCT have been widely used as markers of disease activity for guiding retreatment decisions. Sub-RPE fluid or PED (pigment epithelial detachment) has been considered a less important marker for disease activity, except in PCV. On the other hand, OCTA features have not been consistently incorporated into retreatment assessment. This is due to limitations of repeatability and lack of quantitative comparison. While a progression to a more mature branching pattern within the vascular network has been described, a lack of objective, quantifiable parameters has limited the current application of OCTA in retreatment decisions [13].

28.2.2.3 Geographic Atrophy

Geographic atrophy (GA) appears as a well-defined circular or oval area of depigmentation due to thinning of the outer retina and RPE. The Classification of Atrophy Meeting (CAM) group proposed a classification system of atrophy based on SD-OCT and complimented by CFP (color fundus photo), FAF (fundus autofluorescence), and NIR (near infra-red). Based on CAM classification, GA can be diagnosed in the presence of cRORA (complete RPE and outer retinal atrophy) that is defined by a zone of RPE loss or RPE attenuation of at least 250 μm, a region of choroidal hyper-transmission of at least 250 μm in diameter and loss of the interdigitation zone, ellipsoid zone (EZ), or the external limiting membrane and the absence of scrolled RPE or signs of RPE tear [14]. Alterations in the choriocapillaris have been documented with OCTA in eyes with GA. In addition, OCT can detect EZ disruption, which apparently precedes the development of RPE atrophy. The prediction of individual conversion of early AMD to CNV or GA using Artificial Intelligence (AI) with automated analysis of imaging biomarkers showed that the critical features of conversion to GA were outer retinal thinning with an associated decreased outer nuclear layer thickness and the presence of hyperreflective foci in the outer nuclear layer [15].

28.2.2.4 The Choroid in AMD

EDI-OCT and SS-OCT can penetrate the choroid better than the conventional spectral-domain-OCT, allowing the evaluation of changes in choroidal thickness in AMD. The subfoveal choroidal thickness correlates with the drusen and MNV subtypes. Eyes with thicker choroids tend to develop pachydrusen and PCV; those with thinner choroids tend to develop SDD and type 3 MNV [16]. Besides evaluating subfoveal choroidal thickness, en face OCT and OCTA allow the evaluation of choroidal vasculature noninvasively. These have led to the description of pachyvessels, inter-vortex anastomosis, and unbalanced vortex drainage in eyes with MNV and choroidal congestion. Together with the finding of choriocapillaris flow impairment, the pachychoroid theory has been proposed as a novel mechanism resulting in MNV.

28.3 Retinal Vascular Diseases

28.3.1 Retinal Arteriolar Occlusion or Ischemia

During the acute phase of retinal artery occlusion, there is increased thickness and reflectivity of the inner retinal layers with back-shadowing on OCT. The area of swelling is well-demarcated, which shows the area supplied by the occluded artery. Macular edema, outer retinal layer thickening, and SRF may also be seen. ILM detachment has been recently described as a feature of total retinal artery occlusion and severe retinal ischemia [Fig. 28.6]. In the chronic phase, thinning of the inner and outer retinal layers with loss of stratification of the retinal layers in the area of previous hyperreflectivity can be noted. On OCTA, vessel density is reduced in the SCP and DCP [17].

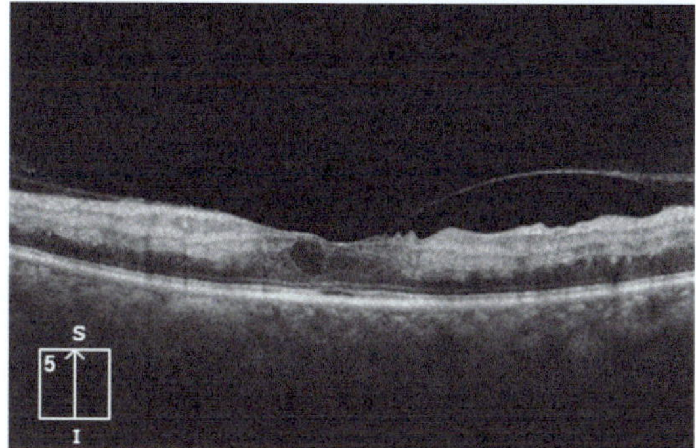

Fig. 28.6 OCT scan of a case of acute central retinal artery occlusion showing the increased retinal thickness and reflectivity of the inner retinal layers with back-shadowing. There is also the presence of cystoid spaces in the inner retina and internal limiting membrane detachment

28.3.2 Retinal Vein Occlusion

In retinal vein occlusion (RVO), OCT is useful in evaluating macular edema, SRF, hemorrhages, and exudates. Macular edema is usually seen as a combination of cystoid edema, sponge-like retinal thickening, and serous retinal detachment [18]. DRIL and disruption of ELM and EZ are associated with a worse visual prognosis. The presence of a prominent middle limiting membrane, a hyperreflective line located in the outer plexiform layer, is a marker of acute ischemia and is also associated with poor visual outcomes [Fig. 28.7].

OCTA can evaluate the presence of a non-perfusion area (NPA) [Fig. 28.8]. The relative degree of NPA between the DCP (deep choroidal plexus) and SCP (superficial choroidal plexus) has been suggested to have prognostic implications. Ischemia affecting both the SCP

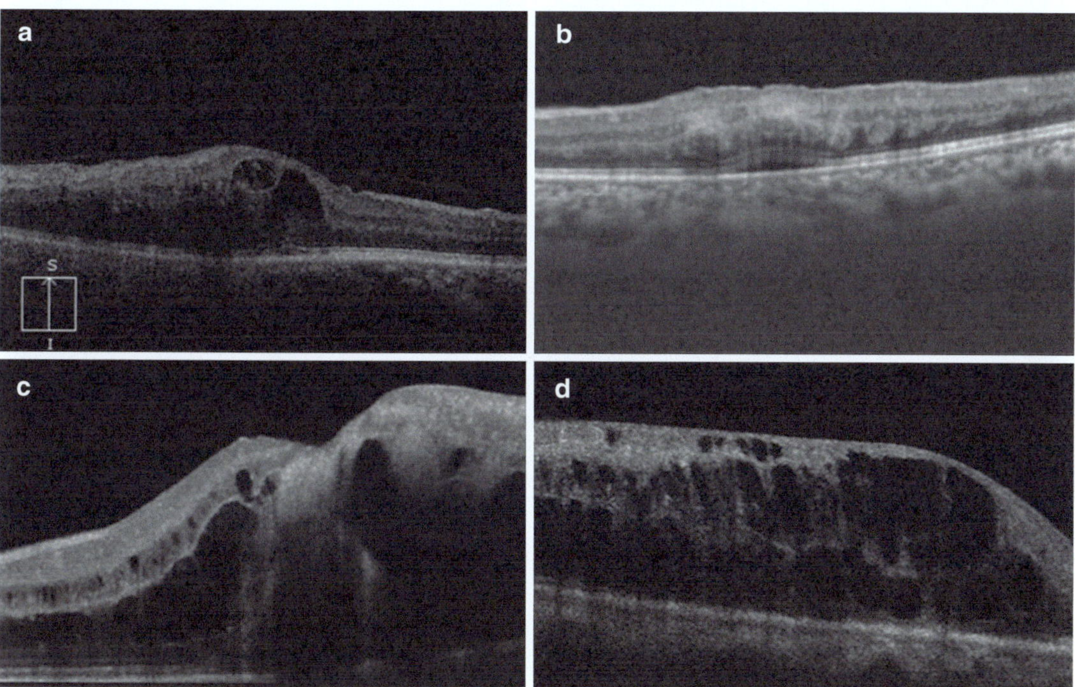

Fig. 28.7 (**a**) Vertical OCT of a case of inferotemporal branch retinal vein occlusion showing increased retinal thickness and cystoid macular edema. (**b**) Prominent middle limiting membrane. (**c**) Disorganization of retinal inner layers. (**d**) Ganglion layer cysts

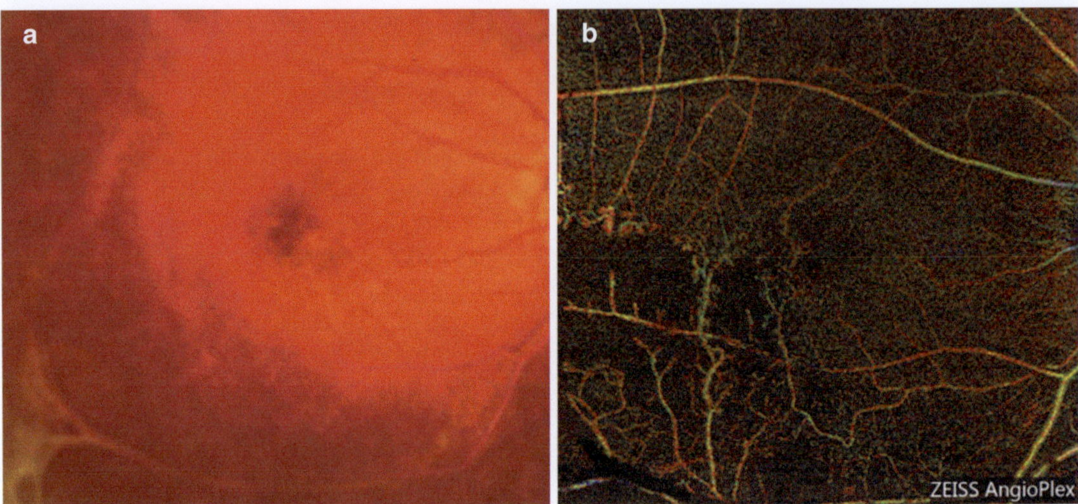

Fig. 28.8 (**a**) Color fundus photo of en face OCTA. (**b**) Image of an eye with inferotemporal retinal vein occlusion. Retinal non-perfusion and disrupted FAZ can be seen on OCTA

and DCP is associated with the development of atrophy. In contrast, eyes with a larger NPA seen in the DCP than SCP may experience recurrent edema due to impaired outflow of fluid through the DCP. The FAZ and acircularity index can also increase in the SCP and DCP. Other features the OCTA can detect are capillary telangiectasias, collateral vessels, microaneurysms, and retinal new vessels [18].

28.3.3 Macular Telangiectasia Type 2 (Mac Tel Type 2)

Mac Tel type 2 is a slowly progressive disease of the macula, primarily involving the Muller cells. In advanced cases, it may be complicated by subretinal neovascularization. The earliest sign of this condition seen on OCT is the temporal widening of the fovea due to thinning of the temporal juxta foveal retina. The hyperreflective middle retinal layer is another early OCT feature, seen as increased reflectivity and thickness between the inner and outer plexiform layers. Other features seen in the nonproliferative stage of the disease include hyporeflective inner and outer retinal cavities, the ILM drape sign, and outward bending of the inner retinal layers. The pigment appears as hyperreflective foci with back-shadowing [Fig. 28.9]. Development of neovascularization may lead to subretinal or intraretinal fluid [19]. Epiretinal neovascularization is a recently described feature which shows communication with the intraretinal abnormal vascular plexus.

Features seen on OCTA include dilated bulbs of perifoveal vessels, dilation of perifoveal vessels, rarefaction and increased intervascular spaces, vessels distorting FAZ, bunching of vessels, and vascular network in the outer retina [Fig. 28.9]. Right-angled veins can be seen associated with pigment plaques.

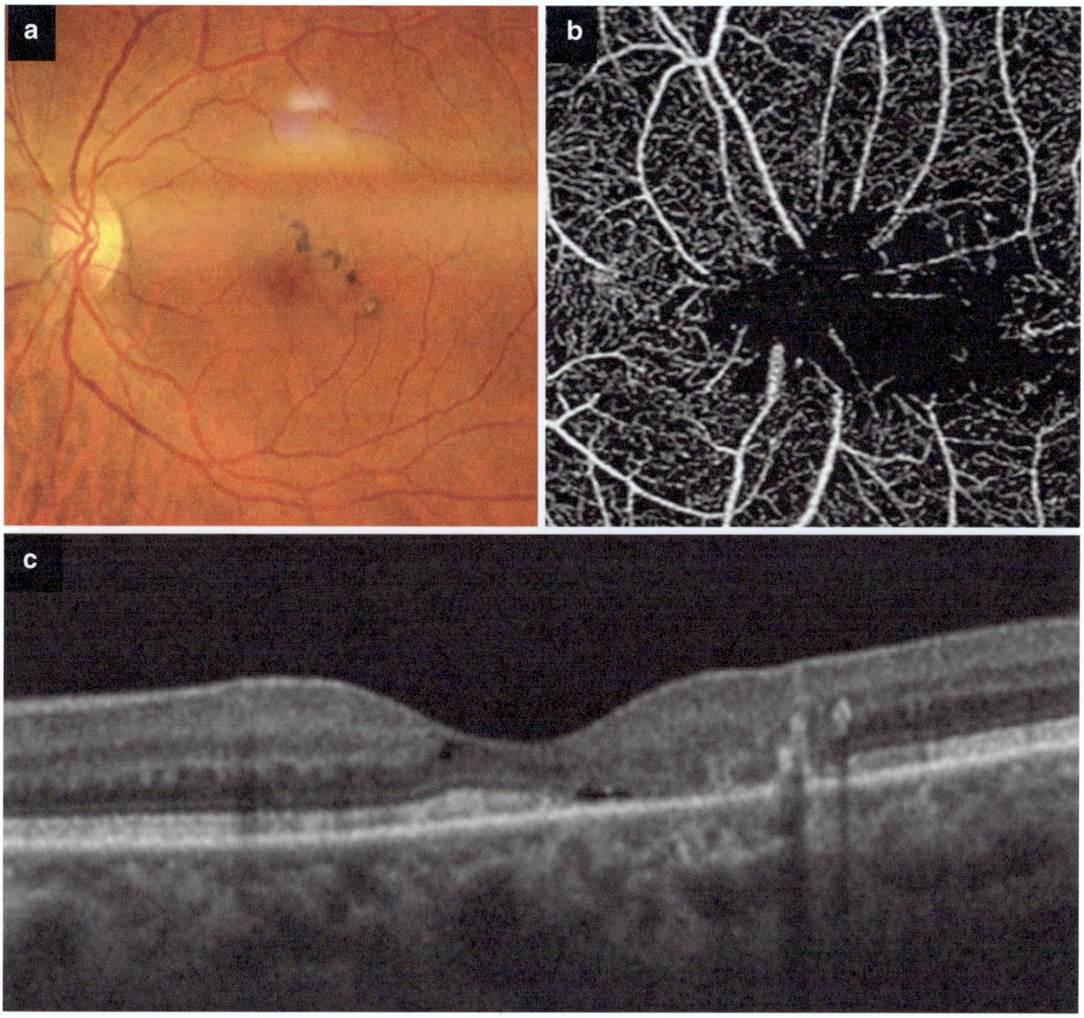

Fig. 28.9 (**a**) Color fundus photograph of the left eye of a patient with Mac Tel type-2. Pigment clumps can be seen temporal to the fovea. (**b**) OCTA showing blunted perifoveal vessels. (**c**) OCT shows a widening of the temporal fovea, hyporeflective space beneath the ILM at the fovea, outward bending of the inner retinal layers, and hyperreflective pigments clumps with back-shadowing

28.4 Vitreomacular Interface Disorders

Vitreomacular interface disorders may cause visual disturbance or loss. OCT is essential in assessing vitreomacular interface disorders and planning surgery. Vitreomacular adhesion (VMA) is defined as a partially detached vitreous in the perifoveal area without retinal abnormalities. There is an elevation of the cortical vitreous above the retinal surface with an area of attachment within the 3 mm radius of the fovea. They can be sub-classified by the size of the adhesion into focal (≤1500 μm) and broad (>1500 μm). Vitreomacular traction (VMT) is present when the attached posterior hyaloid is associated with retinal distortion [Fig. 28.10b] [20]. Visual symptoms may result from further complications such as macular hole formation.

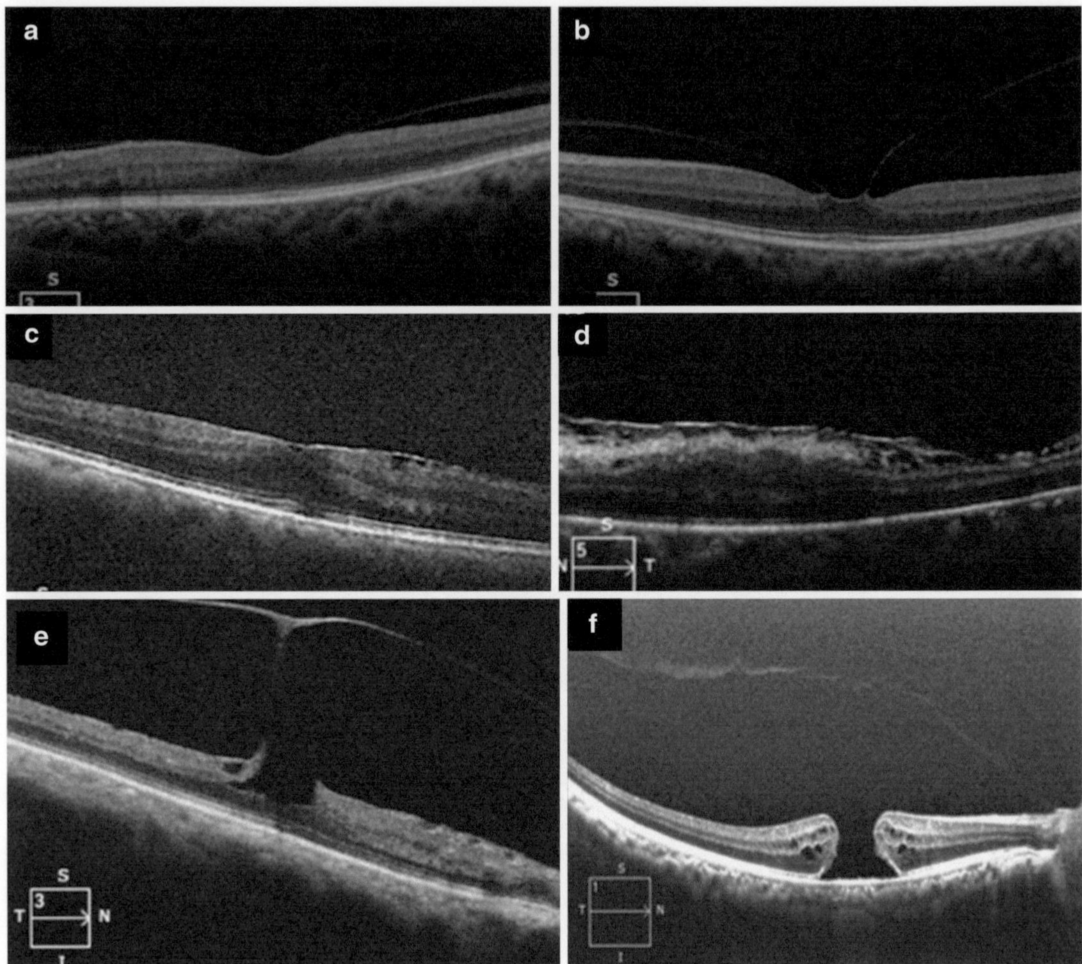

Fig. 28.10 OCT illustrating pathologies related to the vitreoretinal interface. (**a**) Horizontal OCT of vitreomacular adhesion and (**b**) vitreomacular traction. (**c**) A horizontal OCT scan shows a thin hyperreflective membrane suggestive of ERM distorting the normal foveal depression. The outer nuclear layer appears stretched. All retinal layers can be delineated. (**d**) A horizontal OCT shows ERM causing alteration of the normal foveal architecture and ectopic inner foveal layers. Also, the retinal layers cannot be delineated. (**e**) A horizontal OCT scan of a lamellar macular hole shows an irregular foveal contour with loss of foveal tissue. Schitic cavities between the outer nuclear and outer plexiform layers and the inner retinal layers can be seen. The photoreceptor layer appears intact. (**f**) Horizontal OCT shows partial posterior vitreous detachment, with the vitreous cortex still attached to the optic disc margins. A full-thickness defect can be seen in the neurosensory retina with cystic spaces in the outer and inner nuclear layers

28.4.1 Epiretinal Membrane

On OCT, the epiretinal membrane (ERM) is seen as a discrete, irregular, hyperreflective line above the inner retinal surface, usually associated with wrinkling of the retina and hyporeflective spaces between the ERM and ILM. It can be classified into [21] stage 1, where the ERM causes negligible anatomic disruption; stage 2, where the ERM causes stretching of ONL, but all layers can be identified; stage 3, where the ERM is associated with an ectopic inner foveal layer (EIFL), and stage 4 ERM when there is significant retinal thickening, presence of EIFL, and disrupted retinal layers [Fig. 28.10c, d]. On OCTA, the size of the FAZ may be reduced. Also, an increase in foveal vessel density (VD) and a decrease in parafoveal VD at the level of SCP and DCP can be seen.

28.4.2 Lamellar Macular Hole

A lamellar macular hole (LMH) is a defect in the inner fovea with or without actual loss of tissue [Fig. 28.10e]. It can be classified into tractional and degenerative subtypes [22]. Pre-retinal tissue can be seen in both subtypes. In tractional LMH, ERM is seen as a thin, irregular, hyperreflective layer attached intermittently to the retina, and in degenerative LMH, epiretinal proliferation, a thick, homogenous material of medium reflectivity, is seen. On OCTA analysis, a higher foveal VD and lower parafoveal VD are seen at the SCP and DCP level in tractional LMH cases. In degenerative LMH, a lower parafoveal VD can be seen in both SCP and DCP, with no significant difference noted for foveal VD.

28.4.3 Full-Thickness Macular Hole

On OCT, a full-thickness macular hole (FTMH) can be seen as a full-thickness foveal lesion interrupting all macular layers [Fig. 28.10f]. It can be classified based on its size into small (≤250 μm), medium (>250 μm but ≤400 μm), and large (≥400 μm) [20]. Other features that can be seen on OCT include ERM, IRF, and SRF. Following surgery, various closure patterns can be noted on OCT, such as the U, V, and W patterns of closure, and type 0, 1, and 2, and round or linear closure patterns [23].

On OCTA, "vascular sliding" can be seen at the border of the cystoid cavities in FTMH; this suggests the preservation of the microvasculature surrounding the cystoid spaces. Also, following surgery, a decrease in FAZ area and an increase in foveal vessel density and choriocapillaris network are noted.

28.5 Myopia-Related Retinal Diseases

28.5.1 Myopic Macular Degeneration

The META-PM (META-analysis for Pathologic Myopia) study group proposed the classification of myopic macular degeneration (MMD) based on fundus photographs that included atrophic alterations in the macula along with "plus lesions" that included lacquer cracks, Fuchs spot, and myopic choroidal neovascularization (mCNV). Correlation with OCT shows the presence of choroidal thinning with intact RPE in diffuse atrophy and the absence of both RPE and choroid in patchy atrophy [24]. The SFCT (subfoveal choroidal thickness) decreases with worsening MMD. Wong et al. [25] observed that choroidal thinning plays a more crucial role than scleral thinning in the progression of MMD. BM defects also contribute to the progression to macular atrophy.

Posterior staphyloma was classified based on the area of ectasia, shape, margins, and characteristics of the optic disc and retinal vessels. Posterior staphyloma can be observed as a protrusion of the wall of the eye. It can be clearly defined on OCT, characterized by an outpouching area with a radius less than the surrounding curvature of the wall of the eye. Other observations include inward protrusion of the sclera and thinning of the choroid at the edge of the staphyloma.

28.5.2 Myopic Choroidal Neovascularization

One of the complications of high myopia is mCNV (myopic choroidal neovascularization) which can present as sudden, progressive deterioration of central vision if not promptly treated. OCT is useful for detecting and guiding treatment with anti-VEGF (anti-vascular endothelial growth factor) in mCNV (Fig. 28.11). Most mCNVs are typically type 2 lesions that appear as small, flat, grayish lesions; these may be subfoveal, juxtafoveal, or extrafoveal in location. On OCT, mCNV appears as a hyperreflective mound above the RPE. During the active phase, an mCNV exhibits fuzzy edges on OCT, with variable amounts of SRF or IRF. The amount of retinal fluid, in general, is less than that in nAMD and has been attributed to less unhealthy RPE in the myopic population. With treatment, the lesion

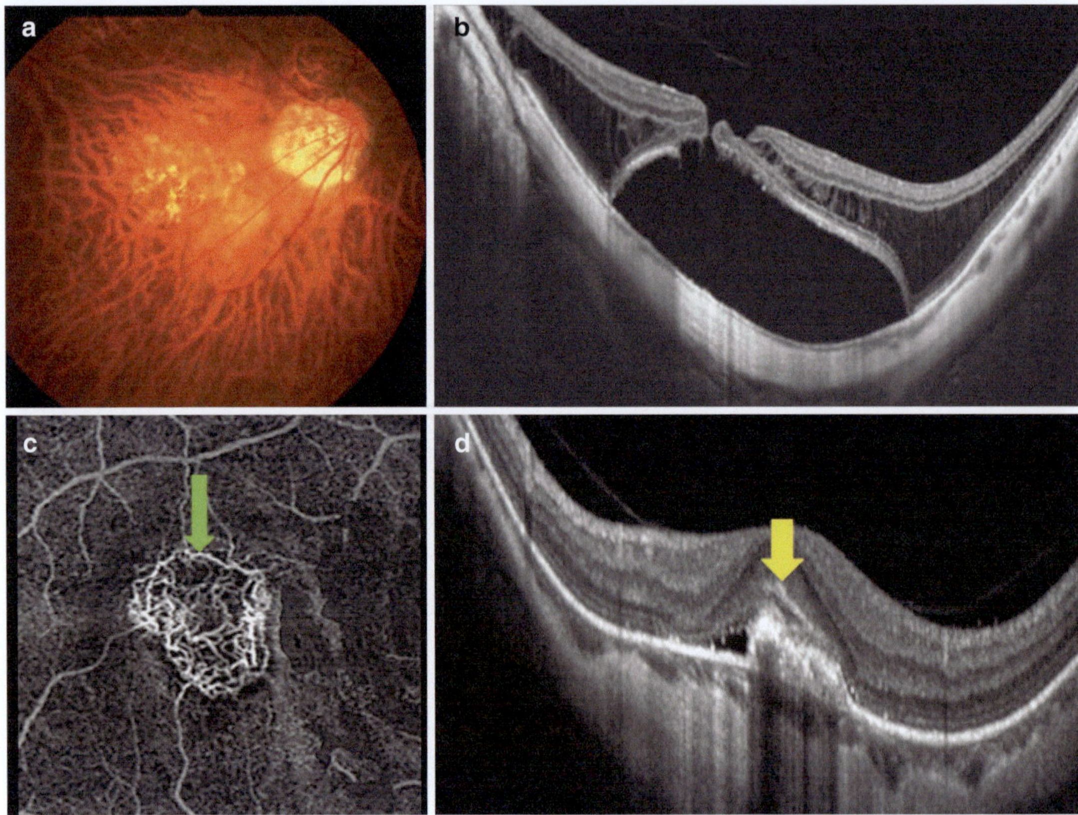

Fig. 28.11 (**a**) Color fundus photo of a myopic patient with a tessellated background, prominent choroidal vessels, and mCNV at the fovea. (**b**) Horizontal OCT scan through the fovea of a myopic patient showing myopic traction maculopathy. (**c**) OCTA of a myopic patient with mCNV showing a prominent network (green arrow). (**d**) Horizontal OCT scan of a myopic patient with mCNV showing subretinal hyperreflective material and subretinal fluid (yellow arrow)

develops a hyperpigmented border and evolves into a Fuchs spot in the scar stage. The corresponding OCT appears as an "encapsulated lesion" with a well-defined, hyperreflective outline and resolution of SRF/IRF. As mCNV regresses, some eyes develop chorioretinal atrophy in the atrophic stage [25, 26]. On OCT, this appears as an area of the outer retina and RPE loss surrounding the mCNV. In the atrophic stage, loss of choriocapillaris and RPE may eventually develop. On OCTA, an mCNV typically appears as vascular nets located above the RPE, in keeping with a type 2 NV [Fig. 28.11]. The lesions were identified as a tight vascular net with a perilesional halo and a visible core on OCTA is considered as an important biomarker in determining the activity of mCNV. Branching with tiny vessels and anastomosis or loops is a sign of neovascular activity. Although changes in shape, size, and flow area in OCTA have been observed with anti-VEGF treatment, there is no standard method to repeatably quantify these parameters. Flow signals may be detected even in treated mCNVs without exudation.

28.5.3 Myopic Traction Maculopathy

Myopic traction maculopathy (MTM) results from vitreomacular traction (VMT) in high myopia and includes myopic foveoschisis, a macular hole with or without RD. The increased rigidity of the retina in the presence of posterior staphyloma contributes to the development of MTM. MTM occurs

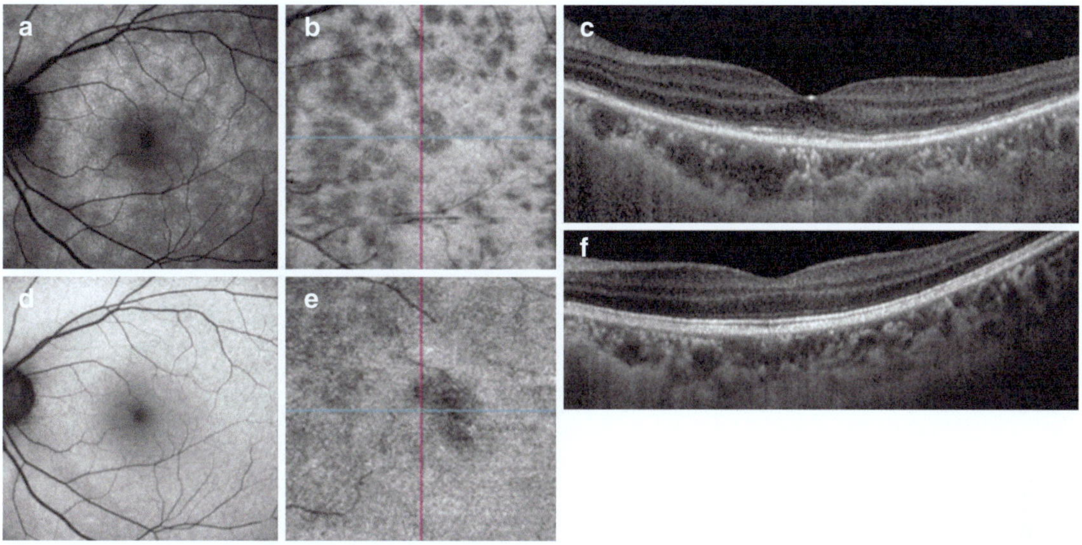

Fig. 28.12 (**a**–**c**)A case of MEWDS at presentation. (**a**) Fundus autofluorescence shows multiple punctate hyper autofluorescent lesions involving the macula. (**b**) Structural en face OCT shows corresponding hyporeflective lesions. (**c**) Structural OCT shows disruption of the ELM and EZ. (**d**–**f**): Case of MEWDS following resolution. (**d**) Most of the initial hyper autofluorescent lesions have completely resolved, with a few foci of consolidated hyper autofluorescent lesions persisting. (**e**) Structural en face OCT shows resolving lesions. (**f**) Structural OCT shows restoration of the ELM and EZ

more frequently in eyes with staphyloma than those without. In addition to detecting MTM, OCT can further delineate the severity of the condition [Fig. 28.11]. Various systems have attempted to classify MTM according to the extent of changes, the level of disruption, and whether or not the fovea is involved. The ATN classification includes the atrophy, traction, and neovascularization components. The traction component was classified based on the size of the macular retinoschisis into absent, extrafoveal, foveal only, and foveal (but not the entire macula), or foveal (entire macula). Parolini et al. identified four retinal stages of MTM that include inner/outer maculoschisis, predominantly outer maculoschisis, maculoschisis-macular detachment, and macular detachment [26, 27]. The foveal stages include normal fovea, inner lamellar macular hole, and full-thickness macular hole. Wang et al. [28] described the imaging characteristics of MTM using OCTA that showed the worse the BCVA, larger retinal volumes, and larger subfoveal choroidal capillary vessel density in retinoschisis.

28.5.3.1 Technical Concerns

Increased axial length, exaggerated curvature deformities, and imaging artifacts can make OCT imaging challenging in highly myopic eyes [27, 29]. SS-OCT offers a higher signal-to-noise ratio, deeper penetration, and longer scan length, resulting in higher resolution in highly myopic eyes than SD-OCT. Magnification correction should be considered when evaluating retinal and choriocapillaris blood flow quantification in myopic eyes.

28.6 Uveitis

28.6.1 White Dot Syndromes

The white dot syndromes comprise a spectrum of inflammatory disorders affecting the retina, including multiple evanescent white dot syndromes (MEWDS), punctate inner choroidopathy (PIC), and multifocal choroiditis (MFC). These may range from self-limiting to recurrent

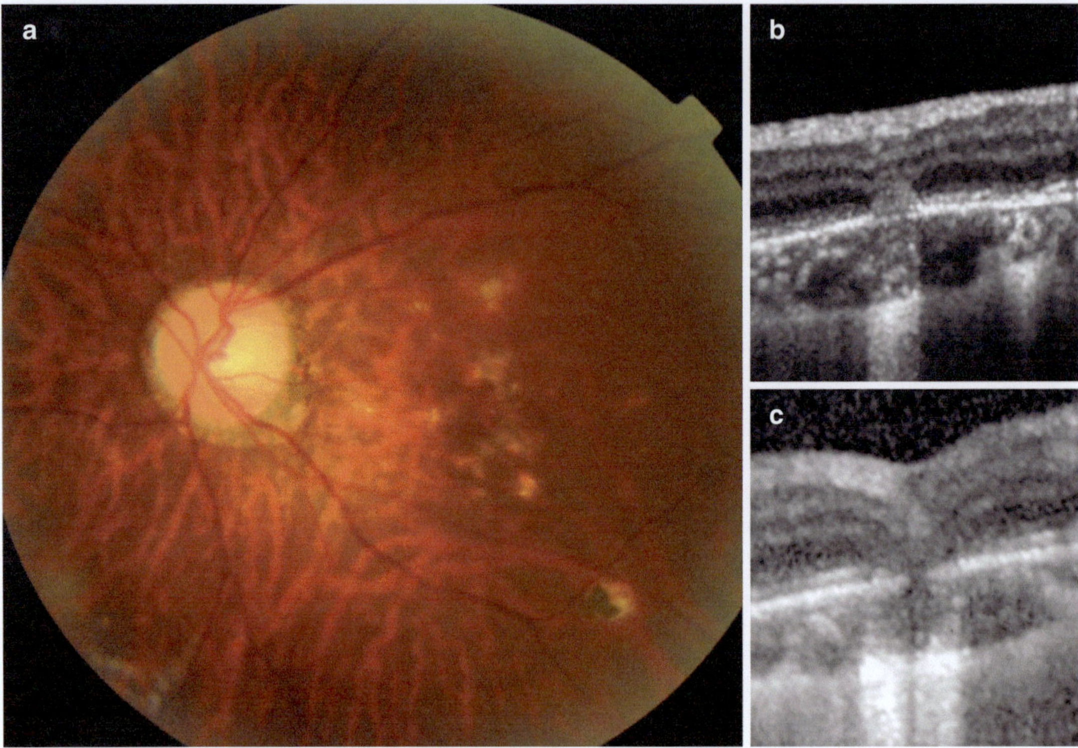

Fig. 28.13 (**a**) Color fundus photograph of a case of multifocal choroiditis (**b**) OCT shows a dome-shaped hyperreflective collection beneath the RPE, with loss of photoreceptors and choroidal hyper-transmissibility (**c**) OCT shows disruption of the outer retina layers with choroidal hyper-transmission

uveitis. Involvement of the choroid and choriocapillaris have also been implicated.

On structural OCT, disruption or loss of EZ is typically seen in MEWDS. These changes usually resolve within weeks, with reconstitution of the EZ band and symptomatic recovery [28, 30]. Thickening of the subfoveal choroid has been described, which suggests some choroidal involvement. Diffuse hyporeflective spots can be seen on en face OCT segmented at the EZ, corresponding to the disrupted EZ seen on OCT B scan [Fig. 28.12].

On OCT, acute MFC/PIC lesions are seen as conical or dome-shaped collections in the sub-RPE space. Widespread loss of outer retinal architecture and localized choroidal hyperreflectivity below the sub-RPE material can also be seen [Fig. 28.13] [29, 31]. Other features include thinning of the choroid, occlusion of the choroidal vessels, and focal choroidal excavation. Active disease can also present as foveal outer retinal hyperreflectivity (FORH), seen as hyperreflective finger-like projections extending from the RPE into the ONL with associated photoreceptor loss, with occasional extension till the ILM. The OCTA evaluation shows the presence of flow voids in choriocapillaris and also helps in the detection of CNVM.

28.6.2 Sympathetic Ophthalmia and Vogt-Koyanagi-Harada Disease

Sympathetic ophthalmia (SO) and Vogt-Koyanagi-Harada disease (VKH) share similar features in OCT. These include multiple serous retinal detachments, bacillary layer detachment, RPE folds, fluctuations of the internal limiting membrane, and subretinal and choroidal hyperreflective dots. Choroidal analysis shows diffuse choroidal thickening with loss of choroidal architecture and increased CVI (choroidal vascularity index) [Fig. 28.14] [30–33]. Dalen-Fuchs nodules are dome-shaped hyperreflective, sub-RPE lesions with associated disruption of the ellipsoid zone and RPE. On OCTA, choriocapillaris flow voids can be seen. With treatment, the neurosensory detachment resolves. Reduced choroidal thickness is a useful measure to assess the improvement of the underlying choroidal inflammation.

28.6.3 Non-infectious Retinitis

Retinal arteriolar and venous circulation can be affected in Behcet's disease. On OCT, superficial retinal infiltrates are seen as focal, hyperreflective thickening of the retina with back-shadowing [Fig. 28.15]. In the case of neuro retinitis, localized vitreous condensation over the inflamed optic disc can be seen, giving a "smoking volcano" appearance. An increase in CMT and macular volume can also be seen. Other features include CME, ERM, serous RD, ELM, and EZ disruption with OPL elevation, INL thinning, VMA/VMT, LMH or FTMH, macular atrophy, and scarring [32, 34]. On OCTA, there is an increase in FAZ with hypo—or non-perfusion in SCP and DCP.

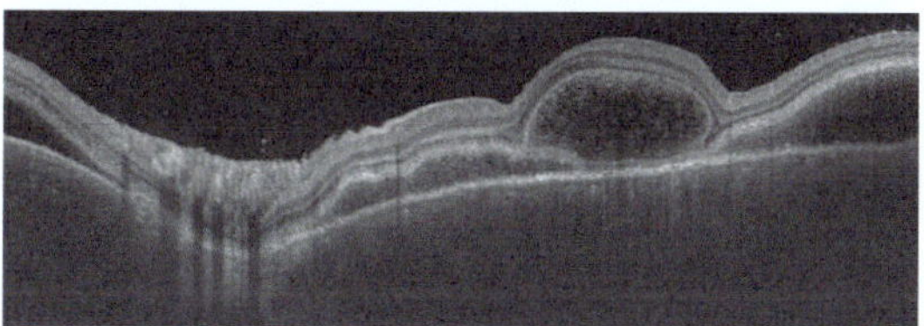

Fig. 28.14 OCT of a patient with Vogt-Koyanagi-Harada disease with increased central macular thickness, bacillary layer detachment, neurosensory layer detachment, and increased choroidal thickness

28.6.4 Infectious Uveitis

28.6.4.1 Toxoplasmosis

The retinitis lesion in toxoplasma retinochoroiditis is seen as an area of increased intraretinal reflectivity and thickness with full-thickness disorganization of the retinal layers [Fig. 28.16]. Posterior hyaloid thickening or detachment may also be seen overlying the lesion. Hyperreflective round-shaped deposits along the posterior hyaloid and hyperreflective dots in the retro hyaloid space are characteristic of the disease. The choroid is hyporeflective below the lesion, and there is diffuse thickening of the choroid with a decrease in the number of hyperreflective septa corresponding to the walls of the choroidal ves-

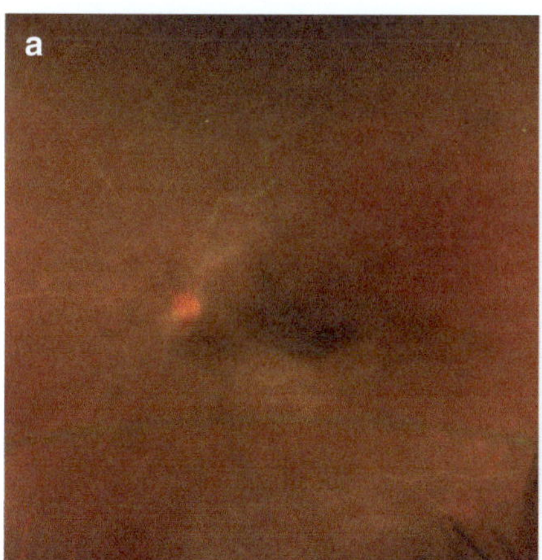

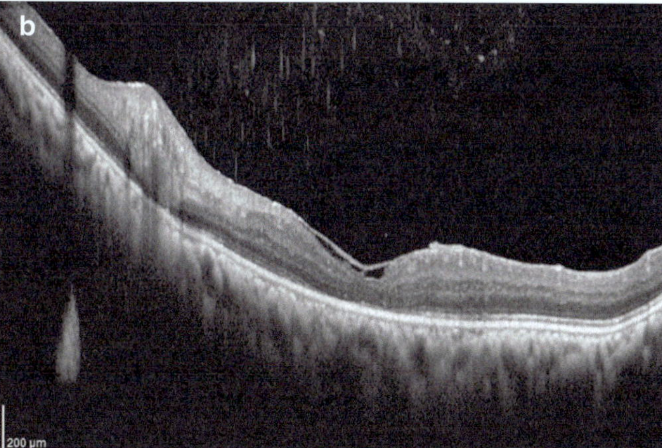

Fig. 28.15 (**a**) Color fundus photo of a case of Behcet's disease showing extensive sclerosed vessels and vitreous hemorrhage. (**b**) Corresponding OCT macula shows hyperreflective lesions in the vitreous cavity suggestive of vitreous hemorrhage, superficial retinal infiltrates seen as hyperreflective lesions in the inner retina, epiretinal membrane, external limiting membrane, and ellipsoid zone disruption

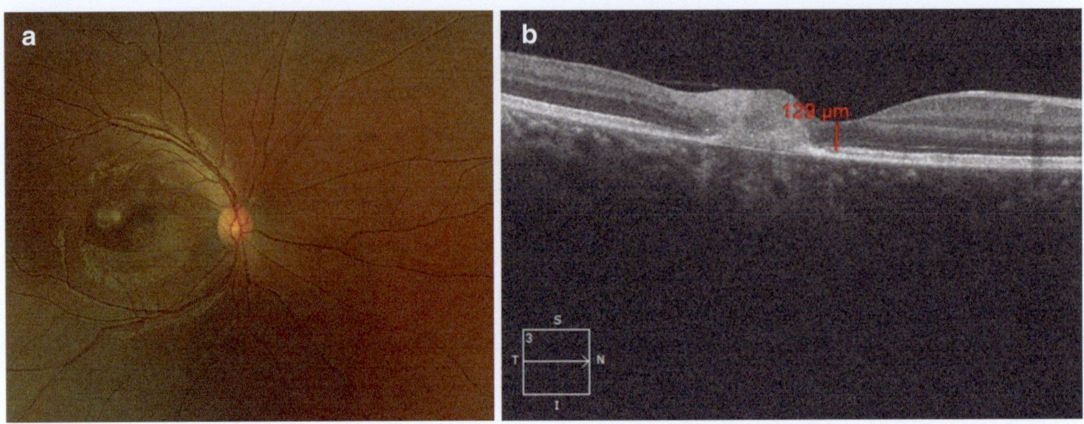

Fig. 28.16 (**a**) Color fundus photograph showing a discrete, well-defined yellowish lesion just temporal to the fovea in a patient with toxoplasma retinochoroiditis. (**b**) Horizontal OCT scan passing through the lesion showing a full-thickness retinitis lesion

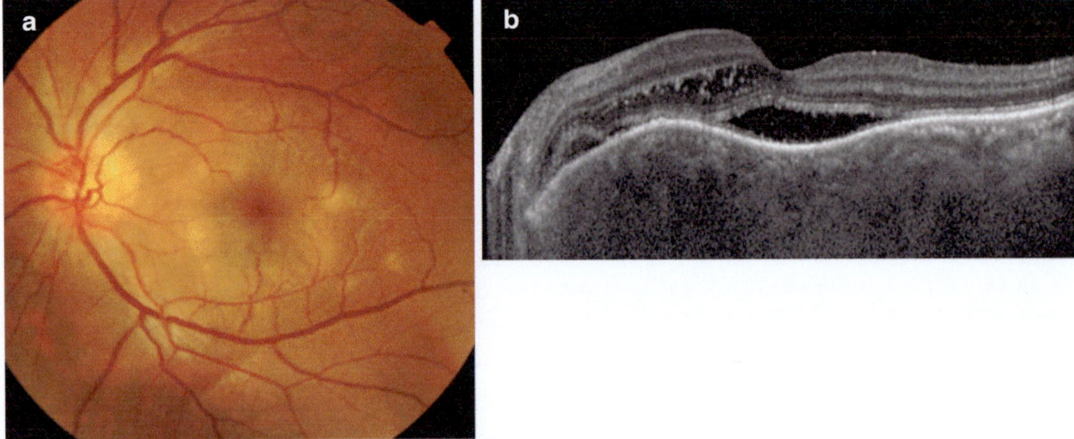

Fig. 28.17 (**a**) Color fundus photograph of a patient with choroidal tuberculoma. (**b**) OCT macula of the patient shows a full-thickness choroidal dome-shaped lesion, "contact sign," and exudative retinal detachment

sels and loss of the dotted physiological pattern of the choriocapillaris. OCTA shows reduced SCP, DCP, and CC flow in the area corresponding to the lesion. It is also useful to diagnose and follow-up cases of CNVM [33, 35].

28.6.4.2 Tuberculosis

Ocular tuberculosis may present as choroidal tubercles, granulomas, occlusive retinal vasculitis, multifocal serpiginoid, or serpiginous-like choroiditis. On OCT, the tubercules are seen as a single, rounded lesion having a hyporeflective core surrounded by a hyperreflective area, in the neurosensory retina, with surrounding SRF. Tuberculous choroidal granulomas are seen as full-thickness choroidal lesions with well-defined margins, having a lobulated shape, non-homogenous internal reflectivity, and hyporeflective compared to the surrounding choroid. It is characterized by a "contact sign," a localized area of adhesion between the RPE-choriocapillaris layer and the neurosensory retina, surrounded by exudative retinal detachment [Fig. 28.17]. In tubercular serpiginous-like choroiditis, the OCT features include ELM and EZ disruption, hyperreflective material over the RPE extending towards the inner retina, RPE elevations, increased choroidal thickness, and choroidal hyperreflective dots. OCTA shows choriocapillaris flow void during the active stage and vascular tufts and tangled vessels in the inner choroid in the healing stage [34–37].

28.7 Retinal and Choroidal Tumors

28.7.1 Choroidal Nevus

Choroidal nevus can be seen as a hyperreflective lesion within the choroid with back-shadowing. They may be flat or associated with mild elevation of the overlying retina [Fig. 28.18a, b]. Associated features which can be imaged with OCT in a case of choroidal nevus are IRF, SRF, photoreceptor loss, EZ irregularity, RPE detachment, atrophy or loss, drusen, and choriocapillaris thinning overlying the drusen. On OCTA, there is fading of the normal homogenous vascular mosaic in CC slab corresponding to the area of the naevus [36, 38].

28.7.2 Choroidal Melanoma

On OCT imaging, the choroidal melanoma lesion shows deep optical back-shadowing. Other features are SRF, subretinal lipofuscin deposition, RPE atrophy, IRF, loss of ELM and EZ and irregularity of GC-IPL [Fig. 28.18c, b]. Shaggy photoreceptors have also been noted, which represent edematous photoreceptors or macrophages with lipofuscin on the posterior surface of the detached retina [37, 39]. Vitreous seeding can be seen as highly reflective spheroidal bodies in the vitreous cavity. Imaging with OCTA shows heteroge-

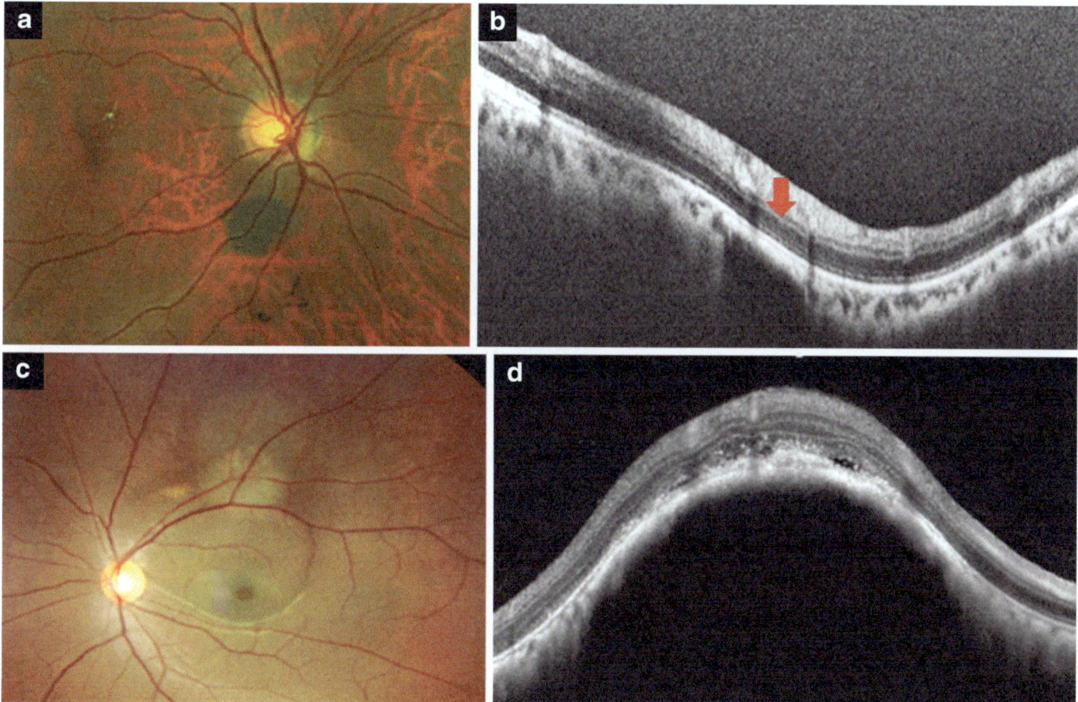

Fig. 28.18 Choroidal mass. (**a**) Color fundus photograph showing a choroidal nevus. (**b**) An OCT scan passing through the lesion shows a flat hyperreflective choroidal lesion with back-shadowing (red arrow). (**c**) Color fundus photograph showing an amelanotic choroidal melanoma along the superotemporal arcade with subretinal fluid extending to the macula. (**d**) An OCT scan passing through the lesion shows an elevated choroidal lesion with deep optical shadowing with overlying subretinal fluid, subretinal lipofuscin, RPE atrophy, and photoreceptor loss

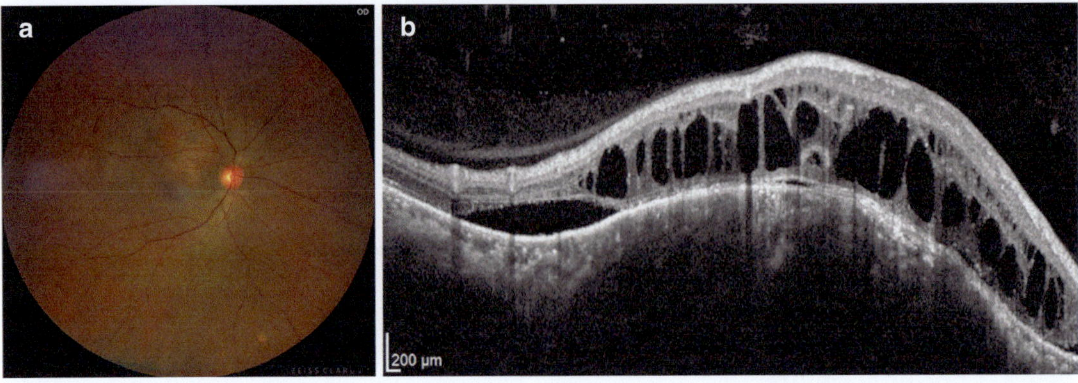

Fig. 28.19 (**a**) Color fundus photograph showing circumscribed choroidal hemangioma along the superotemporal arcade with subretinal fluid extending to the macula. (**b**) An OCT scan passing through the lesion shows a smooth elevated choroidal lesion with dilated Haller and Sattler choroidal vessels. There is overlying subretinal fluid and schitic cavities in the neurosensory retina

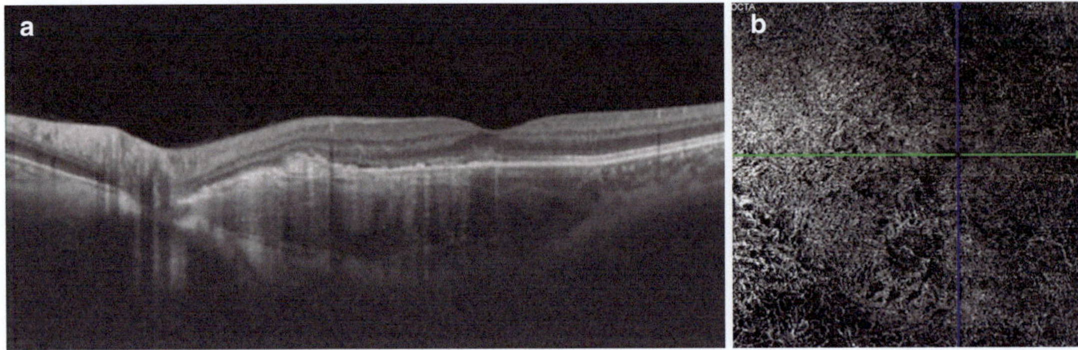

Fig. 28.20 (**a**) SS-OCT scan of a patient with choroidal osteoma showing well-defined choroidal lesion having an intralesional sponge-like appearance. Overlying subretinal hyperreflective material and subretinal fluid can also be seen, which is suggestive of type-2 choroidal neovascular membrane (CNVM). (**b**) Corresponding OCTA through the outer retinal slab shows the presence of fine vascular network confirming the presence of type-2 CNVM

neously distributed small blood vessels and disorganized intratumoral vasculature.

28.7.3 Choroidal Hemangioma

On imaging with EDI-OCT, circumscribed choroidal hemangioma lesions are seen as a smooth, gently sloping anterior contour and gradual choroidal expansion. The lumen of the choriocapillaris, Sattler's, and Haller's layers are expanded. Also, there is partial optical shadowing deep to the lesion, lipofuscin deposition, IRF, retinal schisis, and SRF [Fig. 28.19]. On OCTA, choroidal vessels appear white with few intervening signal void areas. Vessels at the SCP level have a bag of worms appearance, whereas the deeper choroidal vessels demonstrate a club-like appearance [38, 40].

28.7.4 Choroidal Osteoma

With the help of EDI-OCT, an intralesional sponge-like appearance can be seen in cases of choroidal osteoma [Fig. 28.20]. Subtle horizontal hyperreflective lamellar lines representing the bone lamellae and horizontal or vertical tubular channels possibly representing vessels may also be seen. There is marked

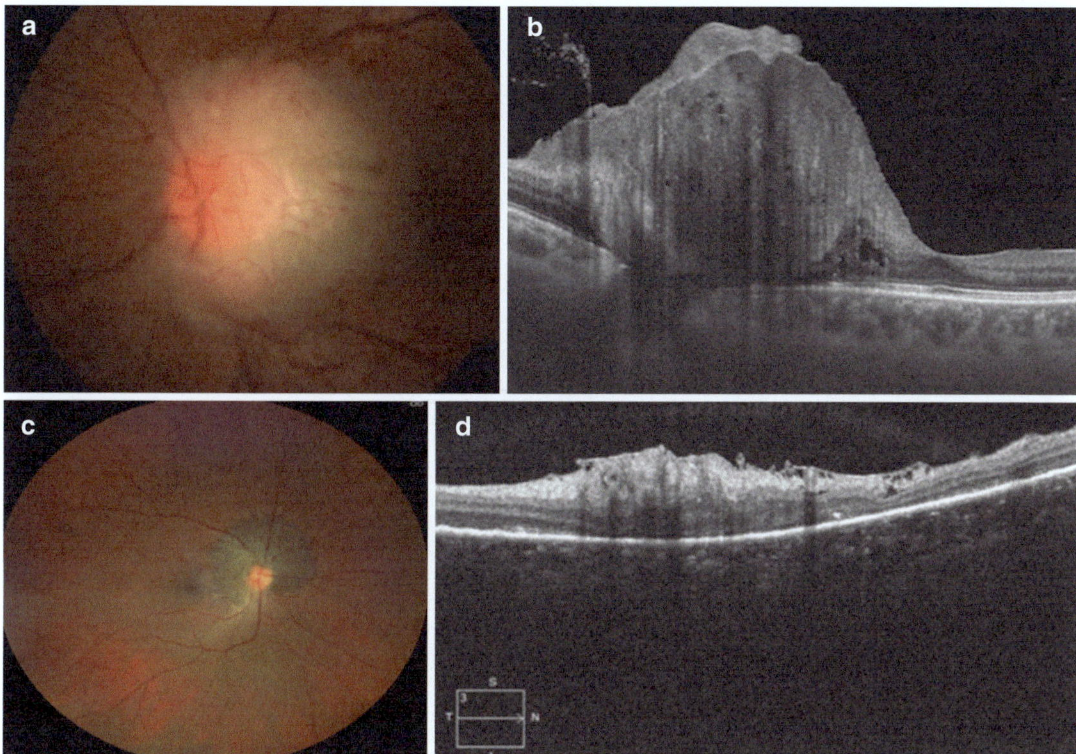

Fig. 28.21 Hamartoma. (**a**) Color fundus photograph of the left eye showing astrocytic hamartoma of the optic disc. (**b**) Corresponding OCT passing through the lesion shows an elevated dome-shaped lesion with intralesional calcifications and back-shadowing. (**c**) Color fundus photograph of the right eye showing combined hamartoma of the retina and retinal pigment epithelium. (**d**) OCT of the same patient shows retinal traction and saw-tooth appearance of the inner retina

thinning of the outer retinal layers with indistinct RPE in areas of the decalcified tumor. On OCTA, blood flow is mainly detected within the choriocapillaries layer and partly within the Sattler's layer. It is also useful in diagnosing and monitoring associated with choroidal neovascular membrane (CNVM) [Fig. 28.20] [39, 41].

28.7.5 Hamartoma

28.7.5.1 Retinal Astrocytic Hamartoma

Retinal astrocytic hamartoma is seen on OCT as a dome/plateau-shaped lesion with the calcified tumors showing high reflectivity and back-shadowing [Fig. 28.21a, b]. There is DRIL with a gradual transition to the adjacent normal retina. Other associated features noted include retinal traction, discrete internal moth-eaten optically empty spaces, adjacent retinal or macular edema, and shallow elevation of the adjacent retina. On OCTA, finely branching tumor vessels can be seen in the superficial and deep retina. Also, the outer retina and choriocapillaris layer show hyporeflective changes due to shadowing caused by calcium or high blood flow within the lesion [40, 42].

28.7.5.2 Combined Hamartoma of the Retina and Retinal Pigment Epithelium

On OCT, focal vitreoretinal traction can be seen and the inner retina shows a "saw-tooth" and "omega sign" pattern [Fig. 28.21c, d]. On OCTA evaluation, a filigree pattern of intratumoral vessels can be identified [41, 43].

28.8 Conclusion

In conclusion, OCT and OCTA provide detailed structural evaluation in a wide range of retinal pathologies. Their use, as part of multimodal imaging strategies, can support the diagnosis and treatment-response evaluation of many retinal conditions. In many cases, the noninvasive nature of OCT and OCTA is significantly advantageous over dye-based angiography.

Funding Hyderabad Eye Research Foundation, Hyderabad, India.

Disclosure GC: Speaker for Zeiss, Topcon

References

1. Popescu DP, Choo-Smith LP, Flueraru C, et al. Optical coherence tomography: fundamental principles, instrumental designs and biomedical applications. Biophys Rev. 2011;3(3):155. https://doi.org/10.1007/s12551-011-0054-7.
2. Bille JF, editor. High resolution imaging in microscopy and ophthalmology: new Frontiers in biomedical optics. Cham: Springer International Publishing; 2019. https://doi.org/10.1007/978-3-030-16638-0.
3. Chhablani J, Krishnan T, Sethi V, Kozak I. Artifacts in optical coherence tomography. Saudi J Ophthalmol. 2014;28(2):81–7.
4. Sadda SVR, Schachat AP, Wilkinson CP, Hinton DR, Wiedemann P, Freund KB, Sarraf D, editors. Ryan's Retina. 7th ed; 2023. https://www.elsevier.com/books/ryan's-retina/978-0-323-72213-1
5. Moir J, Khanna S, Skondra D. Review of OCT angiography findings in diabetic retinopathy: insights and perspectives. Int J Transl Med. 2021;1(3):286–305.
6. Gella L, Raman R, Rani PK, Sharma T. Spectral domain optical coherence tomography characteristics in diabetic retinopathy. Oman J Ophthalmol. 2014;7(3):126–9.
7. Vaz-Pereira S, Morais-Sarmento T, Esteves MR. Optical coherence tomography features of neovascularization in proliferative diabetic retinopathy: a systematic review. Int J Retina Vitr. 2020;6:26. https://doi.org/10.1186/s40942-020-00230-3.
8. Markan A, Agarwal A, Arora A, et al. Novel imaging biomarkers in diabetic retinopathy and diabetic macular edema. Ther Adv Ophthalmol. 2020 Sep;4(12):2515841420950513. https://doi.org/10.1177/2515841420950513.
9. Lazăr AS, Stanca HT, Tăbăcaru B, et al. Quantitative parameters relevant for diabetic macular edema evaluation by optical coherence tomography angiography. Medicina (Mex). 2023;59(6):1120. https://doi.org/10.3390/medicina59061120.
10. Garrity ST, Sarraf D, Freund KB, Sadda SR. Multimodal imaging of Nonneovascular age-related macular degeneration. Invest Ophthalmol Vis Sci. 2018;59(4):AMD48–64. https://doi.org/10.1167/iovs.18-24158.
11. Ambati J, Ambati BK, Yoo SH, et al. Age-related macular degeneration: etiology, pathogenesis, and therapeutic strategies. Surv Ophthalmol. 2003;48(3):257–93.
12. Tsai ASH, Cheung N, Gan ATL, et al. Retinal angiomatous proliferation. Surv Ophthalmol. 2017;62(4):462–92.
13. Al-Sheikh M, Iafe NA, Phasukkijwatana N, et al. Biomarkers of neovascular activity in age-related macular degeneration using optical coherence tomography angiography. Retina Phila Pa. 2018;38(2):220–30.
14. Sadda SR, Guymer R, Holz FG, et al. Consensus definition for atrophy associated with age-related macular degeneration on OCT: classification of atrophy report 3. Ophthalmology. 2018;125(4):537–48.
15. Schmidt-Erfurth U, Waldstein SM, Klimscha S, et al. Prediction of individual disease conversion in early AMD using artificial intelligence. Invest Ophthalmol Vis Sci. 2018;59(8):3199–208.
16. Cheung CMG, Gan A, Yanagi Y, et al. Association between choroidal thickness and Drusen subtypes in age-related macular degeneration. Ophthalmol Retina. 2018;2(12):1196–205.
17. Yang S, Liu X, Li H, et al. Optical coherence tomography angiography characteristics of acute retinal arterial occlusion. BMC Ophthalmol. 2019;19(1):147. https://doi.org/10.1186/s12886-019-1152-8.
18. Hirano Y, Suzuki N, Tomiyasu T, et al. Multimodal imaging of microvascular abnormalities in retinal vein occlusion. J Clin Med. 2021;10(3):405. https://doi.org/10.3390/jcm10030405.
19. Kedarisetti KC, Narayanan R, Stewart MW, et al. Macular telangiectasia type 2: a comprehensive review. Clin Ophthalmol Auckl NZ. 2022;16:3297–309.
20. Duker JS, Kaiser PK, Binder S, et al. The international Vitreomacular traction study group classification of vitreomacular adhesion, traction, and macular hole. Ophthalmology. 2013;120(12):2611–9.
21. Govetto A, Lalane RA, Sarraf D, et al. Insights into Epiretinal membranes: presence of ectopic inner Foveal layers and a new optical coherence tomography staging scheme. Am J Ophthalmol. 2017;175:99–113.
22. Govetto A, Dacquay Y, Farajzadeh M, et al. Lamellar macular hole: two distinct clinical entities? Am J Ophthalmol. 2016;164:99–109.
23. Rossi T, Bacherini D, Caporossi T, et al. Macular hole closure patterns: an updated classification. Graefes Arch Clin Exp Ophthalmol. 2020;258(12):2629–38.

24. Ohno-Matsui K, Kawasaki R, Jonas JB, et al. International photographic classification and grading system for myopic maculopathy. Am J Ophthalmol. 2015;159(5):877–883.e7.
25. Wong CW, Phua V, Lee SY, et al. Is choroidal or scleral thickness related to myopic macular degeneration? Invest Ophthalmol Vis Sci. 2017;58(2):907–13.
26. Cheung CMG, Arnold JJ, Holz FG, et al. Myopic choroidal neovascularization: review, guidance, and consensus statement on management. Ophthalmology. 2017;124(11):1690–711.
27. Parolini B, Palmieri M, Finzi A, et al. The new myopic traction maculopathy staging system. Eur J Ophthalmol. 2021;31(3):1299–312.
28. Wang SW, Hung KC, Tsai CY, et al. Myopic traction maculopathy biomarkers on optical coherence tomography angiography-an overlooked mechanism of visual acuity correction in myopic eyes. Eye. 2019;33:1305–13.
29. Ang M, Wong CW, Hoang QV, et al. Imaging in myopia: potential biomarkers, current challenges and future developments. Br J Ophthalmol. 2019;103(6):855–62.
30. Onal S, Tugal-Tutkun I, Neri P, Herbort P, C. Optical coherence tomography imaging in uveitis. Int Ophthalmol. 2014;34(2):401–35.
31. Spaide RF, Goldberg N, Freund KB. Redefining multifocal choroiditis and panuveitis and punctate inner choroidopathy through multimodal imaging. Retina Phila Pa. 2013;33(7):1315–24.
32. Mahajan S, Invernizzi A, Agrawal R, et al. Multimodal imaging in sympathetic Ophthalmia. Ocul Immunol Inflamm. 2017;25(2):152–9.
33. Liu XY, Peng XY, Wang S, et al. Features of optical coherence tomography for the diagnosis of Vogt-Koyanagi-Harada disease. Retina Phila Pa. 2016;36(11):2116–23.
34. Çakar ÖP. Behçet's uveitis: current diagnostic and therapeutic approach. Turk J Ophthalmol. 2020;50(3):169–82.
35. Brandão-de-Resende C, Balasundaram MB, Narain S, et al. Multimodal imaging in ocular toxoplasmosis. Ocul Immunol Inflamm. 2020;28(8):1196–204.
36. Agarwal A, Mahajan S, Khairallah M, et al. Multimodal Imaging in Ocular Tuberculosis. Ocul Immunol Inflamm. 2017;25(1):134–45.
37. Agarwal A, Pichi F, Invernizzi A, et al. Stepwise approach for fundus imaging in the diagnosis and management of posterior uveitis. Surv Ophthalmol. 2023;68(3):446–80.
38. Ali ZC, Gray J, Balaskas K. Features of choroidal naevi on swept source optical coherence tomography angiography and structural reverse flow optical coherence tomography. Graefes Arch Clin Exp Ophthalmol. 2018;256(7):1319–23.
39. Shields CL, Manalac J, Das C, et al. Review of spectral domain enhanced depth imaging optical coherence tomography of tumors of the choroid. Indian J Ophthalmol. 2015;63(2):117–21.
40. Say EAT, Shah SU, Ferenczy S, Shields CL. Optical coherence tomography of retinal and choroidal tumors. J Ophthalmol. 2011;2011:385058. https://doi.org/10.1155/2012/385058.
41. Olguin-Manríquez F, Enríquez AB, Crim N, et al. Multimodal imaging in choroidal osteoma. Int J Retina Vitr. 2018;4:30. https://doi.org/10.1186/s40942-018-0132-0.
42. Mirzayev I, Gündüz AK. Hamartomas of the retina and optic disc. Turk J Ophthalmol. 2022;52(6):421–31.
43. Arepalli S, Pellegrini M, Ferenczy SR, Shields CL. Combined hamartoma of the retina and retinal pigment epithelium: findings on enhanced depth imaging optical coherence tomography in eight eyes. Retina Phila Pa. 2014;34(11):2202–7.

29 Microperimetry

Kara R. Grimes and Jay Chhablani

29.1 Introduction

Microperimetry, or fundus-tracked perimetry, is a visual field test to assess central retinal function. Current uses of microperimetry have been built on early developments of non-automated fundus-tracked perimetry. These devices have subsequently improved with the innovation of scanning laser ophthalmoscopy. Microperimetry allows for the measurement of fixation stability and topographic characterization of visual function, enabling a correlation between retinal structure and visual function. Using microperimetry, the sensitivity threshold of any point of the retina can be matched with its clinical appearance in real-time. This method can therefore provide insights into disease progression and severity, particularly in conditions that affect the retina. This chapter comprehensively reviews the history, technology, techniques, and clinical application of microperimetry.

K. R. Grimes (✉)
New York Medical College, New York, USA

J. Chhablani
Department of Ophthalmology, University of Pittsburgh, Pittsburgh, PA, USA

29.2 Brief History of Microperimetry

The introduction of perimetry to the field of ophthalmology is credited to Albrecht von Graefe in the mid-nineteenth century, building on the revolutionary work of the founder of the ophthalmoscope, Hermann von Helmholtz [1]. In 1856, these early ophthalmologists used various fixation points during fundus examinations to create a visual field plot [2]. Nearly a century following these experiments, clinicians began publishing documentation of retinal sensitivity while examining the fundus. Early devices permitting static fundus-tracked perimetry were reported in the late 1970s [3]. Subsequent key developments in microperimetry were made following the invention of the scanning laser ophthalmoscope (SLO) by Webb, Hughes, and Pomerantzeff in 1980 [4]. The originally designed SLO used a laser to illuminate a small area of the retina, employing a novel principle in which light was collected from one retinal point at a time [5]. This method facilitates repeated inspection of the retina and allows the exact locus of each point to be viewed directly by the clinician to measure acuity and investigate macular disease [5].

The SLO 101 (Rodenstock Instrument GmbH, Ottobrunn-Riemerling, Germany) was the first commercially available device supporting fundus-tracked perimetry. In the following years, Microperimeter 1 (MP-1, NIDEK, Gamagori,

T. Das, P. Satgunam (eds.), *Ophthalmic Diagnostics*, https://doi.org/10.1007/978-981-97-0138-4_29

Japan) was more often used for fundus-tracked perimetry. The MP-1 had real-time automated full-threshold perimetry software, allowing fundus perimetry in a larger, color-visualized field. Although MP-1 was more reliable than SLO for fixation analysis, limitations of poor infrared image quality and artifacts disrupting the test grid on fundus imaging spurred further developments on this instrument [6]. These technical limitations were addressed by the Macular Integrity Assessment System (CenterVue, Padova, Italy), which provided higher quality images and a dynamic range of 36 dB compared to earlier instruments. The Microperimeter 3 (Mp-3, NIDEK) and Compass (CenterVue) were later adaptations of previous devices that allowed for mesopic (1.27 cd/m^2) and photopic (10 cd/m^2) testing using liquid crystal display (LCD) and light-emitting diode (LED) projectors, respectively. Additionally, various research groups have developed custom-built devices for microperimetry to answer specific research questions [7].

29.3 Technology

The development of commercially available microperimeters over the past 50 years has been largely based on standard automated perimetry and has led to the widespread use of fundus-tracked perimetry. Yet, some factors of fundus-tracking are unique to microperimetry and vary depending on the instrument. Currently, devices used for microperimetry include the MP-1 and MP-3, the Spectral Optical Coherence Tomography (OCT) SLO (OPKO Health, Inc., Miami, FL, USA), the COMPASS, and the Macular Integrity Assessment System (MAIA).

29.3.1 Analysis of Retinal Sensitivity

The principal feature of microperimetry is the ability to present stimuli on a liquid crystal display background at specific locations in the retina, which allows for continuous visualization (Fig. 29.1a and b) of the retina [8]. Retinal sensitivity is measured as the minimal light intensity perceived by the patient when the retina is stimulated by spots of light in specific areas. Each examination can differ with variable numbers of stimuli and different fields of vision. In microperimetry, the stimuli luminance is measured in apostilbs (asb), which is an absolute unit of luminance equal to 0.3183 cd/m^2. The maximum intensity emitted by the fundus-tracking perimeter is then used to create the relative decibel (dB) scale (Fig. 29.1c).

29.3.2 Decibel Scale, Weber's Law, Fechner's Law

Weber's law, Fechner's law, and the decibel scale are used to determine stimulus brightness in microperimetry [7]. Weber's law describes the relationship between the smallest change in the intensity of the light stimulus (ΔI) and the initial stimulus intensity (I). Based on the assumptions

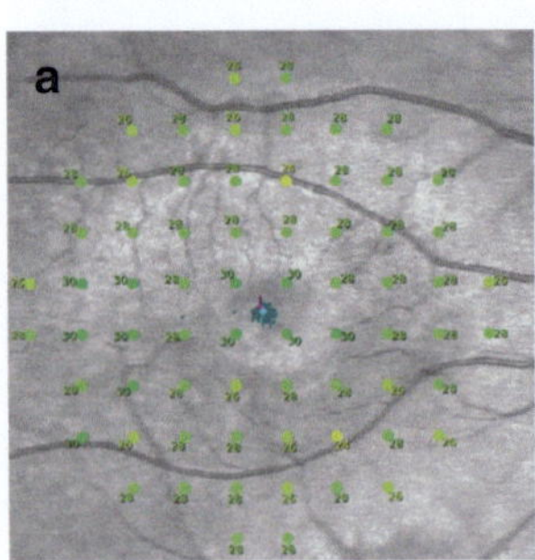

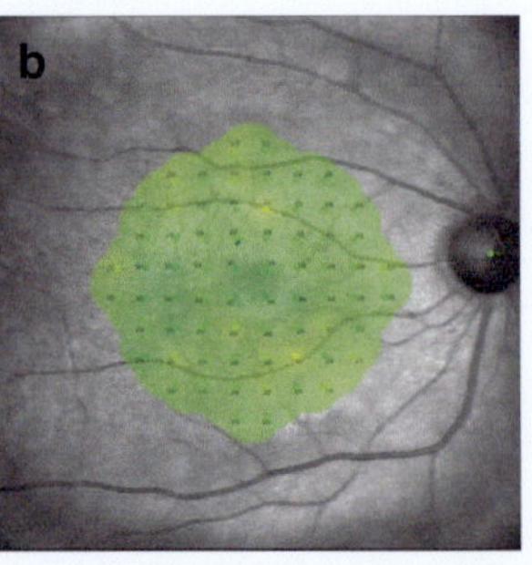

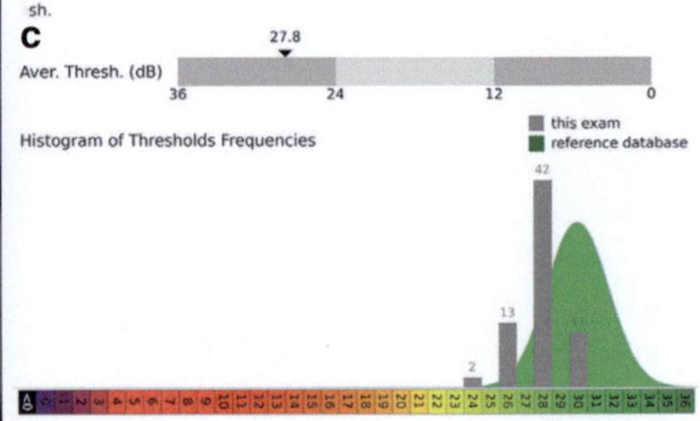

Fig. 29.1 Standard output given by the MAIA microperimeter for a healthy subject. (**a**) Point threshold values overlaid onto a fundus image. (**b**) Heatmap output using a radial interpolation with point threshold values. (**c**) Histogram of point threshold values and a mean sensitivity value for all points. (Reprinted with permission from Josan et al. [8] Copyright 2021, Association for Research in Vision and Ophthalmology)

Table 29.1 Commercially available microperimetry devices

Device	Year; manufacturer	Background luminance	Maximum stimulus luminance	Threshold range	Stimuli Size	Minimum pupil size	Visual field	Tracking frequency
MP-1	2004; Nidek	1.27 cd/m^2	128 cd/m^2	0–20 dB	Goldmann I, II, III, IV eV	4 mm	22.5°	25 Hz
OCT-SLO	2006; Optos	10 cd/m^2	125 cd/m^2	0–20 dB	Goldmann III	4 mm	29.7°	8 Hz
MAIA	2015; CenterVue	1.27 cd/m^2	1000 asb	0–36 dB	Goldmann III	2.5 mm	36°	25 Hz
MP-3	2015; Nidek co.,	31.4 asb	10,000 asb	0–34 dB	Goldmann I-V	4 mm	40°	430 Hz
COMPASS	2016; CenterVue	31.4 asb	10,000 asb	0–25 dB	Goldmann III	3 mm	60°	25 Hz

of Weber's law, Fechner's law describes the proportional relationship between subjective sensation (ΔS) and the logarithm of stimulus intensity. In this equation, the maximal luminance of an instrument (I_{max}) is proportional to the differential luminance ($\Delta I = I_{threshold} - I_{Background}$) [7].

Weber's Law

$$\text{constant}\left(K\right) = \frac{\Delta I}{I}$$

Fechner's Law

$$\Delta S\left(\text{in dB}\right) = 10 \text{ x } \log \frac{I_{max}}{\Delta I}$$

Data are interpreted according to Weber's and Fechner's laws to determine the stimulus brightness in decibels (dB). Zero dB is defined as the brightest stimulus that can be produced. Each 1 dB increment corresponds to an attenuation of the luminance in the stimulus by a factor of 1.26, while 3 dB corresponds to a two-fold attenuation of luminance, and 10 dB corresponds to a ten-fold attenuation as described by Pfau et al. (2021) [7]. In the most widely used commercially available instruments, the stimuli can be presented over a dynamic range of 0–20 dB with a scotopic background luminance of <0.03 cd/m^2, mesopic background luminance of 1.27 cd/m^2, or photopic background luminance of 10 cd/m^2. The decibel scale is not standardized because maximal luminance can vary between instruments (Table 29.1). Additionally, some microperimeters, such as the MAIA, color-code the decibel scale for interpretation, with "green" representing normal, "red" representing abnormal, and "black" representing a scotoma (Fig. 29.1c).

Various stimulus patterns are used to test the central visual field. The fundus image is viewed and tracked using an infrared fundus camera or an infrared SLO throughout perimetric testing. Concurrently, data from the visual field is mapped directly to the fundus image (Fig. 29.1a). The minimal retinal sensitivity over a certain area is then measured by projecting the light stimuli over a specified spot several times at different intensities. Stimuli vary in luminous intensity and size, with the Goldman size III (0.43° and 4.0 mm^2 area) being the most used size (Table 29.1). The Goldman size IV stimulus (1.72 and 64 mm^2 area) is larger and is more often tested in people with low vision or in scotopic conditions in healthy eyes.

29.4 Technique

Microperimetry measures the sensitivity of the macula and allows examiners to perceive changes as a diagnostic tool. Although this process is automatic, the technician can have a substantial impact on the outcome of the examination. The following section will discuss common practices to obtain the best results using microperimetry.

29.4.1 Adaptation of the Retina and Pupil Dilation

Before beginning microperimetry, it is essential to allow the retina to adapt to the changing light conditions. For mesopic (or twilight) testing, 10 minutes of adaptation is sufficient after exposure to a bright stimulus, such as fundus imaging [9]. Contrastingly, adaptation to mesopic lighting is not required following exposure to ambient lighting [10]. Studies have shown that mesopic microperimetry performance does not improve with increasing adaptation time beyond 20 min [10]. Microperimetry in scotopic (or dim-light) conditions requires at least 20 min of dark adaptation, particularly for patients with retinal diseases [11]. Additional time (30–40 minutes) is suggested for older adults and/or those with Bruch's membrane damage [12].

The minimum pupil size needed for adequate testing varies depending on the machine used. Dilation requirements vary from ~2.5 mm to ~6 mm, depending on the instrument (Table 29.1) [13]. The state of the eye must remain consistent across examinations, irrespective of whether the eye is dilated or undilated. No further preparation of the eye is required.

29.4.2 Evaluation, Instruction, and Duration of Testing

During the evaluation, each eye is tested independently by covering one eye first, then the other. A customized stimulus grid may be designed to evaluate a specific number of points located at varying degrees from fixation. The patient must actively collaborate with the provider during the examination by pressing a button each time a light stimulus is perceived in various positions on a screen. Some devices provide auditory feedback if the patient's eyes move out of alignment. Regardless of this feedback, the technician should continue to optimize alignment throughout the examination. This also applies to adjusting the plane of focus. Although many devices will auto-focus, auto-align, and have automatic grid placement, manual input is necessary to ensure the optimal focus and alignment are achieved at the most accurate sensitivity.

The total duration of evaluation (for both eyes) is approximately 25 minutes. If consecutive tests are being performed, a few minutes of rest between the tests may be beneficial to the patient to minimize the effect of fatigue. Additionally, the accuracy of microperimetry can be improved if the patient receives adequate instruction and practice.

29.4.3 Fixation Testing

Microperimetry devices use fixation testing to measure the ability of the eye to fixate on the preferred retinal locus (PRL). In patients who lose central fixation automatically, the next preferred spot is known as the PRL. The provider can instruct the patients to find the PRL quickly (e.g., using flashcards) once the scotoma location, position, and size relative to the PRL have been identified. Providers can then estimate fixation stability at the PRL, which can direct intervention to improve functional vision. Using fixation testing, the precision of eye fixation on a target can be evaluated, and fixation can be measured at a location up to 25 times per second [14]. During testing, landmarks in the retina are tracked and then plotted as fixation points over an image of the fundus, revealing the portion of the retina used to see the stimulus (Fig. 29.2) [15].

29.4.4 Photopic, Scotopic, and Mesopic Conditions

The relative contributions of rods and cones to vision vary across changing light intensities, with most vision being mediated by the cone (photopic) system and the rod (scotopic) system contributing to the low-light vision. However, rods comprise nearly 95% of retinal photoreceptors and cones comprise less than 5%. The properties of rods and cones are isolated in microperimetry by the selection of background luminance. Conventional microperimetry is typically performed under mesopic or twilight conditions in a dim but not completely dark room. The rod versus cone function can be evaluated under photopic, scotopic, or mesopic conditions by selecting the background luminance.

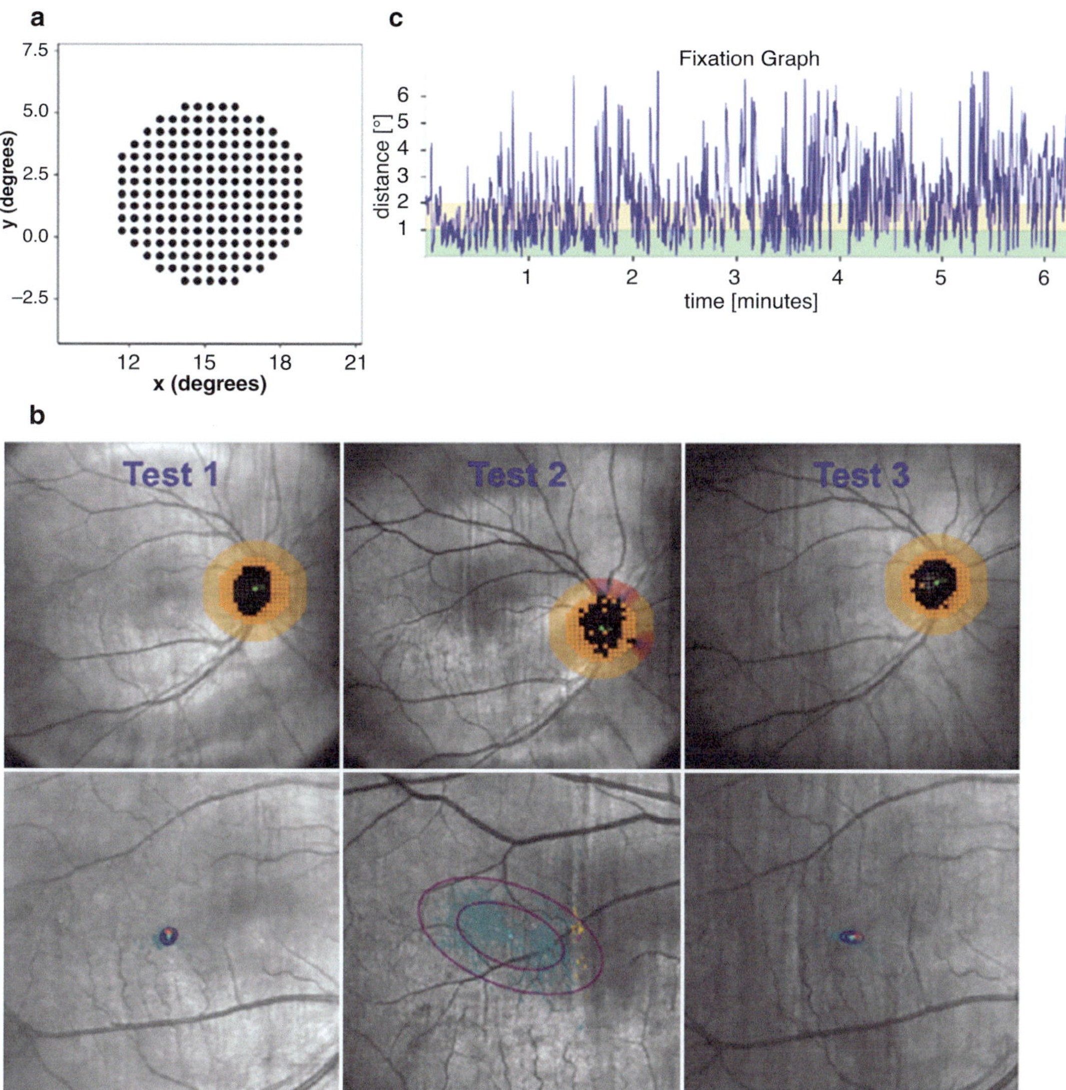

Fig. 29.2 Fixation in a healthy subject. (**a**) Custom 181-point grid pattern with 0.5° spacing. (**b**) Three consecutive examinations for an example participant: *left*, *middle*, and *right* with fixation on the target, fixation off the target, and repeat fixation on the target, respectively. (**c**) Time-series fixation graph detailing eye position throughout testing. (Reprinted with permission from Josan et al. [15] Copyright 2023, Association for Research in Vision and Ophthalmology)

29.4.5 Follow-Up

Follow-up testing can be performed on the same area of the retina using the same parameters as previous tests. By re-measuring the same anatomical locations, changes in sensitivity and fixation allow researchers to evaluate disease progression and/or assessment of treatment outcomes. It is important to remember that comparing fixation stability between machines is unreliable due to inherent differences in stimulus/background contrasts and tracking frequency (Table 29.1).

29.5 Clinical Application and Interpretation

Microperimetry is the technique of choice to assess residual visual function. It has been used to study macular degenerative diseases, including age-related macular degeneration, diabetic macular edema, hereditary retinal dystrophies, and macular dystrophies. This tool is also beneficial for the visual rehabilitation of people with low vision, as its software can be used to train eccentric fixation and stimulate a new preferred point of view [16]. Additionally, microperimetry can quantitatively examine the retina and allow early surgical treatment of macular diseases, such as retinal detachment and epiretinal membrane. In this section, we provide an overview of the clinical application of microperimetry in completed clinical studies and trials.

29.5.1 Age-Related Macular Degeneration

Age-related macular degeneration (AMD) is caused by damage to the macula. Globally, it is the leading cause of blindness in adults over 50 [17]. This disease is categorized into neovascular (wet) and non-neovascular (dry) AMD, with the former referring to the late stage of the disease. The current first-line treatment for neovascular AMD (nAMD) is anti-vascular endothelial growth factor (anti-VEGF) injections. Although OCT has been used to locate fluid in the macula and direct treatment, [18] this technique does not provide information about the retinal function. Microperimetry is a diagnostic technique that can be used to evaluate the function of the retina in people with AMD.

29.5.1.1 Neovascular Age-Related Macular Degeneration

This progressive retinal degenerative disease is characterized by neovascularization of the choroid [19]. The progression of the disease is slow and may not be associated with a loss of vision [20]. Available evidence suggests that an important predictor for visual outcomes in nAMD following treatment with anti-VEGF is the interval between symptom onset and the initiation of treatment [21]. By identifying early changes in the retina, such as fluid in the intraretinal and/or subretinal space, treatments can be initiated earlier, improving the patient's long-term visual outcomes. Microperimetry studies have evaluated improvements in retinal sensitivity and changes in scotoma size following anti-VEGF treatment [22].

An early loss in macular function can be detected by microperimetry before the development of significant visual impairment and has been reported as a predictor of the progression of AMD to the advanced neovascular stage [23]. Other studies have used microperimetry to detect changes in retinal sensitivity in asymptomatic AMD and have measured a statistically significant improvement in retinal sensitivity within treatment-naïve cohorts [20, 22]. These findings, and those reported in anti-VEGF studies, may be subjective because there is a learning curve with microperimetry in which retinal sensitivity can improve with repeat testing [24].

Larger studies, such as the Laser Intervention in Early Stages of AMD (LEAD) study, used microperimetry to detect the onset of nAMD [25]. Although microperimetry was the best method to detect nAMD in this study, further findings revealed no significant difference between microperimetry and best corrected visual acuity in detecting the onset of nAMD due to low sensitivity ranges (between 11% and 35%) [25]. Other studies found that scotopic sensitivity is a better functional indicator for evaluating early and intermediate AMD progression than mesopic sensitivity [26]. Although scotopic microperimetry takes longer and requires prior dark adaptation, this method is more sensitive in detecting and differentiating changes in rod and cone cells [26]. Conversely, mesopic microperimetry was better than scotopic perimetry in predicting AMD progression through morphological changes [27]. Both scotopic and mesopic testing were more sensitive to changes during early AMD than intermediate or advanced AMD [27].

Larger longitudinal studies are needed to continue tracking the progression of AMD using microperimetry. Although it is a useful tool in evaluating changes in the early stages of AMD, the ability to detect such changes using microperimetry can be improved by using patient-tailored perimetry patterns that allow for an increased density of test points [7, 12].

29.5.1.2 Non-Neovascular Age-Related Macular Degeneration and Geographic Atrophy

Microperimetry has frequently been used as an alternative to best corrected visual acuity (BCVA) to measure the foci of geographic atrophy (GA) (Fig. 29.3). These foci often present as foveal-sparing scotomas in non-neovascular AMD [12]. Multiple studies have used this technique to determine the number of scotomatous loci and the mean sensitivity of the macula as an alternative to BCVA [28]. One of the first known studies assessing macular function using microperimetry examined the eye following lutein supplementation in patients with non-neovascular AMD [29]. Microperimetry measurements demonstrated a tendency toward improvement in macular function although the effect did not reach statistical significance [29]. Other assessments of retinal sensitivity using microperimetry are subthreshold laser treatment for GA secondary to AMD, [30] retinal sensitivity at different stages of AMD [31], and following administration of medications such as elamipretide [32].

29.5.2 Diabetic Retinopathy and Diabetic Macular Edema

The long-term effects of diabetes mellitus can lead to diabetic retinopathy (DR), causing damage to the retina and, potentially, blindness [33]. Diabetes is associated with asymptomatic vascular damage that can progress before clinical signs appear. Proposed tests to detect early functional and structural abnormalities in DR include optical coherence tomography (OCT) and OCT-angiography (OCT-A), multifocal electroretinography, contrast sensitivity, low-luminance visual acuity, and microperimetry [34]. Eyes with DR or diabetic macular edema (DME) can have normal visual acuity despite reduced retinal sensitivity, suggesting that changes in sensitivity may precede reductions in visual acuity (Fig. 29.4) [35].

Functional testing of macular sensitivity using microperimetry can assess disease severity and response to therapy by quantifying functional loss due to extrafoveal macular edema or ischemic diabetic maculopathy. Studies using microperimetry have demonstrated that patients with DR have significant loss of retinal sensitivity as compared to healthy individuals ($p < 0.001$); the decrease in sensitivity is more apparent with increasing severity of DR. [36] The decline in retinal sensitivity has been correlated with the decreased thickness of the nerve fiber layer, [37] the photoreceptor layer measured by OCT, [37] and the severity of neuropathy [38]. However, other studies have found only a weak association between the structural and functional deficits in early-stage DR, suggesting that other mechanisms, in addition to retinal thinning, may underlie the functional defects [39].

Most microperimetry studies for DR and diabetic maculopathy are done with pre-established patterns that study 20° of central vision. Other studies created a customized grid that was superimposed with OCT-A. Although this method offers point-to-point structural and functional correlations for a detailed evaluation, the findings have been inconsistent; this may be due to differences in the test populations and the instruments used [40]. Microperimetry can also detect decreased retinal sensitivity in patients without macular edema, without DR, and in pre-diabetics.

29.5.3 Stargardt's Disease

Stargardt's disease type 1 (STGD1) is the most common cause of juvenile macular dystrophy caused by biallelic mutations in the *ABCA4* gene. An early diagnosis may be established using multimodal imaging, but patients can be easily misdiagnosed and subjected to multiple tests and

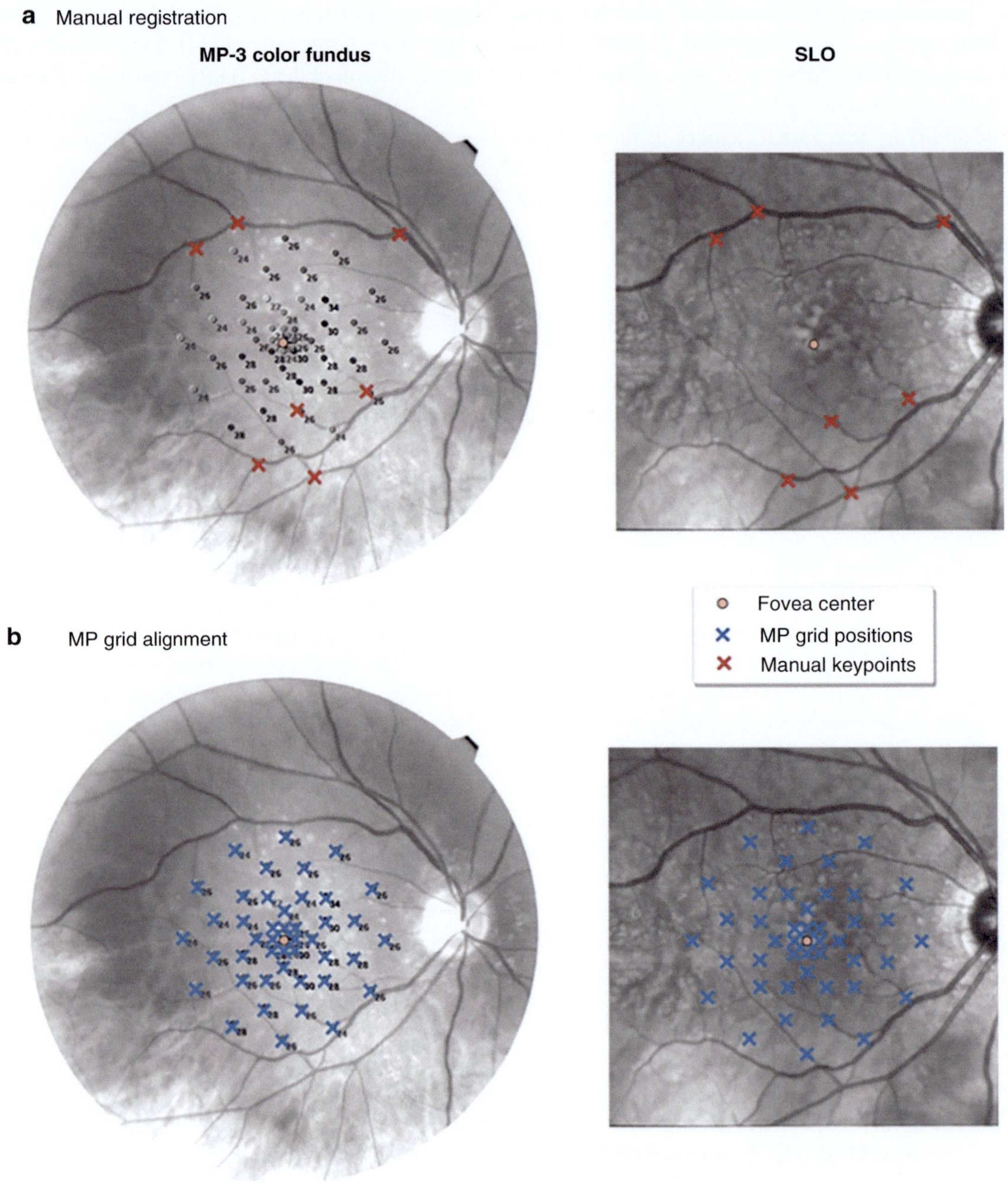

Fig. 29.3 Aligning microperimetry with scanning laser ophthalmoscopy (SLO) image to measure retinal sensitivity in in dry AMD. (**a**) User-selected key points in the color fundus photograph (CFP) and at the same anatomic location in the SLO (red crosses) to align CFP with SLO. (**b**) Fovea center position and scaling of the grid were manually set such that microperimetry measurement locations matched with CFP (left). Final locations are presented on SLO to the user for validation (right). (Reprinted with permission from Reiter et al. [31] Copyright 2023, Springer Nature)

therapies. Typical disease progression spares the peri-capillary and foveal regions and presents with bilateral central vision loss with variable degrees of macular atrophy. As such, BCVA is insufficient in quantifying the functional loss over time. The visual function outcomes generated by microperimetry have been used in Stargardt's disease treatment trials, specifically to

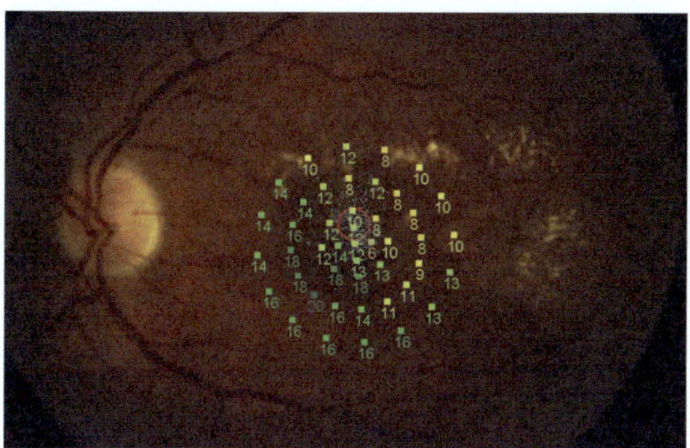

Fig. 29.4 Aligning microperimetry with a scanning laser ophthalmoscopy (SLO) image to measure retinal sensitivity in diabetic macular edema (in decibels). The microperimetry image is superimposed onto the color fundus image in a case of clinically significant diabetic macular edema. A decrease in retinal sensitivity is seen on the temporal side of the macular region (Reprinted with permission from Midena E, and Vujosevic S [35] Copyright 2011, Saudi Ophthalmological Society; Elsevier)

collect data on live eye tracking and to measure macular sensitivity quantitatively [41]. Of these, the Natural History of the Progression of Atrophy Secondary to Stargardt's Disease (ProgStar) studies comprise the largest collection of data evaluating the progression of this disease [42].

Macular sensitivity loss under mesopic conditions has been reported in Stargardt using data from microperimetry [42]. Findings from the ProgStar studies revealed a clinically significant annual change in macular sensitivity of −0.68 dB per year using an MP-1, [42] which was not much lower than the −1.19 dB/year change reported by others [42]. The stability of fixation remained unchanged. Unlike previous studies that have reported associations between early disease onset, long duration, and increasing age with unstable fixation, lower sensitivity, and higher scotoma count, the ProgStar 12-month follow-up study only showed a change in the number of deep scotomas with a decrease in macular sensitivity [42]. The mean reduction in light sensitivity was higher with increasing distance from the fovea, considering the number of regions tested.

Following these reports, the Scotopic Microperimetric Assessment of Rod Function in Stargardt's Disease (SMART) study also used microperimetry to assess macular function loss under scotopic conditions [41]. Data from this study suggested that the loss of scotopic macular function occurs faster (−1.42 dB/year) than mesopic (−0.63 dB/year) macular function in the extrafoveal region, potentially making it a more sensitive outcome measure. As rods progressively decline from the fourth decade of life, studies on AMD have shown dark-adapted dysfunction that can be attributed to the rod system [43]. Although AMD and STGD1 differ, overlapping pathogenic features linked to light exposure suggest potential benefits in testing scotopic visual function using microperimetry for both conditions. As such, specific therapies can have selective effects on the rod versus cone system. Other studies have continued to evaluate the progression of STGD1 using microperimetry. In some of these, high spatial density sampling was used for the functional evaluation of the transition zones between the centrally diseased retina and the less diseased pericentral retina [44]. This may allow for faster detection of the transition zone if there is a statistically significant expansion.

As it most commonly affects children, microperimetry in STGD1 may be challenging to perform in less cooperative patients. However, studies have demonstrated reliable microperimetry values in children above 9 years of age [45]. Challenges with attentiveness and fixation can reduce or remove this reliability. Further studies are needed on optimizing grids, alignment, and eye-tracking systems for accurate co-registration of the retinal examination modalities and microperimetry.

29.5.4 Retinitis Pigmentosa

Retinitis pigmentosa (RP) constitutes a group of retinal disorders that typically presents bilaterally and is caused by mutations in the *RPGR* gene. This condition clinically manifests as nyctalopia due to rode-cone dystrophy, followed by a narrowing of visual fields. Visual acuity is typically preserved due to its dependence on the central fovea. Consequently, BCVA is inadequate in monitoring the progression of this set of diseases.

Instead, microperimetry can be used to isolate the function of rods versus cones by altering background luminance within the photopic (cone function), mesopic (mostly cone function), and scotopic (rod function) ranges. By evaluating rod and cone function throughout the natural history of the disease, the disease response to novel therapies can be compared under mesopic and scotopic conditions.

Data collected in the Photoreceptor Cell Death in Retinitis Pigmentosa Retrospective (PREP-1) study assessed visual acuity, fixation stability, and mean and regional sensitivity annually over 1–4 years [46]. Although no significant changes were detected in visual acuity or fixation stability, all retinal sensitivity parameters showed a significant decline in mean sensitivity of 0.4 dB per year [46]. In this study, the functional features of test loci directly adjacent (horizontally or vertically) to the point of absolute scotoma were measured and referred to as the "edge of scotoma" (ES). Other studies have also used MAIA microperimetry to measure ES sensitivity in *USH2A* retinopathy and have proposed that the greater rates of decline present in ES with a greater area of retinal coverage may require shorter trial periods to optimize the detection of change [28]. The *USH2A*-related Retinal Degeneration (RUSH2A) study compared microperimetry with spectral domain OCT and found that longer disease duration was correlated with more severe retinal structure and function abnormalities such as smaller ellipsoid zone ($p < 0.001$) and lower mean sensitivity ($p < 0.01$) [47].

29.5.5 Other Clinical Applications of Microperimetry

Microperimetry has been widely used to study many retinal disorders in addition to those mentioned in this chapter. This technique has been used to characterize scotoma features in a large cohort with macular telangectasia type 2 (MacTel) as a part of the MacTel Project [48]. Additional studies have used microperimetry to detect anatomical and functional changes in patients with macular epiretinal membrane, macular hole, choroideremia, retinal detachment, retinal vein occlusion, and vitreomacular traction, among others.

29.6 Conclusion

In summary, continuous visualization of the retina using microperimetry allows for (1) the detection of retinal sensitivity in people without stable fixation, (2) the relationship between structure and function, and (3) improved retest reliability at the same location [7]. As a precise diagnostic technique, microperimetry allows the visualization of the 5 mm diameter of the central area of the retina, and small scotomas can be detected. These "blind spots" would otherwise go unnoticed if the retina was visualized using conventional tests. Microperimetry can be a valuable tool for evaluating retinal and macular function, and the field has made great progress over the past 50 years. Current studies have demonstrated the practical applications of this tool in detecting disease onset and progression. However, further research is needed to address present challenges before it becomes a part of routine clinical examinations.

Funding None.

Disclosure None.

References

1. Ivanišević M, Stanić R, Ivanišević P, Vuković A. Albrecht von Graefe (1828–1870) and his contributions to the development of ophthalmology. Int Ophthalmol. 2020;40:1029–33.
2. Fankhauser F, Koch P, Roulier A. On automation of perimetry. Albrecht Von Graefes Arch Klin Exp Ophthalmol. 1972;184(2):126–50.
3. Tagami Y. Correlations between atrophy of Maculopapillar bundles and visual functions in cases of optic neuropathies. In: Greve EL, editor. Third international visual field symposium Tokyo, may 3–6, 1978. Dordrecht: Springer Netherlands; 1979. p. 17–26.
4. Webb RH, Hughes GW, Pomerantzeff O. Flying spot TV ophthalmoscope. Appl Opt. 1980;19(17):2991–7.
5. Mainster MA, Timberlake GT, Webb RH, Hughes GW. Scanning laser ophthalmoscopy. Clin Appl Ophthalmol. 1982;89(7):852–7.

6. Rohrschneider K, Springer C, Bültmann S, Völcker HE. Microperimetry—comparison between the micro perimeter 1 and scanning laser ophthalmoscope—fundus perimetry. Am J Ophthalmol. 2005;139(1):125–34.
7. Pfau M, Jolly JK, Wu Z, Denniss J, Lad EM, Guymer RH, et al. Fundus-controlled perimetry (microperimetry): application as outcome measure in clinical trials. Prog Retin Eye Res. 2021;82:100907.
8. Josan AS, Buckley TMW, Wood LJ, Jolly JK, Cehajic-Kapetanovic J, MacLaren RE. Microperimetry Hill of vision and volumetric measures of retinal sensitivity. Transl Vis Sci Technol. 2021;10(7):12.
9. Han RC, Gray JM, Han J, Maclaren RE, Jolly JK. Optimisation of dark adaptation time required for mesopic microperimetry. Br J Ophthalmol. 2019;103(8):1092–8.
10. Ruofan Connie H, Joanna Monika G, Jennie H, Robert EM, Jasleen KJ. Optimisation of dark adaptation time required for mesopic microperimetry. Br J Ophthalmol. 2019;103(8):1092.
11. Montesano G, Naska TK, Higgins BE, Wright DM, Hogg RE, Crabb DP. Determinants of test variability in scotopic Microperimetry: effects of dark adaptation and test indices. Transl Vis Sci Technol. 2021;10(1):26.
12. Pfau M, Müller PL, von der Emde L, Lindner M, Möller PT, Fleckenstein M, et al. Mesopic and dark-adapted two-color fundus-controlled perimetry in geographic atrophy secondary to age-related macular degeneration. Retina. 2020;40(1):169–80.
13. Wu Z, Ayton LN, Luu CD, Guymer RH. Relationship between retinal microstructures on optical coherence tomography and Microperimetry in age-related macular degeneration. Ophthalmology. 2014;121(7):1445–52.
14. Morales MU, Saker S, Wilde C, Pellizzari C, Pallikaris A, Notaroberto N, et al. Reference clinical database for fixation stability metrics in Normal subjects measured with the MAIA microperimeter. Transl Vis Sci Technol. 2016;5(6):6.
15. Josan AS, Farrance I, Taylor LJ, Adeyoju D, Buckley TMW, Jolly JK, et al. Microperimetry reliability assessed from fixation performance. Transl Vis Sci Technol. 2023;12(5):21.
16. Chiang WY, Lee JJ, Chen YH, Chen CH, Chen YJ, Wu PC, et al. Fixation behavior in macular dystrophy assessed by microperimetry. Graefes Arch Clin Exp Ophthalmol. 2018;256(8):1403–10.
17. Pennington KL, DeAngelis MM. Epidemiology of age-related macular degeneration (AMD): associations with cardiovascular disease phenotypes and lipid factors. Eye Vis (Lond). 2016;3:34.
18. Metrangolo C, Donati S, Mazzola M, Fontanel L, Messina W, D'Alterio G, et al. OCT biomarkers in Neovascular age-related macular degeneration: a narrative review. J Ophthalmol. 2021;2021:9994098.
19. Pugazhendhi A, Hubbell M, Jairam P, Ambati B. Neovascular macular degeneration: a review of etiology, risk factors, and recent advances in research and therapy. Int J Mol Sci. 2021;22(3):1170.
20. Wightman AJ, Abbott CJ, McGuinness MB, Caruso E, Guymer RH, Luu CD. Presymptomatic retinal sensitivity changes in intermediate age-related macular degeneration associated with new retinal fluid. Translational vision. Sci Technol. 2019;8(6):3.
21. Finger RP, Wickremasinghe SS, Baird PN, Guymer RH. Predictors of anti-VEGF treatment response in neovascular age-related macular degeneration. Surv Ophthalmol. 2014;59(1):1–18.
22. Asahi MG, Wallsh J, Onishi SM, Kuroyama S, Gallemore RP. Multifocal ERG and Microperimetry changes in response to Ranibizumab treatment of Neovascular AMD: randomized phase 2 open-label study. Clin Ophthalmol. 2020;14:3599–610.
23. Dinc UA, Yenerel M, Gorgun E, Oncel M. Assessment of macular function by Microperimetry in intermediate age-related macular degeneration. Eur J Ophthalmol. 2008;18(4):595–600.
24. Wu Z, Ayton LN, Guymer RH, Luu CD. Intrasession test-retest variability of microperimetry in age-related macular degeneration. Invest Ophthalmol Vis Sci. 2013;54(12):7378–85.
25. Wu Z, Luu CD, Hodgson LAB, Caruso E, Chen FK, Chakravarthy U, et al. Using microperimetry and low-luminance visual acuity to detect the onset of late age-related macular degeneration: a LEAD study report. Retina. 2021;41(5):1094–101.
26. Madheswaran G, Nasim P, Ballae Ganeshrao S, Raman R, Ve RS. Role of microperimetry in evaluating disease progression in age-related macular degeneration: a scoping review. Int Ophthalmol. 2022;42(6):1975–86.
27. Montesano G, Ometto G, Higgins BE, Iester C, Balaskas K, Tufail A, et al. Structure-function analysis in macular Drusen with Mesopic and scotopic Microperimetry. Transl Vis Sci Technol. 2020;9(13):43.
28. Charng J, Lamey TM, Thompson JA, McLaren TL, Attia MS, McAllister IL, et al. Edge of scotoma sensitivity as a Microperimetry clinical trial end point in USH2A Retinopathy. Transl Vis Sci Technol. 2020;9(10):9.
29. Weigert G, Kaya S, Pemp B, Sacu S, Lasta M, Werkmeister RM, et al. Effects of lutein supplementation on macular pigment optical density and visual acuity in patients with age-related macular degeneration. Invest Ophthalmol Vis Sci. 2011;52(11):8174–8.
30. Querques G, Sacconi R, Gelormini F, Borrelli E, Prascina F, Zucchiatti I, et al. Subthreshold laser treatment for reticular pseudodrusen secondary to age-related macular degeneration. Sci Rep. 2021;11(1):2193.
31. Reiter GS, Bogunovic H, Schlanitz F, Vogl W-D, Seeböck P, Ramazanova D, et al. Point-to-point associations of drusen and hyperreflective foci volumes with retinal sensitivity in non-exudative age-related macular degeneration. Eye. 2023;37(17):3582–8.

32. Allingham MJ, Mettu PS, Cousins SW. Phase 1 clinical trial of Elamipretide in intermediate age-related macular degeneration and high-risk Drusen: ReCLAIM high-risk Drusen study. Ophthalmol Sci. 2022;2(1):100095.
33. Shukla UV, Tripathy K. Diabetic Retinopathy. Treasure Island (FL): StatPearls; 2023.
34. Cheung CMG, Pearce E, Fenner B, Sen P, Chong V, Sivaprasad S. Looking ahead: visual and anatomical endpoints in future trials of diabetic macular ischemia. Ophthalmologica. 2021;244(5):451–64.
35. Midena E, Vujosevic S. Microperimetry in diabetic retinopathy. Saudi J Ophthalmol. 2011;25(2):131–5.
36. Nittala MG, Gella L, Raman R, Sharma T. Measuring retinal sensitivity with the microperimeter in patients with diabetes. Retina. 2012;32(7):1302–9.
37. Orduna-Hospital E, Otero-Rodríguez J, Perdices L, Sánchez-Cano A, Boned-Murillo A, Acha J, et al. Microperimetry and optical coherence tomography changes in Type-1 diabetes mellitus without Retinopathy. Diagnostics (Basel). 2021;11(1):136.
38. Neriyanuri S, Pardhan S, Gella L, Pal SS, Ganesan S, Sharma T, et al. Retinal sensitivity changes associated with diabetic neuropathy in the absence of diabetic retinopathy. Br J Ophthalmol. 2017;101(9):1174–8.
39. Park JC, Chen YF, Liu M, Liu K, McAnany JJ. Structural and functional abnormalities in early-stage diabetic Retinopathy. Curr Eye Res. 2020;45(8):975–85.
40. Cheung CMG, Fawzi A, Teo KYC, Fukuyama H, Sen S, Tsai W-S, et al. Diabetic macular ischaemia—a new therapeutic target? Prog Retin Eye Res. 2022;89:101033.
41. Kong X, Ibrahim-Ahmed M, Bittencourt MG, Strauss RW, Birch DG, Cideciyan AV, et al. Longitudinal changes in scotopic and Mesopic macular function as assessed with Microperimetry in patients with Stargardt disease.: SMART Study Report No. 2. Am J Ophthalmol. 2022;236:32–44.
42. Schönbach EM, Strauss RW, Muñoz B, Wolfson Y, Ibrahim MA, Birch DG, et al. Longitudinal Microperimetric changes of macular sensitivity in Stargardt disease after 12 months: ProgStar report no. 13. JAMA Ophthalmol. 2020;138(7):772–9.
43. Curcio CA, Medeiros NE, Millican CL. Photoreceptor loss in age-related macular degeneration. Invest Ophthalmol Vis Sci. 1996;37(7):1236–49.
44. Cideciyan AV, Swider M, Aleman TS, Feuer WJ, Schwartz SB, Russell RC, et al. Macular function in macular degenerations: repeatability of Microperimetry as a potential outcome measure for ABCA4-associated Retinopathy trials. Invest Ophthalmol Vis Sci. 2012;53(2):841–52.
45. Jones PR, Yasoubi N, Nardini M, Rubin GS. Feasibility of macular integrity assessment (MAIA) Microperimetry in children: sensitivity, reliability, and fixation stability in healthy observers. Invest Ophthalmol Vis Sci. 2016;57(14):6349–59.
46. Iftikhar M, Kherani S, Kaur R, Lemus M, Nefalar A, Usmani B, et al. Progression of retinitis Pigmentosa as measured on Microperimetry: the PREP-1 study. Ophthalmol Retina. 2018;2(5):502–7.
47. Lad EM, Duncan JL, Liang W, Maguire MG, Ayala AR, Audo I, et al. Baseline Microperimetry and OCT in the RUSH2A study: structure−function association and correlation with disease severity. Am J Ophthalmol. 2022;244:98–116.
48. Vujosevic S, Heeren TFC, Florea D, Leung I, Pauleikhoff D, Sallo F, et al. Scotoma characteristics in macular telangiectasia type 2: MacTel project report no. 7—the MacTel research group. Retina. 2018;38:S14–S9.

30 Adaptive Optics

Kara R. Grimes and Jay Chhablani

30.1 Introduction

Adaptive optics (AO) is used for in vivo visualization of individual cells in the retina; historically, this was only possible using in vitro histological methods. Today, AO imaging systems use active optical elements to correct wavefront aberrations in retinal technologies such as the flood-illumination fundus camera, scanning laser ophthalmoscopy (SLO), and optical coherence tomography (OCT). This tool also provides advanced lateral resolution, which facilitates the visualization of photoreceptors, retinal vasculature, and the optic nerve head. This chapter will highlight the history, technology, techniques, and application of AO, as well as the advantages and limitations of implementing AO imaging in a clinical setting.

30.2 Brief History of Adaptive Optics

The principles of AO were devised by the astronomer Horace Babcock in 1953. This wavefront technology was first applied to astronomy to measure distortions in atmospheric light that caused a severe blurring of the images of distant stars captured by the telescope. Images of stars could be refined with diffraction-limited performance through AO [1]. These principles were then used later to correct imperfections in ocular imaging.

In the early 1980s, AO systems were developed to study the human eye with closed-loop controls. These systems helped eliminate aberrations from the eye—such as astigmatisms of the cornea—and made it possible to resolve individual receptors on the fovea. Further research and investigations in the following decade led Liang et al. (1997) to apply these principles to retinal imaging and overcome higher order aberrations, thereby "providing normal eyes with supernormal optical quality." [2] Using AO with Shack-Hartmann wavefront sensors and deformable mirrors, Liang et al. (1997) could visualize single cells in a living human retina [2]. Soon after, AO was used to visualize retinal blood vessels by Burns et al. (2002) and assess cone-rod dystrophy by Roorda (2000) [3, 4]. Currently, AO technology is used to visualize and understand the pathophysiology of diseases that affect the retinal vasculature, individual photoreceptors, retinal pigment epithelial cells, and ganglion cells; it is also used to monitor cellular-level responses to therapeutic interventions.

K. R. Grimes
New York Medical College, New York, USA

J. Chhablani (✉)
Department of Ophthalmology, University of Pittsburgh, Pittsburgh, PA, USA

T. Das, P. Satgunam (eds.), *Ophthalmic Diagnostics*, https://doi.org/10.1007/978-981-97-0138-4_30

30.3 Technology

Optical or wavefront aberrations are irregularities in the eye that can lead to distorted images and decreased visual performance. In recent years, AO has been used to create various measurement devices to assess the refractive properties of the eye [5]. To obtain images with improved resolution and sensitivity, most AO-based devices must contain three main components (Fig. 30.1), namely,

1. *Wavefront sensor*—It is required to measure ocular aberrations. The apparatus will direct a small beam of light into the eye that backscatters off the retina. The resulting light that leaves the eye will be aberrated by the optics of the eye and measured by the wavefront sensor. The most common method for measuring ocular aberrations is with the Shack-Hartmann wavefront sensor, which uses a microlenslet array.
2. *Wavefront corrector*—Typically, it is a deformable mirror based on electromagnetic actuation that can alter its shape to compensate for the measured aberration.
3. *Controller*—The control system is a computer that regulates the interaction between the wavefront sensor and the wavefront collector. The controller can measure and compute signals for the wavefront corrector using the appropriate software.

30.3.1 Quantitative Measurement of Ocular Aberrations

The angular resolution and efficiency of light collection of the optical system are improved with AO. Mathematically, the wavefront aberrations in human eyes are defined by Zernike polynomials. This method classifies the shape of aberration

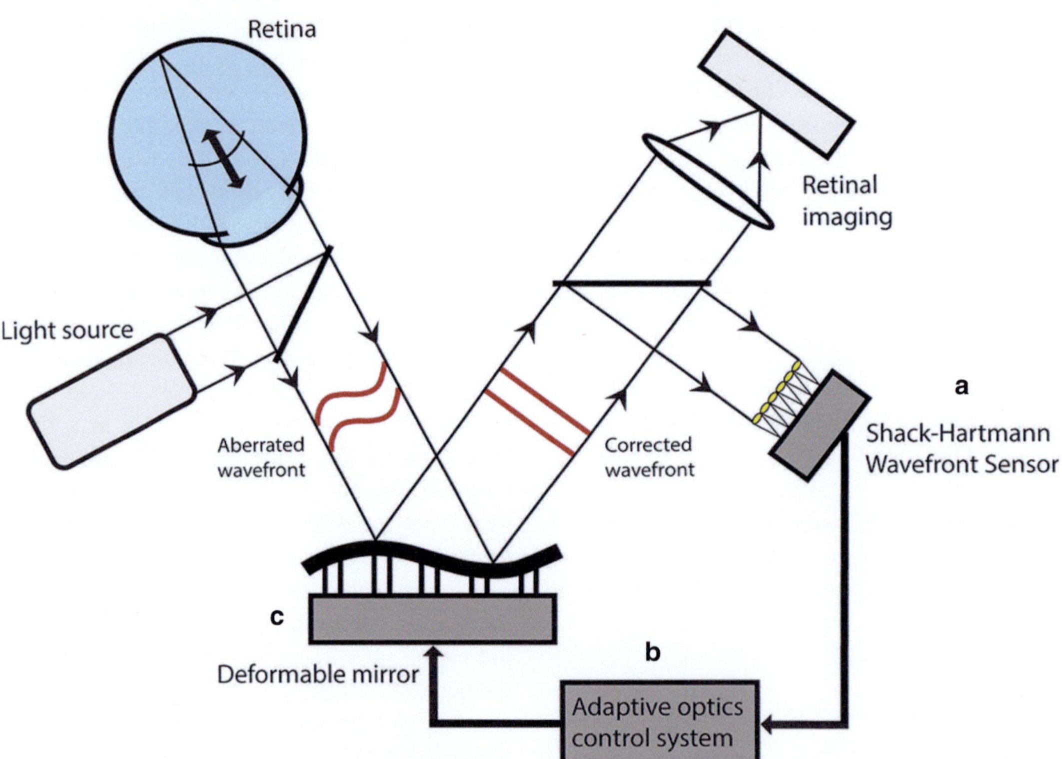

Fig. 30.1 Schematic diagram of an optics-assisted retinal imaging system. The aberrated wavefront is measured using the wavefront sensor (**a**), and the system compensates for the aberration using a wavefront corrector (**c**). The wavefront sensor and corrector are connected by a control system (**b**). (Reprinted with permission from Gill et al. [6] Copyright 2022, Springer Nature)

maps as the sum of fundamental shapes or basic functions and can be further classified into lower order or higher order aberrations. Lower order aberrations make up a majority of aberrations that can be corrected with glasses, contact lenses, or refractive surgery (e.g., myopia, hyperopia, and astigmatism). Higher order aberrations are more complex and can contribute to nyctalopia, glare, and halos. This phenomenon of aberration is simplified into a single number using AO through the calculation of root mean squares (RMS), as described by Jayabalan et al. (2019) [1]. The RMS wavefront error is calculated directly from the Zernike polynomials to find the mean squared value of the wavefront over the pupil. In this equation, A is the area of the pupil, and $\bar{W}$ is the mean wavefront optical path difference to define RMS:

$$RMS = \sqrt{\frac{\iint \left[W(x,y) - \bar{W}\right]^2 dx\, dy}{A}}$$

Additionally, the optical aberration index (OAI) is calculated to determine if the optical system is perfect (OAI = 0) or has infinite aberrations (OAI = 1). The OAI is calculated using the RMS value and is defined as:

$$OAI = 1 - e^{(-RMS)}$$

The point spread function and modulation transfer function are also calculated to measure imaging waves from a point source and to characterize the resolution of an imaging system, respectively [6]. AO can resolve rods and cones in the retina to 2 μm, but there is a substantial difference in determining cones over rods; cones are better resolved, while rods are not, likely due to their smaller size [7]. Typically, the resolution of an imaging system is set by the numerical aperture (NA) of the system, which is defined as:

$$NA = n\sin(\theta)$$

Where n is the index of refraction of the medium and θ is the angle viewed from the retina subtended by distance from the center of the pupil to the pupil margin [8]. The resolution (r) of AO imaging systems is determined using wavelength (λ) and numerical aperture (NA) and is defined as:

$$r = 0.61\lambda / NA$$

The numerical aperture is about 0.23 for a maximally dilated pupil.

30.4 Technique

30.4.1 Retinal Imaging

Imaging the retina using AO is non-invasive but requires a pupillary diameter of at least 4 mm. Most systems require the patient to be positioned comfortably on a conventional chin rest and focus on an internal fixation target. The target can be moved according to the area of interest. Using combined software approaches, this area will then appear on the graphic display, and microscopic structures, such as photoreceptors, may be brought into focus. A template image is used to track relative fine-scale motions of the eye that are captured in each frame of the video [9]. The software will acquire multiple images, of which those with the best contrast are selected and summed together using an auto-correlation algorithm to generate one image [10]. Images with a high signal-to-noise ratio tend to stabilize best [8]. The final image will remove the computed image from the background and be adjusted for brightness and contrast.

30.4.2 Types of AO Imaging Systems

An AO system does not work as a standalone system but operates as a subsystem that must be incorporated into an imaging device. Devices such as SLOs, fundus cameras, and techniques such as OCT have revolutionized in vivo retinal diagnostics to provide a macroscopic view of the retina; this has been invaluable in diagnosing and monitoring the progression of retinal diseases. However, these technologies lack the transverse resolution required to view microscopic retinal structures. Multi-modal imaging combining AO technology with SLO, OCT, and fundus camera systems enables high-fidelity correction of ocular aberration.

30.4.2.1 Adaptive Optics and Flood-Illumination Ophthalmoscopy (AO-FIO)

Fundus photography captures images of the retina in which the illumination and reflectance of the retina occur through the pupil. When combined with AO, flood-illumination ophthalmoscopy (AO-FIO) enables detailed retinal imaging by illuminating the retinal layers with backscattered light. In this technique, a light-emitting diode (LED) is used to illuminate the pupil uniformly, and a guide star (typically a super luminescent diode or SLD) is used to measure and correct aberrations, which are then imaged with a retinal camera.

Using AO-FIO, the contrast is improved, and scanning mirrors are not required to obtain images of retinal microstructures. These images are also acquired in a relatively short time (<10 s), which minimizes the effects of eye movement and operates much faster than the AO-OCT technique. This is especially important when fixation capacity is reduced by retinal disease. Additionally, changing the focus of the camera allows imaging of different layers of the retina by introducing a quadratic phase shift on the deformable mirror [11]. The focus can be calibrated by calculating the average distance between the photoreceptors and the retinal layer of interest [12].

30.4.2.2 Adaptive Optics and Scanning Laser Ophthalmoscopy (AO-SLO)

The AO-SLO system uses confocal laser scanning microscopy to reduce artifacts due to eye motion. In doing so, AO-SLO captures high-resolution motion video of the posterior chamber of the eye using a fast-scanning ophthalmoscope. The advantage of AO-SLO over conventional fundus imaging methods is that it provides a non-invasive method to obtain higher transverse resolution and closer observation of the retina [13].

This technique uses two scanners (one horizontal and one vertical) that are directed to the eye with a photodiode used as the wavefront sensing source. A Shack-Hartmann wavefront sensor and deformable mirror are also present in the optical path for optical aberration correction. Due to its high transverse resolution, this technique can identify/image microscopic structures such as individual photoreceptors, the ganglion cell layer, micro capillaries, and blood flow.

AO-SLO systems can be combined with AO-OCT systems, which obtain images at slower rates (typically several seconds) to create a three-dimensional image. These techniques can be combined with fast-motion videography to capture any eye motion that can be processed post-capture to stabilize the blurring effects that arise during the slower process of capturing AO-OCT images.

30.4.2.3 Adaptive Optics and Optical Coherence Tomography (AO-OCT)

Since OCT provides a scan of the volume of the retina, the combination of AO and optical coherence tomography (AO-OCT) leads to a high transverse and axial resolution. This enables in vivo three-dimensional imaging of cells within the retina with both transverse and axial resolution as small as 2–3 μm, allowing the imaging of individual retina layers [13].

The technique used in AO-OCT is known as low-coherence interferometry, in which a beam of low-coherence light directed at a surface sends reflected light to an interferometer. The major advantage of AO-OCT, when compared to AO-FIO and AO-SLO, is that the axial resolution is determined by the coherence length of the light source and is independent of the system's NA [14]. Additionally, OCT can detect subwavelength changes in the optical path length in the retina that are orders of magnitude smaller than the axial resolution [14]. The benefits of this technique are valuable in studying the pathophysiological process of retinal diseases at the cellular level.

30.4.2.4 Wavefront Sensorless Adaptive Optics (SAO)

In the SAO system, the deformable mirror is not controlled by the measurements of a wavefront sensor; this technique was created to simplify the AO setup. Therefore, SAO uses an adaptive control method of the deformable mirror to determine the aberration and correct turbulence-degraded imaging. Using SAO, the image quality is directly optimized based on the modal deformation of the deformable mirror. The adaptive element is controlled by the image quality metric and search algorithm to change the shape of the mirror [15]. As a result, a compensated wavefront image and fast-adaptive wavefront correction are generated.

The SAO systems have been widely researched in recent years and have been used to study free-space optical communication, inertial confinement fusion, and microscopy. This technique simplifies the optical hardware in AO and reduces equipment costs since the sensor, coupler, and many relay mirrors are not required. However, it requires rapid estimation of the objective function to focus on specific tissue layers. Further applications of SAO have led to the development of handheld AO-SLO systems that enable in vivo imaging of cone photoreceptors (Fig. 30.2) [16]. Handheld systems can also capture retinal images in infants, whereas conventional AO-SLO systems are limited to patients sitting upright and fixating for several minutes.

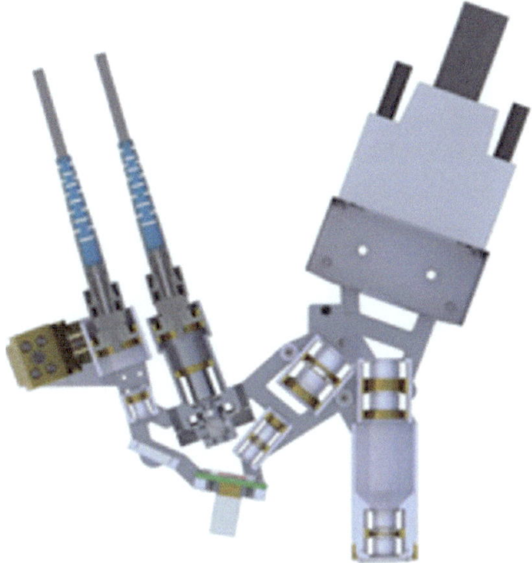

Fig. 30.2 Rendering of the internal skeleton of a handheld sensorless adaptive optics (SAO) system. Dimensions: 10.3 cm × 5.3 cm × 14.4 cm (Reprinted with permission from DuBose et al. [16] Copyright 2018, The Optical Society)

30.5 Clinical Application and Interpretation

Retinal imaging using AO systems allows the direct observation of microscopic structures in the retina. En-face images of the retinal layers show the photoreceptor, retinal vasculature, and retinal nerve fiber layers (Fig. 30.3). Additional image processing methods can be used to improve the quality of these images, and automated routines are continuously being researched to refine the efficiency of these systems.

30.5.1 Healthy Eyes

The early uses of healthy eyes visualized with AO systems included generating a standardized

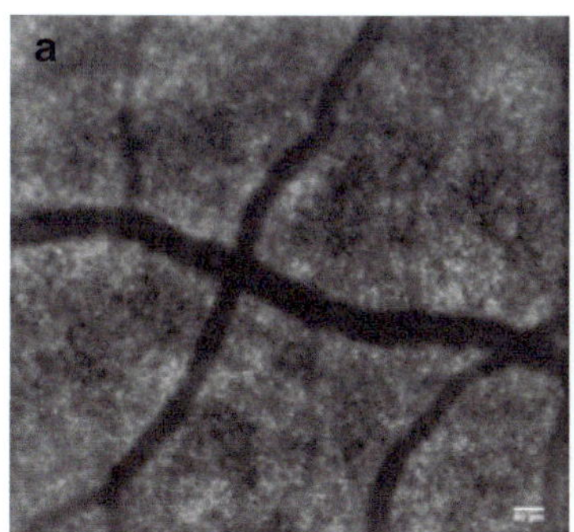

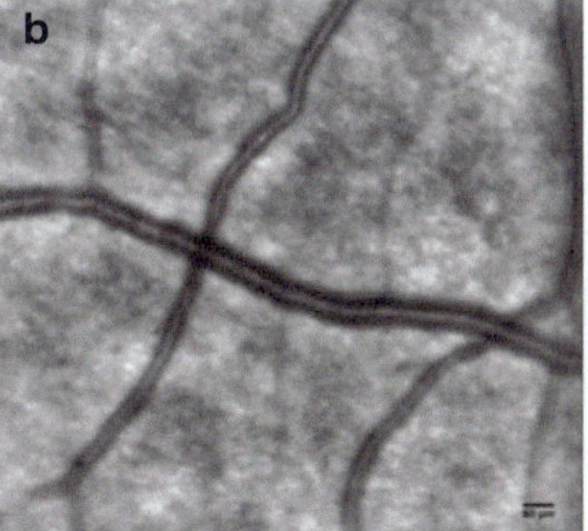

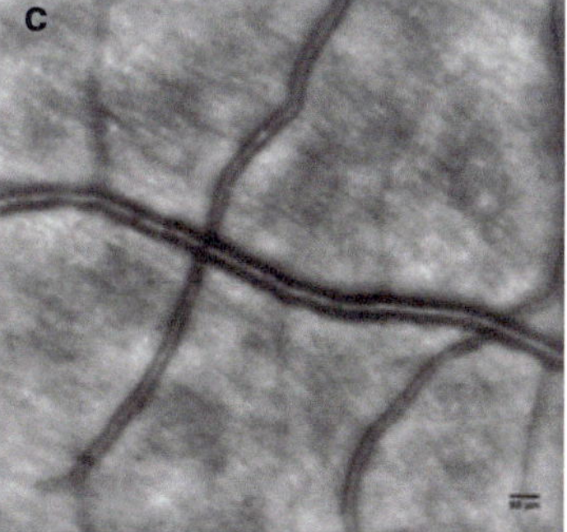

Fig. 30.3 Retinal images obtained using an adaptive optics (AO) system with adaptive compensation of the photoreceptor layer (**a**), vasculature (**b**), and retinal nerve fiber layer (**c**). Scale bars represent 50 μm. Images were captured using a flood-illumination AO retinal camera. (Reprinted with permission from Lombardo et al. [24] Copyright 2013, used under the Creative Commons Attribution 3.0 license)

or normative database. Therefore, any deviations from the norm can be used in clinical practice to describe pathologies. As the techniques using AO continue to improve, additional imaging of healthy eyes is needed to define the evolving norm. Data from healthy eyes are fundamental for characterizing the density, spacing, and brightness of healthy photoreceptor cells in vivo and have been extensively studied in recent years [17, 18]. The AO-OCT system has been used to compare rod and cone morphology in healthy and pathologically aged eyes, revealing the differences in the photoreceptor mosaic. Other studies have used AO-SLO due to its superior spatial resolution compared with perimetry or OCT, to compare retinal nerve fiber bundles in healthy and glaucomatous eyes and the density of foveal cones in healthy eyes and eyes with central serous chorioretinopathy [19]. The following section will discuss some of these.

30.5.2 Age-Related Macular Degeneration (AMD)

Age-related macular degeneration, or AMD, is characterized by the progressive degeneration of photoreceptors and adjacent tissue and the accumulation of extracellular deposits known as drusen bodies in the retinal layers. These characteristics of AMD, in addition to changes in the retinal pigmented epithelium (RPE), can be monitored using AO systems. The promising contributions of AO systems to the diagnosis, monitoring, and research on AMD have helped in exploring the pathophysiology of this condition, identifying novel features in AMD, studying the progression of atrophy, and examining responses to new treatments, particularly for dry AMD.

The AO-FIO system has been used to detect differences in the four main drusen phenotypes: soft drusen, hard drusen, cuticular drusen, and reticular pseudodrusen [20]. Although these drusen bodies are composed of similar components, they are distinguishable through AO imaging due to differences in optical filtering effects, location, and morphology. Research on drusen bodies has also demonstrated that smaller drusen bodies (<30 μm) were more readily detected in gaze-dependent AO images [20] than larger drusen deposits (>30 μm) that could only be seen clinically in fundus photographs. In addition to AO-FIO, AO-SLO has also been used to visualize cone photoreceptors, and these techniques have been used to monitor changes in cone reflectivity with AMD progression [21]. These systems can therefore be used as additional imaging modalities to study visual function in AMD in clinical trials.

Foveal sparing is often observed in AMD when an "island" of intact RPE persists under the fovea amid RPE atrophy. In these cases, slight progression of RPE atrophy towards the fovea can cause severe vision loss. Using AO-FIO, these sensitive areas can be delineated by identifying differences in reflectivity between regions of atrophy and foveal sparing.

The late stage of dry AMD, during which geographic atrophy occurs, is characterized by the degeneration of RPE cells and photoreceptors. As AMD progresses, hyporeflective foci and extensive melanin redistribution occur on OCT angiography (OCTA) and fundoscopic examination, respectively [22]. In AMD, hyporeflective foci are located in atrophic areas and are dispersed along the RPE monolayer. Although functionally and phenotypically normal RPE mosaics can be visualized with current cell culture technology, AO imaging offers useful support in colocalizing lipofuscin and melanin in the transition to geographic atrophy in AMD [23]. The AO system is not yet routinely used to study AMD, but it is useful for visualizing the fate and morphology of individual RPE cells. This can be useful for identifying the origin of hyporeflective foci. However, neovascular (wet) AMD is more difficult to examine with AO systems due to the complex arrangement of lesions and retinal transparency.

30.5.3 Diabetic Retinopathy

The most common and severe complication of uncontrolled diabetes is diabetic retinopathy

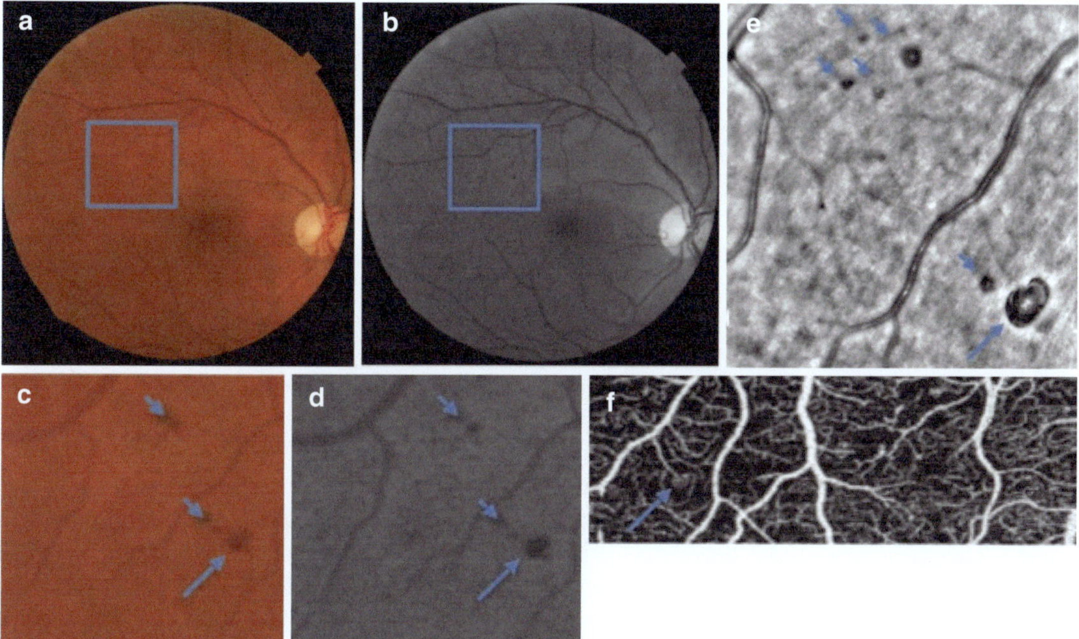

Fig. 30.4 Diabetic retinopathy. Color fundus photo (**a**) and red-free photo (**b**) of a patient with microaneurysms and hemorrhages. Higher magnifications (**c** and **d**) of the area delimited in the previous photos, (**a** and b). The big arrow indicates a microaneurysm, and the arrowheads show hemorrhages. The AO image (**e**) corresponds to (**c** and **d**). The black lesion with inner hyperreflectivity marked by a big arrow is a microaneurysm. The black lesions marked by small arrows are retinal hemorrhages. The OCTA revealed only one lesion (**f**) from the above-mentioned, the microaneurysm. (Reprinted with permission from Cristescu et al. [24] Copyright 2019, used under the Creative Commons Attribution 3.0 license)

(DR), typically characterized by hard exudates, retinal neovascularization, macular edema, and microaneurysms. Fundus photos and OCTA have been used clinically to provide a semi-quantitative assessment of retinal lesions in DR. While these assessments have proved beneficial, optical aberrations from the anterior segment may make viewing small and low-contrast retinal lesions difficult.

Since AO retinal imaging can be used for the precise measurement of photoreceptors, RPE cells, erythrocytes, and ganglion cells, AO-OCT has been used to visualize microvascular lesions, which are the first clinically detectable signs of DR. The technique can also be used to visualize microaneurysms and hemorrhages in patients with DR (Fig. 30.4) [24]. Additionally, AO imaging has been used to visualize hard exudates, decreases in parafoveal cone density (in type 1 DM), [18] and changes in the wall-to-lumen ratios in people with diabetes, but with or without DR. [25]

These imaging techniques, however, are not without their challenges, as confocal AO imaging does not always produce the best structural images of blood vessels. Since AO-FIO produces relatively low-contrast images of the capillaries, this technique makes it challenging to map blood flow [26]. Other methods, such as AO-SLO, have been used to increase the sensitivity of the imaging system to scattered light [26]. In doing so, the use of AO-SLO and motion contrast techniques in people with diabetes (before the onset of DR) has allowed the detection of disruptions in the parafoveal capillaries and arteriovenous channels [27]. Current findings have demonstrated that AO systems may serve as useful screening tools in patients with diabetes mellitus and can also be used in follow-ups to detect the progression of DR by examining changes in the retinal vasculature. Standardized practices, however, are needed to determine the most reliable AO imaging techniques.

30.5.4 Glaucoma

The pathology of glaucoma is complex and multifactorial. One of the earliest detectable changes in glaucoma is axonal tissue loss in the retinal nerve fiber layer (RNFL), which precedes the morphological changes of the optic nerve head. These changes can be detected using OCT. Impaired blood flow to the retina and/or elevated intraocular pressure is associated with damage to the optic nerve and loss of retinal ganglion cells, which can progress to functional defects in the visual field [28]. The sequential order of structural and functional damage in glaucoma suggests that identifying early structural abnormalities in the RNFL or optic nerve using AO imaging can allow an earlier diagnosis of glaucoma [29].

Most commercially available OCT devices cannot discern individual retinal nerve fiber bundles in people with glaucoma. Although AO-SLO, AO-OCT, and AO-FIO [30] have been used to produce high-resolution RNFL and optic nerve images in healthy patients, image resolution in patients with glaucoma is more difficult to obtain [29]. One study has observed the expansion of retinal nerve fiber bundle narrowing in glaucomatous patients using AO-SLO over a short time (1.44 ± 0.42 years) [31]. Despite these findings, fluctuations in the evaluation due to the subjective testing nature of AO require further studies to validate this data. Another study used AO-SLO to distinguish between healthy controls and those with early glaucoma based on RNFL reflectivity. However, there was no clear difference in RNFL damage or RNFL bundles between the controls and patients with early glaucoma in this study. Imaging was moderately successful (in 46% of locations) in patients with moderate to severe glaucoma, but overall, many images across all groups were not discernible [29].

Additional studies using AO-OCT and AO-FIO in people with glaucoma have documented consistent structural changes in cone photoreceptors at locations in the retina where visual sensitivity was compromised. In contrast, another study using AO-SLO demonstrated that cone integrity remained in areas with visual field and nerve fiber loss [32]. The lamina cribrosa is considered the primary site for glaucomatous damage. One study has suggested that quantitative assessment of the lamina cribrosa had good measurement reproducibility (imprecision <4.7% of the mean) to assess longitudinal changes associated with glaucoma [33]. However, as only a few studies have investigated the use of AO imaging in glaucoma, additional research on the use of AO imaging to monitor/study glaucoma is needed.

30.5.5 Retinal Structures Imaged Using Adaptive Optics

Many investigators have used AO to study other retinal diseases. For example, cone photoreceptor loss has been visualized using AO in retinitis pigmentosa, Bietti's crystalline dystrophy, Stargardt's disease, and macular dystrophy. These findings—along with those investigating other retinal structures—have demonstrated the benefits of using AO to stratify patients in clinical trials based on the quantitative or qualitative assessment of retinal structures [7] Table 30.1 shows the clinical significance of imaging various retinal structures using AO systems.

Table 30.1 Clinical significance of AO imaging on the retina

Retinal structure	Clinical significance
Photoreceptors	– Using AO, many retinal diseases show structural changes in the photoreceptor mosaic; these were only detectable at the microscopic level
	Cones – Cones vary in size from ~1.5–8 μm and are specialized for photopic conditions, as well as temporal and spatial high resolution [34] – AO imaging techniques capture the inner segments and improve identification of cone photoreceptors (in comparison to manual processing) [35] – Early detection of retinal pathologies and evaluation of retinal therapies can use cone density and spatial arrangement as promising biomarkers [35]
	Rods – Rods are uniformly sized at ~2 μm and respond to single-photon absorption, comprising scotopic vision [36] – Rods have been more difficult to visualize than cones, probably due to their small size and/or reduced waveguide capabilities, and require optimized confocal AO-SLO, image registration software, and post-imaging processing to be viewed [37] – AO imaging of rods will be useful in pathologies with rod photoreceptor dysfunction (e.g., Usher's syndrome and retinitis pigmentosa)
Retinal vasculature	– The most frequently studied retinal vasculature biomarkers have been the following vessel components: Inner diameter length [38–40] Outer diameter length [38–40] Vessel wall thickness [38] Wall cross-sectional area [38–40] Wall-to-lumen ratio [38–40] – Systemic hypertension is often studied with AO-FIO or AO-SLO Vascular wall is seen more conveniently with AO-FIO than with AO-SLO [41] A meta-analysis showed that inner diameter, vessel wall thickness, and wall-to-lumen ratio were significantly different in hypertensive patients as compared to those in controls [41] – Diabetic retinopathy is most often studied with AO-SLO Capillary diameter and flow velocity are more reliably measured by AO-SLO although AO-FIO can capture images of the capillaries at high speed [41]
Retinal ganglion cells (RGC)/retinal nerve fiber bundles (RNFB)	– RGCs have high optical translucency and have been challenging to image [42] – AO-OCT was the first imaging technique to resolve RGCs in vivo in healthy eyes [42] – Further studies used AO-OCT to demonstrate morphological changes in the RGCs of patients with primary open-angle glaucoma, showing some correlation between structural loss with functional vision loss [43] – AO-SLO has also revealed details of non-homogenous glaucomatous damage in RNFBs [19]
Retinal pigment epithelium (RPE)	– Dysfunction of the RPE is implicated in many retinal diseases, including cone/rod dystrophies, AMD, retinitis pigments, choroideremia, best macular dystrophy, and Stargardt's disease [44] – The first in vivo mosaic of RPE cells was visualized by AO-SLO [44], and other studies have used AO-OCT [45] – Visualizing the RPE and computing the RPE-photoreceptor ratio can help track disease progression and evaluate treatment outcomes in retinal diseases [46]
Lamina cribrosa (LC)	– The LC is a multilayered porous network in the optic nerve head where blood vessels and ganglion cell axons traverse [47] – AO-OCT was used to visualize circular-shaped fenestrations of healthy LCs in vivo due to its high axial resolution [48] – Posterior bowing of the LC is suggested to be the earliest structural change in glaucoma, and a faster rate of retinal nerve fiber layer loss has been significantly associated with a greater curve of the LC [49] – Quantification of pore morphology and density in the LC with predisposing factors can help with the early detection of glaucoma in susceptible individuals [50]

30.6 Limitations

The use of AO imaging equipment may be limited due to its cost, restricted imaging area size, the time needed to image patients, lack of standardized procedures, and image quality [7]. Additionally, most images obtained using AO systems must undergo further processing after being captured, and registration and processing techniques often vary between researchers.

Differences between patients can also impact the quality of images AO systems produce. Image quality may change due to optical abnormalities, uncontrolled eye movements, and other eye conditions such as dry eye or nystagmus. Similarly, healthy eyes do not guarantee a successful scan. Healthy eyes possess more neural tissue and centrally located blood vessels, which can obstruct parts of an image when an attempt to visualize and quantify an entire structure is made. In addition, patient cooperation and stillness are needed to obtain high-quality scans, and once images are obtained, structural observation cannot be assumed to equate to functional changes.

Lastly, although several AO prototypes have been developed, including those by Canon and Boston Micromachines Corporation, these machines are expensive, and few have regulatory approvals. Therefore, in addition to the significant progress made in AO systems over the past 50 years, further research is needed before AO systems become a part of routine clinical practice.

30.7 Future of Adaptive Optics and Conclusion

Imaging with AO is useful for identifying microscopic details of healthy and pathological retinas quickly and effectively. Continuous improvements are being made to AO imaging equipment to enhance our understanding of the early stages of various disease processes and disease progression in conditions such as glaucoma and macular degeneration. A standardized and systematic method to interpret images for diagnosing and monitoring disease progression using AO should be established. Since the current methods of AO imaging are complex, simplified procedures need to be developed for use in clinical practice. In the coming years, the AO systems will continue to be important for monitoring patients in clinical trials to identify early biomarkers of disease, monitor disease progression, and the safety and efficacy of drug treatment.

Funding None.

Disclosure None.

References

1. Jayabalan GS, Bille JF. The development of adaptive optics and its application in ophthalmology. In: Bille JF, editor. High resolution imaging in microscopy and ophthalmology. Cham (CH): New Frontiers in Biomedical Optics; 2019. p. 339–58.
2. Liang J, Williams DR, Miller DT. Supernormal vision and high-resolution retinal imaging through adaptive optics. J Opt Soc Am A Opt Image Sci Vis. 1997;14(11):2884–92.
3. Burns SA, Marcos S, Elsner AE, Bara S. Contrast improvement of confocal retinal imaging by use of phase-correcting plates. Opt Lett. 2002;27(6):400–2.
4. Roorda A. Adaptive optics ophthalmoscopy. J Refract Surg. 2000;16(5):S602–7.
5. Gill JS, Moosajee M, Dubis AM. Cellular imaging of inherited retinal diseases using adaptive optics. Eye. 2019;33(11):1683–98.
6. Jayabalan GS, Kessler R, Fischer J, Bille JF. Compact adaptive Optics scanning laser ophthalmoscope with phase plates. In: Bille JF, editor. High resolution imaging in microscopy and ophthalmology: new Frontiers in biomedical Optics. Cham: Springer International Publishing; 2019. p. 377–94.
7. Akyol E, Hagag AM, Sivaprasad S, Lotery AJ. Adaptive optics: principles and applications in ophthalmology. Eye (Lond). 2021;35(1):244–64.
8. Burns SA, Elsner AE, Sapoznik KA, et al. Adaptive optics imaging of the human retina. Prog Retin Eye Res. 2019;68:1–30.
9. Stevenson S, Roorda A. Correcting for miniature eye movements in high-resolution scanning laser ophthalmoscopy: SPIE; 2005.
10. Mohankumar A, Tripathy K. Adaptive Optics. In: StatPearls. Treasure Island (FL): StatPearls Publishing LLC; 2023.
11. Kunzi M, Laforest T, Kowalczuk L, et al. Transscleral optical phase imaging (TOPI) of human retinal pigment epithelium. Invest Ophthalmol Vis Sci. 2019;60(9):4741.

12. Laforest T, Künzi M, Kowalczuk L, et al. Transscleral optical phase imaging of the human retina. Nat Photonics. 2020;14(7):439–45.
13. Zhang B, Li N, Kang J, et al. Adaptive optics scanning laser ophthalmoscopy in fundus imaging, a review and update. Int J Ophthalmol. 2017;10(11):1751–8.
14. Williams DR, Burns SA, Miller DT, Roorda A. Evolution of adaptive optics retinal imaging [invited]. Biomed Opt Express. 2023;14(3):1307–38.
15. Wahl DJ, Jian Y, Bonora S, et al. Wavefront sensorless adaptive optics fluorescence biomicroscope for in vivo retinal imaging in mice. Biomed Opt Express. 2016;7(1):1–12.
16. DuBose T, Nankivil D, LaRocca F, et al. Handheld adaptive Optics scanning laser ophthalmoscope. Optica. 2018;5(9):1027–36.
17. Mariotti L, Devaney N, Lombardo G, Lombardo M. Analysis of cone mosaic reflectance properties in healthy eyes and in eyes with nonproliferative diabetic retinopathy over time. Invest Ophthalmol Vis Sci. 2017;58(10):4057–67.
18. Lombardo M, Parravano M, Lombardo G, et al. Adaptive optics imaging of parafoveal cones in type 1 diabetes. Retina. 2014;34(3):546–57.
19. Chen MF, Chui TY, Alhadeff P, et al. Adaptive optics imaging of healthy and abnormal regions of retinal nerve fiber bundles of patients with glaucoma. Invest Ophthalmol Vis Sci. 2015;56(1): 674–81.
20. Rossi EA, Norberg N, Eandi C, et al. A new method for visualizing Drusen and their progression in flood-illumination adaptive Optics ophthalmoscopy. Transl Vis Sci Technol. 2021;10(14):19.
21. Wang X, Sadda SR, Ip MS, et al. In vivo longitudinal measurement of cone photoreceptor density in intermediate age-related macular degeneration. Am J Ophthalmol. 2023;248:60–75.
22. Zanzottera EC, Messinger JD, et al. Subducted and melanotic cells in advanced age-related macular degeneration are derived from retinal pigment epithelium. Invest Ophthalmol Vis Sci. 2015;56(5):3269–78.
23. Zanzottera EC, Ach T, Huisingh C, et al. Visualizing retinal pigment epithelium phenotypes in the transition to geographic atrophy in age-related macular degeneration. Retina (Philadelphia, Pa). 2016;36(Suppl 1):S12.
24. Cristescu IE, Ochinciuc R, Balta F, Zagrean L. High-resolution imaging of diabetic retinopathy lesions using an adaptive optics retinal camera. Rom J Ophthalmol. 2019;63(1):29–34.
25. Baltă F, Cristescu IE, Mirescu AE, et al. Investigation of retinal microcirculation in diabetic patients using adaptive Optics ophthalmoscopy and optical coherence angiography. J Diabetes Res. 2022;2022:1516668.
26. Chui TY, Vannasdale DA, Burns SA. The use of forward scatter to improve retinal vascular imaging with an adaptive optics scanning laser ophthalmoscope. Biomed Opt Express. 2012;3(10):2537–49.
27. Tam J, Dhamdhere KP, Tiruveedhula P, et al. Disruption of the retinal parafoveal capillary network in type 2 diabetes before the onset of diabetic retinopathy. Invest Ophthalmol Vis Sci. 2011;52(12):9257–66.
28. Davis BM, Crawley L, Pahlitzsch M, et al. Gaucoma: the retina and beyond. Acta Neuropathol. 2016;132(6):807–26.
29. Choudhari NS, Kumar S, Richhariya A, et al. Adaptive optics scanning laser ophthalmoscopy may support early diagnosis of glaucoma. Indian J Ophthalmol. 2022;70(8):2877–82.
30. Choi SS, Zawadzki RJ, Lim MC, et al. Evidence of outer retinal changes in glaucoma patients as revealed by ultrahigh-resolution in vivo retinal imaging. Br J Ophthalmol. 2011;95(1):131–41.
31. Hasegawa T, Ooto S, Akagi T, et al. Expansion of retinal nerve fiber bundle narrowing in glaucoma: an adaptive optics scanning laser ophthalmoscopy study. Am J Ophthalmol Case Rep. 2020;19:100732.
32. Hasegawa T, Ooto S, Takayama K, et al. Cone integrity in glaucoma: an adaptive-Optics scanning laser ophthalmoscopy study. Am J Ophthalmol. 2016;171:53–66.
33. Nadler Z, Wang B, Wollstein G, et al. Repeatability of in vivo 3D lamina cribrosa microarchitecture using adaptive optics spectral domain optical coherence tomography. Biomed Opt Express. 2014;5(4):1114–23.
34. Wang JS, Kefalov VJ. The cone-specific visual cycle. Prog Retin Eye Res. 2011;30(2):115–28.
35. Bergeles C, Dubis AM, Davidson B, et al. Unsupervised identification of cone photoreceptors in non-confocal adaptive optics scanning light ophthalmoscope images. Biomed Opt Express. 2017;8(6):3081–94.
36. Rieke F, Baylor DA. Single-photon detection by rod cells of the retina. Rev Mod Phys. 1998;70(3):1027–36.
37. Alpern M, Ching CC, Kitahara K. The directional sensitivity of retinal rods. J Physiol. 1983;343:577–92.
38. De Ciuceis C, Salvetti M, Paini A. Comparison of lercanidipine plus hydrochlorothiazide vs. lercanidipine plus enalapril on micro and macrocirculation in patients with mild essential hypertension. Intern Emerg Med. 2017;12(7):963–74.
39. Zaleska-Żmijewska A, Wawrzyniak ZM, Dąbrowska A, Szaflik JP. Adaptive Optics (rtx1) high-resolution imaging of photoreceptors and retinal arteries in patients with diabetic retinopathy. J Diabetes Res. 2019;2019:9548324.
40. Hugo J, Chavane F, Beylerian M, et al. Morphologic analysis of peripapillary retinal arteriole using adaptive optics in primary open-angle glaucoma. J Glaucoma. 2020;29(4):271–5.
41. Bakker E, Dikland FA, van Bakel R, et al. Adaptive optics ophthalmoscopy: a systematic review of vascular biomarkers. Surv Ophthalmol. 2022;67(2):369–87.
42. Liu Z, Kurokawa K, Zhang F, et al. Imaging and quantifying ganglion cells and other transparent neurons in the living human retina. Proc Natl Acad Sci USA. 2017;114(48):12803–8.
43. Liu Z, Saeedi O, Zhang F, Villanueva R, et al. Quantification of retinal ganglion cell morphology

in human glaucomatous eyes. Invest Ophthalmol Vis Sci. 2021;62(3):34.
44. Roorda A, Zhang Y, Duncan JL. High-resolution in vivo imaging of the RPE mosaic in eyes with retinal disease. Invest Ophthalmol Vis Sci. 2007;48(5):2297–303.
45. Liu Z, Kocaoglu O, Turner T, Miller D. Imaging human retinal pigment epithelium cells using adaptive optics optical coherence tomography: SPIE; 2016.
46. Morgan JI, Dubra A, Wolfe R, et al. In vivo autofluorescence imaging of the human and macaque retinal pigment epithelial cell mosaic. Invest Ophthalmol Vis Sci. 2009;50(3):1350–9.
47. Jonnal RS, Kocaoglu OP, Zawadzki RJ, et al. A review of adaptive Optics optical coherence tomography: technical advances, scientific applications, and the future. Invest Ophthalmol Vis Sci. 2016;57(9):51–68.
48. Nadler Z, Wang B, Schuman JS, et al. In vivo three-dimensional characterization of the healthy human lamina Cribrosa with adaptive Optics spectral-domain optical coherence tomography. Invest Ophthalmol Vis Sci. 2014;55(10):6459–66.
49. Kim J-A, Kim T-W, Weinreb RN, et al. Lamina Cribrosa morphology predicts progressive retinal nerve fiber layer loss in eyes with suspected glaucoma. Sci Rep. 2018;8(1):738.
50. Ivers KM, Li C, Patel N, et al. Reproducibility of measuring lamina cribrosa pore geometry in human and nonhuman primates with in vivo adaptive optics imaging. Invest Ophthalmol Vis Sci. 2011;52(8):5473–80.

31 Electroretinography

Amithavikram R. Hathibelagal, Deepika Kommanapalli, Sujoy Mukherjee, Srikanta K. Padhy, and Graham E. Holder

31.1 Introduction

Clinical electrophysiological testing of the retina plays a unique role in patient care. The ability objectively to demonstrate the function of the retina and to localise dysfunction to specific retinal cell types or layers by changing the adaptive state of the eye and/or stimulus characteristics, or possibly specific areas of the retina, can assist diagnosis and inform management. Electroretinography is the recording of the bioelectrical potentials originating in the retina in response to visual stimuli. Electrodes in contact with or in relation to the eye record small electrical biopotentials generated within the retina that can be viewed and analysed following suitable amplification.

There are some fundamental principles. It is essential to understand fully the cellular origins of the signals recorded and to then place those recordings in the context of the underlying pathophysiology of the disorder. It is important to consider the age of the patient, the clinical history, the drug, and surgical history, any possible family history, and the results of ancillary investigations, if any, such as blood tests, psychophysics, or imaging. Only in rare circumstances is electrophysiology diagnostic; it must nearly always be taken in the clinical context, as is the case with most tests in medicine.

This chapter describes the basic testing methods, underlying principles, and clinical implications of standard visual electrophysiological tests. The International Society for Clinical Electrophysiology of Vision (ISCEV) publishes standards documents that provide minimum recording protocols and technical details. All electrophysiology departments should ensure compliance with the standards. This chapter describes the electroretinogram (ERG), multifocal ERG (mfERG), and pattern ERG (PERG) separately.

A. R. Hathibelagal
Brien Holden Institute of Optometry and Vision Sciences, Prof. Brien Holden Eye Research Centre, L V Prasad Eye Institute, Hyderabad, India
e-mail: amithavikram@lvpei.org

D. Kommanapalli
Faculty of Health, Social Care and Education, Anglia Ruskin University, Cambridge, UK

S. Mukherjee
Mithu Tulsi Chanrai Campus, L V Prasad Eye Institute, Bhubaneswar, India
e-mail: sujay@lvpei.org

S. K. Padhy (✉)
Anant Bajaj Retina Institute, Mithu Tulsi Chanrai Campus, L V Prasad Eye Institute, Bhubaneswar, India
e-mail: Srikanta.padhy@lvpei.org

G. E. Holder (✉)
Department of Ophthalmology, Yong Loo Lin School of Medicine, National University of Singapore, Singapore, Singapore
e-mail: ophgeh@nus.edu.sg

T. Das, P. Satgunam (eds.), *Ophthalmic Diagnostics*, https://doi.org/10.1007/978-981-97-0138-4_31

31.2 Electroretinogram (ERG)

31.2.1 Technology

31.2.1.1 Electroretinogram Types

There are three major categories of ERG. Full-field ERG (ffERG or simply ERG) gives the global response of the retina to diffuse flash stimulation that illuminates the entire retina. Although the macula is cone-rich, most retinal cones lie outside the arcades, and disease confined to the macula will not give an abnormal ERG. Testing must, therefore, also be performed of the macula. Multifocal ERG (mfERG) provides a locus-specific function, usually using an approximately 50^0 field with a stimulus consisting of multiple hexagons, each of which flashes on and off in a pseudo-random binary sequence and cross correlational techniques calculate the individual retinal response to each hexagon. The pattern ERG (PERG) uses a constant luminance contrast stimulus, in clinical practice, usually a high contrast reversing black-and-white checkerboard, with the standard stimulated area of $12–15^0$. Although mfERG and PERG both evaluate the macular function, the tests provide different and often complementary information; mfERGs are calculated luminance responses, whereas PERGs are isoluminant contrast responses from different retinal areas.

31.2.1.2 Basic Equipment and Techniques

The basic components of an electrophysiological are usually concerned either with stimulation or recording.

31.2.1.2.1 Stimulation

Full-field ERG requires luminance stimulation. This is best provided by a ganzfeld bowl, which delivers a flash stimulus of uniform strength across the entire visual field. The ganzfeld can also be internally illuminated to provide a photopic environment. There should be an internal fixation light to help the patient maintain fixation, and there should be both forehead and chin rests to ensure a stable head position. An internally mounted infra-red camera allows the technician to monitor the patient during both scotopic and photopic testing, essential to ensure good or recognise poor fixation, incomplete eye opening, etc. The reports of the technician taken during the recording are fundamental to the accurate clinical interpretation of the data.

Pattern ERGs require an isoluminant reversing checkerboard display. There should be no transient luminance spike during pattern reversal. Unfortunately, although that is easily achieved with older technology CRT monitors, there is almost invariably a luminance shift with an LCD monitor as the screen rewrites from a zero "black" state when the pattern reverses. If correctly programmed, this should become less of a problem with OLED (organic light-emitting diode) screens. Although these are expensive at the time of writing, prices could reduce in the future.

Stimulation for mfERG is specific and is dealt with subsequently.

31.2.1.2.2 Recording

Electrodes are required to record the electrical signals. There are both active and reference electrodes and a ground electrode to ensure electrical safety. The selection and quality of electrodes significantly impact the accuracy and reliability of the recorded data. Commonly used electrode types and their characteristics are described below. A common recording setup is also shown.

Electrode placement. Appropriate electrode placement is critical to obtaining reliable and consistent ERG results. There must be active electrodes, optimally corneal or in contact with the bulbar conjunctiva, reference electrodes, and a ground electrode placed on the skin. [Fig. 31.1].

31.2.1.2.3 Active/Recording Electrodes

Contact Lens Electrodes such as Jet and Burian-Allen (BA) electrodes are widely used for ERG [1]. These cannot be used for PERG as they affect the optics of the eye. The BA electrode consists of a conductive material embedded within a contact lens and a lid speculum to help prevent the patient from blinking during recording. They are expensive and intended for multi-

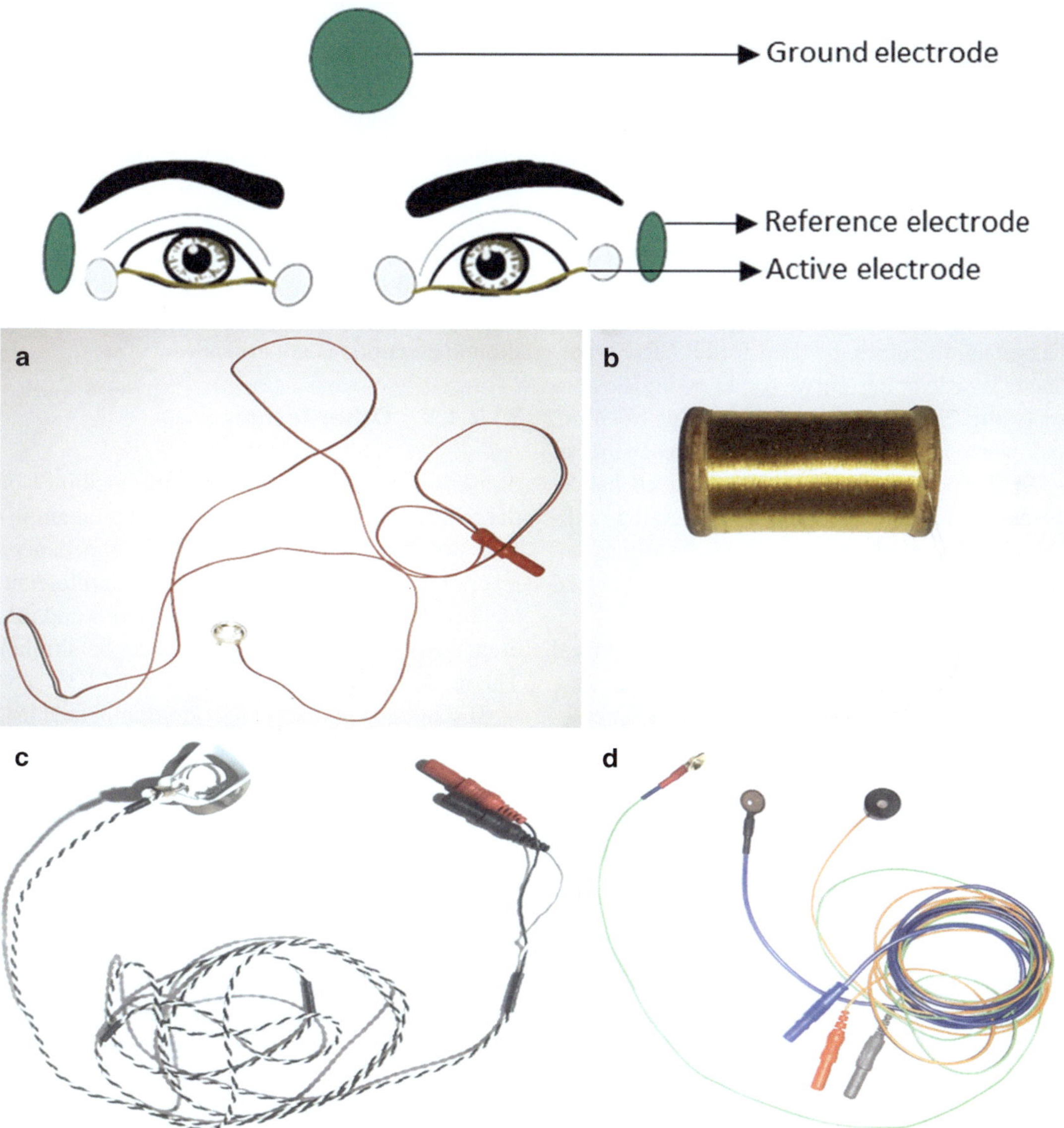

Fig. 31.1 Top Panel. Electrode placement for recording electroretinograms. Bottom Panel. Illustrates a selection of electrodes, including (**a**) Jet electrode, (**b**) LVP-Zari electrode, (**c**) Burian Allen contact lens electrode, and (**d**) skin electrodes

ple uses; hence, appropriate sterilisation techniques must be used, including those recommended by the manufacturers. BA electrodes are not universally well tolerated by patients. A Jet electrode is similar to a BA electrode but smaller in size and does not have a lid speculum. Jet electrodes are intended for single use. Topical anaesthesia is needed for BA and Jet electrodes.

DTL Electrodes (Dawson, Trick, Litzkow) are thin, silver-impregnated threads [2]. These are typically placed in the lower fornix of the eye but can also be placed in relation to the lower lid. When positioned deep in the lower conjunctival fornix, they have better reproducibility but lower recorded ERG amplitudes than when placed at the lower lid margin. DTL electrodes have excellent repeatability when used appropriately by well-trained staff [3, 4] and can be used for all types of electroretinograms (ERG, PERG, mfERG) as they preserve the optics of the eye. They are comfortable and do not require topical anaesthesia. These are often well tolerated by babies or infants. A variant of DTL electrodes, "DTL-plus", is commercially available.

Gold-Foil Electrodes are made of gold leaf attached to a mylar base and loop over the lower eyelid, thus preserving the optics of the eye. These can, therefore, be used for all ERG types. There is a learning curve for knowing how to apply the electrodes to stabilise their position, and inexperienced users often find these slip out when the patient blinks. In experienced hands, the electrodes are stable and well tolerated without topical anaesthesia. Gold-foil electrodes are not recommended if ERGs are only performed occasionally.

LVP-Zari Electrodes, developed at LV Prasad Eye Institute in Hyderabad, India, are fibre electrodes with similar properties to DTL electrodes and can be used for all types of ERG recording.

H-K Loop Electrodes are commercially available electrodes that loop over the lower eyelid. These can be used for all ERG types, but topical anaesthesia is required because they are more rigid than the very flexible gold-foil or DTL electrodes.

Other Types of Electrodes include corneal wick electrodes and skin electrodes. Corneal wick electrodes involve a cotton wick soaked in a conductive gel placed on the cornea to capture the electrical signals. Skin electrodes, such as "Neuroline" or conventional gold electrodes, such as those used for the reference and ground, can be used on or close to the lower lid in young infants or, if it is clinically contraindicated, to use electrodes in contact with the globe of the eye.

Proper care and maintenance of electrodes, including cleaning and replacement as needed, are necessary to ensure optimal performance and signal acquisition. Figure 31.1 (Bottom Panel) depicts various commonly used electrodes.

31.2.1.2.4 Reference Electrode

The reference electrodes are usually conventional gold skin electrodes positioned at the outer canthus for each eye, usually in relation to the zygomatic fossa. They should not be placed on the forehead or ear lobe.

31.2.1.2.5 Ground Electrode

The ground electrode is also placed on the skin, usually on the forehead, but the position of the ground electrode is not critical.

31.2.1.3 Other Technical Considerations

Amplifiers are used to increase the visibility of the recorded signal. These are differential amplifiers with high input and low output impedances receiving inputs from the active and reference electrodes. The impedances of the active and reference electrodes should, if possible, be similar. The reader is advised to consult the ISCEV technical standards publication for further details [5]. In many instances, such as blinking or excessive lateral eye movements, automated artefact rejection of high amplitude artefacts prevents the waveform from being distorted. The level of rejection should be set in consideration of the expected amplitude of the final waveform and the nature of the artefact as recommended by the ISCEV standards. Although full-field ERGs in a normal subject can often be recorded as a single response to a single flash, computerised signal averaging is usually used to increase the signal-to-noise ratio and will inevitably be needed in disease or in the much smaller amplitude signals of the PERG where 100–200 sweeps per average response are commonly used. The improvement in signal-to-noise ratio is related to $1/\sqrt{N}$ where N is the number of repetitions.

Filters are employed to enhance frequencies of interest by discarding unwanted frequencies. Low-pass filters are commonly used, and the choice of any filter will affect signal amplitudes and shape. The relevant ISCEV standards should be consulted. Line frequency "notch" filters should never be used routinely. Line frequency

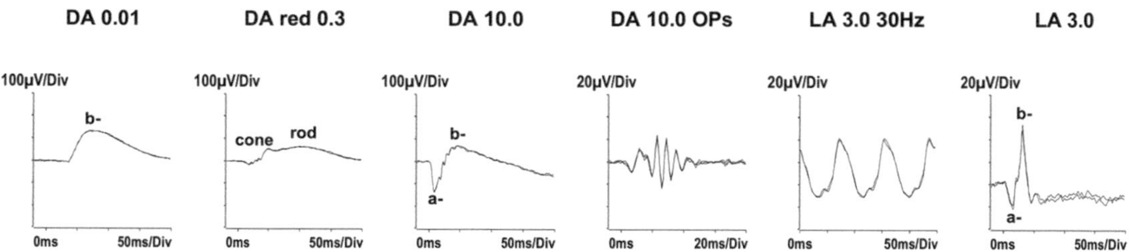

Fig. 31.2 Representative ISCEV Standard ERGs. *DA* dark-adapted, *LA* light-adapted

artefact (50 Hz or 60 Hz, country dependent) is often the first indication of problems with the electrodes; in such cases, the technician should immediately rectify the problem.

Signal Extraction involves extracting the fundamental frequency from the recorded waveform. Fourier analysis is commonly used to break down repetitive patterns and encode the information as sine waves.

31.2.2 Waveform Origins and Characteristics in Full-Field ERG

The external light passes through the ocular media to the retina. As the light reaches the photoreceptors, photoisomerisation of the photopigment, rhodopsin, occurs, initiating the phototransduction cascade resulting in photoreceptor hyperpolarisation. It is beyond the remit of this chapter to address these mechanisms fully, and the reader is referred elsewhere for a more complete description (e.g., Frishman 2006) [6]. The signals are then transmitted to the bipolar cells (which either depolarise [On-bipolar cells, found in association with rods and the three types of cone photoreceptor] or hyperpolarise [Off-bipolar cells, found in association with medium and long wavelength cones; short-wavelength cones, like rods, transmit mainly via On-bipolar cells] depending on the glutamate concentration in the synapses). Horizontal and amacrine cells collate some of the signals across the photoreceptors and bipolar cells, respectively. The impulses are subsequently sent to the retinal ganglion cells, whose axons form the optic nerves, which convey the signal beyond the retina to the brain, where vision occurs.

ERGs can be recorded with different types of electrodes, to flashes of different strengths and colours, and with the retina in different adaptive states. Standardisation is, therefore, essential for meaningful scientific and clinical communication. It also enables the pooling of patients across institutions and ensures the ability of published data directly compared to those recorded in different laboratories worldwide. The ISCEV standards [7–10] exist for all main visual electrophysiology tests and specify the *minimum* for a particular test. It should, however, be noted that minimum standards will not enable an accurate diagnosis in all cases and that additional tests may be needed considering the underlying pathophysiology.

The main ISCEV standard ERGs are shown in Fig. 31.2; all are shown with replication per ISCEV recommendation. Note that all single flash responses (i.e., not the 30 Hz flicker ERG where there is continuous stimulation) have a 20 ms pre-stimulus delay; this helps demonstrate the stability of the baseline.

ISCEV originally defined a standard flash as 3.0 cd.s.m-2 [11]. The response to this flash under scotopic (dark-adapted) conditions, with a fully dilated pupil, is conventionally known as DA 3.0, but more recently, the clinical benefits of a brighter flash strength have been recognised. A brighter DA 10.0 or DA 30.0 response is now required. (Fig. 31.2) This response to a bright flash under dark adaptation is often considered a "typical" ERG. However, it should be remembered that the dark-adapted responses are dominated by rod-driven activity in a normal retina although there is a cone contribution. The brighter flashes (DA 10.0 or DA 30.0) are better used to view and analyse the negative going a-wave, only the initial 8–10 ms of which mainly reflects (rod) photoreceptor hyperpolarisation. The DA 10.0 response thus increases the ability of the ERG to localise disease either to the outer retina (photoreceptors) or the inner nuclear layer and therefore provide anatomical specificity. Indeed, the slope of the a-wave has been related to the kinetics of phototransduction [12]. The dim flash, DA 0.01, sometimes known as a "rod-specific" response, is obtained when the standard flash is attenuated by 2.5 log units to 0.01 cd.s/m^2. With such a stimulus strength, there is insufficient photoactivation to generate a large a-wave (Fig. 31.2) and the positive polarity DA 0.01 response, arising at an inner retinal level. This provides a measure of sensitivity within the rod system as it originates from the rod in relation to the depolarisation of the On-bipolar cells [13]. It cannot distinguish rod photoreceptor dysfunction from primary inner retinal dysfunction. The oscillatory potentials, the small oscillations on the ascending limb of the b-wave, are probably generated in relation to amacrine cell activity but have limited clinical application. They are derived using restricted bandwidth filtering, usually with a low-frequency cut-off of 100 Hz (see Fig. 31.2). Although not formally part of the ISCEV Standard responses, many investigators find the use of a red flash under dark adaptation, in which there is an early component arising in relation to dark-adapted cones and a later component arising from the rod system, to have sufficient clinical value routinely to record the response.

Cone System ERGs are mainly obtained under photopic conditions using a single flash and 30 Hz flicker stimulation superimposed upon a 30 cd/m^2 rod-saturating background. At 30 Hz, the poor temporal resolution of the rod system, in addition to the presence of a rod-suppressing background, enables a cone-specific waveform to be recorded. This response, generated at an inner retinal level, is perhaps a more sensitive measure of cone dysfunction [14]. Localisation within the retina is obtained with the single flash cone response (LA 3.0). Although there is a demonstrated contribution of the hyperpolarising (OFF-) bipolar cells (HBCs) to shaping the photopic a-wave [15], the component is at least partly generated in relation to cone photoreceptor function. The cone b-wave reflects activity arises after phototransduction, and a short duration flash stimulus effectively synchronises on—and off-activity within the photopic system to create the photopic single flash a-wave.

31.2.2.1 Measurement of the ERG Concentrates on Peak Time and Amplitude

The peak time is defined as that from stimulus onset (0 ms in Fig. 31.2) to the peak of the component. In the 30 Hz flicker ERG, the time to the first component is at approximately 25—30 ms in most normal, young adult subjects. The a-wave amplitude is measured from the baseline to the a-wave trough; the b-wave amplitude is measured from the trough of the a-wave to the peak of the b-wave. In the DA 0.01 response, where there is usually no clearly defined a-wave, the b-wave amplitude is measured from the baseline to the peak of the component. Flicker ERG amplitude is measured from trough-peak.

In the rod system, as stimulus intensity increases, the b-wave always remains at a higher amplitude than the a-wave. However, that does not apply under photopic conditions where the so-called "photopic hill" phenomenon occurs [16]. Initially, the photopic b-wave is larger than the a-wave. But as stimulus strength increases, the a-wave, arising from cone photoreceptors and Off-bipolar cells, continues to increase, and the b-wave amplitude, derived from the usually synchronised responses from On—and Off-bipolar cells, declines. This reduction relates to increasing desynchronisation between the On—and Off-bipolar cell responses [17]. The "photopic hill" was first described under photopic conditions, though it is a property of cones, not of the adaptive state of the eye, and can also occur under dark adaptation in disease states in which there are no functioning rods under dark adaptation (see below).

Practical considerations vary, but most laboratories start with scotopic responses and dark adapt the patient (this must be in total darkness) while waiting for the pupils to dilate. The electrodes can be placed before dark adaptation, but many labs prefer to put the electrodes under red-light illumination in scotopic conditions. The red light should not be over-bright, and it is advisable to wait for perhaps 5 min before commencing the recording. Impedances should be checked.

Start with dim flashes. The DA 0.01 response usually consists of 5–10 averaged recordings, with a 2-s interstimulus interval (ISI). As with all steps, it should be repeated. The red flash ERG is best inserted at this stage. If an intensity series is performed (recommended by many labs), the ISI must be increased as the stimulus strength increases to ensure adequate retinal recovery from one flash before delivering the next flash. The details are available in the ISCEV standard document. An ISI of perhaps 20 s will be needed for DA 10 or DA 30 responses, but the number of responses per average will usually be less than the DA 0.01 response. The number of acquisitions per average must be significantly increased in the presence of a major disease or with a poorly cooperative patient, and multiple replications may be necessary to demonstrate reproducible responses. The technician should remain with the patient while the patient is restored to photopic conditions with the background light on in the ganzfeld to ensure that the eyes of the patient remain open (there is a natural tendency to close the eyes). Some equipment comes with suggested protocols that may include a limited number of replications per average. As these are usually based on cooperative normal adult subjects, it is better to set the number of stimuli to a far greater number than considered necessary, and the recording technician stops the recording when the signal-to-noise ratio is acceptable.

31.2.3 Clinical Considerations

31.2.3.1 Photoreceptor Disease

A reduced DA 0.01 (rod-specific) ERG b-wave amplitude is a sensitive indicator of rod system dysfunction, but this does not allow localisation of the defect either to the inner retinal structure or the rod photoreceptors as it is generated in the rod On-bipolar cells. The bright flash DA 10.0 response a-wave, which directly indicates the activity of the rod photoreceptors, allows localisation of the deficit to either the photoreceptors or the inner nuclear layer. The terminology in inherited disease may be determined by the electrophysiology, as shown in Table 31.1.

Table 31.1 Typical photoreceptor diseases

Inherited	Acquired
Rod-cone dystrophy (RP)	Vascular (choroidal circulation)
Cone-rod dystrophy (CORD)	Nutritional
Cone dystrophy (COD)	Toxic
Choroideremia	Inflammatory
Leber congenital Amaurosis	Parasitic
Early onset retinal dystrophy (EORD)	Autoimmune
Others, e.g. RDH5, KCNV2, RGS9, NR2E3, RP1L1	Paraneoplastic (not MAR)

Some rarer genetic disorders may be known by the names of the responsible genes

Representative ERG waveforms in some inherited disorders are shown in Fig. 31.3. Genetically determined retinal photoreceptor degenerations, such as rod-cone (retinitis pigmentosa) and cone-rod dystrophies, and any other disorder that primarily affects photoreceptors, as shown above, thus give overall ERG reduction. The principles of interpretation and localisation of deficit illustrated in these patients may be applied to any aetiology. Please note that replication of the waveform, as specified in the ISCEV ERG standard, is shown for all ERGs in all patients in Fig. 31.3. The retinal origins of the ERG traces (cell types and layers) must be established, and the findings related to the signs, symptoms, history, inheritance, imaging, and presumed underlying pathophysiology before the diagnosis can be established.

With reference to Fig. 31.3, the patient with rod-cone dystrophy (RP) shows a subnormal DA 0.01 response, indicative of rod system sensitivity loss, but the markedly subnormal photoreceptor-derived DA 10 a-wave localises the dysfunction to the photoreceptors. Note the markedly delayed and reduced photopic flicker ERG (*). The delay in the flicker ERG reflects generalised cone system dysfunction. The rod ERGs are more severely

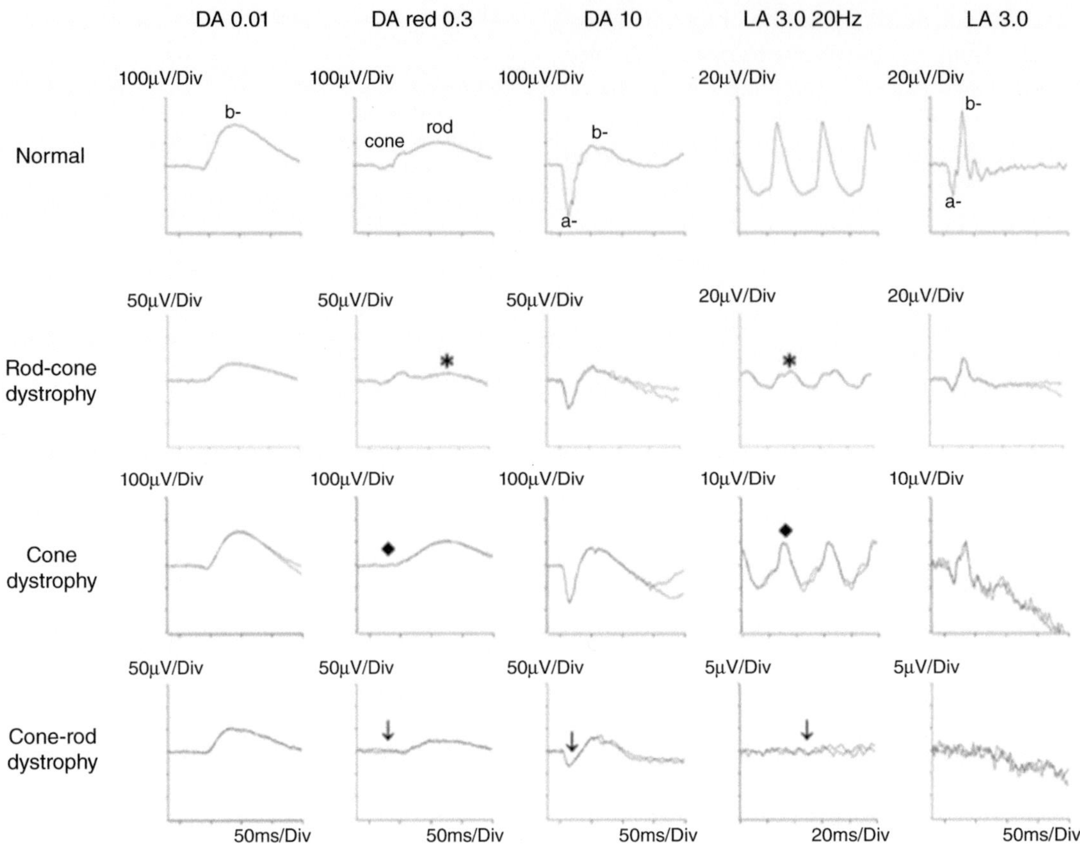

Fig. 31.3 ISCEV Standard ERGs in the main categories of inherited photoreceptor disease (see text for complete details; note variable amplitude calibration scales)

affected than cone-derived ERGs, hence a rod-cone dystrophy. Note the greater effect of the DA red ERG on the rod component than on the cone components (*). RP loss occasionally may only affect rod-derived ERGs, but that is highly unusual and occurs only early in the disease process. True sector (restricted) disease gives amplitude reduction with no peak time change, whereas diffuse or generalised disease is also associated with delayed peak time. The severity or nature of the disorder may not be reflected either in the fundus appearance or on structural imaging such as fundus autofluorescence (FAF) or optical coherence tomography (OCT); the ERG assists in accurate diagnosis and may provide prognostic information. Cone dystrophies have normal rod responses but abnormal cone responses, with the 30 Hz flicker response usually showing both amplitude reduction and delayed peak time, as shown in Figure Fig. 31.3◆. Note that the DA red flash shows a rod component but no cone component (Fig. 31.3◆). This can be particularly useful as cone dystrophy patients are frequently photophobic and may not be able to comply with photopic testing. Under those circumstances, an undetectable cone component in the DA red flash ERG enables the diagnosis. Note that cone ERGs are far more abnormal than rod ERGs in cone-rod dystrophy patients (¯), the subnormal DA 10 a-wave indicating the degree of rod photoreceptor involvement (¯).

A full-field ERG is essential in the workup of a patient with macular dysfunction to determine any generalised retinal involvement and the nature and severity of such involvement. By definition, a patient with pure macular dystrophy has a normal full-field ERG; in these people, PERG and/or mfERG are needed to assess the function of the macula. In ABCA4 disease (Stardgardt, fundus flavimaculatus), for example, which can be associated with generalised retinal involvement, the full-field ERG at presentation has a high prognostic value with only 20% of patients with a normal ERG at presentation showing generalised retinal involvement after 10 years, but 100% of patients with an initial rod system ERG abnormality showing significant clinical and electrophysiological progression after 10 years follow-up. [18].

Delayed 30 Hz flicker ERGs are also a feature of inflammatory disorders such as birdshot chorioretinopathy, but amplitude change may not be present. Indeed, the 30 Hz flicker in birdshot chorioretinopathy is not only a sensitive indicator of generalised retinal dysfunction [19], but can also be used to guide management decisions by objectively assessing retinal function; additionally, this provides an object measure of the response to treatment intervention [20]. Delay in the flicker ERG is also anticipated in AZOOR (acute zonal occult outer retinopathy) [21]. There is a known association between uveitis and multiple sclerosis (MS), and 30 Hz flicker ERG delay can occur in such cases.

31.2.3.2 Inner Retinal Disease

Inner retinal disease is associated with a "negative" or electronegative ERG. A true negative ERG is defined as a selective reduction in the b-wave accompanied by a normal or near-normal a-wave; it indicates dysfunction post-phototransduction, usually in the inner nuclear layer. The term does not mean there is no detectable ERG but that the waveform is dominated by the negative going a-wave. Some causes of negative ERG are listed in Table 31.2.

The "negative" ERG in central retinal artery occlusion (CRAO) reflects the duality of retinal blood supply with RPE/photoreceptors supplied via choroidal circulation and the bipolar cells supplied via the central retinal artery. Again, the principles of interpretation shown in Fig. 31.4 can be applied to any aetiology. As with inherited disease, the retinal origins of the ERG traces (cell types and layers) must be established, and the findings related to the signs, symptoms, history, inheritance, imaging, and presumed underlying pathophysiology before the diagnosis can be established.

Table 31.2 Typical diseases associated with a "negative" ERG

Inherited	Acquired
X-linked retinoschisis (RS1)	Vascular (CRAO, CRVO)
CSNB (NYX, GRM6, TRPM1, etc.)	Nutritional
Batten (CLN3…)	Toxic (includes siderosis)
TRNT1	Parasitic
PMM2-CDG	Inflammatory
Others…	Autoimmune
	Paraneoplastic (MAR; rarely CAR)

CAR Carcinoma-Associated Retinopathy, *CRAO* central retinal artery occlusion, *CRVO* central retinal vein occlusion, *CSNB* congenital stationary night blindness, *MAR* melanoma-associated retinopathy. Some responsible genes are shown in parentheses; rarer genetic disorders may be known by the names of the responsible genes, as shown

In the patient with complete congenital stationary night blindness (cCSNB), there is no rod system activity in the DA 0.01 response, which is usually undetectable as the underlying pathophysiology results in transmission loss from all retinal photoreceptors to On-bipolar cells. The normal a-wave in the DA 10 responses confirms normal rod photoreceptor function, and the waveform, with a normal a-wave but profound relative reduction in the b-wave, is a "negative" ERG. In some cases, a minimal early deflection occurs in the DA 0.01 response (Fig. 31.4*). The early peak time excludes a rod system origin; it suggests dark-adapted cones, confirmed by the DA red flash ERG, but note the preservation of the early negative component in the DA red response and reduction in the positive deflection (Fig. 31.4*), in keeping with inner retinal cone system dysfunction. The photopic ERGs show an a-wave that commences normally (origins in photoreceptors and Off-bipolar cells); there is a broadened trough, a sharply rising b-wave lacking oscillatory potentials, and a reduced b: a ratio (Fig. 31.4*). Such appearances are diagnostic of loss of On-bipolar cell function but preservation of Off-bipolar cell function. The genetic variants responsible for cCSNB result in selective impairment of the function of all On-bipolar cells but spare the Off-bipolar cells.

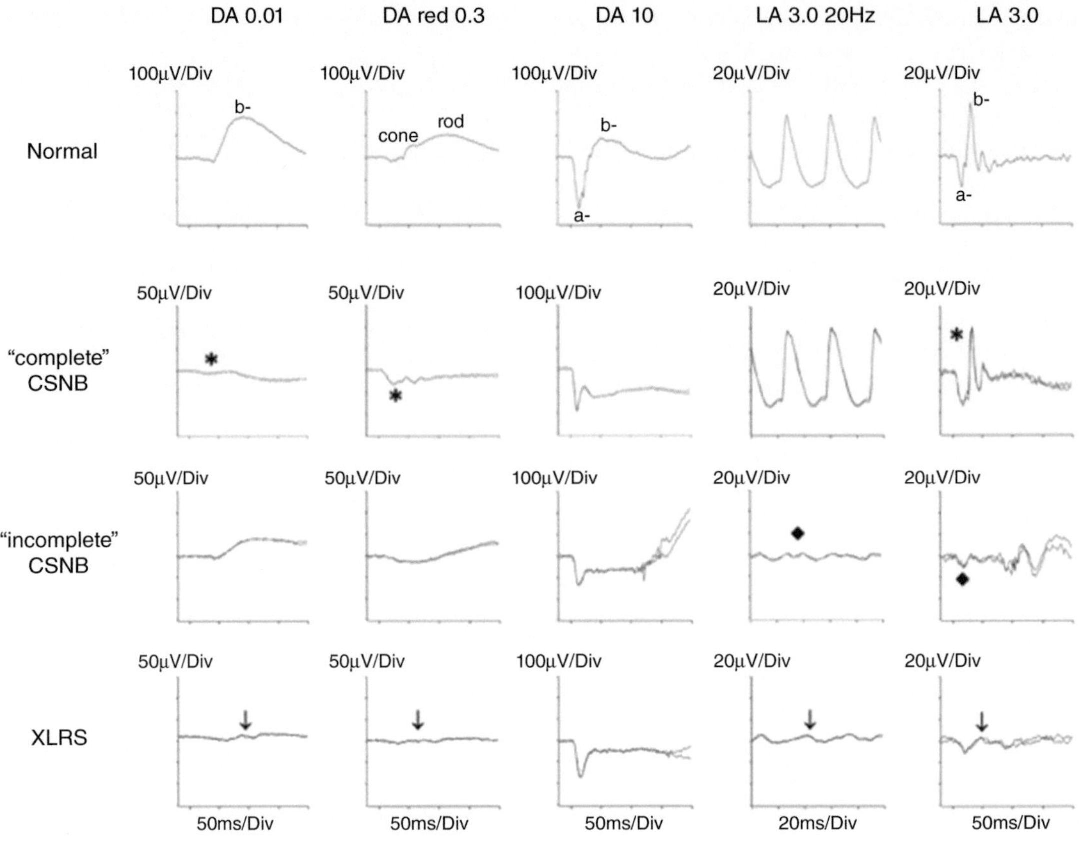

Fig. 31.4 ISCEV Standard ERGs in some inherited disorders of inner retinal function (see text for details; note amplitude calibration scales. *DA* dark adapted, *CSNB*-congenital stationary night blindness, *LA* light adapted, *XLRS* X-linked retinoschisis

The patient with incomplete CSNB (iCSNB) has a detectable but subnormal and delayed DA 0.01 response b-wave and a negative waveform DA 10 response. The latter has a very similar waveform to the patient with cCSNB. It is in the photopic responses that the major differences occur. Note that the 30 Hz flicker ERG is markedly subnormal and has a triphasic appearance (Fig. 31.4♦). Examination of the LA 3 response suggests the pathophysiology. The severe b-wave reduction shows that, unlike cCSNB, where the dysfunction is confined to the On-bipolar cell pathways, there must also be Off-bipolar cell involvement. The loss of the Off-bipolar cell explains why the a-wave is also reduced relative to the normal control, and the very small, almost u-shaped response indicates inner retinal dysfunction involving both on- and off-pathways (Fig. 31.4♦). Cone ERGs are far more abnormal in iCSNB than cCSNB, and this is reflected in the symptomatology; a greater proportion of iCSNB patients have nystagmus or significant visual acuity reduction, and some may even complain of photophobia rather than nyctalopia. Both On- and Off-bipolar cell pathways are affected as the responsible genes encode proteins involved in transmission at the photoreceptor synapse, affecting both on- and off-pathways.

The ERGs in patients with XLRS are severely affected. It demonstrates the effects of inner retinal dysfunction unrelated to the blocking of specific channels. There is profound rod system sensitivity loss indicated by the DA 0.01 responses (ˉ) confirmed to have inner retinal origins by the negative waveform DA 10 ERG (normal a-wave = normal rod photoreceptor function) and the reduction in positive-going components in the DA red ERG(⁻). The cone flicker and single flash ERGs are subnormal and show marked delay with a reduced b: a ratio but do not show the shape changes associated with channel blocking seen in the two cases of CSNB (⁻).

The causes of negative ERG have been extensively reviewed. [22, 23] The findings must always be considered in relation to underlying pathophysiology. The findings in melanoma-associated retinopathy (MAR) are identical to those in "complete" CSNB, reflecting transmission loss across the On-bipolar cell synapse in all retinal cell types. CSNB, however, is a lifelong disorder; MAR presents with a sudden onset of nyctalopia and photopsia in adults who usually have a history of cutaneous malignant melanoma. An accurate history is often essential for an accurate diagnosis. Carcinoma-associated retinopathy (CAR) only rarely gives a "negative" ERG; usually, there is profound, often rapidly progressive, global ERG reduction in keeping with photoreceptor dysfunction. This is mainly related to anti-retinal antibodies to recoverin or enolase. Non-paraneoplastic autoimmune retinopathy (AIR) can also occur; such patients may have a normal fundus but have various electrophysiological features. [24] Paraneoplastic retinopathy can present before the underlying malignancy and calls for a complete systems review.

Some disorders are associated with a "pseudo-negative" ERG where the DA 10 b-wave is of lower amplitude than the a-wave but unrelated to primary inner retinal dysfunction. [25] In pseudo-negative ERG, all signals arise in a dark-adapted cone system in the absence of rod function. Because the "photopic hill" phenomenon described earlier, in which the b-wave in a normal photopic retina becomes of lower amplitude than the a-wave as the stimulus strength increases, is a property of cones rather than the adaptive state of the eye, it can be observed in darkness if there is no or minimal rod system function. This can occur with normal cone function, such as in fundus albipunctatus (RDH5) [26], Oguchi disease [27], or vitamin A deficiency (VAD). [28] The DA red flash adopts critical importance as it shows a normal cone component but no detectable rod component under scotopic conditions.

The restoration of rod function in RDH5 disease by prolonged dark adaptation confirms the diagnosis as one consequence of the RDH5 variant is impaired regeneration of rhodopsin, but rhodopsin levels normalise with extended dark adaptation. This is best performed overnight by sending the patient the necessary materials to patch one eye tightly before sleeping to exclude light. The technician removes the patching under dark adaptation when the patient attends the clinic the following day. ERG recording then proceeds with one eye having had standard dark adaptation and the other overnight dark adaptation. [26].

The accurate diagnosis of vitamin A deficiency is of fundamental importance to management. It is one of the few treatable disorders presenting to an electrophysiologist, usually with full recovery unless it is chronic and is associated with additional nutritional optic neuropathy. A dietary history must be included in any patient with a recent onset of night blindness, in addition to directed questions on previous surgery such as Crohn's disease, a Whipple procedure, or bariatric surgery. Occasionally, patients may present with seeing "white as green" and deny night blindness. Cone dysfunction in VAD is uncommon, but s-cone function is first affected and may give rise to such symptoms. Full recovery from VAD following intramuscular vitamin A therapy is rapid; most symptoms and ERG abnormalities can resolve within 3 days following treatment. [28].

A pseudo-negative ERG can also occur in patients with advanced RP (rod-cone dystrophy), where all rod function is lost, and all signals arise in the remaining cone population. In such a case, the DA 10 a-wave will be profoundly subnormal in accordance with the markedly abnormal cones responsible for all remaining signals. [25].

It is important to be aware that ERGs are rarely diagnostic. In only three rare or relatively rare inherited disorders are ERGs pathognomonic. [29] These relate to variants in KCNV2 (cone dystrophy with supernormal rod ERG), NR2E3 (enhanced S-cone syndrome), and RGS9/R9AP (bradyopsia).

31.2.4 Factors Affecting ERG [Table 31.3]

31.3 The Multifocal ERG

31.3.1 Technology

Developed by Sutter and Tran in 1990 [30], the multifocal electroretinogram (mfERG) is a non-invasive test that objectively assesses the spatial distribution of central retinal cone function. The mfERG uses a stimulus consisting of multiple hexagons, each of which flashes on and off with a pseudo-random binary sequence. Cross correlations between the stimuli and the single recording channel produce a set of traces, each corresponding to one of the stimulus hexagons. The amplitudes and peak times of these small mathematical constructions are then measured similarly to conventional ERG signals and can be compared with age-matched normative data. Given that the mfERG does not test rod function and tests a limited proportion of the retinal cone population, it is usually combined with conventional full-field ERG. If the mfERG is abnormal, it is necessary to examine the full-field responses to determine the nature and extent of generalised retinal involvement.

Table 31.3 Subject-related factors and their effects on the ERG parameters

Feature	Effects on ERG
Age and gender	Neonates have small ERGs that increase rapidly in the first 6 months of life The elderly have lower ERG amplitudes and longer peak times Minimal gender differences between normal ERGs in males and females
Refractive error	Lower ERG amplitudes with increasing myopia. Minor associated peak time change
Interocular asymmetry	An interocular difference in ERG amplitudes is usually considered abnormal if greater than 30% amplitude or > 3 ms in peak times of DA 10 a-wave or flicker ERG
Pupil size	Maximal pupillary dilatation is required. Pupil size must be measured immediately following ERG and given adequate consideration during clinical interpretation
Media opacities	Major lens opacity or vitreous haemorrhage can reduce ERG amplitudes and increase peak times. Mild cataracts have no significant effect on full-field ERGs
Eye-opening	The presence of ptosis or any eye closure during recording must be noted by the technician and considered during interpretation

There are various protocols for mfERG testing, with 61 to 217 hexagon patterns per ISCEV guidelines. [8] Most investigators use either 61 or 103 hexagons for routine clinical applications. These protocols provide good spatial resolution and signal-to-noise ratio. In specific situations, such as children or when targeting light is critical, protocols with fewer than 61 elements, such as 19 and 37 hexagon patterns, may be used. Additionally, there are non-ISCEV protocols for research purposes. These include mfERG scotopic responses, which capture rod-driven responses from multiple retinal areas, and mfERG oscillatory potentials, representing responses from inner retinal cells, particularly the amacrine cells.

31.3.2 The Technique

The test involves presenting a rapid sequence of flashing hexagons arranged in a pattern stimulus. The hexagons have dark and light states, and each hexagon flashes on and off using an m-sequence. The electrical responses to these visual stimuli are calculated, and the standard ERG characteristics of peak time and amplitude are conventionally used for analysis. Additional spatial grouping into rings or quadrants is also enabled.

The choice of stimulus presentation can vary, including regular or scaled hexagons and different numbers of hexagons. Regular hexagons are of consistent size, resulting in larger central responses where there is greater cone photoreceptor density. Most investigators use scaled hexagons that increase in size with increasing eccentricity, thus ensuring that each hexagon stimulates a similar number of photoreceptors.

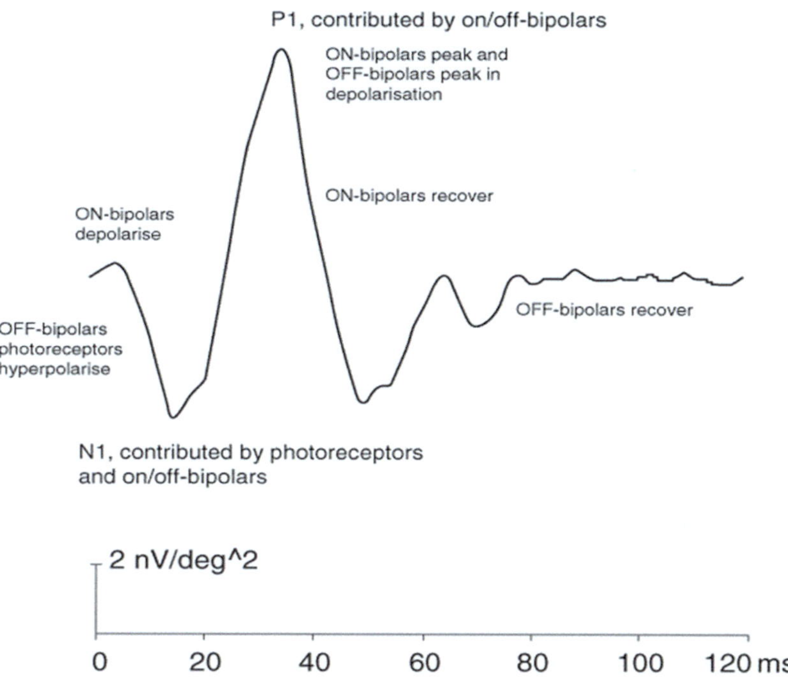

Fig. 31.5 A schematic diagram showing the waveform, timing, and cellular contribution of the first-order kernels of the multifocal electroretinogram. (From Chan et al. [33] reproduced with permission)

The protocol selection depends on the area of interest; 61 and 103-scaled hexagons are commonly used. The higher the number of hexagons, the greater the spatial resolution, but equally, a longer time is taken for the data acquisition. To analyse electrical responses, a mathematical function called a kernel is used. The kernel represents time-domain waveforms from specific retinal areas and is based on age-matched normative data. The first-order response or first-order kernel in mfERG refers to the standard extraction of signals associated with single illumination events. To obtain the first-order kernel, responses following a light stimulus step are added, and those following a dark stimulus step are subtracted. The first-order kernel originates from the outer retina and represents the initial response, usually involving the measurement of the P1 mfERG component. Second - and third-order kernels are averaged responses from bipolar, ganglion, and amacrine cells, providing further information about retinal processing. [31].

Any type of ERG electrode can be used. Reference electrodes are placed at the outer canthi, with the ground electrode commonly on the forehead. The reader is referred to the ISCEV mfERG Standard document for comprehensive information. [8] In the past, mfERG stimuli were often displayed on cathode ray tubes (CRTs). The modern mfERG stimuli can be generated on thin-film-transistor (TFT) liquid crystal displays (LCDs) or other displays such as OLED screens.

The stimuli consist of multiple frames of flickering white and black, with a frame frequency of 75 Hz. The frame rate chosen should be mentioned during interpretation as it can provide information about response time and amplitude height. During the test, the patient focuses on a cross target in the centre of the pattern of hexagons; pupillary dilation is usually used. The recordings are often obtained binocularly.

A typical mfERG result consists of well-formed bi-phasic waveforms with components including N1 (first trough), P1 (peak), and N2 (second trough) [Fig. 31.5]. The N1 component is the initial downward deflection observed after the onset of the visual stimulus. It is primarily generated by the activity of cone photoreceptors. The P1 component mainly relates to inner retinal activity in the on- and Off-bipolar cells. Finally, the N2 component appears as a second downward deflection after the P1, and it may arise from the activity of the amacrine cells, which integrate signals from the photoreceptors, bipolar cells, and ganglion cells. [32] The waveforms represent the mathematical extraction of retinal responses in a mapped manner.

31.3.2.1 Patient Preparation Tips

The preparation begins with documenting the patient's demographic information and refractive correction. The appropriate protocol must be chosen, including the number of hexagons required for the test. Binocular recording enables the better eye to maintain fixation in a patient with monocularly reduced visual acuity, but some laboratories use monocular stimulation routinely. As accurate fixation is essential to obtaining meaningful mfERG data, caution must be exercised when recording monocularly from an eye with a central scotoma or markedly reduced visual acuity. Monocular stimulation must, however, be performed if there is strabismus. The procedure is explained to the patient, and the nature of the stimulus is demonstrated before commencing. Correcting any refractive error using the patient's current glasses or wide-aperture trial frames is used when appropriate. The patient should be instructed to maintain fixation on the centre of the screen, usually marked by intersecting diagonal lines to assist those with a central scotoma; an eye gaze tracker may be used.

31.3.2.2 Recording Procedure

The mfERG test results can be shown in either the "field" or the "retina" view. Further display options are available, such as responses per ring, distribution per quadrant, and maps of amplitudes and peak time. Results can be visualised in 2D or 3D, with the 3D view showing response density using hot colours to indicate high-density areas. All results should include the standard trace array and never have only the scalar product image.

Maintaining stable fixation is crucial. Eccentric fixation shifts the waveforms either laterally or vertically. Improper trial frame placement reduces amplitudes throughout the periphery; wide-aperture trial frames are necessary. Noise can arise from micro-eye movements, improperly placed or loosely connected electrodes, muscle artefact, excessive blinking, etc. These factors can introduce artefacts and disrupt the reliability of the mfERG waveform.

31.3.2.3 Response Analysis

The mfERG analysis involves assessing the amplitude and peak time of the main components. The amplitude is usually measured in nanovolts (nV), and the peak time is in milliseconds (ms). As the mfERG test result display may utilise both microvolts (μV) and nanovolts (nV), it is important, as with all electrophysiological recordings, to be aware of the calibration scale.

During mfERG analysis, several observations are considered, including absolute rejects, relative rejects, and noise levels. Absolute reject refers to high amplitude artefacts that are rejected by the system. Relative reject involves excluding signal-to-noise ratios that are deemed noisy. A low signal-to-noise ratio indicates a high noise level, making it challenging to detect meaningful responses, and such data may not be useful. Steady and accurate fixation is important, as is the ability of the patient as much as possible to refrain from blinking during recording; excessive ocular movements result in increased noise levels and poor-quality recordings that may not be fit for purpose.

Figure 31.6 provides a visual representation of important features and parameters in mfERG analysis. Average responses from different locations within each ring in response to visual stimuli can be depicted in colour-coded graphs, the colour of the responses corresponding to specific zonal rings. The panel of average responses shows the mean responses from each ring. Average RMS (root mean square) amplitudes provide information on the strength of the electrical responses evoked in the retina. These responses may be accompanied by artefacts highlighted in black. Average N1, P1, and N2 amplitudes depict the mean response of each component in each ring, free from artefacts and filtering.

In mfERG analysis, average response values, RMS amplitudes, individual amplitudes, and peak times are compared with normative data. The ring ratio, which represents the ratio of the response amplitudes at the central ring compared to the peripheral rings, is an important parameter.

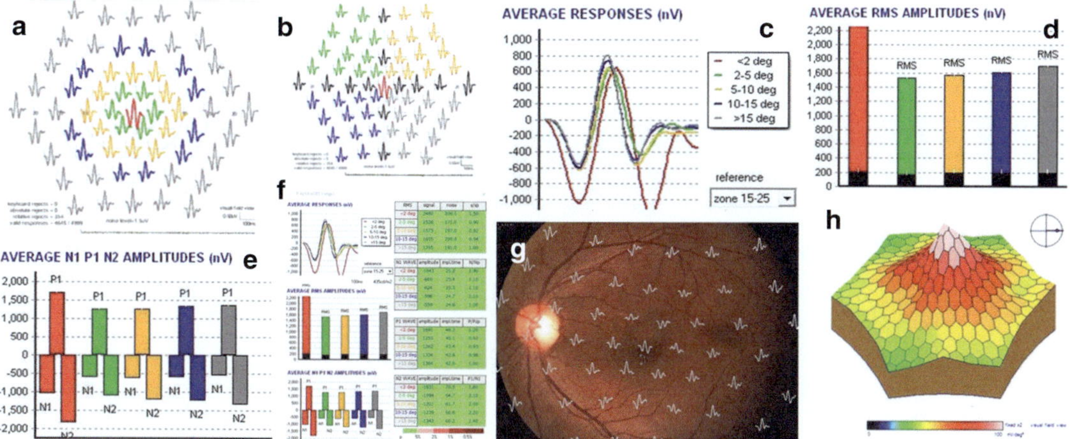

Fig. 31.6 Illustration of various components and analysis of mfERG responses. (**a**) Field view of extracted mfERG responses represented in a ring pattern used for calculating ring ratios. The colour of the responses corresponds to specific zonal rings. For example, at the 0–2° level, the response from the fovea is depicted in red. At the 2–5° level, the responses are represented in green. Similarly, the 5–10, 10–15, and > 15° regions from the fixation area are shown in yellow, blue, and grey, respectively. (**b**) Responses were obtained from each quadrant of the retina. (**c**) Summation of coded responses within a specific region. (**d**) True response and noise levels, where coloured histograms represent the true response (per rings or quadrants) and the black region at the bottom indicates the amount of generated noise. (**e**) Individual components of N1, P1, and N2 responses are displayed in amplitudes based on the region of interest (by ring or quadrant). (**f**) Composite view presenting the responses along with scalar values, compared with age-matched controls and colour-coded (green: within normal range, warm colours towards red indicating reduced response compared to normal). (**g**) Merged responses overlaid on a fundus image, known as the retina view. (**h**) Three-dimensional view of response density providing insights into sensitivity. These visual representations aid in analysing and interpreting mfERG data for assessing retinal function

Artefacts can arise from the patient (eye movements, muscle, etc.) or environmental factors (electrical contamination due to induced or inherent line frequency noise) and should be minimised to obtain a satisfactory signal: noise ratio. Therefore, available systems often provide options to filter out noise or artefacts, and repeating the test is recommended if the artefact values exceed a certain level. In general, it is best practice to determine the source of artefacts and eliminate these at the source instead of filtering. Testing should never routinely be performed using a 50/60 Hz line frequency notch filter; it should be remembered that line frequency artefact is often the first sign of electrode problems, alerting the technician to intervene.

31.3.2.4 Artefacts

Several artefacts can impact the mfERG recordings. [Fig. 31.7] These include line frequency interference, eye movements, eccentric fixation, positioning errors, central peak artefact, and waveform distortions. Careful inspection of trace arrays is crucial for correctly identifying and interpreting these artefacts. Reports should mention all recording issues that could impact reliability and interpretation, such as media opacities, pseudophakia, refractive correction problems, blocked view, unstable fixation, and frequent blinking. Repeat recordings, using monocular fixation or adjusted trial frames, may be necessary to rule out artefactual causes of abnormal mfERG results. [34].

31.3.2.5 Interpretation of Data

Interpreting mfERG test results involves careful analysis and comparison with normative data; each laboratory should establish its normative values. The main components (N1, P1, and N2) can be evaluated, but many investigators focus on P1; amplitude and peak time values are measured and compared against age-matched controls. Reporting should include demographic details, visual acuity, pupil status, noise level, compliance, and protocol. Normative data can be pro-

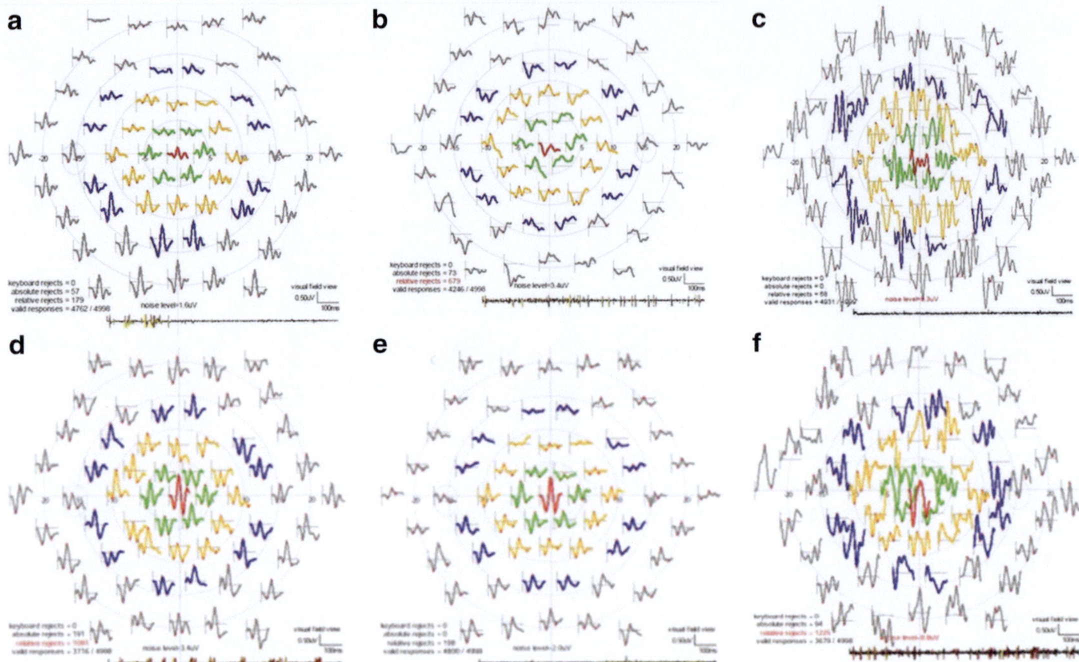

Fig. 31.7 Examples of artefacts and their impact on mfERG results. (**a**) Sloping effect observed in the test result, indicating improper fixation during the procedure. Eccentric fixation can lead to trace arrays and topographic 3-D plots that exhibit central depression or a "sloping" appearance, characterised by low signals on one side and high signals on the other. (**b**) A case demonstrating no fixation, resulting in erratic and unreliable responses. (**c**) Test results are affected by loosely connected electrodes, leading to distorted waveforms and unreliable data. (**d**) Eye gaze tracker at the bottom indicates intermittent eye movement, which can introduce artefacts and affect the accuracy of the results. (**e**) Positioning errors or rim artefacts observed in the test result causing localised irregularities in the response pattern. The trial frame's rim obstructed the view, causing a reduction in the eccentric superior responses. (**f**) Excessive blink artefacts affect the test result, characterised by abrupt disturbances in the waveform due to blinking during the recording

vided in a tabular format if an available option on the equipment is used.

31.3.2.6 Clinical Applications of Multifocal ERG [Table 31.4]

31.4 The Pattern ERG

The pattern ERG is the retinal response to an isoluminant contrast reversing stimulus. In clinical practice, it is usually a reversing black-and-white checkerboard. It is a small signal compared to full-field ERGs, and computerised signal averaging is essential to obtain clinically usable data. As a small signal, technical factors are important, but when given due consideration, test-retest and trial-to-trial variability are like full-field ERG. Practitioners should perform testing per the ISCEV Standard recommendations. A minimum of 100 averages per trial will be needed and usually far more in patients with significant disease. The standard field is usually ~15^0x 12^0, which measures central macular function; doubling the stimulus size from 15^0 to 30^0 allows an objective measure of peripheral macular function. [38] With a high contrast stimulus reversing at 4/s, the waveform consists of two main components [Fig. 31.8]: a positive component at approximately 50 ms, P50, and a larger negative component at approximately 95 ms, N95. [39] A small early

Table 31.4 Depicts clinical applications of multifocal ERG

Disorder	Multifocal ERG changes
Glaucoma	Some authors find mfERG useful in glaucoma [33], but in general, PERG or PhNR recording may be of more value
Drug toxicity	mfERG is useful in determining central retinal involvement in suspected drug toxicity. It can assist in long-term monitoring of disease progression or improvement [35]
Age-related macular degeneration (ARMD)	The extent and severity of macular dysfunction in ARMD can be assessed with mfERG. It provides insights into disease progression and response to interventions. It can reveal localised areas with reduced amplitudes or delayed implicit times that may not be evident in overall averaged results (flash electroretinogram) [36]
Diabetic retinopathy	Some authors find mfERG useful in diabetes, showing delayed timing in retinal locations with vascular lesions and in some locations outside of lesions. Amplitude remains relatively normal. It may reveal abnormalities in people with diabetes without retinopathy [37]
Inherited retinal disease (IRD)	Many patients with IRD have generalised retinal dysfunction, and the nature of the disorder (rod-cone dystrophy, cone-rod dystrophy, etc.) may be defined by the electrophysiological features. The mfERG can help quantify the severity and spatial extent of macular involvement. For example, in "classical retinitis pigmentosa (RP)" where the patient has very constricted visual fields but normal Snellen visual acuity, full-field ERGs may be virtually undetectable, but PERGs or the central mfERG responses may be normal or near-normal. Equally, the full-field ERG is normal if dysfunction is confined to the macula; in these cases, testing of macular function with PERG and/or mfERG is essential to determine the nature and severity of macular involvement. Such patients may have normal macular structure, and normal macular optical coherence tomography (OCT) or fundus autofluorescence imaging should not be assumed to be normal macular function
Macular oedema	mfERG may be unaffected in cystoid macular oedema as the elevated photoreceptors are still capable of phototransduction, and thresholds may be normal on microperimetry
Central serous Chorioretinopathy	mfERG may help define the extent and severity of the disorder
Retinal vascular disorders	mfERG is used in conjunction with full-field ERG and may be useful in branch artery occlusions in demonstrating the extent of dysfunction, particularly after re-perfusion
High myopia	Many high myopes will show mfERG abnormalities, particularly in a peripapillary distribution
Neuro-ophthalmic disorders	The presence of a normal mfERG, when it is clinically challenging to differentiate between macular or optic nerve dysfunction (both can have delayed pattern VEP), PERG is preferred as it provides the retinal responses to the same reversing checkerboard pattern used for evoking the pattern VEP, and in addition, the N95 component indicates central retinal ganglion cell function directly

negative component, N35, can be seen at approximately 35 ms in most subjects. From clinical practice [40], confirmed by pharmacological blocking experiments [41], it has been established that N95 arises exclusively in the retinal ganglion cells (RGCs). Much of P50 arises in the RGCs, perhaps 70%, with the remainder arising in pre-ganglionic structures that have not been fully elucidated. From a clinical point of view, P50 is generated via stimulation of the macular photoreceptors and objectively reflects the function of the macula. PERG measurement usually focuses on the peak time and N35 trough-to-peak amplitude for P50, and the amplitude of N95 measured from the peak of P50 to the trough of N95. It is often difficult to accurately measure N95 peak time as it is often broadened, and many workers do not routinely address that parameter.

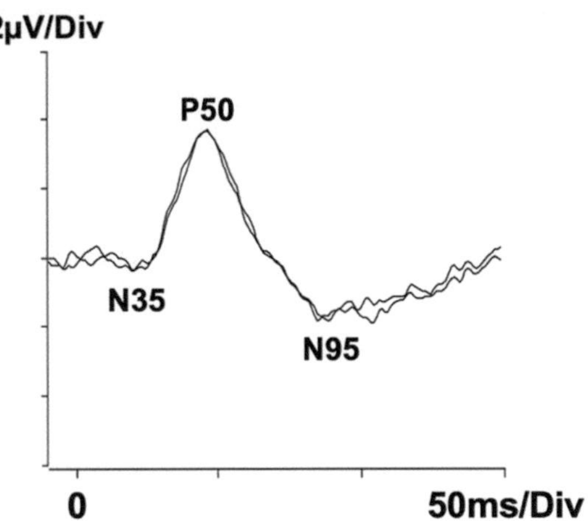

Fig. 31.8 The normal PERG

31.4.1 Clinical Applications

The PERG in clinical practice is usually combined with full-field ERG and/or pattern VEP.

Retinal Diseases: The ERG assesses global retinal function (the peripheral retina), and the PERG assesses the degree of macular involvement. This enables the distinction between macular dystrophy, cone dystrophy, and cone-rod dystrophy in a patient with clinically abnormal appearing macula. For example, primary macular dysfunction is characterised by a normal ERG and an abnormal PERG, a common combination in ABCA4 retinopathy (Stargardt-fundus flavimaculatus; (Fig. 31.9). As described above, the full-field ERG is of prognostic value in ABCA4 disease, which is not necessarily progressive, and the PERG helps delineate the extent and severity of macular involvement. Indeed, it can demonstrate early macular involvement at a stage when fundus examination may not reveal a significant abnormality.

Patients with rod-cone dystrophy (RP) may have spared central retinal function, and in such cases, the PERG may be normal even when the ERG is almost undetectable. Further, the objective index of macular function provided by the PERG can demonstrate early central retinal abnormalities before the symptoms or signs of macular involvement appear (Fig. 31.10).

Optic Nerve Diseases. The clinical distinction between maculopathy and optic neuropathy can be difficult as both are associated with reduced visual acuity, a central visual field defect, and may have a relative afferent pupillary defect. A delayed pattern VEP is very common in people with macular dysfunction [40] and must never in itself be considered to indicate optic nerve disease. The ability of the PERG to detect macular dysfunction, even in the presence of normal macular anatomy, or to demonstrate retinal ganglion cell dysfunction directly makes it an invaluable adjunct to the PVEP in assessing people with suspected or possible optic nerve dysfunction. The P50 component is affected in macular disease, whereas a delayed PVEP with a normal PERG or a PERG with a normal P50 but N95 component reduction indicates optic nerve disease. Providing the patient can maintain reasonably good fixation, even an eye with no light perception from optic nerve disease will have a detectable pattern ERG; it is a macular disease that is associated with an undetectable PERG. There is eventual P50 involvement with increasing severity of retinal ganglion cell dysfunction. There would be some P50 amplitude reduction (never extinction), which is usually associated with a shortening of P50 peak time. The shortening reflects the exposure of the contribution to P50 of pre-ganglionic structures by the loss of the ganglion cell-derived N95 component. Some clinical PERG examples are shown in Fig. 31.11.

The PERG is also important in primary retinal ganglion cell disease such as Leber Hereditary Optic Neuropathy (LHON) or Kjer type dominantly inherited optic atrophy (DOA; OPA1 variant). Figure 31.12 data are from an LHON patient.

The delayed VEP in primary retinal disease can be distinguished from optic neuropathy using the PERG (Fig. 31.13).

The pattern ERG is of great clinical value in the objective assessment of macular function and retinal ganglion cell function. It is fundamental to the accurate clinical interpretation of a pattern VEP delay as delay in the VEP is non-specific, and major delay can occur due to macular dysfunction. [40] The PERG is also of value in glau-

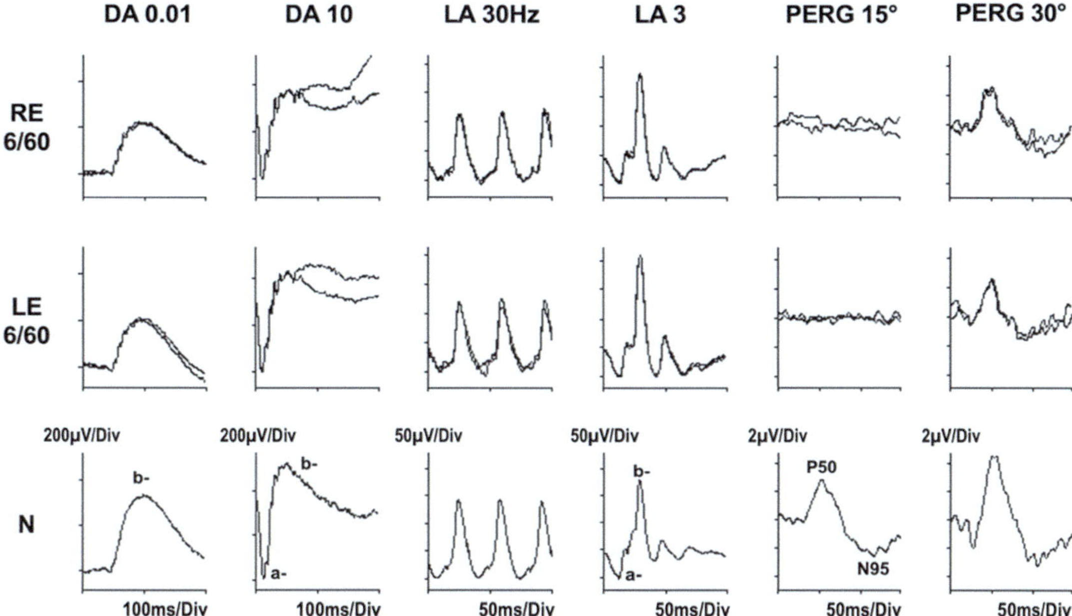

Fig. 31.9 Electrophysiology in Group 1 ABCA4 retinopathy. A patient with bilaterally reduced visual acuity due to ABCA4 retinopathy (Stardgardt disease). All full-field ERGs from each eye are normal. The standard field PERG is bilaterally undetectable, but the large field PERG, although subnormal, is present

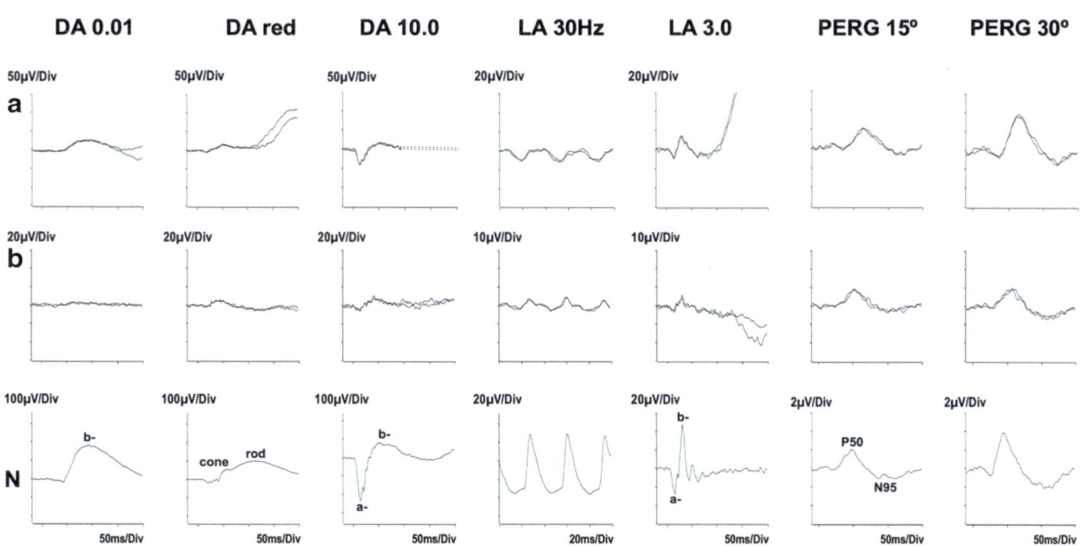

Fig. 31.10 Use of PERG in retinitis pigmentosa (rod-cone dystrophy). Data from two patients with retinitis pigmentosa (**a**, **b**). The ERGs in each patient show marked generalised impairment of retinal photoreceptor function, severe for patient **b** (please note amplitude calibrations). The appearances in patient **b** suggest that most, if not all, of the ERGs are arising in the small residual cone population. The 15^0 and 30^0 PERGs from patient **a** are normal, showing the expected doubling in P50 amplitude in the 30^0 field response relative to the 15^0 response. Patient **b** shows a detectable standard 15^0 field response, but there is only minimal increase with the large field stimulus, confirming that function has been lost between 15^0 and 30^0 eccentricity. Please compare the above findings in ABCA4 disease (Fig. 31.9), where the 30^0 field response is preserved, albeit subnormal, but the 15^0 field response is undetectable

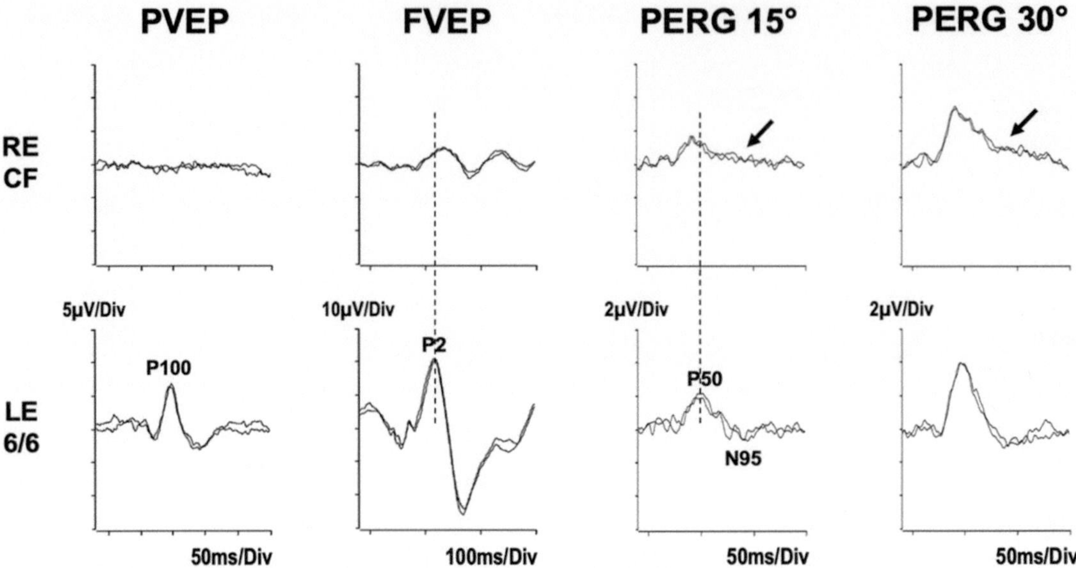

Fig. 31.11 Longstanding optic nerve disease. These data are from a patient with an optic nerve glioma. The right eye (RE) pattern VEP is undetectable. Right eye flash VEP is delayed and markedly subnormal. Both standard (15^0) and large field (30^0) pattern ERGs show a good P50 component but with a shortening of P50 peak time in keeping with marked retrograde degeneration of the retinal ganglion cells. All left eye (LE) findings are normal

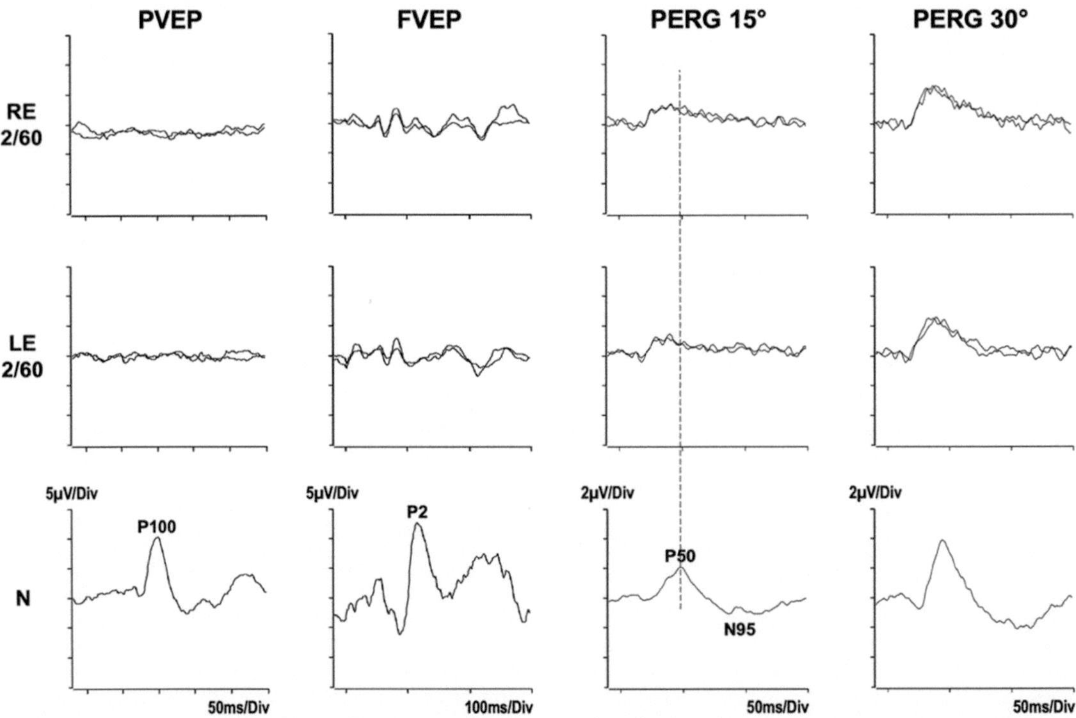

Fig. 31.12 Leber Hereditary Optic Neuropathy. VEP and PERGs from a teenage patient with a 16-month history of LHON. Pattern VEPs are bilaterally undetectable. Flash VEPs are profoundly subnormal and of the altered waveform, precluding accurate component identification. Both standard and large field (15^0 and 30^0) PERGs show significant N95 component reduction. Note there is a mild effect on P50 amplitude and a marked shortening of P50 peak time, in keeping with severe retinal ganglion cell dysfunction

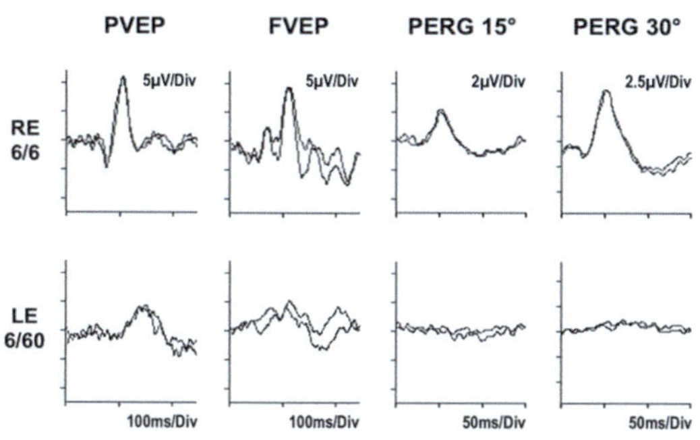

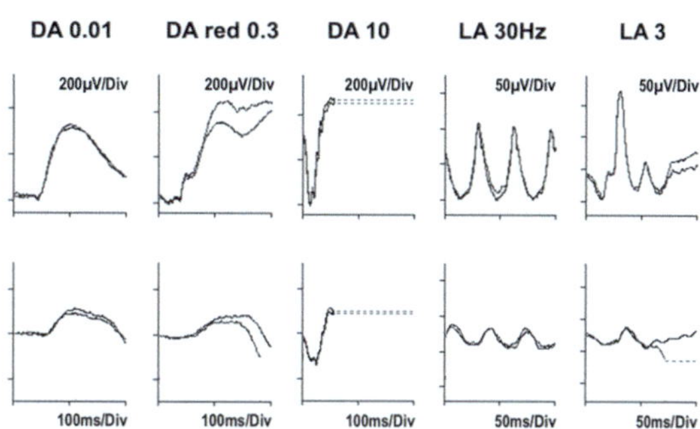

Fig. 31.13 Electrophysiological findings in a patient with reduced left visual acuity and a relative afferent pupillary defect initially thought to be secondary to optic nerve disease. Neuroimaging could not assign a cause. All right eye (RE) findings were normal. There are clear pattern VEP and flash VEP abnormalities from the left eye (both delayed and reduced), but PERGs indicate marked left macular dysfunction as a cause of the delayed pattern VEPs. Right eye ERGs are unremarkable; in the left eye (LE), the DA 0.01 response is subnormal—loss of rod system sensitivity; the DA red flash lacks a discernible cone component; the bright flash a- and b-waves are subnormal, with additional delay, confirming the rod system defect to have a photoreceptor origin; and cone ERGs are markedly delayed and subnormal. The findings, therefore, indicate generalised left retinal photoreceptor dysfunction, with cones more affected than rods, with PERGs showing global left macular involvement

coma, where ganglion cell-related N95 abnormalities can occur, but in which VEP delays are uncommon and usually minor. [42] Further, while most optic nerve disorders are associated with N95 loss, acute demyelinating optic neuritis can show P50 abnormalities, suggesting that macular involvement may contribute to the acute visual loss [43], and they may possibly be prognostic for the degree of visual acuity recovery. [40] It is also important to realise that as a contrast response requiring the optics of the eye to be preserved, media opacities and refractive error. Multifocal ERGs, which are luminance responses, are used in conjunction with PERGs as the two tests provide complementary information.

31.5 Other Tests

The ISCEV Standard recommendations are intended as minimum standards, and additional testing may be needed to make an accurate diagnosis. Examples of some of these refinements have been noted, such as the dark-adapted red flash, additional large field for PERG, extended dark adaptation in RDH5 variant testing, etc. ISCEV publishes "extended protocols" that include long-duration stimulation to separate the function of the on- and off-pathways and protocols for recording the activity of short-wavelength cones. It is beyond the remit of this chapter to address these in detail, and the reader is referred to the ISCEV website for further details (www.iscev.org). In addition, the reader is referred to two main documents that address the clinical issues. ([7, 44]).

Recent developments in electrophysiology include the use of hand-held stimulators and recording devices that have a valuable role in screening and some clinical applications. These can be very useful for recording at the bedside, in intensive care, etc. and may provide a rapid assessment for retinal screening in a paediatric patient. Such devices will likely expand in the future, but at the time of writing, these are unable to perform a comprehensive range of tests and are, therefore, limited in application.

31.6 Conclusion

Electrophysiological recording provides objective, non-invasive functional data. This short review has addressed some of the basics of acquisition and interpretation. All data should be obtained in consideration of existing International Standards, with the recognition that as minimum standards, the data may not be sufficient to make an accurate diagnosis in all circumstances. Additional testing may be needed. It is usually the integration of the different test protocols available to the electrophysiologist that enables an accurate diagnosis, but the importance of a comprehensive clinical history cannot be underestimated. The data should always be placed in full clinical context, with the origins of the signals identified and the abnormalities observed related to the presumed underlying pathophysiology. Electrophysiology aims to answer clinical questions, and a complete knowledge of the tests helps choose the appropriate tests to answer those questions.

Funding Hyderabad Eye Research Foundation.

Disclosure None.

References

1. Burian HM, Allen L. A speculum contact lens electrode for electroretinography. Electroencephalogr Clin Neurophysiol. 1954;6(3):509–11.
2. Dawson WW, Trick GL, Litzkow CA. Improved electrode for electroretinography. Invest Ophthalmol Vis Sci. 1979;18(9):988–91.
3. Zrenner E, Holder GE, Schiefer U, Wild JM. Quality control procedures and baseline values for electroretinography, Perimetry, color vision, and visual acuity in an international multicenter study: observations from a safety trial in chronic stable angina pectoris. Transl Vis Sci Technol. 2020;9(8):38.
4. Zrenner E, Holder GE, Schiefer U, Wild JM. Three-year changes in visual function in the placebo Group of a Randomized Double-Blind International Multicenter Safety Study: analysis of electroretinography, Perimetry, color vision, and visual acuity in individuals with chronic stable angina pectoris. Transl Vis Sci Technol. 2022;11(1):2.
5. McCulloch DL, Bach M, Brigell M, et al. ISCEV guidelines for calibration and verification of stimuli and recording instruments (2023 update). Doc Ophthalmol. 2023;146(3):199–210.
6. Frishman L. Principles and practice of clinical electrophysiology of vision. MIT Press; 2023. https://mitpress.mit.edu/9780262083461/principles-and-practice-of-clinical-electrophysiology-of-vision/.
7. Robson AG, Nilsson J, Li S, Jalali S, et al. ISCEV guide to visual electrodiagnostic procedures. Doc Ophthalmol Adv Ophthalmol. 2018;136(1):1–26.
8. Hoffmann MB, Bach M, Kondo M, et al. ISCEV standard for clinical multifocal electroretinography (mfERG) (2021 update). Doc Ophthalmol. 2021;142(1):5–16.
9. Bach M, Brigell MG, Hawlina M, et al. ISCEV standard for clinical pattern electroretinography (PERG): 2012 update. Doc Ophthalmol. 2013;126(1):1–7.
10. Robson AG, Frishman LJ, Grigg J, et al. ISCEV standard for full-field clinical electroretinography (2022 update). Doc Ophthalmol. 2022;144(3):165–77.
11. Marmor MF, Arden GB, Nilsson SEG, Zrenner E. Standard for clinical electroretinography: international standardization committee. Arch Ophthalmol. 1989;107(6):816–9.
12. Hood DC, Birch DG. Rod phototransduction in retinitis pigmentosa: estimation and interpretation of parameters derived from the rod a-wave. Invest Ophthalmol Vis Sci. 1994;35(7):2948–61.
13. Shiells RA, Falk G. Contribution of rod, on-bipolar, and horizontal cell light responses to the ERG of dogfish retina. Vis Neurosci. 1999;16(3):503–11.
14. Bush RA, Sieving PA. Inner retinal contributions to the primate photopic fast flicker electroretinogram. J Opt Soc Am A Opt Image Sci Vis. 1996;13(3):557–65.
15. Bush RA, Sieving PA. A proximal retinal component in the primate photopic ERG a-wave. Invest Ophthalmol Vis Sci. 1994;35(2):635–45.
16. Wali N, Leguire LE. The photopic hill: a new phenomenon of the light adapted electroretinogram. Doc Ophthalmol Adv Ophthalmol. 1992;80(4):335–45.
17. Ueno S, Kondo M, Niwa Y, et al. Luminance dependence of neural components that underlies the primate Photopic Electroretinogram. Invest Ophthalmol Vis Sci. 2004;45(3):1033–40.
18. Fujinami K, Lois N, Davidson AE, et al. A longitudinal study of Stargardt disease: clinical and Electrophysiologic assessment, progression, and genotype correlations. Am J Ophthalmol. 2013;155(6):1075–1088.e13.
19. Zacks DN, Samson MC, Loewenstein J, Foster SC. Electroretinograms as an indicator of disease activity in birdshot retinochoroidopathy. Graefes Arch Clin Exp Ophthalmol. 2002;240(8):601–7.
20. Holder GE, Robson AG, Pavesio C, Graham EM. Electrophysiological characterisation and monitoring in the management of birdshot chorioretinopathy. Br J Ophthalmol. 2005;89(6):709–18.
21. Francis PJ, Marinescu A, Fitzke FW, et al. Acute zonal occult outer retinopathy: towards a set of diagnostic criteria. Br J Ophthalmol. 2005;89(1):70–3.
22. Audo I, Robson AG, Holder GE, Moore AT. The negative ERG: clinical phenotypes and disease mechanisms of inner retinal dysfunction. Surv Ophthalmol. 2008;53(1):16–40.
23. Jiang X, Mahroo OA. Negative electroretinograms: genetic and acquired causes, diagnostic approaches and physiological insights. Eye. 2021;35(9):2419–37.
24. Mantel I, Ramchand KV, Holder GE, et al. Macular and retinal dysfunction of unknown origin in adults with normal fundi: evidence for an autoimmune pathophysiology. Exp Mol Pathol. 2008;84(2):90–101.

25. Holder GE, Mahroo O. Electronegative ERG or pseudo-negative ERG? Doc Ophthalmol. 2022;145(3):283–6.
26. Sergouniotis PI, Sohn EH, Li Z, et al. Phenotypic variability in RDH5 retinopathy (fundus Albipunctatus). Ophthalmology. 2011;118(8):1661–70.
27. Miyake Y, Horiguchi M, Suzuki S, et al. Electrophysiological findings in patients with Oguchi's disease. Jpn J Ophthalmol. 1996;40(4):511–9.
28. McBain VA, Egan CA, Pieris SJ, et al. Functional observations in vitamin a deficiency: diagnosis and time course of recovery. Eye Lond Engl. 2007;21(3):367–76.
29. Vincent A, Robson AG, Holder GE. Pathognomonic (diagnostic) ERGs. A review and update. Retina. 2013;33(1):5–12.
30. Sutter EE, Tran D. The field topography of ERG components in man—I. The photopic luminance response. Vis Res. 1992;32(3):433–46.
31. Marmor MF, Tan F. Central serous chorioretinopathy: bilateral multifocal electroretinographic abnormalities. Arch Ophthalmol Chic Ill 1960. 1999;117(2):184–8.
32. Hood DC, Odel JG, Chen CS, Winn BJ. The multifocal electroretinogram. J Neuroophthalmol. 2003;23(3):225–35.
33. Chan HHL, Ng Y, fai, Chu PH wai. Applications of the multifocal electroretinogram in the detection of glaucoma. Clin Exp Optom. 2011;94(3): 247–58.
34. Hood DC, Bach M, Brigell M, et al. International society for clinical electrophysiology of vision. ISCEV standard for clinical multifocal electroretinography (mfERG) (2011 edition). Doc Ophthalmol. 2012;124(1):1–13.
35. Tsang AC, Ahmadi S, Hamilton J, et al. The diagnostic utility of multifocal electroretinography in detecting chloroquine and Hydroxychloroquine retinal toxicity. Am J Ophthalmol. 2019;206:132–9.
36. Gin TJ, Luu CD, Guymer RH. Central retinal function as measured by the multifocal Electroretinogram and flicker Perimetry in early age-related macular degeneration. Invest Ophthalmol Vis Sci. 2011;52(12):9267–74.
37. McAnany JJ, Persidina OS, Park JC. Clinical electroretinography in diabetic retinopathy: a review. Surv Ophthalmol. 2022;67(3):712–22.
38. Lenassi E, Robson AG, Hawlina M, Holder GE. The value of two-field pattern electroretinogram in routine clinical electrophysiologic practice. Retina. 2012;32(3):588–99.
39. Holder GE. Significance of abnormal pattern electroretinography in anterior visual pathway dysfunction. Br J Ophthalmol. 1987;71(3):166–71.
40. Holder GE. Pattern electroretinography (PERG) and an integrated approach to visual pathway diagnosis. Prog Retin Eye Res. 2001;20(4):531–61.
41. Viswanathan S, Frishman LJ, Robson JG. The uniform field and pattern ERG in macaques with experimental glaucoma: removal of spiking activity. Invest Ophthalmol Vis Sci. 2000;41(9):2797–810.
42. Grippo TM, Hood DC, Kanadani FN, et al. A comparison between multifocal and conventional VEP latency changes secondary to glaucomatous damage. Invest Ophthalmol Vis Sci. 2006;47(12):5331–6.
43. Kleerekooper I, Del Porto L, Dell'Arti L, et al. Pattern ERGs suggest a possible retinal contribution to the visual acuity loss in acute optic neuritis. Doc Ophthalmol. 2022;145(3):185–95.
44. Holder GE, Celesia GG, Miyake Y, et al. International Federation of Clinical Neurophysiology. International Federation of Clinical Neurophysiology: recommendations for visual system testing. Clin Neurophysiol. 2010;121(9):1393–409.

The Visual Evoked Potential

32

Oliver R. Marmoy

32.1 Introduction

The visual evoked potential (VEP) was one of the first time-locked electroencephalographic potentials recorded in humans. Seminal works first demonstrated that a series of positive and negative potentials could be recorded from the human scalp following flash stimulation, demonstrating the recording of a flash VEP for the first time. Along with technological developments in visual display units (VDUs), the VEP to structured stimuli (i.e., patterns, gratings) was soon developed. These were found to have more reproducible and predictable waveforms than that produced to flash stimuli. Following its conception, the pattern VEP has subsequently been used in assessment visual pathway dysfunction, particularly for optic nerve disease. Much of its application was used to discover "clinically silent" lesions of the optic nerve in patients with demyelinating disease [1]. However, it is now known that the pattern VEP can be affected in a range of conditions affecting the visual apparatus from the macula to the primary visual cortex, and the flash VEP is less sensitive in the disorders of the visual pathway. As such, the clinical practice encourages the complementary use of the pattern and flash VEPs with a pattern electroretinogram (PERG) or full-field electroretinogram (FFERG) [2]. These allied electrophysiological tests provide specificity in the locus of visual pathway dysfunction and complement normal or abnormal VEP findings.

The VEP can often be overlooked in clinical practice, yet it provides a unique and valuable addition to ophthalmic diagnoses in the modern age. The pattern VEP can be used in disease monitoring, outcome measurements in clinical trials, or estimation of vision levels in people unable to comply with subjective testing. In the era of genetic testing, phenotyping, and novel treatments or therapies for eye disease, the VEP will likely provide an objective functional measure of the visual pathway.

32.2 Technology

Recording the VEP requires two major technological considerations: the recording equipment and stimuli to elicit a visually evoked response.

O. R. Marmoy (✉)
Great Ormond Street Hospital for Children NHS Foundation Trust , London, UK

GOS-ICH University College London, London, UK
e-mail: o.marmoy@nhs.net

T. Das, P. Satgunam (eds.), *Ophthalmic Diagnostics*, https://doi.org/10.1007/978-981-97-0138-4_32

32.2.1 Recording Equipment

32.2.1.1 Electrodes

Electrodes to record the VEP are typically Cl-Cl-chloride, gold cup, or surface electrodes applied to the occipital scalp. According to the international 10–20 system, at a minimum, the electrode should be placed at the mid-occiput (Oz) and is typically referred to as the mid-frontal region (Fz), with a ground placed around the central scalp (Cz), to record a single channel VEP. As these are a minimum requirement, additional electrodes placed laterally (i.e., O1/O2, or even T5/T6) can be used to identify the contributions from each hemisphere to a stimulus. The latter is useful in evaluating hemianopic or bi-temporal/bi-nasal field deficits [3]. Furthermore, in pediatric practice, an electrode placed inferiorly to the Oz over the inion (Iz) provides larger amplitudes for those under 8 years of age for a standard check width (50′) and for those under 12 years of age for a small check width (12.5′) [4]. An illustration of these electrode positions is seen in Fig. 32.1.

Before applying the electrodes, the application site should be prepared using an abrasive gel. This is typically performed using a cotton tip, which can also be used to part the hair, depending on the location. Electrode impedance (measured by passing a low voltage signal through the electrodes to observe their respective resistance) should then be measured to ensure that these are balanced (typically within 20%) and maintained below 5 kOhms. It is the author's practice to wrap a Coban strip around the electrode sites following electrode application to minimize movement (including coiling of wires) and potential shift of electrodes during testing to minimize external noise intrusion.

32.2.1.2 Signal Acquisition

The VEP is a time-locked subtraction of the background electroencephalographic signal. As such, this is an analog signal arising from cortical neurons. Modern systems require digitization of the signals to enable processing on software and potential post-hoc analysis or modification. To achieve this, the incoming ongoing electro-

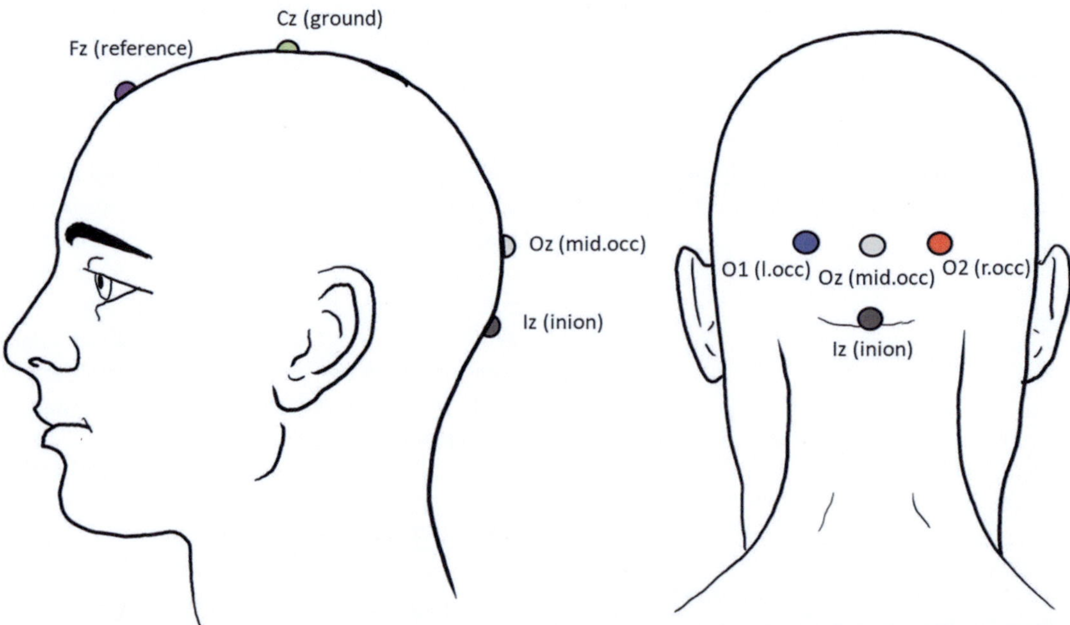

Fig. 32.1 Illustration of electrode positions for the VEP. Electrodes are placed according to positions defined in the international 10–20 system. The left illustration shows the side view of the head, with active electrodes positioned at Oz (middle of the occiput), Iz (inion), with the reference electrode placed anteriorly over Fz (mid-frontal) and ground around the center of the head (Cz). The posterior view of the head shows the multichannel VEP electrode array, with the Oz and Iz electrodes, but also lateral electrodes placed over the left (O1) and right (O2) occiput

graphic signal is sampled at a high rate (at a minimum, twice the frequency of the signal of interest according to the Nyquist-Shannon theorem) in the order of <1 kbps. All signals will have a form of differential amplification of the signal prior to signal analysis.

Differential amplifiers work in a manner whereby the difference between two inputs is calculated. Therefore, a large signal in one electrode and a minimal signal in another will produce a large amplitude output. An example of this would be the Oz electrode being an active electrode over the visual cortex and the Fz electrode being a relatively inactive electrode over the anterior scalp; therefore, the VEP produced is due to a difference in signal strength between these electrodes. Signals of the same size and temporal profile, when they enter both electrodes, are said to be in *common mode*, which typically results in minimal signal output and highlights the importance of balanced electrode inputs. The amplified signals are then subject to filtering, typically used to attenuate frequency bands, allowing one to eliminate unwanted signals (i.e., noise). For the VEP, this is typically set as a 0.3–100 Hz band-pass filter as per the ISCEV (International Society for Clinical Electrophysiology of Vision) standards.

The size of the incoming signal can be automatically rejected in some software programs by determining a rejection criterion based on amplitude. For most instances, this is 100–200 μV (signals above this are automatically rejected).

As the VEP is a time-locked signal of the background electroencephalogram (EEG) signal, averaging is required to improve the signal–noise ratio. Typically, 100 trials are used to constitute an average response, which is then repeated to demonstrate reproducibility. The number of trials may be reduced in people with poorer fixation and compliance but should be repeated to confirm the reproducibility of the response.

32.2.1.3 Display and Software Requirements

Display requirements for the analysis of the VEP should allow analysis of the entire waveform on a high-resolution monitor. The software should enable measuring the peak-time and amplitude of the VEP, ideally with enabled post-hoc manual or automatic rejection of trials to improve the signal–noise ratio.

32.2.2 Stimuli

A VEP can theoretically be elicited to a variety of visual stimuli, for example, color, motion, contrast, luminance, or in some circumstances, an event related to particular stimuli. Despite this, the major clinical applications of the VEP relate to luminance and contrast through the flash (f-) and pattern reversal (pr-) or pattern onset-offset (po-) stimuli, respectively. Accordingly, there are ISCEV standards for these flash and pattern stimuli [3].

The prVEP, poVEP, and f-VEP show different waveforms, which are typically named according to their respective polarity (P for positive and N for negative), timing (i.e., P100 = positivity at 100 ms), or order of presentation (i.e., P1 or P2). These waveforms are illustrated in Fig. 32.2.

For patterned stimuli, there should be an abrupt change of contrast at the stimulus onset without any significant alterations in mean luminance. This is easily achieved with the older visual display units (VDU), such as plasma display panels or cathode-ray tube devices; however, at the time of writing, these devices are obsolete and not widely manufactured. Unfortunately, common alternatives such as liquid crystal display monitors are usually unsuitable as these have a detrimental luminance artifact with pattern reversals [5, 6]. Modern devices such as digital light projection (DLP) systems or organic light-emitting diode (OLED) devices may be able to overcome these issues, but these are still under review [7, 8]. Any transient luminance artifacts can be easily visualized by darkening the room and placing a piece of paper before the observer's eyes, facing toward the stimulus, to monitor for any transient luminance alterations visually. Otherwise, these can be measured formally with a photodiode. Any individuals setting up laboratories should be aware of these potential VDU limitations and their confounding effects on the PVEP or PERG.

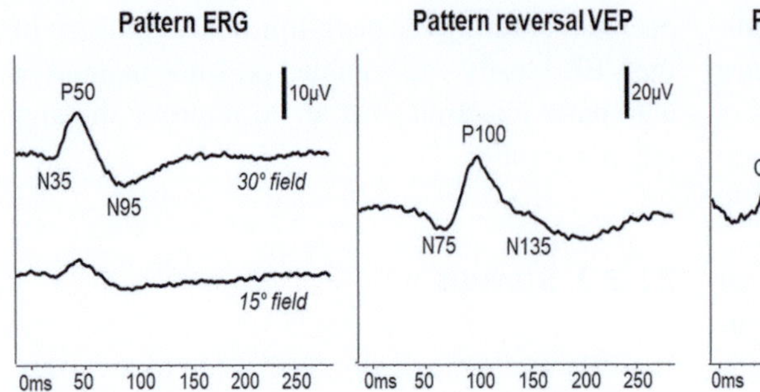

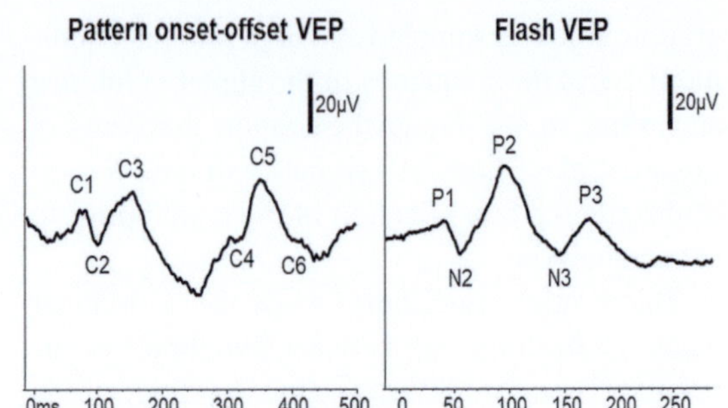

Fig. 32.2 Typical waveforms of the pattern electroretinogram (PERG), pattern reversal visual evoked potential (prVEP), pattern onset-offset VEP (poVEP), and flash VEP (f-VEP). The waveforms are plotted by amplitude and time and labeled according to the conventional nomenclature consistent with the ISCEV standards

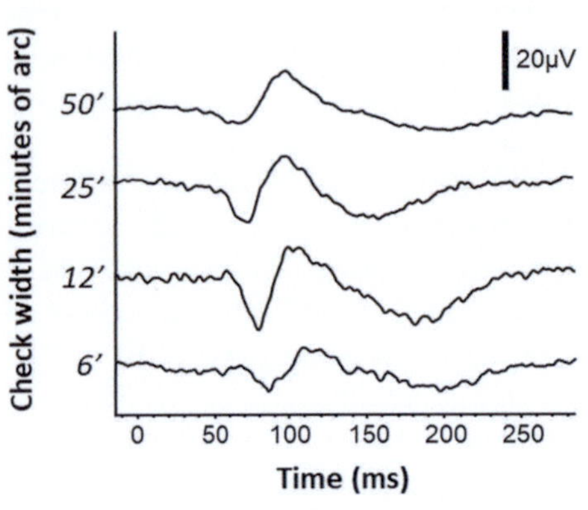

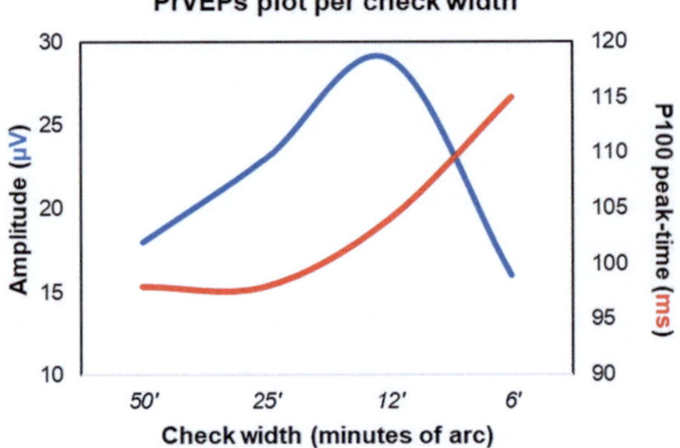

Fig. 32.3 The effect of check width on the pattern reversal VEP. The figure on the left shows the waveform alterations with check width, with the top (large check) showing the earliest peak-time, with the amplitude then showing an inverse U-shaped function with decreasing check width, with increasing peak-time. These data are plotted according to the check width in the right panel (amplitude in blue, peak-time in red)

The temporal frequency of the stimulus can either be transient or steady-state. The former is most common in clinical practice, as this allows the isolation of individual waveform components, which can be measured for their peak-time, amplitudes, and shape to identify dysfunction. Steady-state responses are those recorded at higher temporal frequencies (typically >10 Hz). These have been utilized in clinical practice with varying purposes; the most commonly used is a sweep VEP to provide an objective estimation of visual acuity [9].

The stimulus field size should subtend at least 15° of the visual field, typically viewed at around 1 m, per the ISCEV VEP standards [3]. It is the author's practice to have a larger field size, which is advantageous for pediatric patients whose fixation and eye position may be more variable; it is increased to around 30° to allow for variable fixation. However, with increasing field size, one must be more aware of the alterations in the prVEP morphology. Typically, with larger field sizes, there are larger contributions from paramacular prVEP components, which is discussed later in this chapter.

Check width is an important factor for performing the VEP. The ISCEV VEP standard specifies that the prVEP should be recorded with a large (1°) and small (0.25°) check width. Importantly, the amplitude typically shows an inverse U-shaped function with the peak amplitude around 15 min of arc (0.25°), while the amplitude shows a more linear increase with decreasing check width (Fig. 32.3). Expanding the number of check widths used in clinical practice can reveal macular pathway dysfunction where small check widths are affected first [10] and can give more consistency to a response. Therefore, while a minimum of two check widths should be used, additional check widths are beneficial to characterize macular pathway function in practice.

32.3 Technique

A typical recording setup would have a patient seated comfortably in a chair, preferably with a high back and headrest. Electrodes would be applied with low, balanced impedances. During application, a discussion on how the test is performed and what is needed from the patient can be initiated, and any questions can be answered. It is essential to ensure that the patient is relaxed to minimize muscle artifacts (i.e., chewing, neck straining, etc.) and ensure their comfort as best possible (i.e., with neck pillows, adjustment of seating position, etc.).

The patient should wear their most recent spectacles for testing. If these are unavailable, trial frames can be used, or if unavailable, a note made in the report that the tests were performed uncorrected (and define their correction). The pattern VEP can withstand a significant degree of optical blur but is dependent on test strategy and other patient factors, the degree of which should be noted.

For children, alternating the stimulus checkerboard with a video of their choosing will most likely result in better testing conditions and a happier child! The prVEP depends on fixation and attention; therefore, this should be monitored closely for fixation loss, deliberate mis-fixation, or fixation drift. One way this can be achieved is by simultaneously using camera systems (i.e., CCTV, IP cameras) to monitor the patient's fixation during signal acquisition. Thus, in periods of fixation loss, signal acquisition can be paused and resumed once fixation has returned. In younger children, larger field sizes are necessary to attract attention and account for some unavoidable fixation variance. In these circumstances, it is best to work with colleagues as a pair, one to "distract and interact" with the child and the other to focus solely on signal acquisition. Fixation can be encouraged using small toys or fingers at the top of the stimulus screen. As the prVEP is dominated by the inferior field, small obscurations in the superior field have negligible impacts on the PVEP and enable more reliable fixation on the stimulus. Intermittent averaging is required to allow for the patient's attention. Prolonged presentation of a checkerboard stimulus will lead to tiredness, habituation, or defocus, even in the most enthusiastic of adults.

32.4 Clinical Application and Interpretation

The typical responses to flash, pattern reversal, pattern onset-offset stimuli are illustrated in Fig. 32.2. To interpret the VEP waveform, the acronym "PAST" (Peak-time, Amplitude, Shape, Transoccipital asymmetry) can be used to evaluate the response.

32.4.1 Peak-Time

The peak-time of the waveform signifies the time taken for cortical activation following afferent pathway stimulation. The peak-time is most conventionally measured from the major positive peak of the respective VEP waveform, for example, the P100 of the prVEP, C1 of the poVEP, and P2 of the flash VEP [3]. A delay in peak-time (i.e., a peak-time exceeding the laboratory reference range) can result from dysfunction of the physiological substrates underlying the response. For example, a delay of the prVEP P100 can be due to a dysfunction of the macular, retinal ganglion cells, optic nerve, or chiasmal/retro chiasmal visual pathway. To elaborate on the dysfunction site, a PERG is required to delineate between macular, retinal ganglion cell, or optic nerve/pathway dysfunction. While prVEPs to standard check widths are fairly resistant to an optical blur of <5 D, the interpretation of peak-time delays to smaller check widths must be cautiously made, as this may result from uncorrected refractive error, reduced contrast (i.e., from anterior segment disease such as cataract) or poor fixation/blurring. Another important consideration is the maturation of the VEP. The VEP to standard (large) check widths is typically within 10% of adult peak-times by 6 months of age, but younger people may have longer peak-times due to the immaturity of their visual pathways.

Similarly, poVEPs can show shape-dependent changes with maturation [11]. This is an important consideration for interpreting the PVEP, as these factors should be excluded before attributing a peak-time delay to macular pathway dysfunction, including age-matched reference data. Simultaneous PERG and PVEP recordings can elaborate on an abnormal VEP, particularly for suspected optical blur or defocus, as the PERG is far more sensitive to uncorrected refractive error and contrast alterations [12].

Peak-time delays of the prVEP with normal amplitude most commonly signify conduction delay but are not specific to demyelinating disease. In demyelinating disease, a conduction delay can be observed even following the resolution of visual symptoms or, in some cases, may show abnormality as a "clinically silent" lesion, providing paraclinical evidence of demyelination in conditions such as multiple sclerosis [1]. Importantly, peak-time delay is not specific to demyelination but can be observed in various optic nerve diseases, albeit to varying degrees. Typically, with severe forms of demyelinating optic neuropathies, PERG N95 loss and amplitude reduction of the VEP following the acute phase are often associated with poorer visual outcomes (Fig. 32.4).

While peak-time delay is most common, in some pathologies, one can expect an atypically early peak-time. Such abnormalities are usually associated with an alteration in waveform morphology, such as bifid or double-peaked waveform, discussed in the "shape" analysis below.

32.4.2 Amplitude

Reduced amplitude of a VEP suggests poor signal strength; as such, this is associated with macular pathway dysfunction. Reduced amplitude is also a relatively non-specific indication of macular pathway abnormality. It is often observed in conditions with reduced physiological signal generation; for example, this may be reduced in retinal disease, optic atrophy (whereby fewer axons are functioning), or optic nerve hypoplasia. It is beneficial to record pattern VEPs to larger check widths to observe the alterations with changes in spatial frequency. Recording to a range of check widths is also useful, as it can help with the monitoring of the disease, whereas those for standard or small checks may progressively diminish in amplitude; therefore, the larger check widths may sometimes be the only means by which disease progression can be monitored [13].

While reduced amplitudes are most commonly observed in diseases of the macular pathway, in rarer circumstances, VEPs may be atypically large or "giant." This may occur with normal peak-time of the response in patients with chronically raised intracranial pressure, perhaps due to thinning of the skull, reduced cerebrospinal fluid thickness, or cortical hyperexcitability [14]. Similarly, atypically large VEPs can occur with cortical hyperexcitability in epileptic disorders such as neuronal ceroid lipofuscinosis battens disease, where a "spike and wave" type paroxysmal VEP response is observed, often with an early peak-time [15]. In such circumstances, VEP testing may be halted to minimize the risk of pattern or flash-related seizure induction.

The pattern VEP can be a useful addition in monitoring retinal disease, particularly in those with rod–cone photoreceptor dystrophies. As field size reduces from the periphery and encroaches upon the macula, the full-field ERG can be reduced or extinguished, albeit with vestigial PERG responses. As the fovea is often more preserved during the later disease stages, the prVEP recorded to a range of check widths can provide information on the remaining integrity of the macular pathway and be used for monitoring disease progression. This is likely due to the expanded foveal representation of the PVEP due to cortical magnification, but it is particularly useful to apply this when the ERG or PERG is extinguished to provide a functional outcome measure in disease [16]. An example of this is shown in Fig. 32.5.

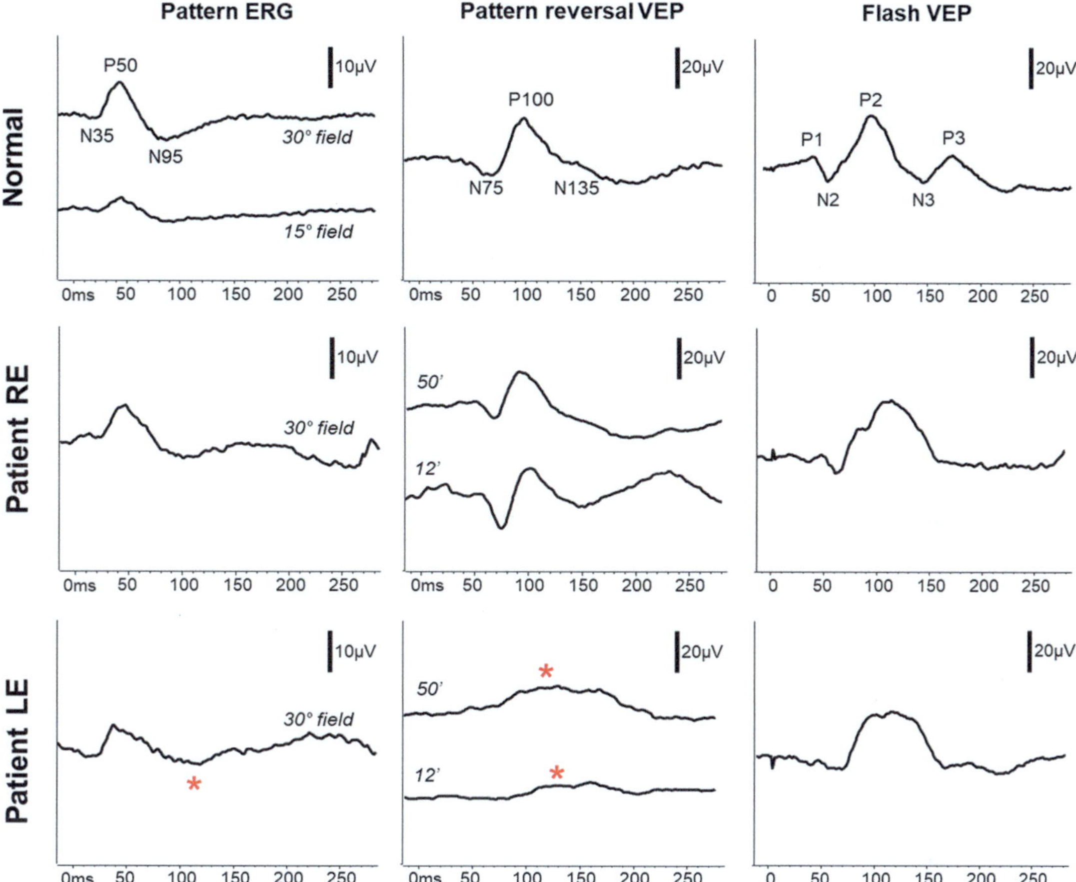

Fig. 32.4 An example of the waveforms seen in a patient with left eye (LE) optic neuritis is associated with myelin oligodendrocyte glycoprotein antibody-associated disease (MOGAD). The normal waveforms of the pattern ERG, VEP, and flash VEP are shown in the top panels. The patient's (unaffected) right eye (RE) shows normal PERG findings, with normal prVEP to large and small check widths and normal flash VEP. The patient's affected LE shows N95 amplitude loss and shortening of P50 peak-time, associated with retinal ganglion cell dysfunction. The patient's prVEP is reduced and delayed in the LE relative to the RE to both large and small check widths. The flash VEP is slightly simplified relative to the RE but is of similar amplitude and peak-time

32.4.3 Shape

The morphology of the VEP can be altered in disease states and so can be used to delineate visual pathway dysfunction. The most common abnormality in the VEP is a broadened or bifid VEP waveform.

A broadened prVEP can occur with macular pathway abnormalities, likely due to temporal dispersion of the afferent signal to the striate cortex. This has been reported in grading schemes of VEPs in craniosynostosis [13], alongside other pathologies. This has been proposed as a waveform N75-N135 peak-time difference exceeding 90 ms [13, 17]. The significance of a broadened prVEP likely reflects mild macular pathway dysfunction in the absence of amplitude or peak-time anomalies. Nonetheless, these changes are worth monitoring as they may suggest an early manifestation of visual pathway dysfunction.

A bifid VEP is a waveform which adopts a P-N-P morphology, opposite to the typical configuration of N-P-N. This can be associated with optic nerve or demyelinating disease, and it is the author's experience that these changes are due to

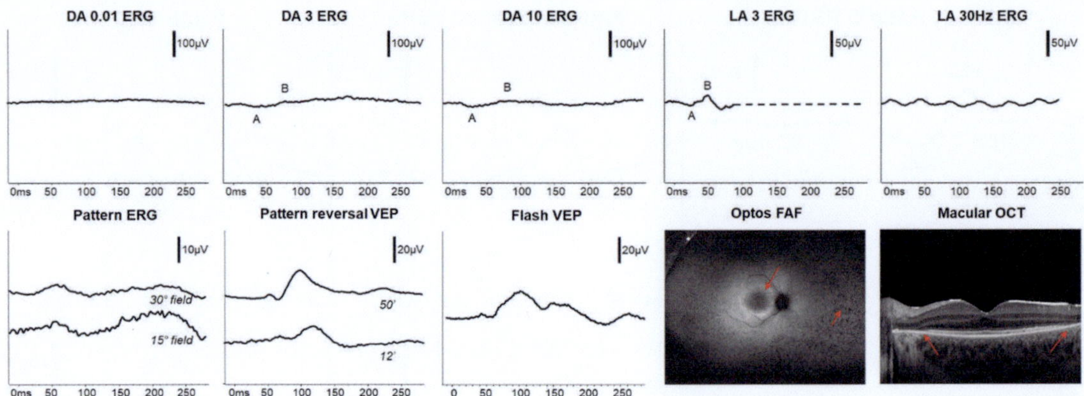

Fig. 32.5 Electrophysiological findings in a patient with retinitis pigmentosa. The full-field ERGs show severely reduced DA a - and b-wave amplitudes, with preserved but significantly reduced amplitudes of the LA cone-mediated responses indicative of severe rod–cone dystrophy. The pattern ERG was reduced, and the amplitude did not increase substantially between the 15° and 30° fields, indicating distal retinal (cone-driven) dysfunction affecting the 15°–30° field. Despite these findings, the prVEPs and fVEPs are within the reference range. The ultra-widefield (Optos) fundus autofluorescence shows pigmentary changes in the periphery (red arrow) alongside a hyperfluorescent ring around the macula. The macular OCT shows IS/OS loss around the macular periphery, with relative foveal sparing. The preservation of the prVEPs is likely due to the relative foveal sparing

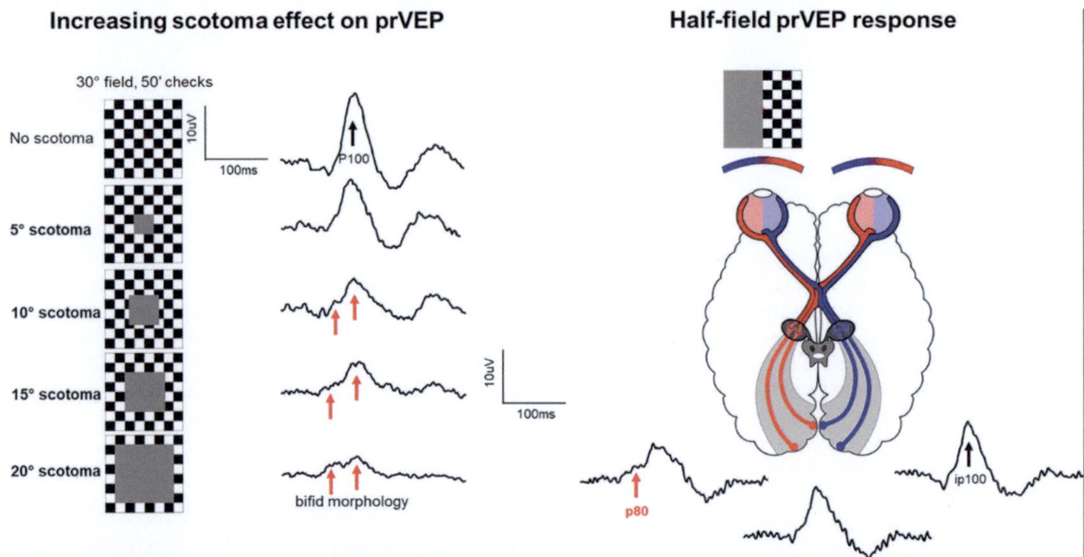

Fig. 32.6 The prVEPs in a healthy participant were recorded with increasing central scotoma size (0–20°). The waveform alterations can be observed with increasing scotoma size to exhibit a bifid morphology of the waveform with two positive peaks (red arrows). These peaks correspond to the paramacular components of the half-field prVEP (right panel, red arrow)

an enhancement of the paramacular prVEP components and a reduction of the major P100 peak [12]. Accordingly, the finding of a bifid prVEP often suggests reduced central field sensitivity or central scotoma, meaning that the paramacular retinal generators predominate the resultant VEP. This is illustrated in Fig. 32.6 in a healthy individual; an increasingly larger scotoma alters the prVEP morphology to adopt a bifid waveform. As can also be seen, this waveform is similar to the paramacular components (p80) observed contralaterally in the half-field prVEP. As such,

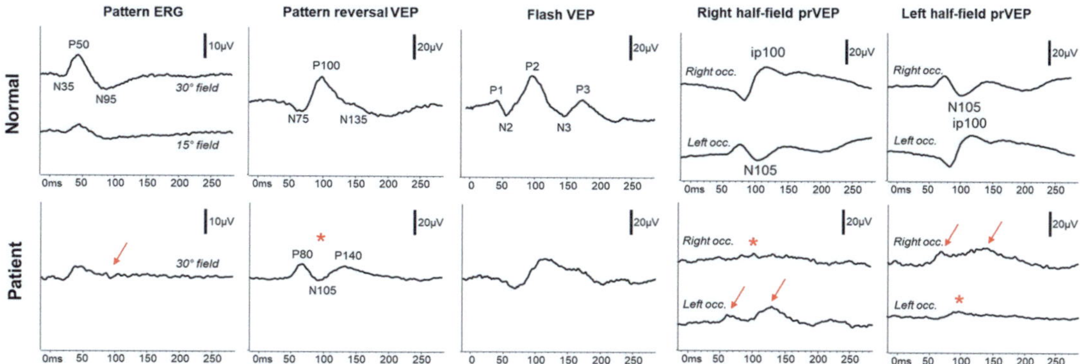

Fig. 32.7 Electrophysiological findings in a patient with Leber's hereditary optic neuropathy. The pattern ERG shows early P50 peak-time and N95 amplitude loss indicating severe retinal ganglion cell disease. The prVEP shows an abnormal morphology (red asterisk) with atypical bifid morphology. The half-field prVEPs show attenuation of the ipsilateral major ip100 component (red asterisks), yet the contralateral paramacular components remain and correspond to the P80/P140 peaks observed in the full-field prVEP. This patient was later detected to have a central scotoma on visual field testing

recording half-field prVEPs in patients with bifid prVEP waveforms helps one understand if these components truly arise from a paramacular origin or are caused by an alteration in the macular VEP waveform (Fig. 32.7).

32.4.4 Transoccipital Asymmetry

Transoccipital asymmetries can be investigated when one extends the electrode montage to include a multichannel recording. This typically uses additional lateral electrodes, "O1" or "O2," according to the international 10–20 system. An asymmetry across the occiput can define transoccipital asymmetries. While individual laboratory reference ranges will determine the limits for a significant transoccipital asymmetry (which may depend on the check width and the field size), it is the author's experience that a transoccipital asymmetry (i.e., a difference between the lateral electrodes) for an amplitude of >30% is considered suspicious, and those with amplitudes >50% are considered significant. Similarly, a peak-time difference exceeding 6 ms across the transoccipital array is also considered significant.

A transoccipital asymmetry is typically suggestive of a chiasmal, post-chiasmal, or relative field defect, depending on the pattern of abnormality and if confirmed with appropriate testing. The localization of the lesion can be achieved with half-field VEPs although knowledge of the underlying neural substrates generating the responses is crucial to determine the site of the dysfunction accurately.

When using a large field, with standard (or large) check widths, with a mid-frontal reference electrode, prVEPs demonstrate a phenomenon known as paradoxical lateralization [18]. This phenomenon means that responses generated to the right half-field stimulation (corresponding to the left hemisphere) are "paradoxically" observed over the right occipital electrode (Fig. 32.6, right panel). This is likely due to the oblique orientation of the cortical prVEP generators within the calcarine sulcus. Conversely, pattern onset VEPs do not exhibit paradoxical lateralization, yet pattern offset VEPs do, similar to prVEPs [19]. Abnormalities of the prVEP transoccipital distribution can therefore be elaborated upon using half-field stimulation of the left or right-half field of each eye. The abnormalities may be "crossed," meaning that the distribution of the transoccipital asymmetry will be altered depending on which eye is stimulated (e.g., in chiasmal dysfunction or disproportion), or can be "un-crossed" in homonymous hemianopia (i.e., post-chiasmal lesions). Half-field testing can be used to elaborate on full-field prVEP distributions, to identify whether the transoccipital asymmetry is due to a relative deficit of one half-field or whether this is instead due to individual cortical architecture or

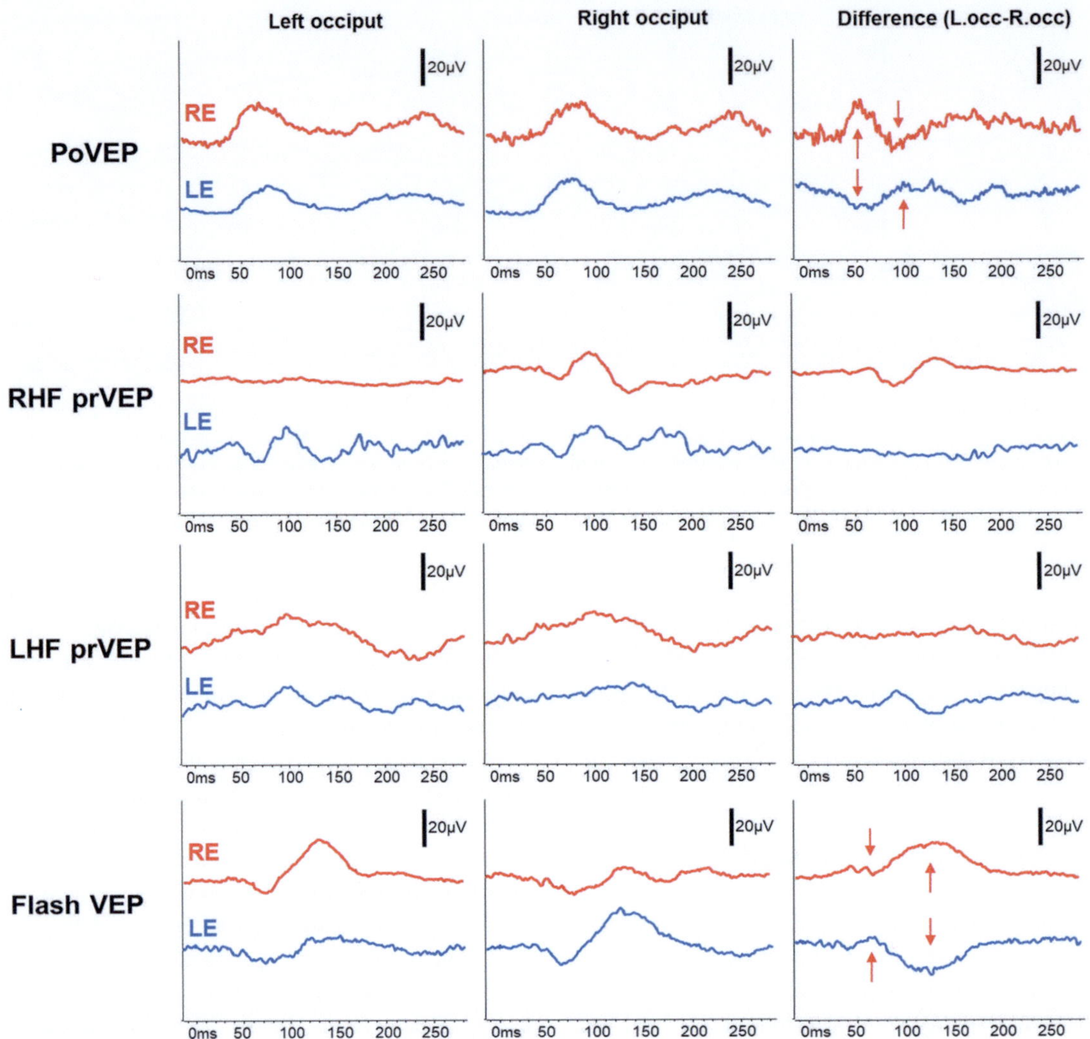

Fig. 32.8 A patient with genetically confirmed oculocutaneous albinism. Data for the pattern onset (poVEP) VEP, half-field pattern reversal VEP (RHF prVEP/LHF prVEP), and flash VEP are presented for electrodes overlaying the left occiput (left panels), right occiput (middle panels), and a difference of these two (right panels). The RE (red) and LE (blue) data are illustrated. The pattern onset VEP shows that the major positive peak was largest over the contralateral occiput, which when compared from each eye in the difference channel shows a phase reversal (red arrows). The half-field prVEPs show a normal distribution of the bi-temporal fields but an atypically symmetrical distribution of the bi-nasal fields. The fVEPs show a clear difference in lateralization between eyes, with a contralateral predominance of the major negativity (~70 ms) and positivity (~120 ms) from each eye, which is observed as a clear crossed asymmetry in the difference channel (red arrows)

VEP generator orientation. If half-field testing is not possible due to poor fixation or cooperation, the poVEP can be used to corroborate any potential field defect. If the major pattern onset VEP positivity is largest over the same lateral electrode as the prVEP, this likely reflects individual cortical architecture/VEP generator orientation, whereas if the laterality is opposite between prVEPs and pattern onset VEPs, this is suggestive of a relative deficit of a half-field [19]. For crossed asymmetries (i.e., where the direction of the lateralization depends on the stimulated eye), a virtual channel subtracting the difference between the right and left occipital electrode is useful to visualize the transoccipital symmetries between the eyes (Fig. 32.8). Some centers also perform a "chiasmal coefficient" calculation [20], in which the difference between the left and right electrodes from each eye are quantified for a significant correlation (negative or positive). Such differences are usually utilized to investigate chiasmal misrouting associated with albinism although these may also be used to identify patients with chiasmal dysfunction (i.e., space-occupying lesions or chiasmal hypoplasia).

32.5 Pitfalls and Pearls in Recording VEPs

The VEP can be an easily accessible and efficient technique for assessing macular or generalized pathway function and investigating visual pathway integrity. However, there are some circumstances where one must be aware of the limitations or pitfalls of recording VEPs.

Perhaps one of the major misconceptions of the VEP is that a normal VEP is equivalent to normal sight. As the VEP only assesses the visual pathway from the retina to the primary striate cortex, disorders of higher visual processing (e.g., cerebral visual impairment) may not appear as abnormalities in the VEP. Similarly, the VEP cannot be used in isolation to determine normal acuity in people with functional disease. An otherwise normal patient with organically reduced visual acuity would be less likely to have a normal VEP. However, it should be investigated with a sweep VEP to estimate visual acuity (Fig. 32.9) objectively.

An important technical consideration for recording the VEP is the importance of good fixation and attention. The VEP can be easily altered due to poor attention or fixation on the stimulus. Therefore, it is often advantageous to simultaneously monitor the patient's fixation with an infrared camera to perform intermittent averaging (e.g., stimulus averaging is performed when the patient's fixation is verified by viewing corneal reflections). This is particularly beneficial in pediatric or non-compliant people so that any erroneous fixation is accounted for when recording the VEP.

Lastly, an important note for recording the VEP is to remain aware of the principles of VEP signal acquisition. The VEP is an averaged response from the time-locked background EEG. As such, in people with abnormal posterior EEG activity (i.e., due to seizure disorders or encephalopathies), the signal-to-noise ratio of the VEP may be too poor to obtain a consistent or repeatable response. In such circumstances, the VEPs elicited can be easily distinguished from erroneous EEG activity by recording non-stimulus trials. To perform this, one typically runs the VEP recording without presenting a stimulus (i.e., by turning off the monitor or facing the flash strobe down). If the non-stimulus and stimulus trials are comparable, this suggests that any recorded waveform is artifactual, whereas if these show a distinct difference, then it provides confidence in its authenticity.

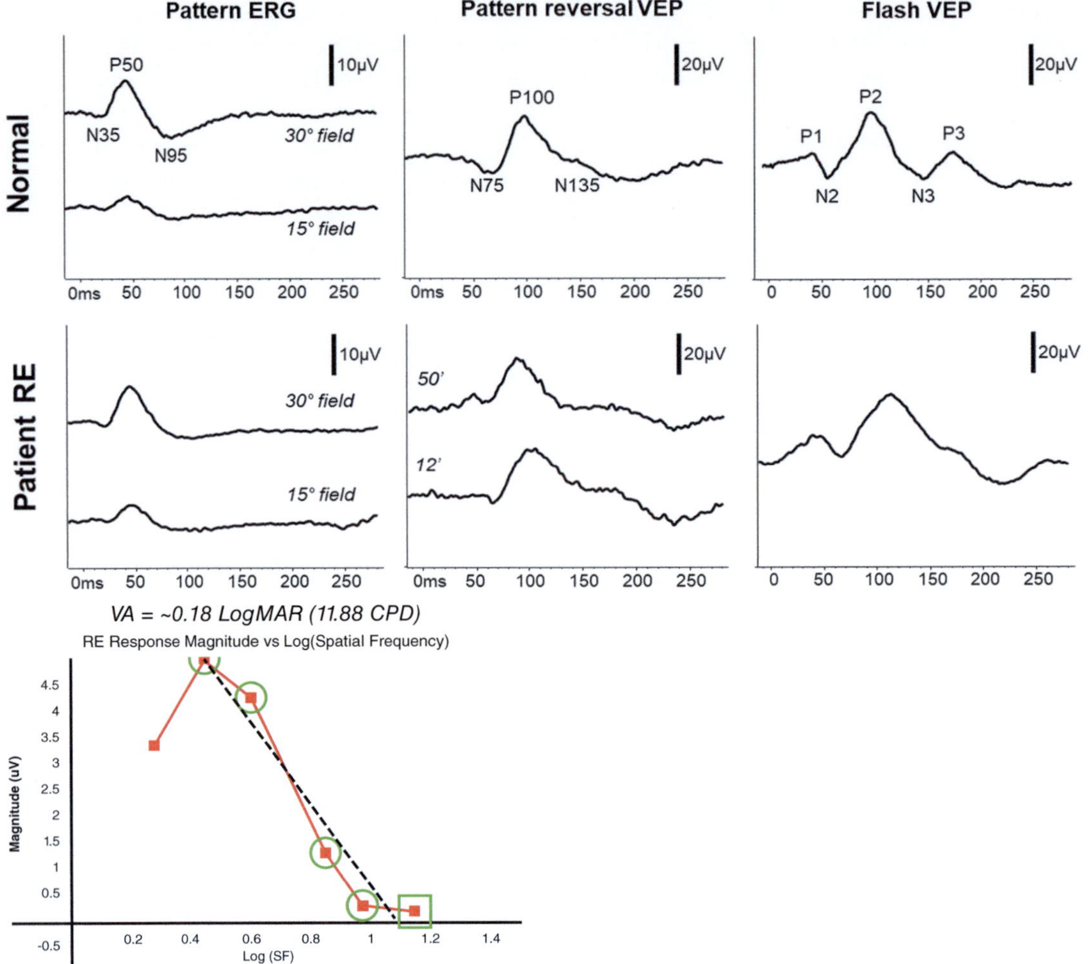

Fig. 32.9 A teenage patient presented with only light perception in the right eye (RE) following an assault on the right side of the face. The clinical impression was that the patient was functional, but this could not be objectively determined. Typical electrophysiological data (PERG, prVEP, flash VEP) were within the reference range, indicating normal macular, retinal ganglion cell, and pathway function in the affected eye. A sweep VEP showed a spatial threshold of 11.88 CPD (~0.18 LogMAR), suggesting that the objective visual acuity estimate was far better than the patient's reported visual acuity, consistent with the clinical impression of functional visual loss

32.6 Summary

The VEP is an incredibly valuable tool in assessing the visual pathway. It is easily performed and provides complementary information not only in neuro-ophthalmic and neurological diseases but also in primary diseases of the eye itself. The VEP is a robust method for assessing visual pathway integrity, but as described in this chapter, its uses are often complementary to other structural or functional techniques. One must remain aware of the potential caveats to an abnormal VEP response or the limitations of a normal VEP, including the prompts for further investigation of function.

Funding None.

Disclosure None.

References

1. Walsh P, Kane N, Butler S. The clinical role of evoked potentials. J Neurol Neurosurg Psychiatry. 2005;76: Suppl 2(Suppl 2):ii16-22. https://doi.org/10.1136/jnnp.2005.068130.
2. Robson AG, Nilsson J, Li S, et al. ISCEV guide to visual electrodiagnostic procedures. Doc Ophthalmol. 2018;136(1):1–26. https://doi.org/10.1007/s10633-017-9621-y.
3. Odom JV, Bach M, Brigell M, et al. ISCEV standard for clinical visual evoked potentials: (2016 update). Doc Ophthalmol. 2016;133(1):1–9. https://doi.org/10.1007/s10633-016-9553-y.
4. Marmoy OR, Horvat-Gitsels LA, Cortina-Borja M, Thompson DA. Pattern visual evoked potentials show an inferior-superior topographic shift through maturation in childhood. J Physiol. 2023;601(10):1869–80. https://doi.org/10.1113/jp283408.
5. Ghodrati M, Morris AP, Price NS. The (un)suitability of modern liquid crystal displays (LCDs) for vision research. Front Psychol. 2015;6:303. https://doi.org/10.3389/fpsyg.2015.00303.
6. Matsumoto CS, Shinoda K, Matsumoto H, et al. Liquid crystal display screens as stimulators for visually evoked potentials: flash effect due to delay in luminance changes. Doc Ophthalmol. 2013;127(2):103–12. https://doi.org/10.1007/s10633-013-9387-9.
7. Marmoy OR, Thompson DA. Assessment of digital light processing (DLP) projector stimulators for visual electrophysiology. Doc Ophthalmol. 2023;146(2):151–63. https://doi.org/10.1007/s10633-022-09917-4.
8. Matsumoto CS, Shinoda K, Matsumoto H, et al. Pattern visual evoked potentials elicited by organic electroluminescence screen. Biomed Res Int. 2014;2014:606951. https://doi.org/10.1155/2014/606951.
9. Hamilton R, Bach M, Heinrich SP, et al. VEP estimation of visual acuity: a systematic review. Documenta Ophthalmologica. 2021;142(1):25–74. https://doi.org/10.1007/s10633-020-09770-3.
10. Thompson DA, Kriss A, Taylor D, et al. Early VEP and ERG evidence of visual dysfunction in autosomal recessive osteopetrosis. Neuropediatrics. 1998;29(3):137–44. https://doi.org/10.1055/s-2007-973550.
11. Thompson DA, Fritsch DM, Hardy SE. The changing shape of the ISCEV standard pattern onset VEP. Doc Ophthalmol. 2017;135(1):69–76. https://doi.org/10.1007/s10633-017-9596-8.
12. Marmoy OR, Viswanathan S. Clinical electrophysiology of the optic nerve and retinal ganglion cells. Eye. 2021;35(9):2386–405. https://doi.org/10.1038/s41433-021-01614-x.
13. Rufai SR, Marmoy OR, Thompson DA, et al. Electrophysiological and fundoscopic detection of intracranial hypertension in craniosynostosis. Eye. 2023;37(1):139–45. https://doi.org/10.1038/s41433-021-01839-w.
14. Thompson DA, Marmoy OR, Prise KL, et al. Giant pattern VEPs in children. Eur J Paediatr Neurol. 2021;34:33–42. https://doi.org/10.1016/j.ejpn.2021.07.008.
15. Thompson DA, Handley SE, Henderson RH, et al. An ERG and OCT study of neuronal ceroid lipofuscinosis CLN2 battens retinopathy. Eye (Lond). 2021;35(9):2438–48. https://doi.org/10.1038/s41433-021-01594-y.
16. Slotnick SD, Klein SA, Carney T, Sutter EE. Electrophysiological estimate of human cortical magnification. Clin Neurophysiol. 2001;112(7):1349–56. https://doi.org/10.1016/s1388-2457(01)00561-2.
17. Thompson DA, Liasis A, Hardy S, et al. Prevalence of abnormal pattern reversal visual evoked potentials in craniosynostosis. Plast Reconstr Surg. 2006;118(1):184–92. https://doi.org/10.1097/01.prs.0000220873.72953.3e.
18. Barrett G, Blumhardt L, Halliday AM, et al. A paradox in the lateralisation of the visual evoked response. Nature. 1976;261(5557):253–5. https://doi.org/10.1038/261253a0.
19. Marmoy OR, Handley SE, Thompson DA. Pattern-onset and OFFset visual evoked potentials in the diagnosis of hemianopic field defects. Doc Ophthalmol. 2021;142(2):165–76. https://doi.org/10.1007/s10633-020-09785-w.
20. van Genderen MM, Riemslag FC, Schuil J, et al. Chiasmal misrouting and foveal hypoplasia without albinism. Br J Ophthalmol. 2006;90(9):1098–102. https://doi.org/10.1136/bjo.2006.091702.

33 The Clinical Electro-Oculogram

Paul A. Constable

33.1 Introduction

The clinical electro-oculogram (EOG) measures the electrical activity of the retina and retinal pigment epithelium (RPE) in response to light stimulation. The test is especially useful in conditions affecting the structural integrity of the rods and the RPE. At rest, there is a positive "standing potential" of the eye that is maintained by differences in the ionic conductance of the apical and basal membranes of the RPE. Changes in the flow of ions across these membranes alter the standing potential of the eye; these can be recorded from horizontal saccadic eye movements under dark - and light-adapted intervals. Clinically, the standing potential falls during the dark adaptation phase and increases during the light-adapting phase. The ratio of the recorded saccadic amplitudes during these phases is used as a clinical index for the functional integrity of the rods and the RPE. The EOG may be abnormal in conditions affecting bestrophin, a calcium and chloride regulator localized in the RPE. Mutations in the gene encoding bestrophin (*BEST1*) result in conditions such as Best's vitelliform macular dystrophy.

P. A. Constable (✉)
Flinders University, College of Nursing and Health Sciences, Caring Futures Institute, Adelaide, SA, Australia
e-mail: paul.constable@flinders.edu.au

33.2 History

The clinical utility of the EOG was first described by Geoffrey Arden, who recorded changes in the standing potential of the eye as a measure of retinal function in response to light [1]. Arden found that the standing potential was reduced in conditions where the retina was not in contact with the RPE, such as retinal detachment, retinal hypoxia following retinal artery occlusion, and in inherited retinal dystrophies such as retinitis pigmentosa [2, 3]. These clinical observations suggested that the EOG largely depends on normal RPE and rod function and when the RPE and the retina remain in contact. Using micro-electrode recordings in retina-RPE whole mounts of geckos, Griff and Steinberg later demonstrated that the standing potential originated in the RPE [4]. The standing potential of the eye was later shown to be due to the difference in the basal and apical membrane potentials of the RPE (termed the transepithelial potential) and depended upon the integrity of the tight junctions; these junctions maintain the difference in the electrical potentials between the basolateral and apical membranes [5]. An increase in basolateral chloride conductance produced a basolateral membrane depolarization that increased the transepithelial potential that could be recorded as changes in the standing potential of the eye [6, 7]. Further studies have identified a large potassium conductance in the apical membrane with voltage-gated potassium

T. Das, P. Satgunam (eds.), *Ophthalmic Diagnostics*, https://doi.org/10.1007/978-981-97-0138-4_33

channels and active and passive co-transporters regulating potassium and pH within the subretinal space and RPE, respectively [8, 9]. One does not know how light could change the basolateral chloride conductance of the RPE, several hypotheses have been proposed.

Based on the slow time course and spectral properties of the light-rise [3], Arden proposed that a "light-rise" substance is released from the rods; this substance then binds to an apical RPE receptor that initiates an intracellular secondary messenger cascade to open basolateral chloride channels. Based on this model, several molecules were proposed as candidates for the elusive "light-rise" substance, including cyclic nucleotides [10], dopamine [4], epinephrine [11], and adenosine triphosphate [12]; but to date, no definitive human studies have identified the "light-rise" substance. One suggestion was that light might act directly on the apical phospholipid bilayer of the RPE, resulting in direct biosynthesis of the intracellular secondary messenger molecule, inositol 1,4,5-trisphosphate (IP_3); however, this model is also unconfirmed in human [13]. The photosensitive protein, melanopsin is also a possible candidate, given its expression in the RPE, but it has been reported that knock-out *opn4*$^{-/-}$ mice exhibit a normal light-rise suggesting that this protein is not involved in the generation of the light-rise [14]. Despite this evidence, IP_3 is still implicated in the process due to its role in the release of calcium from the endoplasmic reticulum and the involvement of calcium in the generation of the changes in basolateral chloride conductance [11, 15]. In addition, studies on humans have shown that individuals with cystic fibrosis have a normal light-rise [16], but a decrease in the light-rise following pharmacological blockade of L-type Ca^{2+} channels with nifedipine supports the hypothesis that calcium signaling is involved in the light-rise [17].

Even though the identity of the trigger for the light-rise has not yet been confirmed, a greater understanding of the mechanism for the basolateral depolarization has been developed. The reduced light-rise in patients with Best's disease [18] led to the identification of the gene *BEST1* or *VMD2* that encodes bestrophin. Mutations in this gene cause Best's vitelliform macular dystrophy [19]. Although bestrophin is known to be involved in the generation of the light-rise, it is also known to play a central role in the pathogenesis of Best's vitelliform macular dystrophy, the precise function and location of this protein within the RPE remains unclear [20]. Early studies suggested that bestrophin could either be a calcium-gated chloride channel or a regulator of intracellular calcium stores [21–23].

Strauss and co-workers resolved these conflicts by demonstrating that bestrophin was localized in the endoplasmic reticulum and not the basolateral membrane of the RPE, as previously thought [24]. At this location, bestrophin could regulate intracellular calcium through direct interactions with the basolateral L-type calcium channel [15, 25] and thereby help regulate intracellular calcium stores. The transmembrane calcium-gated (Transmembrane 16 A, TMEM16A; also known as anoctamin1) chloride channel [26–28] was then shown to be the ion channel responsible for changes in the basolateral membrane potential and, ultimately, the generation of the light-rise. Thus, mutations affecting bestrophin result in a reduced light-rise and abnormal EOG [29]. Fig. 33.1 is a schematic outline of the mechanism of the light-rise of the EOG secondary to basolateral membrane depolarization.

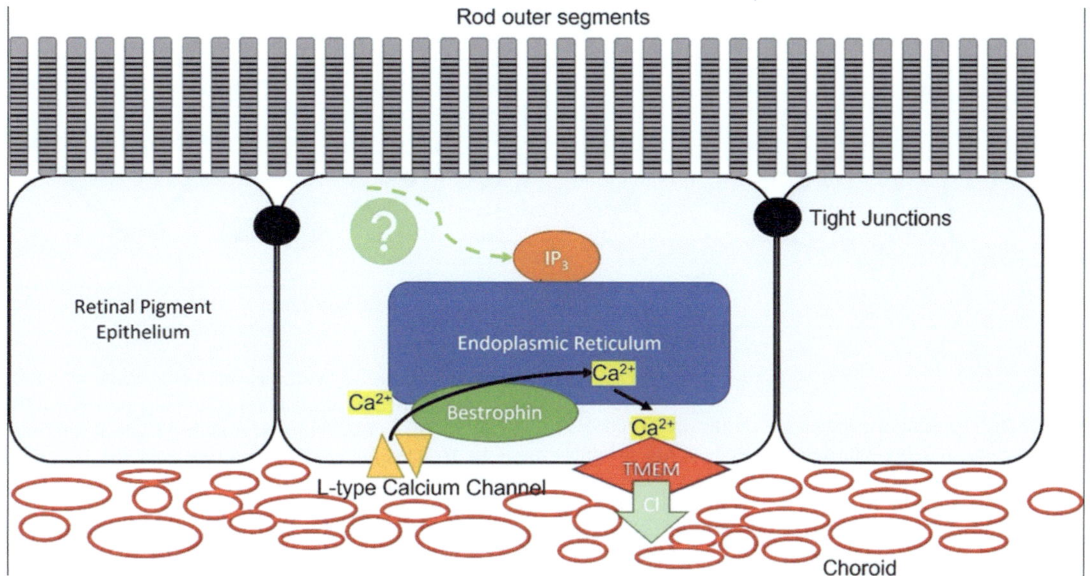

Fig. 33.1 The complete mechanism of the light-rise of the EOG (EOG). The main pathways involved in the generation of the intracellular secondary messenger molecule, inositol 1,4,5-trisphosphate (IP_3). The rod photoreceptors may be a likely source of the "light-rise" substance that triggers IP_3 synthesis and release from the phospholipid bilayer. IP_3 releases calcium from intracellular stores that open the transmembrane (TMEM16A) chloride channel to depolarize the basolateral membrane and increase the transepithelial potential of the retinal pigment epithelium (RPE). These changes are recorded from horizontal saccadic eye movements in the dark and light as changes in the standing potential of the eye. Bestrophin, localized in the endoplasmic reticulum, regulates intracellular calcium stores and concentrations through direct interactions with the voltage-gated L-type calcium channels that contribute to the slow oscillations of the standing potential. (Schematic, not to scale)

33.3 Technology, Physics, and Mechanics of Electro-Oculogram

The clinical EOG has two main components that reflect changes in the standing potential of the eye during dark adaptation (dark phase) and light adaptation (light phase). In the dark phase, the recorded standing potential of the eye falls to a minimum value after 10–15 min and is known as the dark trough (DT). In the light phase, the standing potential peaks at approximately 7–12 min after light onset and is known as the light peak (LP) before falling again and continuing in a slow-damped oscillation. The ratio of the LP:DT is a measure of the integrity of the photoreceptor/rod-RPE complex and is known as the LP:DT ratio as defined by the current standards of the International Society for Clinical Electrophysiology of Vision (ISCEV) [30]. The slow-damped oscillations under dark or light conditions will continue for 120 min [2]. But the dark and light slow oscillations may have different origins, with an unknown mechanism for the dark oscillations; however, it is suspected that these oscillations may be caused due to volume changes in the RPE [31]. The slow oscillations represent the slow changes in intracellular calcium concentrations driven by the L-type voltage-gated calcium channel. Figure 33.2 shows the slow dark and light-damped oscillations of the standing potential.

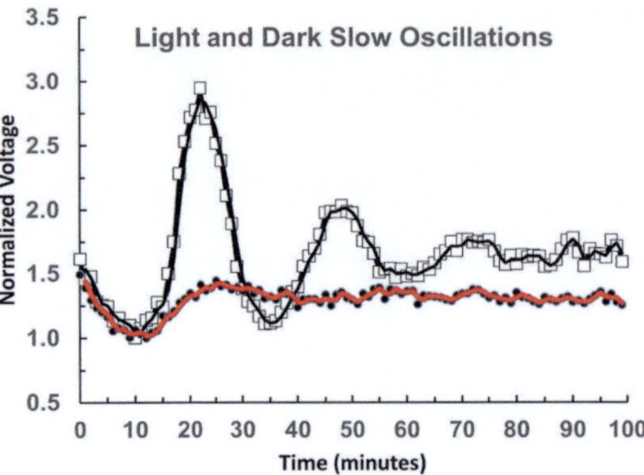

Fig. 33.2 The standing potential of the eye recorded under prolonged light—and dark-adapted periods exhibits a slow-damped oscillation. In the dark, the oscillations form the first negative trough, known as the dark trough. The first of the light oscillations form the light peak. Although the mechanism underlying the dark oscillations is unclear, the slow light oscillations are known to reflect changes in intracellular calcium concentrations that drive an increase in chloride conductance across the basolateral membrane, resulting in changes in the standing potential of the eye. The squares represent the slow light oscillations, and the black circles represent the dark oscillations; the dark oscillations are smaller than the light oscillations. The plots represent the averages of values obtained from 11 normal human subjects

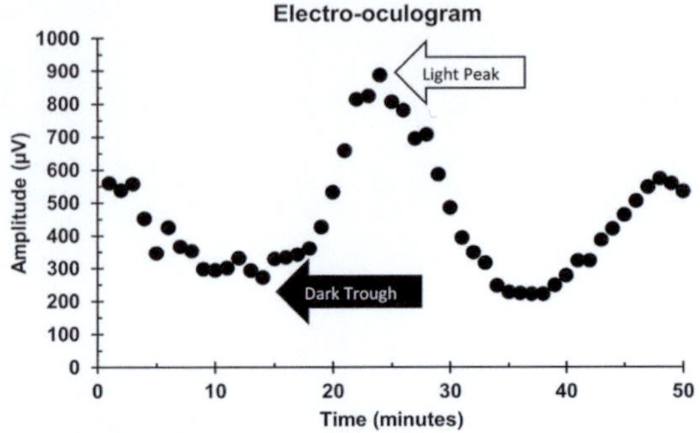

Fig. 33.3 The EOG with measurements made at 1-min intervals during the dark phase (20 min) and the light phase (20–50 min). The dark trough occurs at approximately 10–15 min of dark adaption, and the light-rise commences at the light onset with a gradual increase in the recorded potential; it reaches a peak at approximately 7–12 min following light onset before falling again in a slow-damped oscillation. The ratio of the amplitude at the light peak (LP) to the amplitude at the dark trough (DT) or the LP:DT ratio is a measure of the photoreceptor/rod-RPE integrity

The fast oscillations of the EOG are not generally clinically recorded. They represent changes in the apical membrane potential in response to potassium currents during brief 1-min alternating intervals of light and dark, which are reduced in early diabetes [32, 33]. However, these fast oscillations are preserved in Best's vitelliform macular dystrophy, which supports the hypothesis that the fast oscillations of the EOG are caused by mechanisms different from those responsible for the slower changes in the potential that characterize the EOG [18]. The fast oscillations affect the standing potential in a manner opposite to that of the slower changes, with a fall during the light phase and a rise in the dark phase [30]. The readers are encouraged to review section on "fast oscillations" in "The electro-oculogram" by Arden and Constable (2006) [34].

Incidentally, non-photic substances may also change the standing potential, with ethanol mimicking the light-EOG that presumably triggers the same intracellular pathways as light [35]. The ethanol-induced EOG may help identify RPE stress in early age-related macular degeneration [36]. Other non-photic stimuli such as hypoxia, hypercapnia, and hyperosmolarity have also been evaluated as potential clinical tests for detecting RPE stress, but these do not demonstrate any potential as clinical tests despite their ability to change the standing potential of the eye [37, 38]. Fig. 33.3 shows a typical raw clinical recording of the EOG from a normal subject.

33.4 Technique

ISCEV has developed guidelines on the methods used for recording clinical EOGs and fast oscillations, which are updated as required [30]. Recordings are performed in people with dilated pupils to ensure standard retinal illumination with a ganzfeld stimulator to obtain responses from the entire retina. The patient must avoid bright lights before recording. The patient should be allowed to practice eye movements beforehand and avoid talking during the recording phases to minimize muscle artifacts. The patient must be informed of the test procedure, and they will be asked to look left and right (horizontal

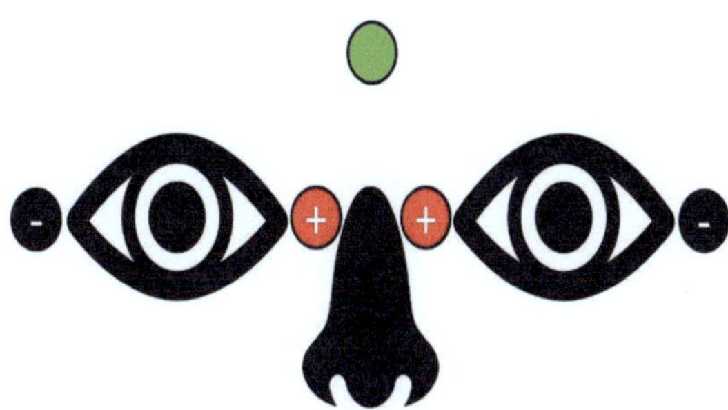

Fig. 33.4 An illustration of the positioning of the electrodes with a central forehead earth electrode (green) and recording electrodes (red and black) at the inner and outer canthi, respectively. As the eyes move to the left and right, the red and black electrodes measure the amplitude of the standing potential as the positively charged cornea moves from the positive to the negative electrode

saccades) for 10 s at 1-s interval or on an auditory/verbal cue at 1-min intervals with 15 min in the dark and 15 min in the light. White light is used as the stimulus with a luminance of 100 cd. m^{-2} ± 10%. The patient should be in a dimly lit room, and their skin should be cleaned to reduce impedance to <5 kΩ. The electrodes (usually gold cups) include two surface electrodes placed on the skin—one on the outer canthus (the bony part of the eye at the corner closest to the ear) and one on the nose near the inner canthus. A third reference electrode can be placed on the center of the forehead or earlobe. Care should be taken to avoid any contact between the nasal electrodes. In cases where the patient cannot execute a horizontal saccade, such as in strabismus, then the EOG cannot be recorded from that eye. Figure 33.4 shows the typical electrode placement for recording an EOG.

The EOG signals are amplified using a biological amplifier with a high input impedance and are filtered between 0.1 and 30 Hz with a sampling rate of >1 kHz to record the saccades. The horizontal saccades have a 30° amplitude; dim red light-emitting diodes (LEDs) mounted in the ganzfeld dome are typically used to aid with fixation. Averages of the saccadic amplitudes are taken as the standing potential of the eye during the dark and light phases. Fig. 33.5 shows a typical averaged series of saccades with a cursor mark indicating the measured amplitude.

Modifications to the ISCEV standard protocol have been proposed to improve patient comfort by not dilating their eyes and reducing the periods of dark and light adaptation [30]. Türksever et al. [39] proposed using a higher luminance of 450 cd.m^{-2} if dilation is not possible; this gives a quantitatively similar LP:DT ratio to that obtained from a subject exposed to a luminance of 100 cd. m^{-2} with dilated eyes. In addition, the authors proposed a shortened protocol with 10 min of the dark phase followed by 14 min of the light phase. Any variations from the ISCEV standard protocol should be noted in any reporting of the EOG findings and should include the LP:DT ratio, the time to peak of the light-rise (taken from the time of the light phase onset to the light peak), and the dark trough amplitude [30]. The dark trough can be variable between subjects, and hence, care should be taken to ensure that the patient is comfortable during the recordings. In the initial minute of the light phase, the patient may be uncomfortable owing to the large change in luminance and pupil dilatation. It is important to inform them that the initial phase could be uncomfortable, but that they must keep their eyes open, as the light entering the eye is required to initiate the light-rise. During recordings, it is important to monitor the subject's eye position to ensure that they remain correctly centered and have their eyes open during the recordings. Typically, an infrared camera is mounted within the ganzfeld dome in a recording instrument to enable this.

Once the recordings are complete, a plot of the saccadic amplitudes and time is made, as shown in Fig. 33.3. The "raw" values characterize the physiological shape of the changes in the standing potential and identify the dark trough from the light peak. Although several smoothing or averaging strategies of the recorded saccadic amplitudes are possible, the ISCEV standard does not have a preferred method [30]. The physiological response may be identified by simply fitting a curve using the line of best fit or using a moving average to smoothen the curve first, or by averaging values around the light peak and dark trough. Smoothing using a moving average can be applied using Eq. 33.1, where the amplitude

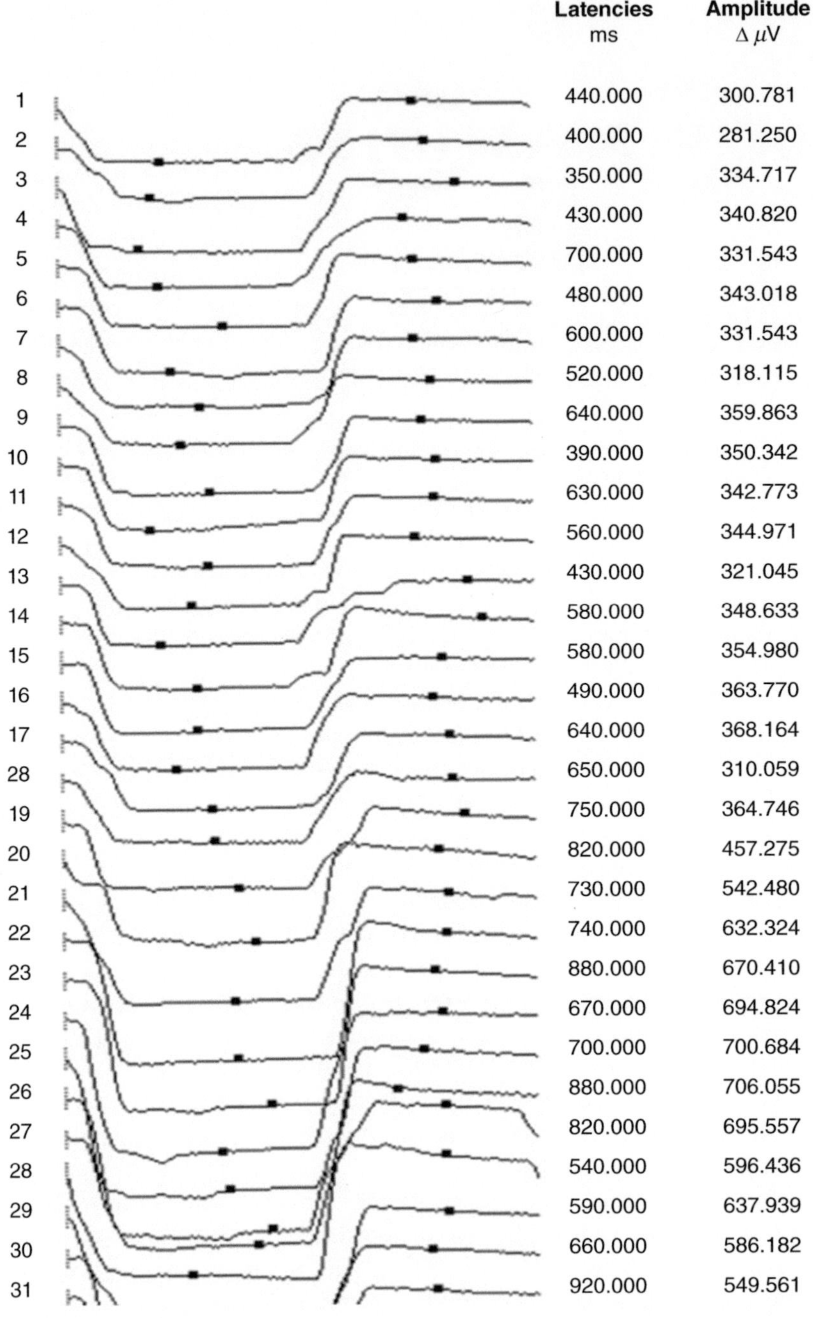

Fig. 33.5 A series of averaged saccades during a 10-s recording epoch for one eye, recorded at 1-min intervals. Note the smaller amplitudes in the initial 15 min of the dark phase and with the dark trough minimal amplitude (321 μV) occurring at $t = 13$ min and the maximal amplitude at $t = 26$ min (11 min after light onset with a saccadic amplitude of 706 μV)

for each standing potential voltage (V_t) at time (t) can be weighted by 0.5 times the value of the preceding and subsequent standing potential voltage.

$$V_t = \frac{\left[V_t + \left(0.5.V_{t+1}\right) + \left(0.5.V_{t-1}\right)\right]}{2} \quad (33.1)$$

This method results in a slight change to the time axis as the first and last recordings are lost because of the averaging. Figure 33.6 shows a raw and smoothed EOG using a moving average of the recorded time interval values as described initially by Arden and Wolf for the amplitude of the measured saccades [35, 36]. In addition, the

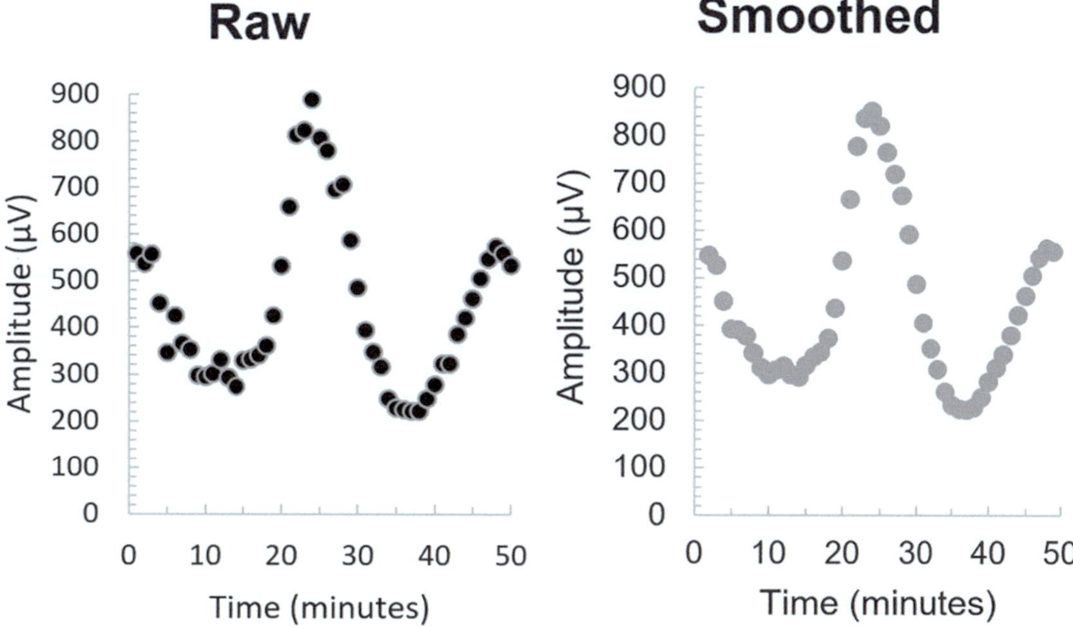

Fig. 33.6 The raw and smoothed values of the saccadic amplitudes (using Eq. 33.1) recorded during the 20-min dark and 30-min light phase. The main objective in the interpretation of the plots is to define the physiological response, and so a line of best fit or averages of the points at the peak and trough may be used to define the light peak and dark trough to calculate the LP:DT ratio. Since there is no defined or preferred method, clinicians are advised to report the method (if any) of smoothing or averaging

y-axis may be plotted as a normalized voltage to the light peak maximum, or sometimes as µV/degree with the recorded voltage divided by the saccadic amplitude of typically 30°so that a potential of 300 µV would be recorded as 10 µV/degree.

Typical measures for the EOG clinical parameters are summarized in a meta-analysis of clinical values in subjects with a mean age of 34.1 ± 12.9 years [40]. The reported mean (95% confidence interval, CI) from the meta-analysis of studies were as follows: for dilated pupil, LP:DT ratio = 2.35 (2.28–2.42); dark trough amplitude = 358 µV (292–424 µV), and time to peak of the light-rise was 8.2 min (7.7–8.7 min) with amplitude = 835 µV (631–1039 µV); for non-dilated pupil, LP:DT ratio = 2.37 (2.28–2.45), and the fast oscillation peak to trough ratio was 1.13 (1.11–1.16).

Thavikulwat et al. [41] performed one of the largest clinical studies to study the impact of age and gender on the EOG parameters in 121 subjects aged 7–72 years. The study found that the LP:DT ratio decreased at a rate of 0.13 per decade, and the lower fifth centile of the LP:DT ratio decreased from 2.0 to 1.7 between the ages of 10 and 60 years. In addition, the time to peak of the light-rise was 2 min slower in subjects aged 55 years or older, and that female subjects had a higher absolute amplitude for the light peak.

Artifacts can be caused by blinks or under or overshoots of the target LED. One should carefully observe these in the saccadic recordings so that the true saccade amplitude is noted when placing the cursors. Automatic cursor placement by in-built algorithms may misplace the cursors. Figure 33.7 shows a representation of an undershoot, then a corrective saccade to the target, and a distinctive blink artifact in the saccadic recording. Generally, some practice runs are recommended to ensure that the patient knows what to do. They should always be requested to refrain from blinking during the 10-s recording interval.

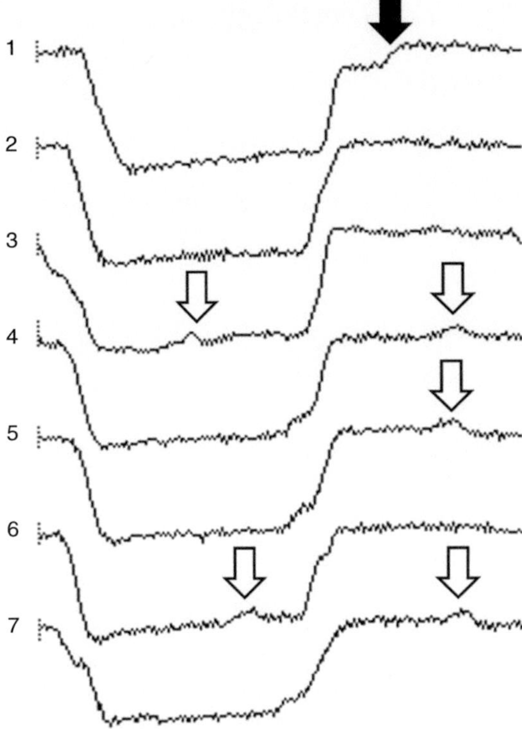

Fig. 33.7 Illustrative artifacts in the saccades. In the recording at $t = 1$ min, there is an undershoot and correction to the LED (filled arrow). In the recordings at $t = 3–7$ min, there are blink artifacts during the recordings (unfilled arrows). Care should be taken to ensure that measurements of the saccadic amplitudes are not taken from blinks or under/overshoots

33.4.1 Clinical Applications

The main clinical application of the EOG is to diagnose and monitor conditions where mutations occur in the *BEST1*/*VMD2* gene that encodes bestrophin (the calcium and chloride regulator of the RPE). Collectively these conditions are referred to as bestrophinopathies (for reviews on these, see Johnson et al. [42] and Toto et al. [43]). The most common of these conditions is the autosomal dominant condition, Best's vitelliform macular dystrophy, where the light-rise is reduced or absent, but the fast oscillations of the EOG are preserved [18]. This condition may present in any decade of life, but is characterized by a central vitelliform lesion on the macula, that degenerates over time, leading to macular degeneration [19, 44]. The macula is selectively affected owing to the low expression of bestrophin in this area of the retina [45]. Fig. 33.8 shows the fundus, optical coherence tomography (OCT) images, and EOG in a patient with Best's vitelliform macular dystrophy. In cases where EOG cannot be performed (e.g., in a child suspected of having Best's macular dystrophy), testing the parents may show a reduced EOG owing to the autosomal dominant inheritance pattern of this condition.

In autosomal recessive bestrophinopathies, [46] the EOG is typically abnormal, with a normal electroretinogram in the early stages of the disease. The typical age of onset ranges from 4 to 35 years (mean = 18.6 years); the common ocular findings are hyperopia and narrow anterior chamber angles with increased risk of angle closure glaucoma. The fundus appearance may vary, but consists of vitelliform lesions in the retina, subretinal deposits with central serous retinopathy, or a macular hole [47, 48]. Fig. 33.9 shows a 25-year-old male with autosomal recessive bestrophinopathy with a homozygous splice variant in exon 4 of the *BEST1* gene. In this case, the subject had reported reductions in vision over 5 years with nyctalopia and had a normal anterior segment and color vision; the visual acuities of the right and left eyes were 6/12 and 6/6, respectively. Light—and dark-adapted full-field electroretinograms were reduced with an absent light-rise in the EOG. The fundus had a central macular edema (right>left) with a mid-peripheral band of hyper-fluorescence corresponding to increased pigmentation in the RPE.

In autosomal dominant vitreoretinochoroidopathy [49] linked to mutations in *BEST1* [50], the EOG is also abnormal with an initially normal electroretinogram; however, central cone dysfunction can develop [51]. Typically, the ocular findings include short axial length with hyperopia and small angles, and a typically hyperpigmented band at the equator with some white dots and a cystoid macular edema [42]. In diseases affecting the integrity of the RPE tight junctions, such as Danon's disease (where there is a loss of regulation of lysozyme function), the dark trough

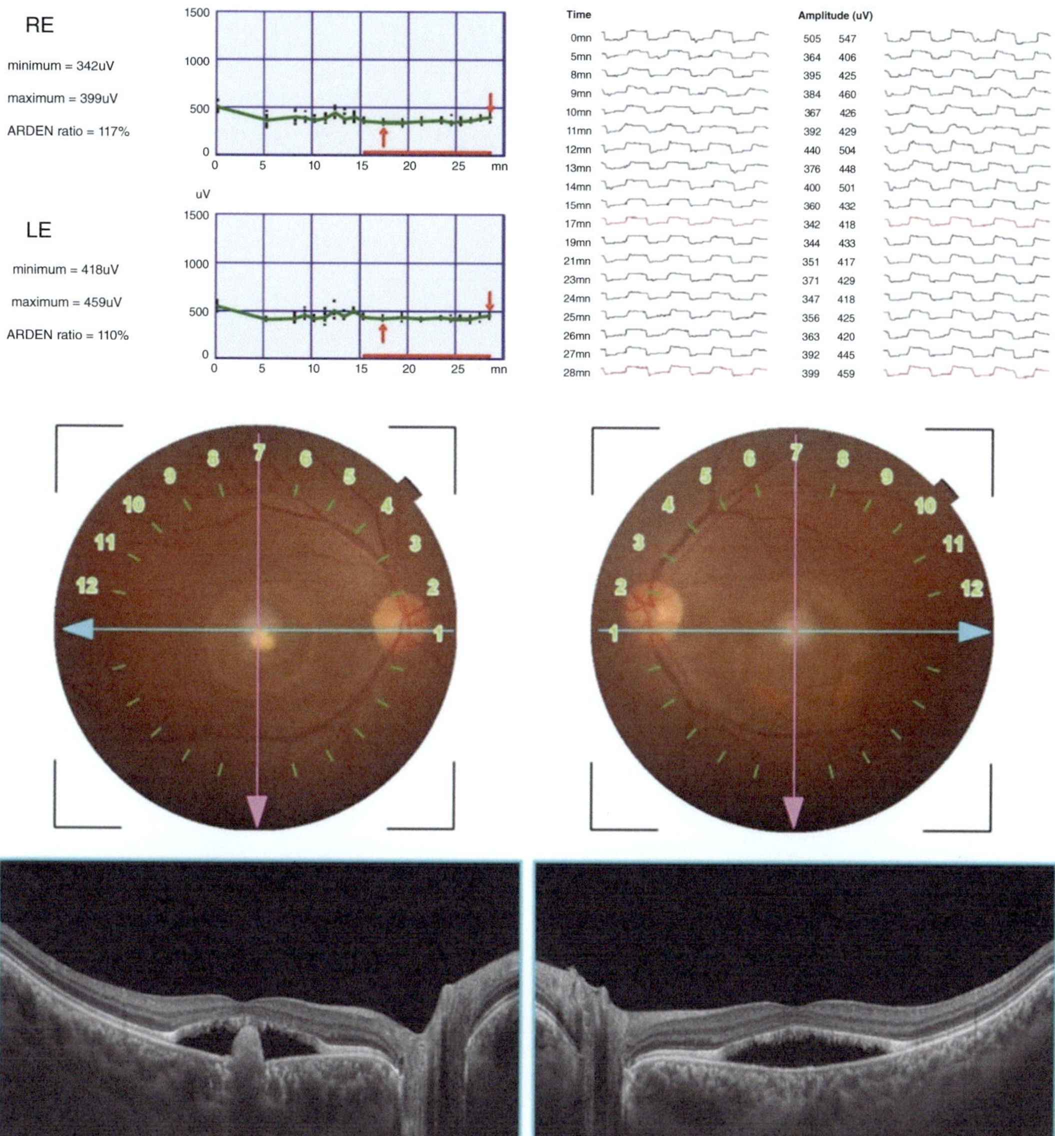

Fig. 33.8 Best's vitelliform macular dystrophy. Upper panel-The EOG recordings for the right and left eyes show a marked reduction in the Arden or LP:DT ratio of approximately 1.1; Middle panel-color fundus image with characteristic central vitelliform lesions; Lower panel-Ocular coherence tomography (OCT) images of the macula show a central pigmented area (with lipofuscin) of the detached epithelium, which will eventually degenerate. Images courtesy: Srikanta Padhy, MD

of the EOG can be abnormally low, resulting in a paradoxically normal or elevated LP:DT ratio [52].

Systemic drugs affecting the outer retina or RPE are also associated with a reduced or absent light-rise of the EOG [53]. Chloroquine retinopathy is associated with a reduced light-rise but may not be detected through multi-focal electroretinography or color vision testing [54]. The iron chelator, deferoxamine, can cause a reduction in the light-rise and dark trough amplitudes as it can damage the RPE [55]. The anti-epileptic

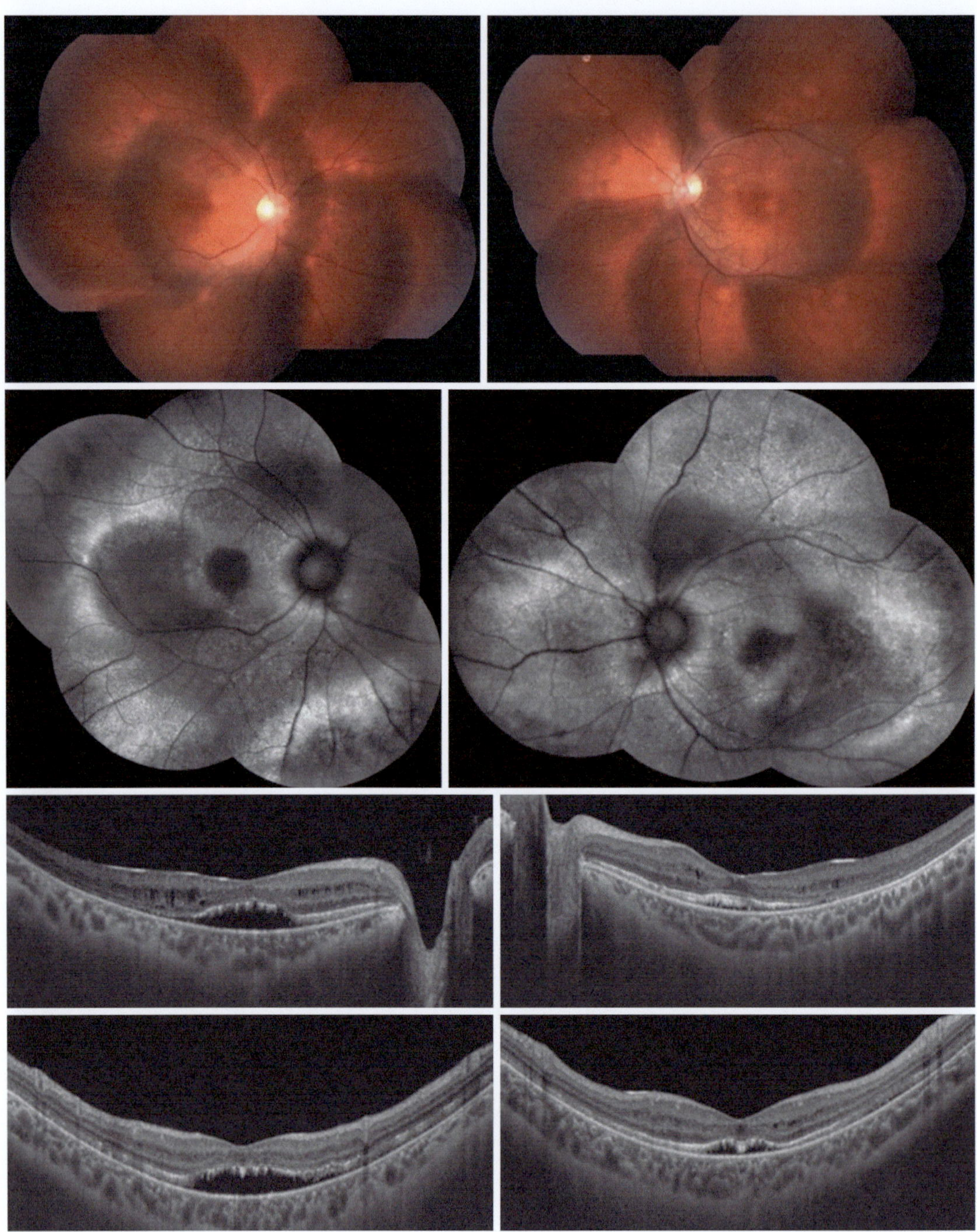

Fig. 33.9 Images and EOG of autosomal recessive bestrophinopathy (confirmed via genetic tests) in a 25-year-old male. The first and second panels show a montage of the fundi with a hyperpigmented ring at the equator corresponding with hyper-fluorescence of the RPE. The third panel shows OCT scans of the horizontal and vertical meridians through the macula with a hypo-reflective region in the right and left eyes corresponding with a separation of the RPE from the Bruch's membrane. The fourth panel shows reduced or absent light-rise in the EOG, implicating the *BEST1* gene in the potential differential diagnosis. Images courtesy: Srikanta Padhy, MD

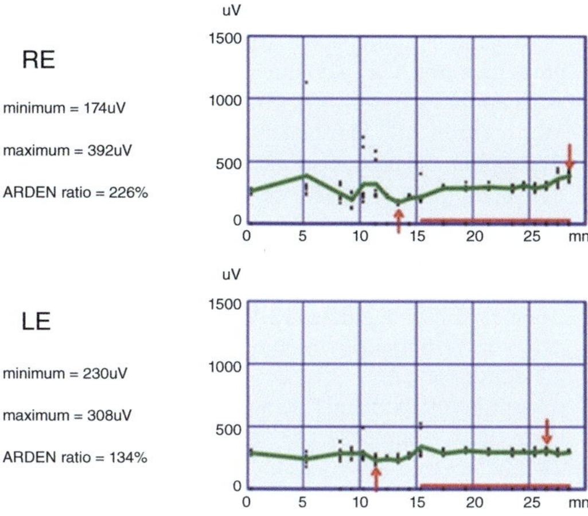

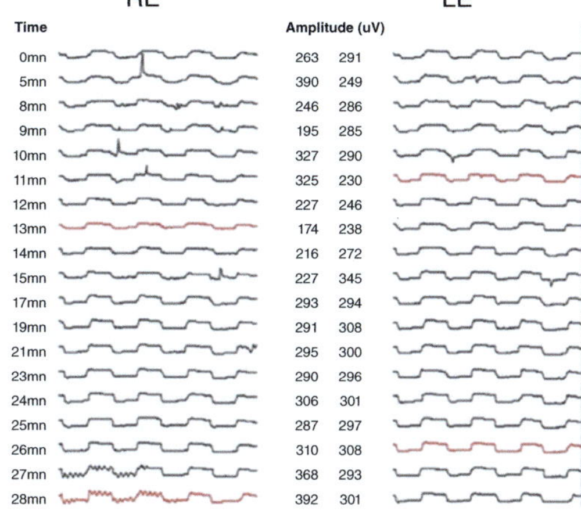

Fig. 33.9 (continued)

drug, vigabatrin, is also linked to visual field loss and reduced EOGs in children due to its toxicity to the outer retina [56]. Other drugs that change the EOG are: digoxin (elevates EOG), cisplatin (reduces the EOG), ethambutol (elevates the LP:DT ratio), and isotretinoin (reduces LP:DT ratios) [53]. A reduced light-rise has also been reported in tamoxifen retinopathy [57]. EOGs are not routinely performed to monitor the toxic effects of drugs since electroretinograms and retinal imaging can identify functional or structural changes in the retina ahead of any marked reductions in the EOG. Incidentally, the LP:DT ratio is reduced in seasonal affective disorder, which is characterized by depression in the wintertime [58], and Parkinson's Disease [59].

33.5 Clinical Interpretation

Clinically, the main utility of an EOG is in diagnosing and monitoring conditions caused by mutations in the *BEST1* gene, which lead to a functional loss of bestrophin in the RPE. The ratio of the light-rise peak to the dark trough minimum is the main clinical measure. The ratio is reduced where there is a disruption to the rod-RPE interface, when bestrophin function is affected, and there is a reduction in the basolateral chloride conductance. However, care must be taken to observe the amplitude of the dark trough as a reduced dark trough amplitude and a relatively normal LP:DT ratio may indicate disruptions in the tight junctions. The timing of the light peak is slower in those aged 55 years and older, and the LP:DT ratio also reduces at a rate of 0.13 units per decade; these measures must be considered when recording/interpreting the EOG in older subjects [41]. Typically, the EOG is interpreted in conjunction with additional imaging and visual electrophysiological tests such as the electroretinogram; these, combined with genetic information and family history, are used to make a clinical diagnosis.

References

1. Arden GB, Barrada A, Kelsey JH. New clinical test of retinal function based upon the standing potential of the eye. Br J Ophthalmol. 1962;46:449–67.
2. Arden GB, Kelsey JH. Changes produced by light in the standing potential of the human eye. J Physiol. 1962;161:189–204.
3. Arden GB, Kelsey JH. Some observations on the relationship between the standing potential of the human eye and bleaching and regeneration of visual purple. J Physiol. 1962;161:205–26.
4. Gallemore RP, Griff ER, Steinberg RH. Evidence in support of a photoreceptoral origin for the "light-peak substance". Invest Ophthalmol Vis Sci. 1988;29:566–71.

5. Griff ER, Steinberg RH. Origin of the light peak:in vitrostudy of *Gekko gekko*. J Physiol. 1982;331:637–52.
6. Gallemore RP, Steinberg RH. Effects of DIDS on the chick retinal pigment epithelium. II. Mechanism of the light peak and other responses originating at the basal membrane. J Neurosci. 1989;9:1977–84.
7. Bialek S, Miller SS. K^+ and cl^- transport mechanisms in bovine pigment epithelium that could modulate subretinal space volume and composition. J Physiol. 1994;475:401–17.
8. Wimmers S, Karl MO, Strauss O. Ion channels in the RPE. Prog Retin Eye Res. 2007;26:263–301.
9. Strauss O. The retinal pigment epithelium in visual function. Physiol Rev. 2005;85:845–81.
10. Nao-i N, Gallemore RP, Steinberg RH. Effects of cAMP and IBMX on the chick retinal pigment epithelium. Membrane potentials and light-evoked responses. Invest Ophthalmol Vis Sci. 1990;31:54–66.
11. Rymer J, Miller SS, Edelman JL. Epinephrine-induced increases in $[Ca2+]_{in}$ and KCl-coupled fluid absorption in bovine RPE. Invest Ophthal Visual Sci. 2001;42:1921–9.
12. Mitchell CH. Release of ATP by a human retinal pigment epithelial cell line: potential for autocrine stimulation through subretinal space. J Physiol. 2001;534(Pt 1):193–202.
13. Constable PA. A perspective on the mechanism of the light-rise of the electrooculogram. Invest Ophthalmol Vis Sci. 2014;55:2669–73.
14. Constable PA, Kapoor G. Is white the right light for the clinical electrooculogram? Doc Ophthalmol. 2021;143:297–304.
15. Wimmers S, Coeppicus L, Rosenthal R, Strauss O. Expression profile of voltage-dependent Ca2+ channel subunits in the human retinal pigment epithelium. Graefes Arch Clin Exp Ophthalmol. 2008;246:685–92.
16. Constable PA, Lawrenson JG, Arden GB. Light and alcohol evoked electro-oculograms in cystic fibrosis. Doc Ophthalmol. 2006;113:133–43.
17. Constable PA. Nifedipine alters the light-rise of the electro-oculogram in man. Graefes Arch Clin Exp Ophthalmol. 2011;249:677–84.
18. Weleber RG. Fast and slow oscillations of the electro-oculogram in Best's macular dystrophy and retinitis pigmentosa. Arch Ophthalmol. 1989;107:530–7.
19. Petrukhin K, Koisti MJ, Bakall B, et al. Identification of the gene responsible for best macular dystrophy. Nat Genet. 1998;19(3):241–7.
20. Marmorstein AD, Kinnick TR. Focus on molecules: bestrophin (best-1). Exp Eye Res. 2007;85:423–4.
21. Rosenthal R, Bakall B, Kinnick T, et al. Expression of bestrophin-1, the product of the *VMD2* gene, modulates voltage-dependent Ca^{2+} channels in retinal pigment epithelial cells. FASEB J. 2006;20:178–80.
22. Wu J, Peachey NS, Marmorstein AD. Light-evoked responses of the mouse retinal pigment epithelium. J Neurophysiol. 2004;91:1134–42.
23. Marmorstein AD, Kinnick TR, Stanton JB, et al. Bestrophin-1 influences transepithelial electrical properties and Ca^{2+} signaling in human retinal pigment epithelium. Mol Vis. 2015;21:347–59.
24. Marmorstein AD, Marmorstein LY, Rayborn M, et al. Bestrophin, the product of the best vitelliform macular dystrophy gene (*VMD2*), localizes to the basolateral plasma membrane of the retinal pigment epithelium. Proc Natl Acad Sci USA. 2000;97:12758–63.
25. Yu K, Xiao Q, Cui G, et al. The best disease-linked cl^- channel hBest1 regulates ca V 1 (L-type) Ca^{2+} channels via src-homology-binding domains. J Neurosci. 2008;28:5660–70.
26. Barro-Soria R, Aldehni F, Almaça J, et al. ER-localized bestrophin 1 activates Ca^{2+-}dependent ion channels TMEM16A and SK4 possibly by acting as a counter-ion channel. Pflugers Arch. 2010;459:485–97.
27. Cordeiro S, Strauss O. Expression of Orai genes and I_{CRAC} activation in the human retinal pigment epithelium. Graefes Arch Clin Exp Ophthalmol. 2011;249:47–54.
28. Kunzelmann K, Kongsuphol P, Aldehni F, et al. Bestrophin and TMEM16-Ca^{2+} activated cl^- channels with different functions. Cell Calcium. 2009;46:233–41.
29. Marmorstein AD, Cross HE, Peachey NS. Functional roles of bestrophins in ocular epithelia. Prog Retin Eye Res. 2009;28:206–26.
30. Constable PA, Bach M, Frishman LJ, et al. ISCEV standard for clinical electro-oculography (2017 update). Doc Ophthalmol. 2017;134:1–9.
31. Constable PA, Ngo D. The slow light and dark oscillation of the clinical electro-oculogram. Clin Exp Optom. 2018;101:786–92.
32. Schneck ME, Shupenko L, Adams AJ. The fast oscillation of the EOG in diabetes with and without mild retinopathy. Doc Ophthalmol. 2008;116:231–6.
33. Mergaerts F, Daems E, Van Malderen L, Spileers W. Recording of the fast oscillations in the human electro-oculogram. Doc Ophthalmol. 2001;103:63–72.
34. Arden GB, Constable PA. The electro-oculogram. Prog Retin Eye Res. 2006;25:207–48.
35. Arden GB, Wolf JE. The human electro-oculogram: interaction of light and alcohol. Invest Ophthalmol Vis Sci. 2000;41:2722–9.
36. Arden GB, Wolf JE. Differential effects of light and alcohol on the electro-oculographic responses of patients with age-related macular disease. Invest Ophthalmol Vis Sci. 2003;44:3226–32.
37. Gupta LY, Marmor MF. Sequential recording of photic and nonphotic electro-oculogram responses in patients with extensive extramacular drusen. Doc Ophthalmol. 1994;88:49–55.
38. Marmor M, Donovan W, Gaba D. Effects of hypoxia and hyperoxia on the human standing potential. Doc Ophthalmol. 1985;60:347–52.
39. Türksever C, Orgül S, Todorova MG. Comparing short-duration electro-oculograms with and with-

out mydriasis in healthy subjects. Klin Monatsbl Augenheilkd. 2015;232:471–6.
40. Constable PA, Ngo D, Quinn S, Thompson DA. A meta-analysis of clinical electro-oculography values. Doc Ophthalmol. 2017;135:219–32.
41. Thavikulwat AT, Lopez P, Caruso RC, Jeffrey BG. The effects of gender and age on the range of the normal human electro-oculogram. Doc Ophthalmol. 2015;131:177–88.
42. Johnson AA, Guziewicz KE, Lee CJ, et al. Bestrophin 1 and retinal disease. Prog Retin Eye Res. 2017;58:45–69.
43. Toto L, Boon CJ, Di Antonio L, et al. Bestrophinopathy: a spectrum of ocular abnormalities caused by the c.614T>C mutation in the *BEST1* gene. Retina. 2016;36:1586–95.
44. Guziewicz KE, Sinha D, Gómez NM, et al. Bestrophinopathy: an RPE-photoreceptor interface disease. Prog Retin Eye Res. 2017;58:70–88.
45. Mullins RF, Kuehn MH, Faidley EA, et al. Differential macular and peripheral expression of bestrophin in human eyes and its implication for best disease. Invest Ophthalmol Vis Sci. 2007;48:3372–80.
46. Burgess R, Millar ID, Leroy BP, et al. Biallelic mutation of *BEST1* causes a distinct retinopathy in humans. Am J Hum Genet. 2008;82:19–31.
47. Khojasteh H, Azarmina M, Ebrahimiadib N, et al. Autosomal recessive bestrophinopathy: clinical and genetic characteristics of twenty-four cases. J Ophthalmol. 2021;2021:6674290.
48. Fouad YA, Tawfik CA, Nowara M. Autosomal recessive bestrophinopathy presenting with a macular hole retinal detachment. J Vitreoretin Dis. 2022;6:312–5.
49. Kaufman SJ, Goldberg MF, Orth DH, et al. Autosomal dominant vitreoretinochoroidopathy. Arch Ophthalmol. 1982;100:272–8.
50. Yardley J, Leroy BP, Hart-Holden N, et al. Mutations of *VMD2* splicing regulators cause nanophthalmos and autosomal dominant vitreoretinochoroidopathy (ADVIRC). Invest Ophthalmol Vis Sci. 2004;45:3683–9.
51. Chen CJ, Goldberg MF. Progressive cone dysfunction and geographic atrophy of the macula in late stage autosomal dominant vitreoretinochoroidopathy (ADVIRC). Ophthalmic Genet. 2016;37:81–5.
52. Thompson DA, Constable PA, Liasis A, et al. The physiology of the retinal pigment epithelium in Danon disease. Retina. 2016;36:629–38.
53. Chiang TK, White KM, Kurup SK, Yu M. Use of visual electrophysiology to monitor retinal and optic nerve toxicity. Biomol Ther. 2022;29(12):1390.
54. Neubauer AS, Samari-Kermani K, Schaller U, et al. Detecting chloroquine retinopathy: electro-oculogram versus colour vision. Br J Ophthalmol. 2003;87:902–8.
55. Haimovici R, D'Amico DJ, Gragoudas ES, Sokol S. The expanded clinical spectrum of deferoxamine retinopathy. Ophthalmology. 2002;109:164–71.
56. Besch D, Kurtenbach A, Apfelstedt-Sylla E, et al. Visual field constriction and electrophysiological changes associated with vigabatrin. Doc Ophthalmol. 2002;104:151–70.
57. Wang L, Miao H, Li X. Tamoxifen retinopathy: a case report. Springerplus. 2015;4:501.
58. Lam RW, Beattie CW, Buchanan A, et al. Low electrooculographic ratios in patients with seasonal affective disorder. Am J Psychiatry. 1991;148:1526–9.
59. Economou SG, Stefanis CN. Changes of electrooculogram (EOG) in Parkinson's disease. Acta Neurol Scand. 1978;58:44–52.

34 Computed Tomography: Dacryocystography

Nandini Bothra and Suryasnata Rath

34.1 Introduction

A century ago, in 1909, Ewing performed the first dacryocystography (DCG) to visualize the lacrimal abscess cavity and passages using X-rays. He used bismuth subnitrate as the contrast material. However, the surrounding bone and soft tissue details were not discernible in this DCG [1, 2]. A modification of this technique, namely, digital subtraction, made the lacrimal passage stand out but failed to show the surrounding details. Nevertheless, details of the common canaliculus and nasolacrimal duct could be seen, making it a useful tool in cases with stenosis. Using X-rays was a disadvantage due to the dangers of radiation exposure [1]. This was overcome to some extent by the advent of computed tomography dacryocystography (CT-DCG) in 1990. This allowed the documentation of the bone and soft tissue anatomy and the lacrimal drainage system (LDS) [3]. The most important use of CT-DCG was in complex nasolacrimal duct obstructions (NLDO) in craniofacial trauma. It is also useful in diagnosing and monitoring tumors and masquerades involving the LDS [1]. Magnetic resonance dacryocystography (MR-DCG) was first performed in 1993 to study the functional and morphological aspects of the lacrimal pathways. Although the adverse effects of radiation exposure were nullified, the high cost, longer acquisition time, and motion artifacts were the limitations [4]. CT-DCG is currently the most used technique because of its distinct advantages in delineating details of the LDS, adjacent bone and soft tissue anatomy, low acquisition time, and relatively low radiation exposure.

34.2 Indications of Dacryocystography

It delineates the following in the lacrimal drainage system:

1. Position and size of the lacrimal sac with respect to the bony landmarks.
2. Abnormalities like lacrimal sac diverticula.
3. Filling defects caused by mucopeptide concretions.
4. Functional passage of tears in the lacrimal system.
5. Lacrimal sac tumours.
6. Partial nasolacrimal duct obstructions.
7. Differentiate masquerading conditions from LDS abnormalities.

N. Bothra
Govindram Seksaria Institute of Dacryology, Kallam Anji Reddy Campus L V Prasad Eye Institute, Hyderabad, India

S. Rath (✉)
Mithu Tulsi Chanrai Campus, L V Prasad Eye Institute, Bhubaneswar, India
e-mail: suryasnata@lvpei.org

T. Das, P. Satgunam (eds.), *Ophthalmic Diagnostics*, https://doi.org/10.1007/978-981-97-0138-4_34

34.3 Dyes Used in Dacryocystography

There are oil-soluble and water-soluble dyes available for conventional DCG and CT-DCG. The ideal dye must be radio-opaque, non-irritant, non-toxic, homogenous, with optimal viscosity, and should not cause adverse reactions [1]. Oil-soluble dyes like lipiodol provide significantly better images than water-soluble dyes like iohexol, iopamidol, sinografin, and omnipaque; however, these are also very viscous, immiscible with tears, and carry a risk of tissue reaction or granuloma formation [5–7]. This makes water-soluble dyes preferable over oil-soluble counterparts. Water-soluble dyes can have a high (iohexol, iopamidol 300) or low (omnipaque) iodine content. Those with high iodine content provide better images but may cause more patient discomfort [5–7]. For patients allergic to iodinated substances, gadobutrol can be used [8]. MR-DCG uses a gadolinium solution as a contrast medium [4]. The authors use iohexol dye in a 50:50 dilution with normal saline for CT-DCG.

34.4 CT-DCG Scan Requisition

A request for CT-DCG should ideally fulfil a few prerequisites for optimal information. These include:

1. Region of interest: computed tomography scans of the orbit + dacryocystography.
2. Slice thickness: typically, 2 mm cuts (sections) are preferred for the orbit.
3. Imaging plane: Coronal, axial, three-dimensional volumetric reconstruction (3-DR), and parasagittal views are requested. Coronal and axial views demonstrate the passage of the LDS in the lacrimal sac fossa and a small portion of the NLD (nasolacrimal duct) and surrounding bony canal. The 3-DR scans provide a view of the LDS in three dimensions and determine the position of the LDS with respect to the bony structures. The parasagittal view shows the bony segment of NLD in its entirety.
4. Tissue windows: The bone windows help delineate the relationship of a dye-filled LDS with the surrounding bony structures, and the soft tissue windows show the position of the dye-filled LDS within the surrounding soft tissues.

34.5 Methods

1. Drop method: The dye is instilled in the inferior cul-de-sac, and the passage of the dye is monitored on serial scans. This technique is mainly used to assess the functional capacity of the LDS.
2. Injection method: The dye is directly injected into the system using an irrigation cannula. This method is faster and serial scans are not needed.

34.5.1 Patient Stories

Patient 1

A 27-year-old male presented with complaints of watering from his left eye and double vision for 2 months. He had sustained a road traffic accident 4 months before, followed by a maxillofacial repair of facial fractures. The irrigation of the left LDS showed complete regurgitation of mucoid discharge from the opposite punctum, and the right side was patent. CT-DCG 3-DR scans showed a large dilated sac on the left side with a block at the junction of the lacrimal sac and nasolacrimal duct with minimal spillover of the dye and patent system on the left side. The sac was fairly in position on the left side. There was an inferior rim fracture with plates on the maxillary bone just short of the expected area of surgery. Coronal CT scans of the orbit showed an associated large floor fracture on the left side involving the strut. The nasal anatomy and cribriform plate position appeared normal (Fig. 34.1).

Inference: CT-DCG helped delineate the anatomy of the bones in relation to the lacrimal system, which was relatively preserved. This allowed the surgical team to decide on an external or endoscopic dacryocystorhinostomy. An orbital

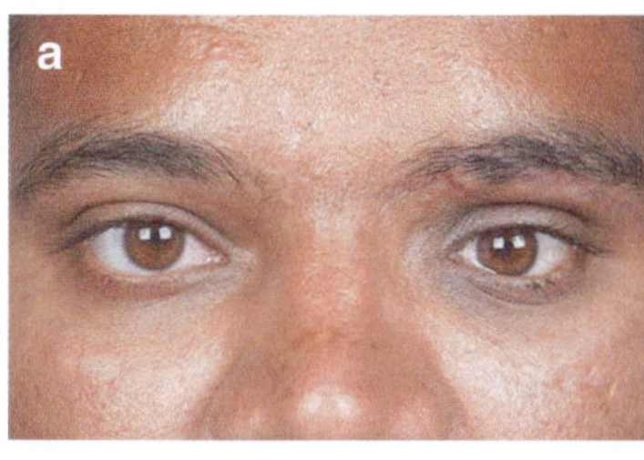

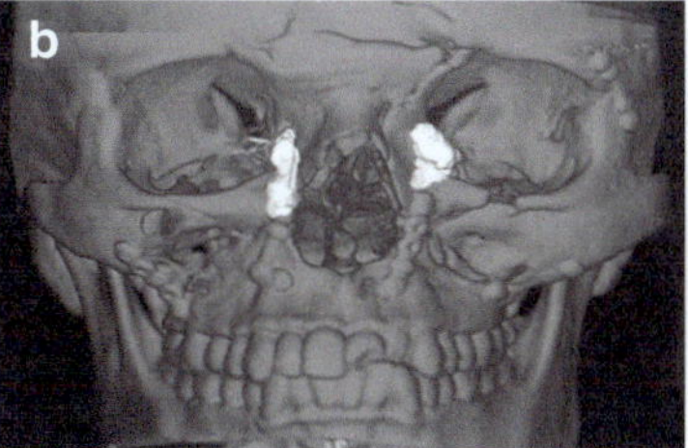

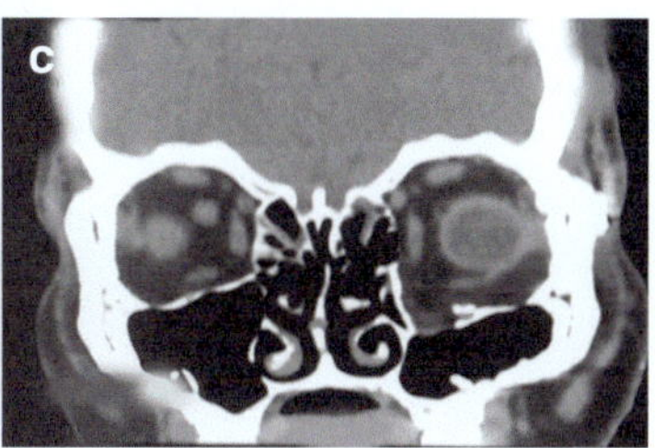

Fig. 34.1 Clinical photograph showing minimal pigmentation of the medial canthal region with mild telecanthus on the left side (Panel A). Computed tomography scans with dacryocystography and 3D reconstructed images demonstrate a dilated sac on the left side with obstruction at the sac-duct junction; the right side shows drainage of the dye to the inferior meatus; left inferior orbital rim fracture, screws and plates on the maxillary and zygomatic bones on both sides (Panel B) and coronal scans showing left-sided orbital floor and medial wall fracture involving the strut, with the cribriform plate having a normal position and normal nasal anatomy (Panel C)

fracture repair could be planned during the same sitting.

Patient 2

A 30-year-old gentleman with a history of blunt trauma to the forehead and upper part of his nose with a cricket bat 4 years ago complained of right eye watering after trauma. A CT-DCG scan and 3-DR images showed a small shrunken lacrimal sac on the right side and an obstruction at the lacrimal sac-nasolacrimal duct junction. On rotating the 3-DR images, the right-side sac position could be confirmed with respect to the underlying lacrimal sac fossa. The coronal images, bone windows depicted a normal relationship between the dye-filled sac with the lacrimal sac fossa and a shrunken sac compared to the left side. The parasagittal cuts showed no evidence of any bony fractures in the bony NLD canal. The remaining orbital and nasal anatomy appears normal (Fig. 34.2).

Inference: External or endoscopic approach could be attempted. Expect the sac to be small, fibrosed, and slightly higher in position.

Patient 3

A 38-year-old male sustained multiple facial fractures after a road traffic accident. He complained of epiphora on both sides. He underwent a maxillofacial repair after the accident. On looking at the CT-DCG scans, gross lacrimal sac malposition was noted (left, more than right). The right lacrimal sac was almost completely scarred. The left sac was displaced postero-superiorly in orbit beneath the ipsilateral frontal sinus. Damage to the horizontal plate of the cribriform and other fractures of the orbital walls were also noted (Fig. 34.3).

Inference: An osteotomy at this location could lead to a significant risk of injury to the skull base. In addition, maneuvering the canalicular- lacrimal sac anatomy in such a malposition would be challenging. In this scenario, DCT (dacryocystectomy) may be a safer option. Alternatively, if attempted, a staged approach with the reconstruction of the naso-ethmoid fracture and correction of the medial canthal dystopia may need navigation guidance to decrease the risk of CSF (cerebrospinal fluid) leak. Subsequently, a conjunctival DCR with a Jone's tube may be considered for intractable epiphora.

Patient 4

After a road traffic accident, a young male presented with a red, inflamed, and tender swelling below the right lower eyelid medially with complaints of epiphora. Irrigation revealed total regurgitation of the fluid from the opposite punctum, with the swelling becoming more tense and pronounced. The CT-DCG scans showed a minimally displaced sac with a large postero-lateral diverticulum, partially filled with diluted dye (Fig. 34.4).

Inference: While trying to do a dacryocystorhinostomy surgery, one has to ensure that the diverticula are either completely excised or internalized into the ostium created to prevent recurrences of the problem and failure of the procedure.

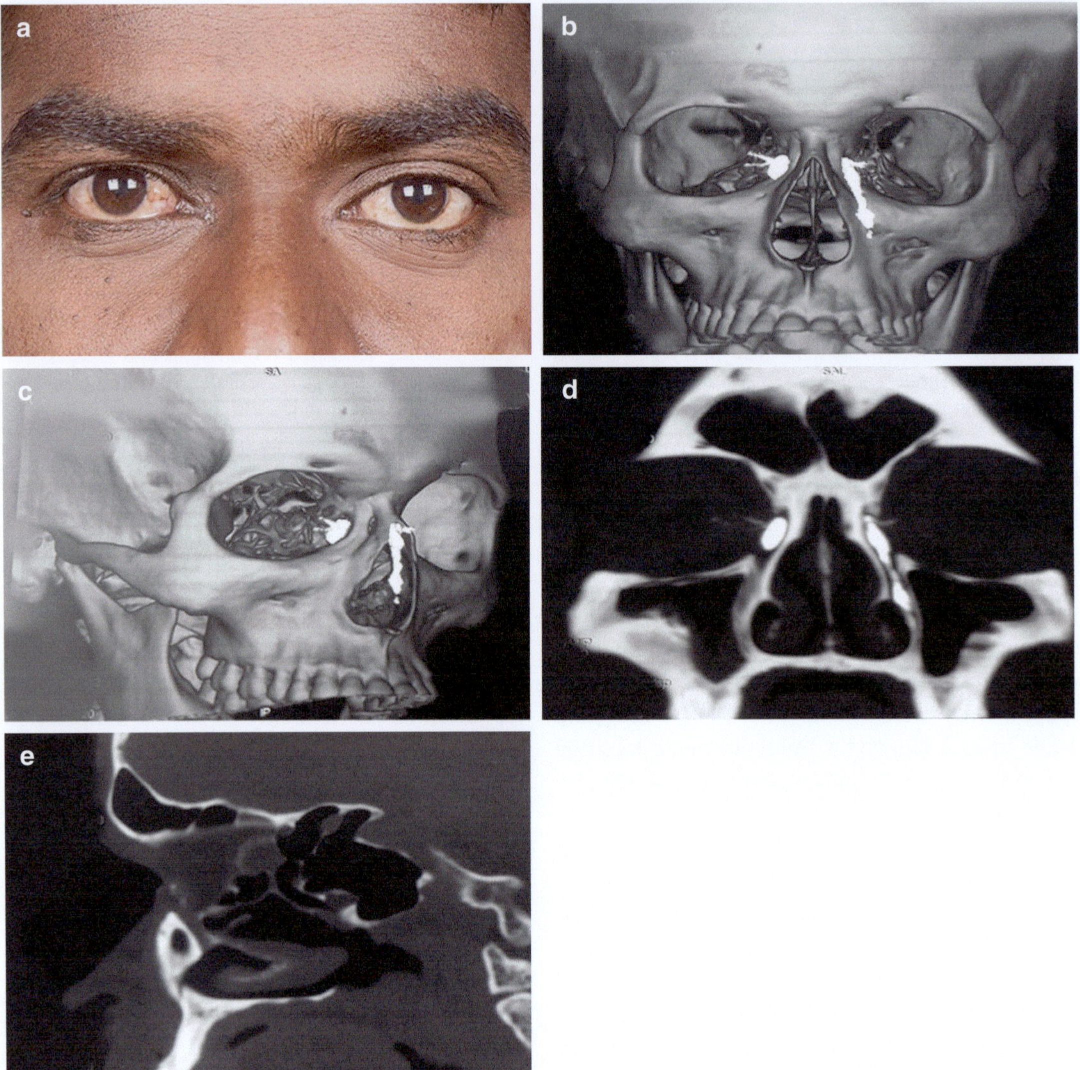

Fig. 34.2 Clinical photograph demonstrating a raised tear meniscus height and minimal discharge medially in the right eye (Panel A). The CT-DCG and 3DR images show a small shrunken sac with obstruction at the sac-duct junction (Panel B). The 3-DR image, right-sided view, and maximum intensity projection sequence (MIPS) show the sac is within the lacrimal sac fossa with the obstruction at the sac-duct junction (Panels C and D). The parasagittal cuts demonstrate a normal bony nasolacrimal duct with no drainage (Panel E)

The position of the diverticula noted on the scans will help take the appropriate surgical steps. A posterior diverticulum can be managed to a large extent during an endoscopic DCR, but a large anterolateral diverticulum is best approached via an external approach.

Patient 5

A 10-year-old boy was scratched by a dog in the medial part of the right eye about a year ago. He has had complaints of epiphora for the past 10 months. There was scarring in the mid-canalicular area. On probing and irrigation, the

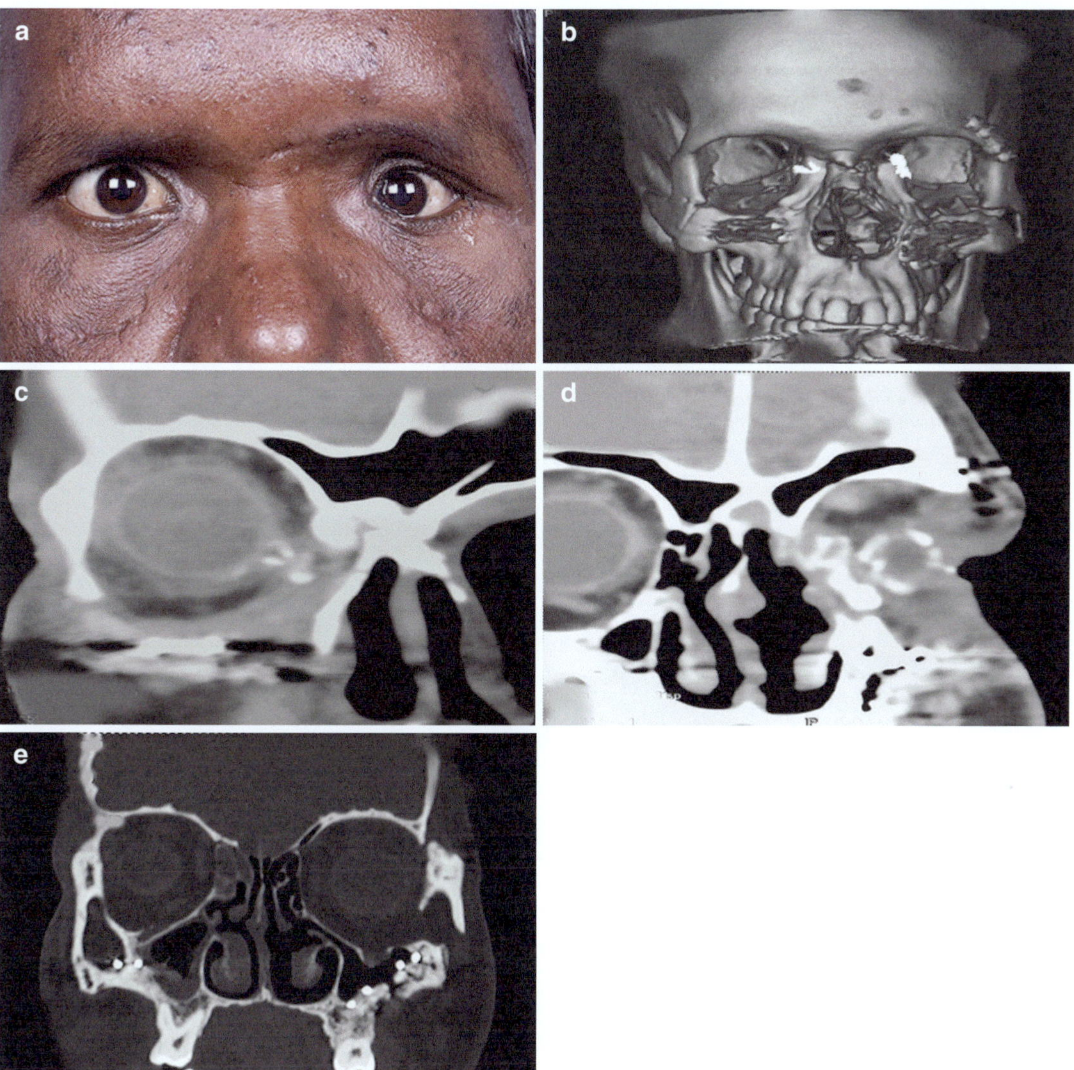

Fig. 34.3 Clinical photograph showing traumatic telecanthus on the left side (Panel A). The 3D CT-DCG showed a shrunken, fibrosed sac on the right side and a postero-superiorly displaced sac on the left side (Panel B). The CT-DCG scans, coronal cuts demonstrate the orbital fractures on the right side a displaced, shrunken sac and a damaged cribriform plate (Panel C) and naso-orbito-ethmoid fracture, postero-superior dislocation of the sac, and damaged cribriform plate on the left side (Panel D). The CT scan orbit, coronal cuts, bone windows demonstrate the presence of orbital fractures and cribriform plate damage on both sides (Panel E)

upper and lower canaliculus on the right side showed a mid-canalicular obstruction, but the child was certain he could appreciate minimal fluid in the nasal cavity. The CT-DCG scans confirmed the mid-canalicular obstruction with no evidence of any trace of dye in the remaining LDS (Fig. 34.5).

Inference: Considering the scarred tissue on the conjunctival side of the medial eyelid and the obstruction precisely at the same spot, one can explore the area with a guarded prognosis or convince the patient to undergo a conjunctival-dacryocystorhinostomy since the remaining anatomy is unaffected.

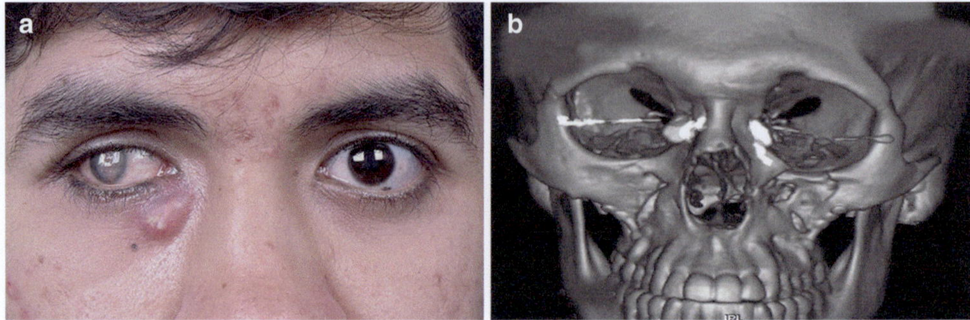

Fig. 34.4 A clinical photograph showing an inflamed swelling on the lower eyelid extending lateral to the lacrimal sac position with a pus point along with corneal scarring and exotropia (Panel A). The 3D CT-DCG scan demonstrates a minimally superiorly displaced sac on the right side with a postero-lateral sac diverticulum (Panel B)

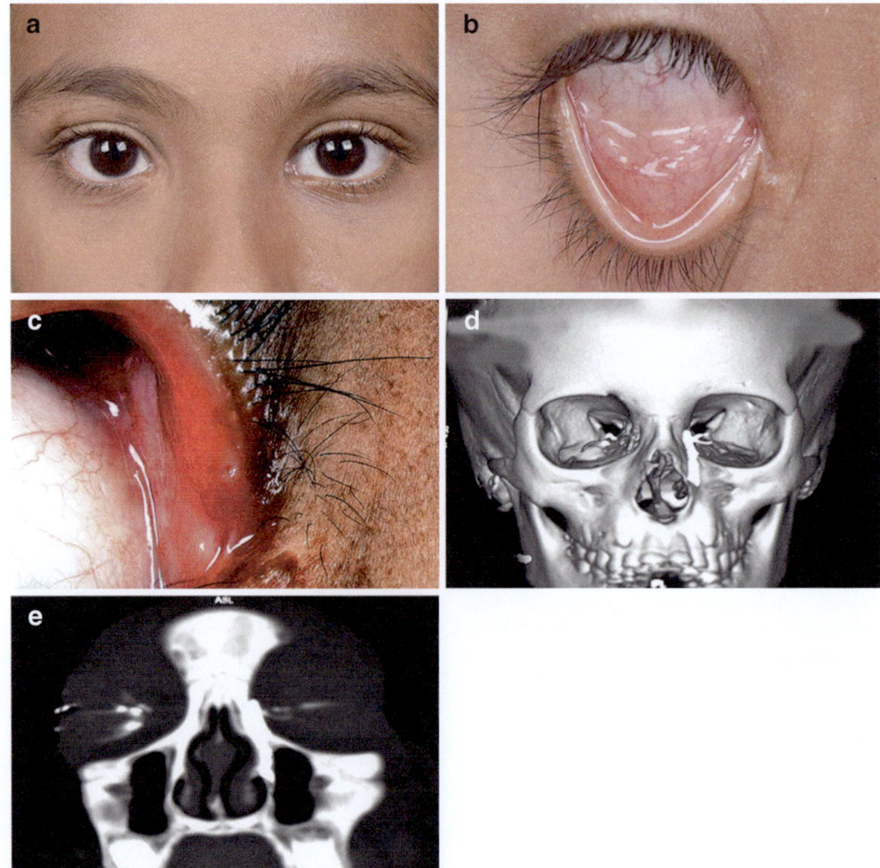

Fig. 34.5 The clinical photograph demonstrates telecanthus on the right side (Panel A) and normal lower and upper puncta (Panels B and C). The 3D CT-DCG and maximum intensity projection sequence demonstrate a canalicular obstruction involving the upper and lower canaliculus on the right side and a patent lacrimal drainage system on the left side (Panels D and E)

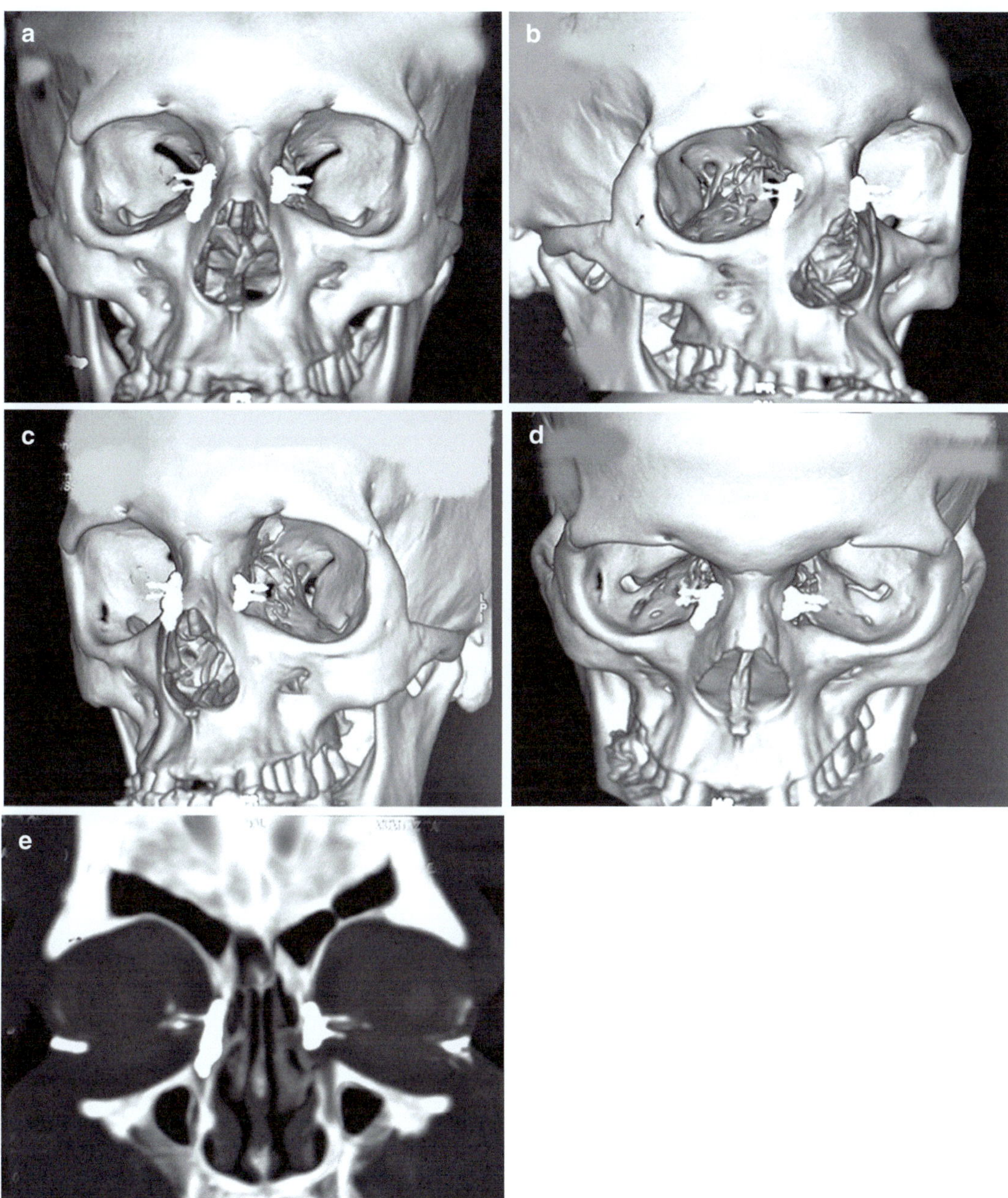

Fig. 34.6 The 3D CT-DCG scans demonstrated a dilated sac on the right side and an inferiorly fibrosed sac on the left side, in the lacrimal sac fossa (Panels A, B, C, and D), and the maximum intensity projection sequence showed a bilateral incomplete, inferior osteotomy indicative of a previous surgery (Panel E)

Patient 6

A 48-year-old female had undergone bilateral endonasal endoscopic DCR elsewhere 3 years ago. A month after surgery, she had watering and discharge from both eyes. Endoscopic examination revealed complete scarring anterior to the middle turbinate in the sac-duct junction (inferior scarring). The CT-DCG scans showed a dilated sac on the side and a comparatively shrunken sac on the left side with an underlying incomplete bony osteotomy (Fig. 34.6).

Inference: During the revision DCR surgery, the osteotomy should be enlarged (Right eye more than Left eye) to open the sac completely into the nasal cavity. It also identifies that the failure of the previous surgery was due to inadequate osteotomy, which was mainly inferior. The area opposite the common canaliculus was still covered with bone and could likely cause failure.

34.6 Conclusion

Dacryocystography can be an adjunct to diagnosing and managing complex and complicated cases. It cannot be used as a single modality to understand the case scenarios. It has to be combined with a proper history, clinical examination, and other corroborative tests. Also, it provides a clear picture and helps make appropriate decisions on further management.

Funding Hyderabad Eye Research Foundation.

Disclosure Receives royalties from Springer for his treatise *The textbook Surgery in Thyroid Eye Disease: A Conceptual Approach.*

References

1. Singh S, Ali MJ, Paulsen F. Dacryocystography: from theory to current practice. Ann Anat. 2019;224:33–40.
2. Ewing AE. Roentgen ray demonstrations of the lacrimal abscess cavity. Am J Ophthalmol. 1909;26:1–4.
3. Zinreich SI, Miller NR, Freeman LN, et al. Tomographic dacryocystography using topical contrast media for lacrimal system visualization. Orbit. 1990;9:79–87.
4. Goldberg RA, Heinz GW, Chiu L. Gadolinium MR imaging dacryocystogra-phy. Am J Ophthalmol. 1993;15:738–41.
5. Munk PL, Burhenne LW, Buffam FV, et al. Dacryocystography: comparison of water-soluble and oil-based contrast agents. Radiology. 1989;173:827–30.
6. Mansfield DC, Zeki SM, Mackenzie JR. Case report: extravasation of lipiodol—a complication of dacryocystography. Clin Radiol. 1994;49:217–8.
7. Delaney Y, Khooshabeh R. Lipogranuloma following traumatic dacryocystography in a 4-year-old boy. Eye (Lond). 2001;15:683–4.
8. Priebe M, Mohr A, Brossman J, et al. Gadobutrol: an alternative contrast agent for digital subtraction dacryocystography. Eur Radiol. 2002;12:208386.

Home Care and Teleophthalmology

35

Taraprasad Das, Debananada Padhy, Kalpa Negiloni, Jenil Sheth, Sanil Joseph, Suryasnata Rath, and Ramesh Kekunnaya

35.1 Introduction

Family medicine comprises comprehensive health care for people and their families and provides continuing health care to everyone across all ages, genders, and diseases [1]. Although family medicine has been an age-old practice globally and in India, it has slowly given way to specialist medical care. While it is not practiced as much in eye care as it is for systemic care, even in the latter, it is decreasing. Despite its dwindling popularity, one of the key advantages of family medicine is last-mile access, especially to vulnerable individuals, due to their age, sickness, and/or mobility constraints.

Home care emerged as an acute need during the SARS-CoV-2 pandemic, forcing people to stay indoors for several months. As a result, various technologies for keeping patients safe and healthy emerged. Tools that enabled home care and were a matter of convenience and compliance at one point have now become a critical need. Moreover, home care has become essential, with the WHO reaffirming the criticality of prioritizing primary health care to ensure that people receive comprehensive promotive, preventive, curative, rehabilitative, and palliative care as close to their everyday environments as possible [2, 3]. However, to be acceptable, home care must be technologically safe, scientifically sound, socially acceptable, easily accessible, and financially affordable.

Eye disease and visual impairment are frequently seen in older adults. Although ophthalmic pathology is rarely life-threatening, the

The original version of this chapter has been revised by author's name. A correction to this chapter can be found at https://doi.org/10.1007/978-981-97-0138-4_36

T. Das (✉)
Anant Bajaj Retina Institute, Srimati Kanuri Santhamma Centre for Vitreoretinal Diseases, Kallam Anji Reddy Campus, L V Prasad Eye Institute, Hyderabad, Telangana, India
e-mail: tpd@lvpei.org

D. Padhy
Gullapalli Pratibha Rao International Centre for Advancement of Rural Eye Care, L V Prasad Eye Institute, Hyderabad, India

K. Negiloni
Remidio Innovative Solutions Pvt Ltd, Bengaluru, India

J. Sheth
Shantilal Shanghvi Eye Institute, Mumbai, India

S. Joseph
Lions Aravind Institute of Community Ophthalmology, Aravind Eye Care System, Madurai, India

S. Rath
Mithu Tulsi Chanrai Campus, L V Prasad Eye Institute, Bhubaneswar, India
e-mail: suryasnata@lvpei.org

R. Kekunnaya
Child Sight Institute, Jasti V Ramanamma Children's Eye Care Center, Kallam Anji Reddy Campus, L V Prasad Eye Institute, Hyderabad, India
e-mail: rameshak@lvpei.org

T. Das, P. Satgunam (eds.), *Ophthalmic Diagnostics*, https://doi.org/10.1007/978-981-97-0138-4_35

Table 35.1 Teleophthalmology methods

Modality	Parameters	Description
Store and forward	Process	Patient information, such as medical images, is acquired and sent to the specialist as needed.
	Advantage	Medical practitioners need not meet the patient in person. It saves time and is convenient for the physician.
	Disadvantage	Given that it relies on history and documented information or images rather than a physical examination, it has the potential for misdiagnosis.
Remote monitoring (self-testing)	Process	Remote monitoring uses various technological devices to remotely monitor a patient's health and clinical signs.
	Advantage	It is cost-effective; hence, more frequent monitoring is possible, and there is greater patient satisfaction.
	Disadvantage	Given that it is patient-dependent, the tests conducted by the patients may not always be accurate.
Real-time interactive asynchronous	Process	It utilizes several different media, including phones, online consultations, and home visits by technicians of the field team.
	Advantage	A video/audio interaction between the patient and physician occurs after the field team has visited the individual's home, either on the same or another day.
	Disadvantage	Relatively expensive and time-consuming.
Real-time interactive synchronous	Process	While it is similar to the asynchronous modality, the main difference is the live consultation by an ophthalmologist/an eye care personnel.
	Advantage	A real-time video/audio interaction between the patient and physician occurs immediately after the field team completes the eye examination.
	Disadvantage	Relatively expensive and time-consuming; logistic challenge of coordinating the video call at the time of the home visit. Needs a reliable network connection.

consequences of visual impairment are wide-ranging. Visual impairment may be associated with social and functional decline, depression, falls, and increased mortality. These could be partly met with telemedicine and home care. Telemedicine is an exchange of medical data by electronic telecommunication technology that allows a remotely located physician to evaluate and monitor the patient's medical problems. Ophthalmology being highly visual and image intensive is uniquely suited for telemedicine. There are three main types of telemedicine: (1) store-and-forward, (2) remote monitoring, and (3) real-time synchronous and asynchronous interactive services. Each one has its advantages and disadvantages. (Table 35.1).

This chapter describes the ophthalmic devices and technology of home eye care and teleophthalmology. Table 35.2 lists the eight eye examinations for which teleconsultation and home care are available for adults.

Table 35.2 Eight eye examinations

Sr. No.	Parameter	Device
1	Visual acuity	Web-based/smartphone-based (PEEK)
2	Refraction	Folding Phoropter, autoref (e-see; InstaRef)
3	Intraocular pressure	Rebound tonometer, modular slit lamp with applanation
4	External eye	Pocket flashlight
5	Visual field	Head-mounted device, virtual reality-based perimetry
6	Anterior segment	Modular slit lamp, an anterior imaging system (Grabi ™)
7	Pupil	Pupillometer
8	Fundus	Direct and indirect ophthalmoscopy, non-mydriatic fundus camera

35.2 Visual Acuity

Visual acuity (VA) is essential for assessing a patient's eye health. It is conventionally measured using a printed Snellen or ETDRS (Early Treatment Diabetic Retinopathy Study) chart placed at a 6-m (20 ft) distance under a standard illumination of 300 lux. With the introduction of digital charts, the distance for visual acuity measurement is now reduced to 3–4 m. Historically, while VA testing has been done exclusively in a clinical setting under the guidance of a trained professional, in recent years, various options have been created for testing VA outside of the clinic, using web-based (e.g., www.smart-optometry.com) or smartphone-based (e.g., PEEK; https://peakvision.org) tests. These devices are validated against the standard visual acuity charts [4].

35.2.1 PEEK is one of the popular VA measurement devices. (Fig. 35.1)

Technology: It is a smartphone-based vision check app that allows anyone to check VA using an Android smartphone. The advantages of PEEK include a visual representation of results for easy explanation to patients, and it provides standard units of Snellen acuity.

Technique: A "Tumbling E" is used in PEEK. Only the letter "E" appears on the smartphone, but it has a different orientation each time it appears. Once this has been explained to the patient, the smartphone is held at a distance of 1 m. One eye is examined at a time, with the other eye covered.

Clinical Application: PEEK helps screen and identify people who need further examination. It is not intended to replace detailed examinations from a qualified eye health professional.

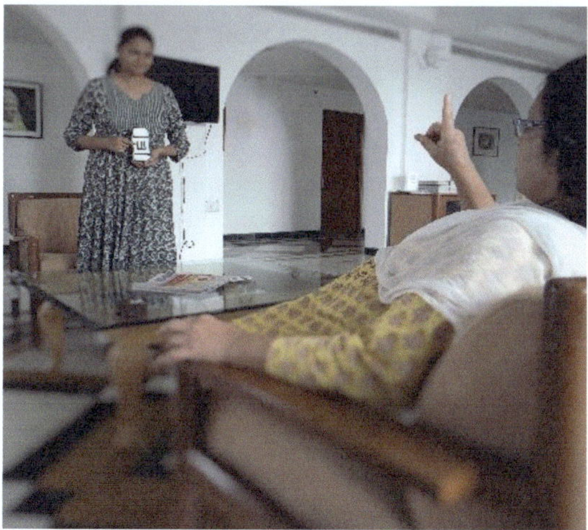

Fig. 35.1 Visual acuity testing using PEEK. A new letter appears when the phone is swiped in the direction the patient identifies the letter. (Photo courtesy: Krishnaveni & Monika, LV Prasad Eye Institute, Hyderabad, India)

35.3 Refraction

The global burden of uncorrected refractive error is high. Refraction is the first essential step in the correction of refractive error. The patient can be refracted at home by traditional retinoscopy using a streak retinoscope, followed by a subjective correction with a series of trial lenses. While ideal, this requires an elaborate setup, including a skilled workforce. De-skilling the refraction process would reduce the cost of training. This will help increase efficiency and improve the quality of spectacle prescriptions and the cost of care. Although autorefraction is an alternative option that can be performed at home, the autorefractometer must be portable, lightweight, reliable enough to avoid a subjective correction, and able to transfer data to an eye clinic or optical outlet. We will describe three such devices in the following section.

35.3.1 Folding Phoropter (FoFo) (Fig. 35.2)

Technology: The Folding Phoropter is a foldable paper device comprising two retractable paper tubes with a converging and diverging lens on each tube. (Fig. 35.2; Left panel) Like a telescope, the user can move the tubes while looking through them and stop when the target is viewed clearly. The target image becomes clear by adjusting the distance between the lenses. A scale

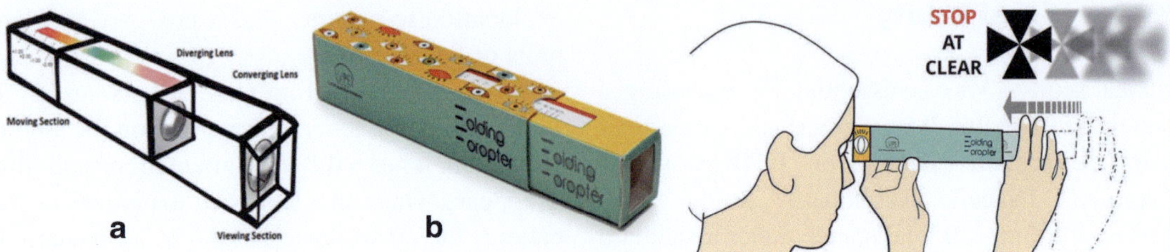

Fig. 35.2 Left panel: (**a**) optics; (**b**) the FoFo device. Right panel: schematic diagram describing how the FoFo is operated. (Copyrights Padhay D et al., 2023 [5] under Creative Common Attribution License)

embedded into the device approximates the refractive error when a clear image is obtained and gives the spherical equivalent of the refractive error. The refractive error range for the FoFo is +4.00 to–7.00 D. It is user-dependent since it relies on a subjective assessment of refractive error.

Technique: The FoFo is held at eye level in the non-dominant hand. The subject focuses on a distance target of 6/60 level at 3 m. The height or level of the eye is aligned parallel with the distance target. The subject then focuses on the letter/image (Fig. 35.2; right panel). The target image becomes clear by adjusting the distance between the lenses. The dominant hand slides the outer tube to find the point where the target appears clear. With one eye, the user looks through the FoFo and moves the tubes while fixating on the distant target. The measurement of refractive error for each eye is done separately. When the endpoint for each eye is obtained, the scale on the FoFo gives the spherical equivalent of the refractive error.

Clinical Application: The FoFo is useful in screening during home visits. It could be used for screening children at schools as well. It is valuable for refractive error assessment in low-resource settings. Its relative advantages and disadvantages are shown in Table 35.3 [5].

Table 35.3 Advantages and disadvantages of the FoFo

Advantages	Disadvantages
Easy to understand and use	Difficult to measure the refractive error in people in extremes of age—Very elderly and young children
Requires less time	Findings are not reliable if used improperly
Inexpensive	Cannot measure astigmatism
Lightweight	Breaks easily
Portable	Works well with literate people
No need for electricity/ battery	Cannot determine higher refractive errors

35.3.2 QuickSee (e-See)

Technology: The QuickSee is a portable open-view wavefront aberrometer capable of conducting binocular autorefraction. There is also a monocular model of the QuickSee, the "QuickSee Flip" or "e-see," specifically designed to market at a lower price to increase accessibility in low- and middle-income countries [6]. (Fig. 35.3).

Technique: The subject holds the autorefractor to the face and looks through the device at a back-lit VA chart placed at 3 or 6 m. The interpupillary distance wheel on the autorefractor and the pitch of the instrument are manually adjusted until one sees a red spot on the autorefractor. A trained technician is usually required to guide the subjects using it. The device illuminates the eye using a low-power laser diode through the pupil, and the light captured by the inbuilt wavefront sensor provides an estimate of the magnitude of various aberrations in the subject's eye. An approximately 10-s video of the captured light is recorded for each eye. The device then uses this information to estimate the subject's refraction and generate the spectacle prescription on a laptop [7, 8].

Clinical Application: The e-see provides glass prescriptions that satisfy most individuals without requiring highly trained personnel to perform subjective refraction.

35.3.3 InstaRef

Technology. InstaRef R20™ is a portable, Hartmann Shack wavefront aberrometer-based autorefractometer. It is a monocular handheld

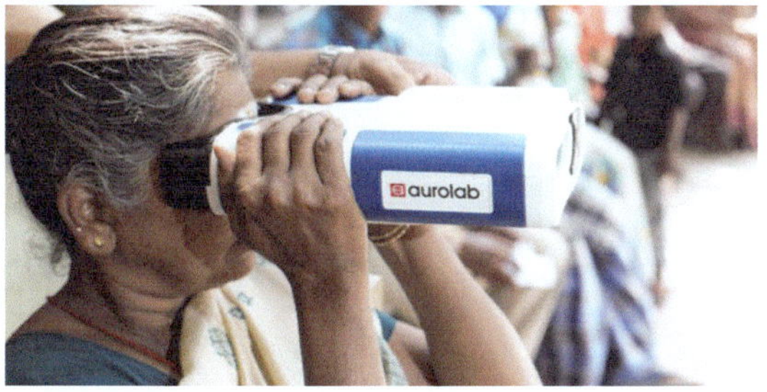

Fig. 35.3 The e-See is used to refract one eye at a time

device weighing 400 g, allowing monocular refractive error measurements. (Fig. 35.4) A specific point on the retina is illuminated using an Infrared (IR) beam (Fig. 35.4c-red) with a wavelength of 850 nm, emitted from a laser module. The reflected IR laser beam (Fig. 35.4c-blue) passes through the lens system. The wavefront sensor comprises a micro lenslet array measuring 12.92 × 8.75 mm and 1.55 mm thick. This array confines the reflected light to a pattern of spots, which are detected by an image sensor measuring 4.76 × 5.61 mm. (Fig. 35.5) The tilt of the wavefront that enters each lenslet corresponds directly to the position of each spot on the image sensor. By determining the positions of the spots, the phase of the wavefront, which relates to the ocular aberrations, is calculated. Using standard mathematical calculations, these spot-position coordinates are used in modal reconstruction to approximate the three-dimensional wavefront

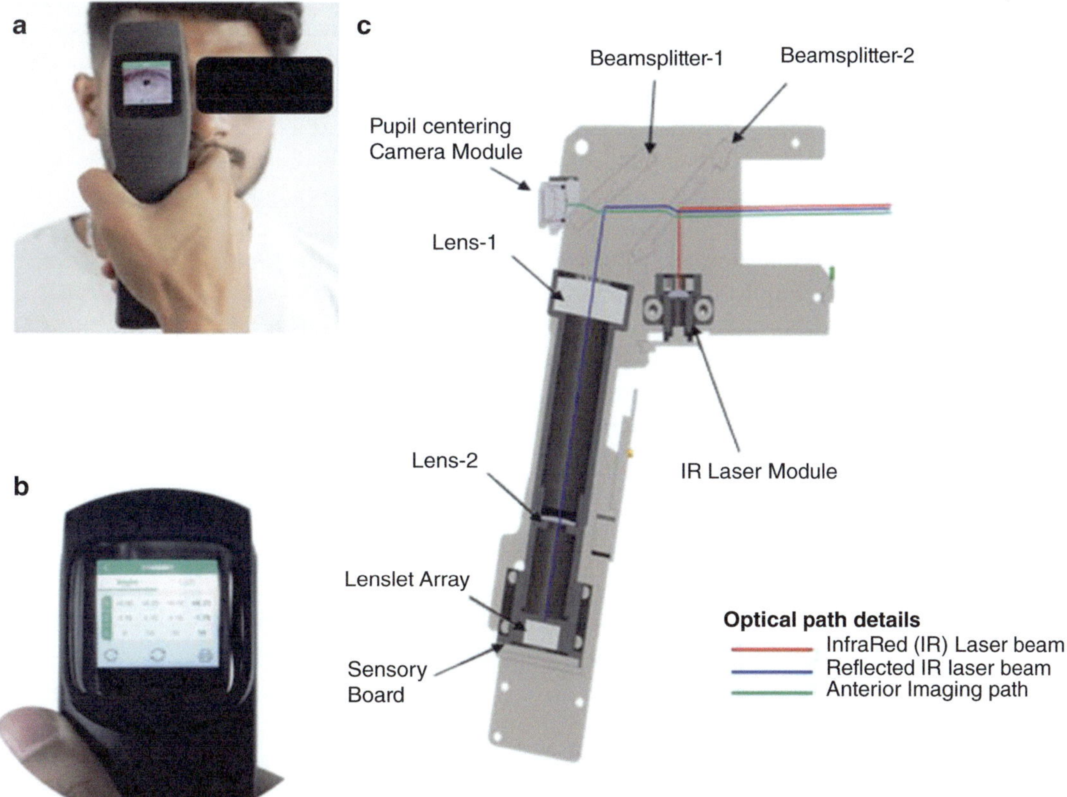

Fig. 35.4 InstaRef: (**a**) monocular device capture mode, (**b**) measurement recordings, and (**c**) optical components of the system. (Source: Rao DP, et al. [9])

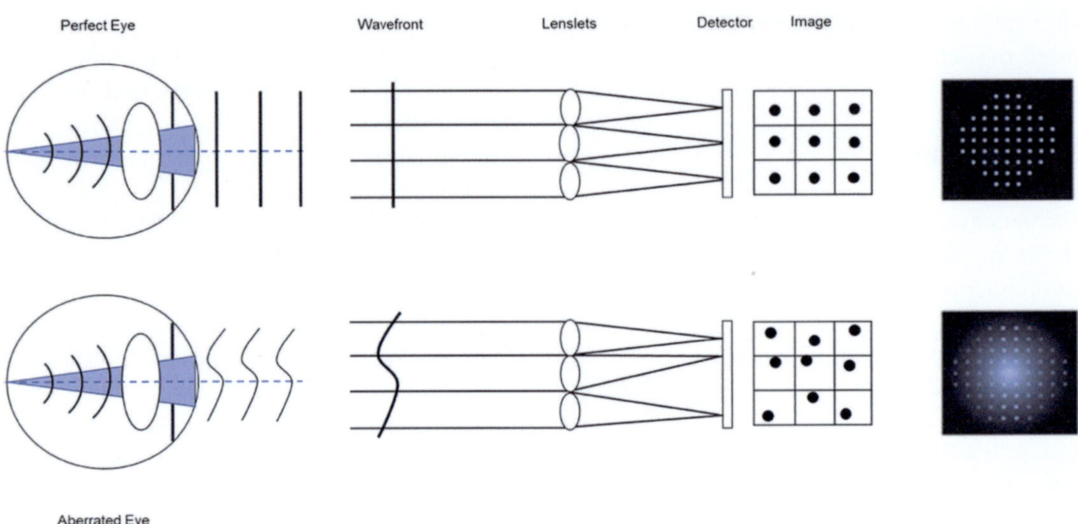

Fig. 35.5 Optics of the InstaRef. (Kalpa-more details)

topology for lower order aberrations. The device also includes a pupil-centering module and an audible tilt warning system. The refractive error range is −10.0 D to +10.0D sphere and − 5.0D to +5.0D cylinder.

Technique. Using the non-testing eye, the subject is instructed to fixate on a distant target (~20 feet). This can eliminate the influence of accommodation on measurement. The examiner places the device in front of the testing eye (Fig. 35.4a). It is advisable to test under dim illumination so that the pupil diameter is large and the wavefront-based measurements are more reliable. The pupil-centration crosshair in the device is aligned with the center of the subject's pupil. The device alerts the examiner if there is any significant tilt in the device through a tilt warning system. Once the crosshair is centered and after ensuring that the fellow eye is fixed for the distance, the examiner triggers the measurement button. The device lets the examiner capture three readings per eye in 3 s. Based on the three readings, the device automatically calculates the average of spherical, cylindrical, and axial values. It also allows the negative and positive representations of the cylindrical values. The same procedure is followed for refractive error measurement in the other eye. The results can be immediately printed using Bluetooth-enabled printers or accessed on an electronic medical record system.

Clinical Applications. The InstaRef is a good starting point for subjective refraction in all age groups and is useful in clinical and community vision screening as a quick and reliable tool. The advantages of this tool are: it requires less clinical space, provides a quick reading, requires less training, and has electronic compatibility. Compared with the open-field autorefractometer (OFAR), the device works well in adults [9], can be used pre- and post-cycloplegic treatment, and can be used for subjective refraction in children older than 8 [10].

35.4 Intraocular Pressure

Glaucoma is one of the leading causes of visual impairment and blindness globally. Increased intraocular pressure (IOP) is one of the signs of glaucoma. The development and progression of glaucoma can be slowed only by controlling the IOP. Therefore, accurate measurement of IOP is of paramount importance. It can be measured at home by allied ophthalmic personnel using a handheld device. One such device is described below.

35.4.1 Rebound Tonometer

The Goldman applanation tonometer (GAT) is the current reference standard in IOP measurement. However, it requires a slit lamp, topical anesthesia, and sodium fluorescein dye; it can only be measured with the patient in a sitting posture. Other ocular tonometers, such as the rebound tonometer, are comparable to the GAT [11] while also portable, lightweight, easy to use, and do not require topical anesthesia.

Technology: The rebound tonometer consists of a tiny probe (of variable length) made of stainless steel with a 1.8 mm diameter plastic ball. The probe is held in the device by an electromagnetic field powered by a battery. When the button on the device is pushed, a spring drives the probe with its plastic ball to hit the corneal surface. The speed of deceleration of the probe when it hits the corneal surface is measured and converted into an IOP measurement. (Fig. 35.6) The speed of deceleration depends on the IOP; it is rapid for high IOPs and slow for low IOPs. The motion parameter (probe deceleration) and contact time (when the probe hits the cornea) are measured by an induction-based coil system and analyzed by an advanced algorithm in the device. The rebound tonometer was introduced as the Icare TAO1i (Helsinki, Finland) device in 2003. Updated versions of the rebound tonometer, i.e., the Icare Pro, Icare 100, and Icare 200, were introduced subsequently. It weighs around 250–400 g. It is handheld, rechargeable battery-operated, lightweight, and portable.

Technique: For recording the IOP, the patient sits upright, looks straight ahead, and keeps his/her eyes steady (the device can also be used on the subject in a supine position). The device is held in front of the eye so that the ball of the probe is around 4–8 mm from the center of the cornea and is perpendicular to the corneal surface. When the push button of the device is pressed, the probe touches the center of the cornea rapidly. Six consecutive measurements are taken, and the result is displayed on an LCD screen facing the examiner. The IOP measurement in the rebound tonometer does not need any prior eye preparation and does not need corneal anesthesia.

Unlike the first-generation rebound tonometer, the current versions have magnetized probes and position sensors; these allow IOP measurements only if the probe is perpendicular to the center of the cornea (in sitting or supine positions), thereby improving the reliability and repeatability of the IOP recordings.

Clinical Application: The rebound tonometer is particularly useful for recording IOP in conditions like corneal scarring, active inflammatory and infectious corneal conditions, where other tonometers cannot record the IOP reliably. Additionally, in post-refractive surgery, for patients where an air-puff and/or applanation tonometer is contraindicated due to the risk of flap displacement, a rebound tonometer would be very useful for measuring IOP. However, its reliability decreases with increasing corneal thick-

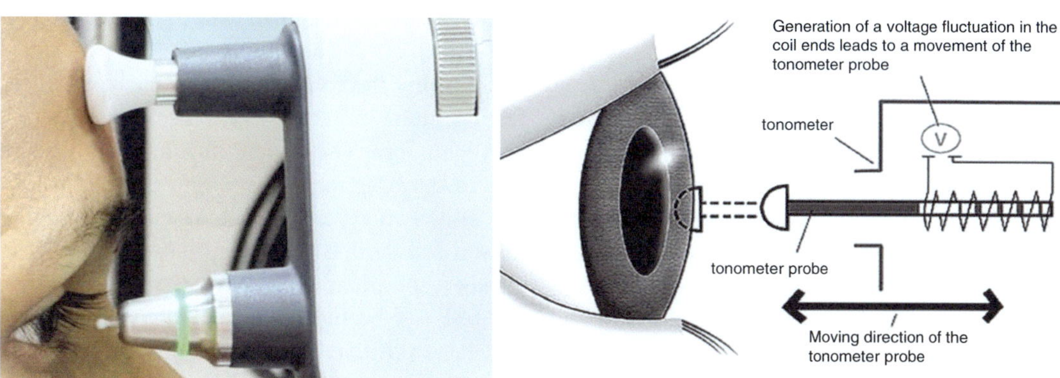

Fig. 35.6 Rebound tonometer. Left: the device in use; the green circle indicates correct alignment; Right: the principle of the rebound tonometer works; (Reprinted with permission from Ruokonen PC et al. [12] Copyright, 2007, Springer Nature)

ness [12]. Given its portability, ease of use, and non-requirement of local anesthesia, a rebound tonometer is also useful for monitoring IOP in children and mass screening for glaucoma.

35.5 External Eye Examination

The external eye structures include the eyelids, tissues surrounding the eyes, conjunctiva, and lacrimal apparatus. A pocket flashlight is usually sufficient to conduct an external eye examination.

Technique: One looks for asymmetry of the eyes, prominence of one/both eyes, improper closure of the eyelids, eye alignment and ocular motility and any unusual eyeball movements, the health of lid margins (mucus or pus discharge, scales, or lumps), conjunctiva of both lids (upper lid conjunctiva can only be observed by everting the upper lid), lacrimal apparatus (tearing, discharge on pressure over the lacrimal sac), or any other eye defects, such as anophthalmia, microphthalmia, coloboma, or any mass lesions during an external examination of the eye.

Clinical Application: Many systemic diseases manifest in the eyes. Metabolic disorders such as hyperthyroidism cause changes in the tissues surrounding the eye, thereby altering their appearance and functionality. Changes in the autonomic nervous system alter the position of the eyelids. While abnormal lipids may be deposited on the lids, abnormal heavy metal deposits may be seen in a specific ring near the edge of the cornea. Abnormalities of the lacrimal system may produce either tearing or dry eyes. Rheumatoid arthritis or collagen diseases may decrease tear and mucus production, causing dry eyes. There could also be localized bacterial, viral, or fungal infections of the lids, conjunctiva, and cornea.

35.6 Visual Field

Visual field testing is integral to diagnosing glaucoma and a few neuro-ophthalmic conditions. It is also used for follow-ups and monitoring of these conditions. Standard automated perimetry (SAP) is the current gold standard of visual field testing. This technique quantitatively assesses an individual's visual function across the field of vision. It determines sensitivity thresholds (ST) at specific retinotopic locations to measure the visual field. However, it is not without limitations. In addition to its cost, SAP acquisition takes around 6–8 min for each eye, during which the patient is required to maintain high levels of concentration [13]. Such long acquisition times, combined with the slight forward-leaning position of the subject, can be uncomfortable and taxing. Some of these limitations can be overcome by using portable alternatives. One such modality is the head-mounted device (HMD) system. The HMD, along with its accompanying tablet PC and handheld controller, has the advantage of being low cost, having a shorter testing time (under 3 min for each eye), being portable (can be used in an examination chair), and a having more flexible options than the traditional method of visual field testing. The HMD can also perform 10–2, 24–2, and 30–2 visual fields in addition to contour stereo testing [14]. The Order of Magnitude (OM) is an HMD device described below.

35.6.1 Order of Magnitude

Order of Magnitude is a virtual reality-based perimetry device.

Technology: The OM allows static automated perimetry using a customized supra-thresholding algorithm. The test is very similar to a conventional perimetry test using a Humphry Field Analyzer (HFA) machine, where patients respond using a clicker. The test is done in two steps: determining the fovea threshold and visual field testing. (Fig. 35.7).

Technique: The fovea thresholding uses a staircase testing method and finalizes the threshold after two reversals. The visual field testing uses a standard 24–2 test grid with 54 testing points (each point is 6° apart). The reliability of the test can be monitored using fixation losses and false positives, which are tested during the visual field testing. The device uses Heijl-Krakau blind spot tracking to check for fixation losses. While the OM tests for false positives by giving a blank or no stimulus and checks for a click

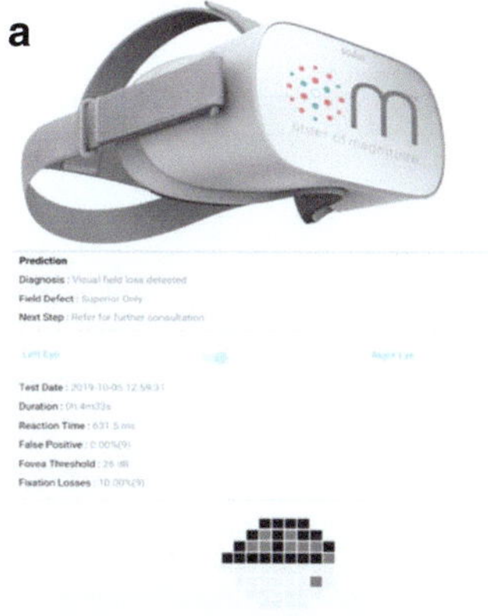

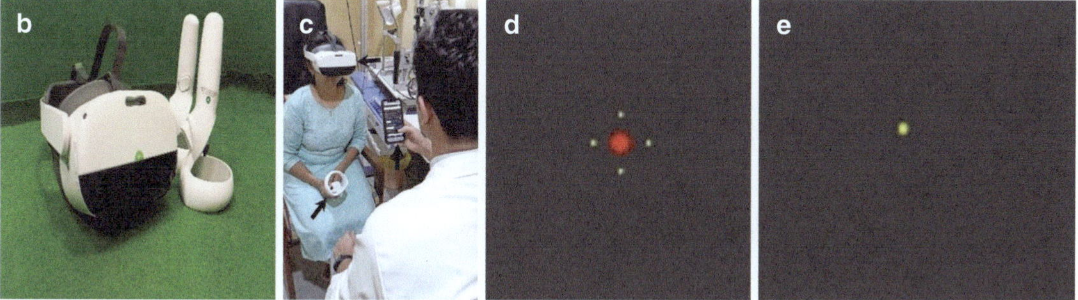

Fig. 35.7 (**a**) The OM visual field showing superior altitudinal field defect. (**b**) VR-based OM visual field analyzer device. (**c**) A patient wearing the headset and the examiner pairing the device to the smartphone. (**d**) Fixation target. (**e**) High decibel stimulus

response, it does not check for false-negative responses as the testing algorithm takes the best two-of-three responses for a light stimulus level.

Clinical application: On comparing a custom-designed VR perimeter with a conventional visual field-testing device (Octopus 900; Haag-Streit, Bern, Switzerland), the VR perimeter slightly underestimated the visual field defects in glaucoma subjects (1.4 dB). However, there was no significant bias with respect to eccentricity or subject age [14]. The OM can be used reliably to detect visual field defects caused by glaucoma and other neuro-ophthalmic conditions [15, 16].

35.7 Examination of the Anterior Segment

A detailed examination of the anterior segment is best performed with a slit lamp. A slit lamp is a stereoscopic biomicroscope that emits a focused beam of light with variable height, width, and angle. It allows three-dimensional visualization and measurement of the fine anatomy of the adnexa and anterior segment of the eye. It is a mainstay of the comprehensive eye examination. Documenting slit lamp images can help in furthering patient care. Typically, a slit lamp is a tabletop device housed in an eye clinic with large spaces. The new portable slit lamps are as versatile as the tabletop ones but less expensive. This has largely benefitted teleophthalmology and home care. A description of a modular portable slit lamp and anterior segment imaging device follows.

35.7.1 HOLDEN ™ (Modular Slit Lamp with Applanation is a Handheld Slit Lamp)

Technology: This compact and adaptable handheld ophthalmic device operates with a smartphone. It consists of multiple modules, such as anterior segment imaging with slit functionality, tonometry

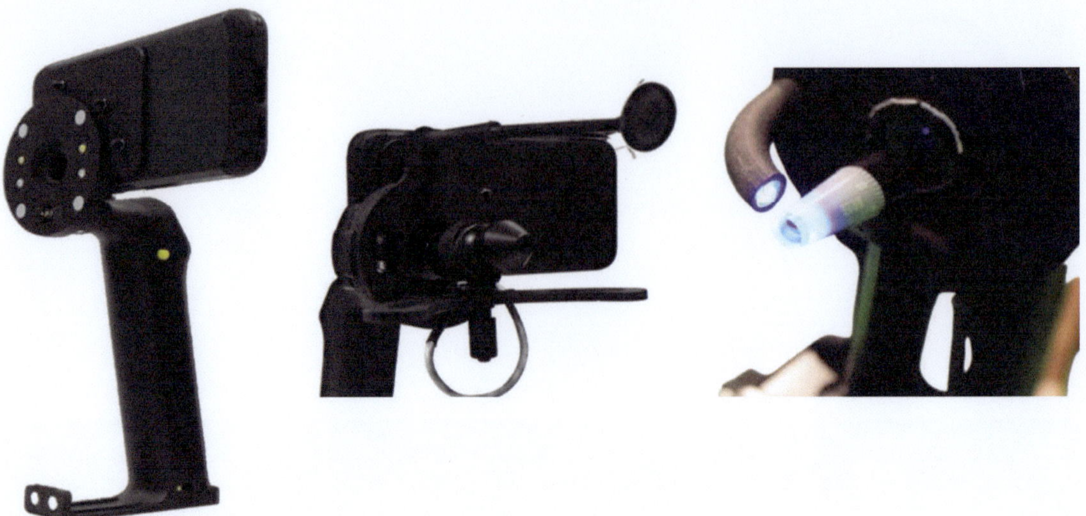

Fig. 35.8 Left: modular slit lamp; Middle: slit module; Right: tonometer module

based on the Goldmann applanation mechanism, and corneal topography, among others. (Fig. 35.8) These modules can be effortlessly interchanged using high-power neodymium magnets, facilitating seamless, and comprehensive eye examinations. The slit module width is 0.2 mm, and the tonometry module incorporates the standard applanation bi-prism technique. Additionally, the device offers a corneal topography module capable of generating axial and tangential heat maps.

Technique: Modular slit lamp is held against the forehead (Fig. 35.8, middle panel) for anterior segment examination, IOP measurement, and corneal topography as an optional attachment.

Clinical Application: The modular slit lamp has the advantage of storing the images while performing the anterior segment examination. This handheld device can also be used in people in a supine position. It is useful for home care, teleophthalmology, and primary and secondary care level centers.

35.7.2 Grabi ™ is a Device to Image the Anterior Segment of the Eye

Technology: Smartphones have powerful cameras for general photography. But the variability in their features and lack of appropriate tuning makes them unsuitable for macro-ophthalmic photography. Grabi images the anterior segment of the eye, mainly the conjunctiva and cornea. It can be operated directly by the patients, irrespective of the kind of smartphone they possess (Fig. 35.9). The Grabi has specifically designed hardware and a specifically configured app. The app fine-tunes the native smartphone camera and flashes by adjusting the magnification, illumination, and focus to get a good-quality image of the cornea, limbus, iris, and lens.

Technique: The spacer device is mounted on the smartphone, as shown in the figure by the user (patient's relative or caretaker), in such a way that it does not obstruct the camera lenses and fits snugly. The distal end of the spacer should touch the forehead of the patient; this acts to provide mechanical support to stabilize the hand and smartphone and also align the camera at a set distance from the eye of the patient. The app is then engaged so that the user aligns the cornea and iris within the center of the screen. To help in this process, a simple white circular graticule appears on the screen as a guide, assisting the users in aligning the cornea and iris within it and tapping on the screen to capture the image. The process is simplified and user-friendly because the user is trained to obtain images of the patient's eye on their smartphone camera. This simplifies

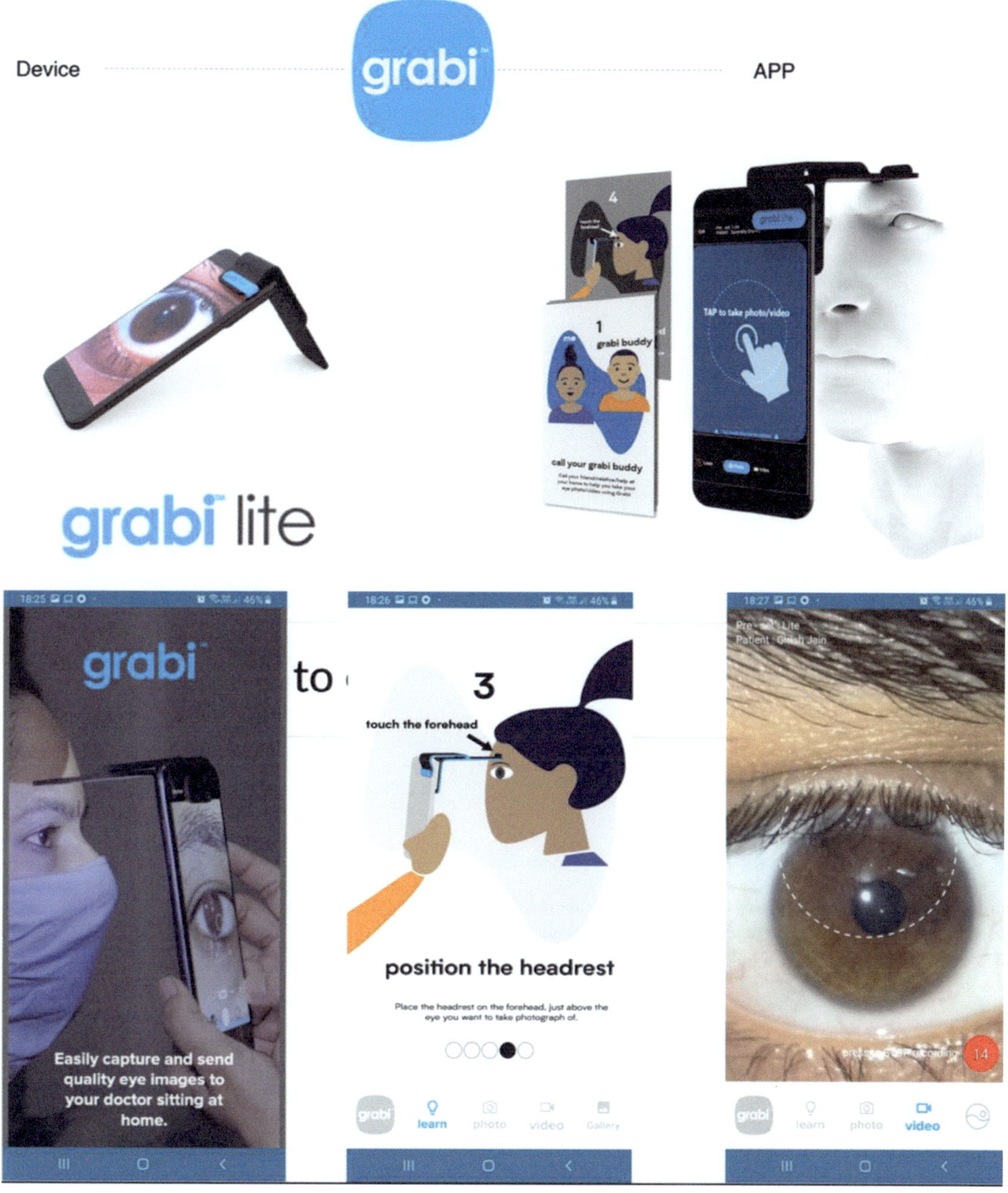

Fig. 35.9 Upper panel: left-Grabilite™ device; Upper right: Grabi app must be paired to the smartphone. Lower panel: Left and Middle: the guide must be fixed to the forehead above the eyebrow. Right: the dotted circle shows the area of interest for photography

the learning curve, and users can acquire good anterior segment images.

Clinical Application: These images are sent to the consulting clinician via the teleconsultation platform, which helps manage the follow-ups and medications more effectively. These images are also stored in the cloud. Further applications include utilizing AI, deep learning algorithms,

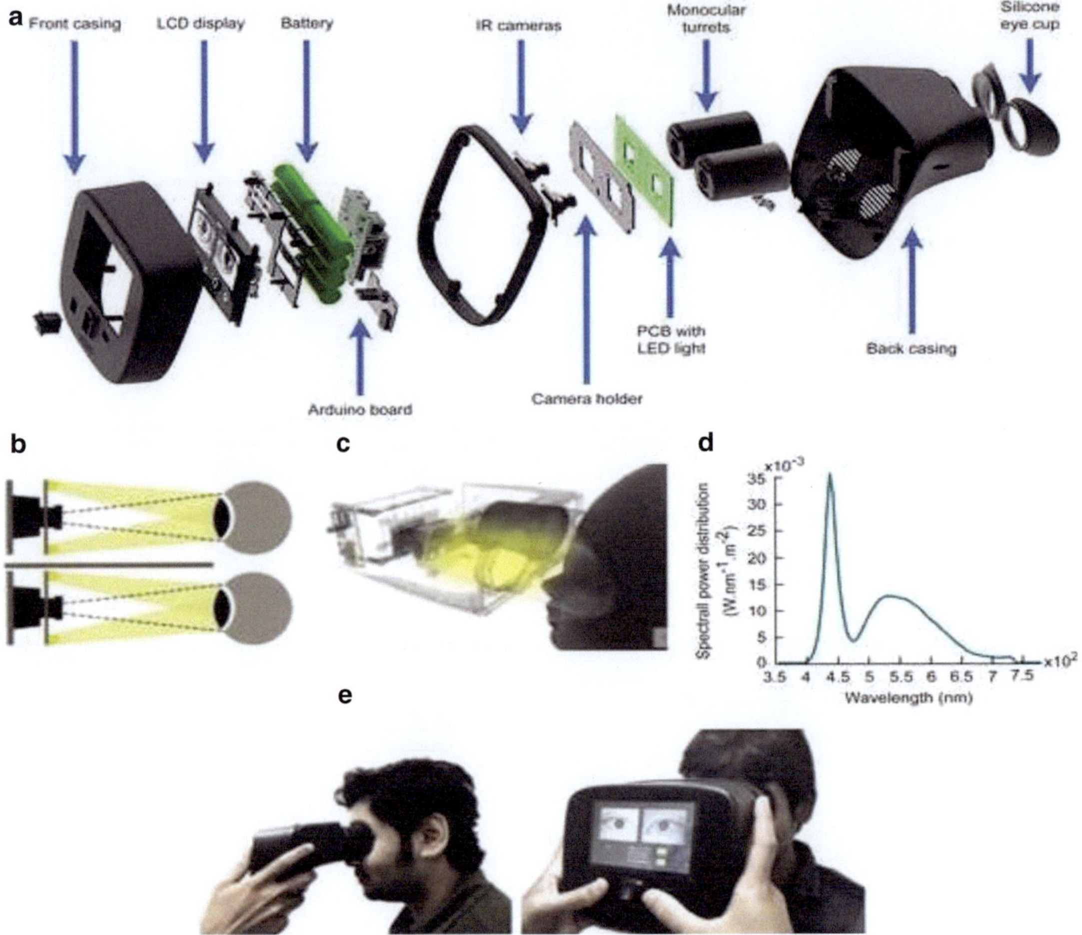

Fig. 35.10 Left Panel (**a**) shows the segmented diagram of the key elements of the custom-designed dynamic pupillometer. (**b** and **c**) Light stimulation channel used in the 488 Pupil+ device. (**d**) Plots the spectral power distribution as a function of the wavelength of the LED used in the device for stimulating the pupillary light reflex. (**e**) The device in use and the LCD screen-based user interface for initiating the test; observing the progress of the test in real-time

and computer vision to improve the quality of the images, helping patients obtain better images, and identifying the at-risk signs to be flagged for further medical or surgical intervention.

35.7.3 Pupil

Examination of the pupil is important to monitor the health of the eye. Testing for relative afferent pupillary defect (RAPD) is an important test. The RAPD grading can be automated using the concept of the swinging flashlight test, and the pupil response can be quantified to reduce subjectivity and test variability.

35.7.3.1 Pupil-Lite (Device for Assessing the Pupil)

Technology: The device uses image processing to acquire the raw diameter of the pupil and then runs through the algorithm in the cloud to estimate the pupillary parameters. It uses an edge identification algorithm. (Fig. 35.10).

Technique: The device is held up to the patient's face, and the patient is instructed to look into it like they would look into a pair of binoculars. The device is connected to a computer that displays live video feeds from the two cameras. When the device is in place, the person administering the test clicks on the center of each pupil.

This allows the image processing algorithm to use edge identification techniques to identify the pupil diameter for each frame. The rest runs at a speed of 30 frames per second. Once the test begins, the cameras start recording.

Clinical applications: [17] (1) Grading of RAPD; (2) monitoring the pupil size before and after any intervention, including neurological interventions; (3) documenting pupil size and shape.

35.8 Fundus

Classically, fundus examination is done by a handheld direct or head-worn indirect ophthalmoscope. While pupil dilatation may not be necessary for fundus examination with a direct ophthalmoscope, it is nearly always required for indirect ophthalmoscopy. However, one should remember that an undilated eye exam is not complete.

35.8.1 Direct Ophthalmoscope

Technology: The direct ophthalmoscope (Fig. 35.11) contains a handle with a battery and a head. The head contains a bulb, a set of apertures for the light source, and a set of lenses. The light source is bright enough to evaluate the pupil. A cobalt blue filter is often built into the instrument for use with fluorescein staining of the cornea. The direct ophthalmoscope provides a monocular, non-stereoscopic, narrow field of view, but it is magnified. Light from a bulb is reflected at right angles and projected as a spot through the patient's pupil to illuminate the retina. The illuminated retina is seen directly by the examiner.

Technique: Using mydriatics for direct ophthalmoscopy is generally unnecessary, but a weak mydriatic agent (0.5% or 1% tropicamide or 2.5% phenylephrine) is a good choice when required. The patient must sit in a comfortable position so that his/her head is at the level of the examiner. A dim light helps. The patient then fixes his/her gaze on an object across the room without looking directly at the light. When the patient is comfortable, the examiner should start at a distance of at least arm's length. The examiner looks through the hole in the ophthalmoscope and approaches the patient's eye gradually until the red reflex of the retina is visible. Once the retina is in good focus, it is critical to then maintain this axis of alignment. The −3 to −4 D lens on the ophthalmoscope usually generates a comfortable view of the fundus. The examiner's left eye is examined by the patient's left eye, standing on the patient's left side, and vice versa. Usually, removing the examiner's eyeglasses is unnecessary, but one must remove the patient's

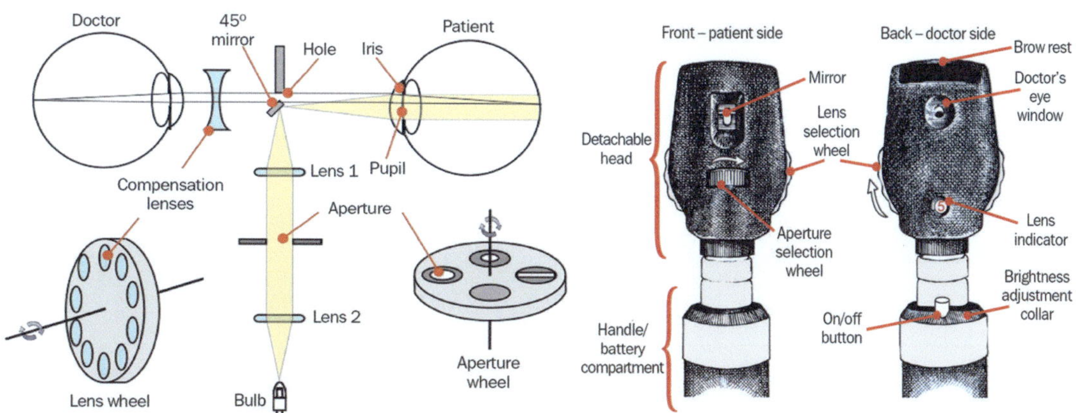

Fig. 35.11 Direct ophthalmoscope. Left: optics; Right: the device. (Source: Ismael Cordero. Copyright 2016, used under the Creative Common Attribution 2.0 license) [18]

glasses (no need to remove contact lenses, if any).

Clinical Application: Even in undilated eyes, examination with the direct ophthalmoscope can give useful information on the clarity of the ocular media and refractive error. A diminished red reflex or irregularities might result from cloudy media (e.g., corneal or lens opacities, blood in the vitreous) and unusual/high refractive errors. The direct ophthalmoscope evaluates the optic nerve head, retinal vessels, and macula.

35.8.2 Indirect Ophthalmoscope

The (binocular) indirect ophthalmoscope is worn on the examiner's head, and it is sometimes attached to spectacles for fundus examination. It produces a stereoscopic image of the fundus.

Technology: The viewing system of the instrument (Fig. 35.12) consists of a pair of low-powered convex lenses. This design affords the examiner a stereoscopic view of the virtual image. The lens condenses light from the illumination system towards the patient's pupil. Light reflected from the retina passes back through the lens, creating a real, horizontal, and laterally inverted image of the fundus between the lens and the examiner. A + 20 D lens is the standard lens for general examination offering 3× magnification and approximately 45° fields of view. A + 30 D lens is sometimes used for small children and/or in eyes with small pupils; it provides 2× magnification and approximately 65° fields of view.

Technique: In a dark room, the examiner orientates his/her head so that light from the internal light source is directed into the patient's eye. The examiner then holds a positive-powered condensing lens from the patient's eye at its focal length. (Fig. 35.12) The patient's pupils must be dilated for retinal examination using an indirect ophthalmoscope. The patient is asked to look straight up at the ceiling if supine or over the examiner's shoulder if seated. The condensing lens is grasped with the index finger and thumb. The examiner uses one or more of the spare fingers of the same hand to brace against the patient's forehead to steady the lens. The right eye is examined by holding the lens in the right hand, with the examiner standing on the patient's right side, and vice versa. The other hand is used for scleral indentation as and when required. Typically, the extreme periphery is examined first, working towards the equator along the 12 o'clock meridian. Having examined the entire retina from the equator to the ora serrata in each quadrant, the procedure is completed by examining the posterior pole. When seeking to sweep the view across the retina (e.g., from the extreme periphery to the equator), it is vital to maintain a direct line between the observation system, the center of the condensing lens, and the patient's pupil, referred to as the "common axis principle."

Clinical Applications: The indirect ophthalmoscope is exceptionally valuable for detecting retinal detachments, retinal holes, and retinal tears. The comparison of indirect and direct ophthalmoscopy is shown in Table 35.4.

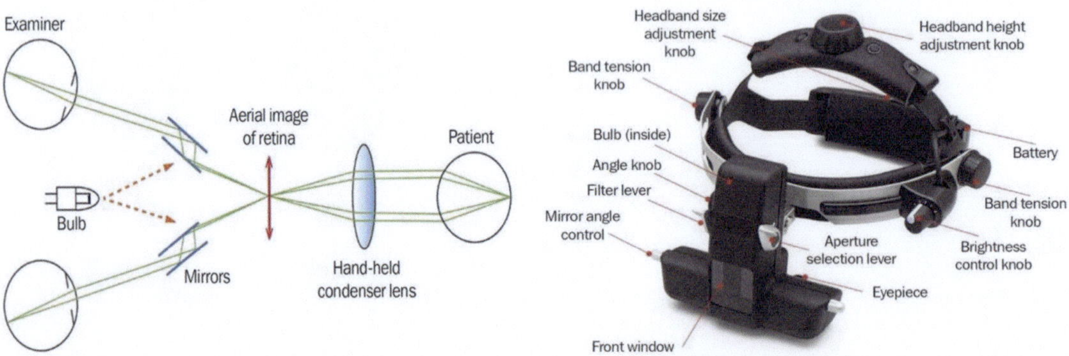

Fig. 35.12 Indirect ophthalmoscope. (Source: Ismael Cordero. Copyright 2016, used under the Creative Common Attribution 2.0 license) [19]

Table. 35.4 Comparison between indirect and direct ophthalmoscopy

Parameter	Indirect Ophthalmoscopy	Direct Ophthalmoscopy
Condensing lens	Required	Not required
Examining distance	Arm's length	As close to the patient as possible
Field of view (diameter)	20D—45°; 30D—65°	Small (approximately 10°)
Magnification	20D—3x; 30D—2x	Approximately 15x
Structures viewed	Peripheral retina seen	Only the central retina seen
Brightness	More	Less
Stereopsis	Binocular—Superior stereopsis	Uniocular—Non-stereoscopic
Image of fundus	Inverted and virtual image	Erect and real image
Scleral indentation	Easily achieved	Difficult
Retina anterior to the equator	More easily seen	Can be seen with difficulty
Visibility in hazy media	Better	Poor

35.8.3 Integrating Teleophthalmology with Home Eye Care

Technology is increasingly important to reach the last mile in eye care [20]. In addition to improving accessibility, it also reduces the cost of care [21]. To reach the unreached and meet the 2030 sustainable development goals, the World Health Organization has suggested adopting an integrated, people-centered eye care (IPEC) model that caters to eye care from primary to tertiary levels [22]. Vision centers are part of one such model adopted in India that provides in-person services to around 50,000 people in remote rural and tribal regions [23]. Using newer technology, these vision centers can connect to secondary and tertiary care, and one could expand teleophthalmology from the vision center to home care [24].

Another method is the use of mobile services for home eye care. All devices used in home care are lightweight and portable. These are packed in a box, and typically one allied ophthalmic personnel trained explicitly for home care drives a two-wheeler carrying the box. (Fig. 35.13) Mobile home eye care generally is a hybrid teleophthalmology asynchronous/synchronous model. In this model, a field team visits the individual's home, records vision, performs refraction, measures intraocular pressure, obtains high-resolution anterior and posterior segment images, and uploads these to the electronic medical record in the examination site (possibly cloud-based). This facilitates the ophthalmologist's video consult in real-time (synchronous) or at a pre-decided time (asynchronous) to treat the patients. Medical prescriptions reach the individual electronically, and the patients are invited to visit fixed eye care facilities for investigations and/or surgery as needed.

The advantages of integrating home eye care with fixed eye care centers include:

- Suited for individuals of vulnerable age groups (extremes of age) and those who are sick and/or homebound. Following the tests at home, the individuals can be referred for specific investigations to fixed eye care facilities where these could be fast-tracked for comfort and convenience.
- Reduce the number of visits for those suffering from chronic eye conditions like glaucoma, uveitis, and diabetic retinopathy.
- Avoids over-crowding at fixed-capacity eye care facilities.
- Continuity of care is maintained as data points recorded at the home visit get integrated into the individual's medical record.
- Scalability: Home eye care (synchronous or asynchronous) is offered within 10–20 km of the fixed eye care centers. Integration with eye care at the district, state, or national level can ensure that eye care is delivered at the last mile across the region and reach all those who cannot reach a hospital.

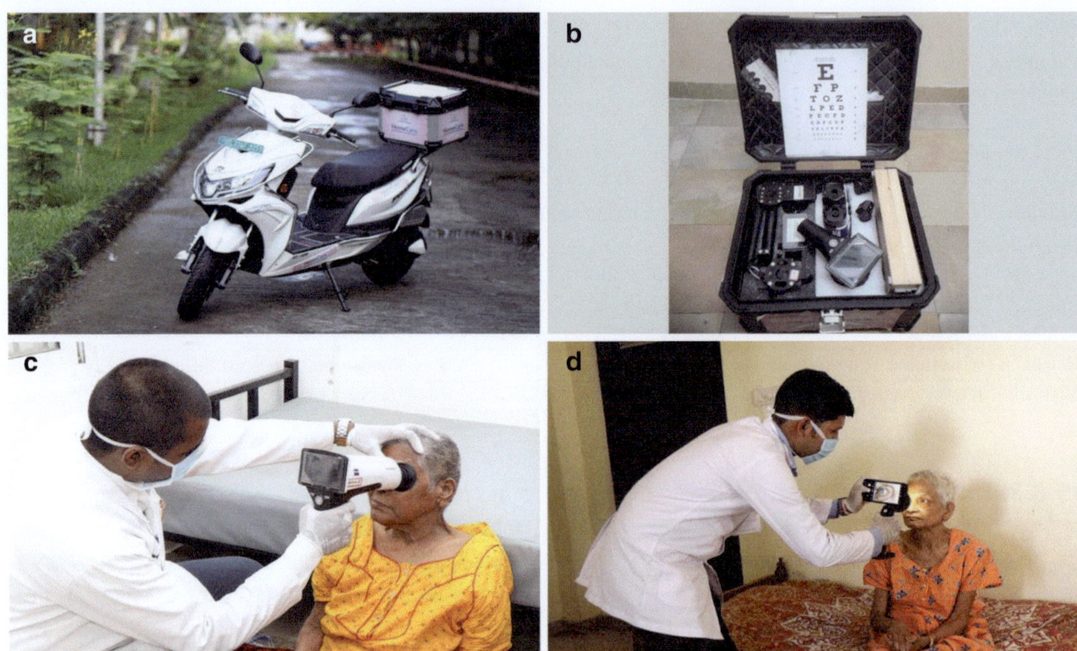

Fig. 35.13 (**a**) Electric scooter with a box containing the ophthalmic devices used in home eye care. (**b**) The devices inside the box; (**c**) fundus photography; (**d**) slit lamp examination and imaging. (Images "c" and "d" are reproduced after signed written consent

35.9 Conclusion

There are two compelling reasons for the increasing use of teleophthalmology. These are population growth and population aging. The Global Burden of Disease has estimated that nearly one-fourth (2.2 of 8 billion) of the world population needs eye care for distance and/or near vision [25]. Thus, one would expect more people to need ophthalmologists for their eye care. However, there are insufficient human resources for health to meet this demand [26]. In five decades (1970–2022), the global mean age has increased from 20 to over 30 years [27]. Most eye diseases that require medical/surgical attention beyond a pair of spectacles occur in the elderly, and approximately 10% of the world population is 65 years or older [27]. Thus, an increasing number of older adults will need eye care. However, many of them do not have timely access to eye care either because of other ailments such as multimorbidity and/or multi-disability (in one elderly residential care study in India, these were 37.6% and 23.6%, respectively [28]). In addition, these older adults could be too old to reach the eye care facility independently due to low/no family support. In these instances, teleophthalmology and home eye care would be useful. Although technology has now made this more accessible and safer than before, it is only the beginning to reach the last mile.

Acknowledgments Kartikesh Anche, Rahul Negi, Amir Ali, Vineet Joshi, and all members of Center for Technology Innovation, LVPEI, Hyderabad, India.

Funding Hyderabad Eye Research Foundation, Hyderabad, India.

Disclosure KN: Employee of Remidio Innovative Solutions Pvt Ltd, Bangalore, India.

Others: None.

References

1. Kumar R. Frequently asked questions about family medicine in India. J Family Med Prim Care. 2016;5(1):3–6.
2. World Health Organization. Report of the international conference on primary health care Alma Ata, USSR, 6–12 September. Geneva: World Health

Organization; 1978. https://bit.ly/3vqrZfZ. Accessed 3 Jun 2023

3. World Health Organization. Global conference on primary health care: from Alma-Ata towards universal health coverage and the sustainable development goals, Astana, Kazakhstan, 25 and 26 October 2018. Astana: World Health Organization; 2018. https://www.who.int/teams/primary-healthcare/conference. Accessed 3 Jun 2023.
4. Bellsmith KN, Gale MJ, Yang S, et al. Validation of home visual acuity tests for telehealth in the COVID-19 era. JAMA Ophthalmol. 2022;140:465–71.
5. Padhy D, Das T, Majhi D, et al. Prevalence of Refractive error among *Dongarias* and Use of Folding Phoropter (FoFo) as a field device enabling implementation research in this indigenous community. tribal Odisha eye disease study (TOES) Report # 13. PLoS One. 2023;18:e0284790. https://doi.org/10.1371/journal.pone.0284790.
6. Padhy D, Bharadwaj S, Nayak S, Rath S, Das T. Does the accuracy of refractive error estimates depend on the measurement principle of autorefractors? Trans Vis Sci Tech. 2021;10(1):2. https://doi.org/10.1167/tvst.10.1.2.
7. Durr NJ, Dave SR, Lim D, et al. Quality of eyeglass prescriptions from a low-cost wavefront autorefractor evaluated in rural India: results of a 708-participant field study. BMJ Open Ophthalmol. 2019;4(1):e000225. https://doi.org/10.1136/bmjophth-2018-000225.
8. Joseph S, Varadaraj V, Dave SR, et al. Investigation of the accuracy of a low-cost, portable autorefractor to provide well-tolerated eyeglass prescriptions: a randomized crossover trial. Ophthalmology. 2021;128:1672–80.
9. Rao DP, Negiloni K, Gurunathan S, et al. Validation of a simple-to-use, affordable, portable, wavefront aberrometry-based auto refractometer in the adult population: a prospective study. BMC Ophthalmol. 2022;22:498. https://doi.org/10.1186/s12886-022-02684-5.
10. Rao DP, Negiloni K, Gurunathan S, et al. Validation of a simple-to-use, affordable, portable Wavefront Aberrometry-based auto refractometer in a Paediatric population. Clin Ophthalmol. 2022;16:4281–91. https://doi.org/10.2147/OPTH.S387831.
11. Nakakura S, Asaoka R, Terao E, et al. Evaluation of rebound tonometer iCare IC200 as compared with IcarePRO and Goldmann applanation tonometer in patients with glaucoma. Eye and vision (London). 2021;8(1):25. https://doi.org/10.1186/s40662-021-00249-z.
12. Ruokonen PC, Schwenteck T, Draeger J. Evaluation of the impedance tonometers TGDc-01 and iCare according to the international ocular tonometer standards ISO 8612. Graefes Arch Clin Exp Ophthalmol. 2007;245:1259–65.
13. Marra G, Flammer J. The learning and fatigue effect in automated perimetry. Graefes Arch Clin Exp Ophthalmol. 1991;229:501–4.
14. Stapelfeldt J, Kucur SS, Huber N, et al. Virtual reality–based and conventional visual field examination comparison in healthy and glaucoma patients. Transl Vis Sci Technol. 2021;10:10. https://doi.org/10.1167/tvst.10.12.10.
15. Baskar J, Ali M, Choudhary N S, Senthil S. Order of magnitude (OM): virtual reality-based visual field examination to detect glaucomatous field loss, eye. 2023.
16. Badakere A, Kekunnaya R, Sachdeva V. Agreement between Virtual reality (VR) perimetry vs. Static automated perimetry (SAP) in various Neuro-ophthalmological conditions: a pilot study. Neuro-Ophthalmol. 2023;47(5-6):255–61.
17. Negi R, Raviselvan M, Divyank Y, et al. Severity of relative afferent pupillary defect is dependent on the intensity of pupillary light stimulation. Optom Vis Sci. 2023;
18. Ismael C. Understanding and caring for the direct ophthalmoscope. Comm Eye Health J. 2016;29(93):17.
19. Ismael C. Understanding and caring for an indirect ophthalmoscope. Community Eye Health. 2016;29(95):57.
20. Das T, Sapkota YD. Promoting technology-enabled primary eye care in South-East Asia. Community Eye Health. 2021;34(111):s7–8. PMID: 36033409
21. Das T. Reaching the last mile in eye care. Indian J Ophthalmol. 2020;68:s3–5.
22. World Report on Vision. https://www.who.int. Accessed 3 Jun 2013.
23. Rao GN, Khanna RC, Athota SM, et al. Integrated model of primary and secondary eye care for underserved rural areas: the L V Prasad eye institute experience. Indian J Ophthalmol. 2012;60:396–400.
24. Aruljyothi L, Bavishi A, Balasundaram MB, et al. Expanding the scope of tele-ophthalmology from vision centers to home. Indian J Ophthalmol. 2021;69:442–6.
25. GBD 2019 Blindness and Vision Impairment Collaborators. Causes of blindness and vision impairment in 2020 and trends over 30 years, and prevalence of avoidable blindness in relation to VISION 2020: the Right to Sight: an analysis for the Global Burden of Disease Study. Lancet Global Health. 2021;9(2):e144–60. https://doi.org/10.1016/S2214-109(x)30489-7.
26. Ravilla T, Karumanchi S, Das T. Health management and information: key principles and enablers in eye health program. In: Das T, Nayar PD, editors. South-East Asia eye health. Singapore :p23–50: Springer; 2021. https://doi.org/10.1007/978-981-16-3787-2_2.
27. Ritchie H, Roser M. Age structure. www.oneworlddata.org. Accessed 19 Jun 2023.
28. Marmamula S, Kumbham TR, Shidhaye R, et al. Multimorbidity and multi-disability among the elderly in residential care in India: the Hyderabad ocular morbidity in elderly study (HOMES). Sci Rep. 2022;12(1):11779. https://doi.org/10.1038/s41598-022-15943-8.

Correction to: Home Care and Teleophthalmology

Taraprasad Das, Debananada Padhy, Kalpa Negiloni, Jenil Sheth, Sanil Joseph, Suryasnata Rath, and Ramesh Kekunnaya

Correction to:
Chapter 35 in: T. Das, P. Satgunam (eds.), *Ophthalmic Diagnostics*, https://doi.org/10.1007/978-981-97-0138-4_35

This book was inadvertently published with an incorrect spelling of the author's last name in Chapter 35 as Sanil Jospeph, whereas it should be Sanil Joseph.

The updated version of this chapter can be found at https://doi.org/10.1007/978-981-97-0138-4_35

T. Das, P. Satgunam (eds.), *Ophthalmic Diagnostics*, https://doi.org/10.1007/978-981-97-0138-4_36

Index

T. Das, P. Satgunam (eds.), *Ophthalmic Diagnostics*, https://doi.org/10.1007/978-981-97-0138-4

M

O

P

R

S

T

U

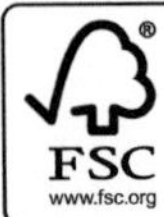

MIX
Papier aus verantwortungsvollen Quellen
Paper from responsible sources
FSC® C105338

If you have any concerns about our products, you can contact us on
ProductSafety@springernature.com

In case Publisher is established outside the EU, the EU authorized representative is:
Springer Nature Customer Service Center GmbH
Europaplatz 3, 69115 Heidelberg, Germany

Printed by Libri Plureos GmbH
in Hamburg, Germany